PY

PDxMD

Cardiology

PDxMD
An Imprint of Elsevier Science
Philadelphia ■ St Louis ■ London ■ Sydney ■ New York ■ Toronto

PDxMD Medical Conditions Series is dedicated to health and healing professionals everywhere. We are privileged to be in your service and hope our efforts help you in your quest for better quality-of-life and optimized outcomes for all your patients.

PDxMD
An imprint of Elsevier Science

Publisher:	Steven Merahn, MD
Project Managers:	Caroline Barnett, Lucy Hamilton, Zak Knowles
Programmer:	Narinder Chandi
Production:	Aoibhe O'Shea – GMS UK, Alan Palfreyman – PTU
Designer:	Jayne Jones
Layout:	The Designers Collective Limited

NOTICE
Medicine is an ever-changing field. Standard safety precautions must be followed, but as new research and clinical experience broaden our knowledge, changes in treatment and drug therapy may become necessary or appropriate. Readers are advised to check the most current product information provided by the manufacturer of each drug to be administered to verify the recommended dose, the method and duration of administration, and contraindications. It is the responsibility of the licensed prescriber, relying on experience and knowledge of the patient, to determine dosages and the best treatment for each individual patient. Neither the publisher nor the editor assumes any liability for any injury and/or damage to persons or property arising from this publication.

All PDxMD contributors are participating in the activities of PDxMD in an individual capacity, and not as representatives of or on behalf of their individual affiliated hospitals, associations or institutions (where indicated herein), and their participation should not be taken as an endorsement of PDxMD by their individual affiliated hospitals, associations or institutions. Individual affiliated hospitals, associations or institutions are not responsible for the accuracy or availability of information on the product.

Printed in China by RDC Group

PDxMD
Elsevier Science
The Curtis Center
625 Walnut Street,
Philadelphia, PA 19106

The Publisher's policy is to use **paper manufactured from sustainable forests**

ISBN 1-932141-01-4

Contents

Contents

Introduction

What is PDxMD?

PDxMD is a new, evidence-based primary care clinical information system designed to support your judgment with practical clinical information. The content is continuously updated by expert contributors with the latest on evaluation, diagnosis, management, outcomes and prevention – all designed for use at the point and time of care.

First and foremost, PDxMD is an electronic resource. This book gives you access to just a fraction of the content available on-line. At www.pdxmd.com, you will find:

- Over 1400 differential diagnoses for you to search for information according to your patient's chief complaint via a unique signs and symptoms matrix
- Information on more than 450 medical conditions and more than 750 drugs and other therapies, organised in condition-specific 'MediFiles'
- Patient information sheets on 300 topics for you to customize and hand to your patient during consultation

About This Book

The PDxMD Medical Conditions Series is a print version of the comprehensive approach offered on line. Concise information on medical conditions is systematically organized in a consistent MediFile format, our electronic equivalent of chapters.

Each MediFile covers summary information and background on each condition, and comprehensive information on diagnosis, treatment, outcomes, and prevention, and other resources, especially written and designed for use in practice. Each MediFile is organized identically to allow you to find information consistently and reliably for every condition. See the MediFile 'Road Map' inside the back cover for more information.

Ranging from epidemiology to risk assessment and reduction, from diagnostic evaluation and testing to therapeutic options, prognosis and outcomes - you'll find the information that you need is easier to locate with this methodical approach.

How to Use This Book

Find the MediFile for any specific medical condition in the Contents list. Familiarize yourself with the MediFile Road Map (see inside back cover) to rapidly find the precise information you require.

Information on drugs and tests are found within the MediFiles for the specific conditions. For an overview, see the 'Summary of options' sections under DIAGNOSIS and under TREATMENT in the relevant MediFile. Details of tests, drugs and other therapies then follow.

PDxMD believes that physician clinical judgment is central to appropriate diagnostic and therapeutic decision-making. The information is designed to support professional judgment and, accounting for individual patient differences, does not provide direct answers or force specific practices or policies.

How is PDxMD created?

PDxMD is created through Collaborative Authoring. This process allows medical information to be reviewed and synthesized from multiple sources – including but not limited to peer-reviewed articles, evidence databases, guidelines and position papers – and by multiple individuals. The information is organized around and integrated into a template that matches the needs of primary care physicians in practice.

Professional medical writers begin the process of reviewing and synthesizing information for PDxMD, working from core evidence databases and other expert resources and with the guidance of Editorial Advisory Board (EAB) members. This first draft is sent to a physician 'clinical reviewer', who works with the writer to make sure the information is accurate and properly organized. A second review by the physician clinical reviewer ensures that appropriate changes are in place.

After these first two levels of clinical review, the files are reviewed and edited by the relevant specialist member of the Editorial Advisory Board. A primary care member of the EAB, who has final sign-off authority, then conducts the final review and edit. Editorial checks are conducted between all review stages and, after primary care sign-off, a pharmacist double checks the drug recommendations prior to a final editorial review.

There are a minimum of three and as many as five physicians involved in each MediFile, and additional clinical reviewers and/or EAB members are added when appropriate (e.g., alternative/complementary medicine experts, or conditions requiring multi-disciplinary approaches). The contributor team for each MediFile is listed in the Resources section.

A complete list of Editorial Faculty and staff of PDxMD is provided below. All Editorial Faculty, and specifically the Editorial Advisory Board members, participate in PDxMD as individuals and not as representatives of, or on behalf of, their affiliated institutions or associations and any indication of their affiliation with a specific institution or association should not be taken as an endorsement of PDxMD or any participation of their institution or association with PDxMD.

Continuous Product Improvement

PDxMD is committed to continuous quality improvement and welcomes any comments, suggestions and feedback from the professional community. Please send any ideas or considerations regarding this volume or any other volume in the PDxMD series via e-mail to feedback.pdxmd@elsevier.com or to PDxMD, Elsevier Science, The Curtis Center, 625 Walnut Street, Philadelphia, PA 19106.

Evidence-Based Medicine Policies

PDxMD is committed to providing available and up-to-date evidence for the diagnostic and therapeutic recommendations provided in our knowledge base. All MediFiles begin with a core set of evidence-based references from recognized sources. These are supplemented with extensive searches of the literature and reviews of reference books, peer-reviewed journals, association guidelines and position papers, among others.

Criteria for Evidence-Based Medicine

Evidence Sources

PDxMD has taken the best evidence currently available from the following:

Published Critically Evaluated Evidence

- Cochrane Systematic Reviews – respected throughout the world as one of the most rigorous searches of medical journals with highly structured systematic reviews and use of meta-analysis to produce reliable evidence
- Clinical Evidence – produced jointly by the British Medical Journal Publishing Group and the American College of Physicians–American Society of Internal Medicine. Clinical Evidence provides a concise account of the current state of knowledge on the treatment and prevention of many clinical conditions based on the search and appraisal of the available literature
- The National Guideline Clearinghouse – a comprehensive database of evidence-based clinical practice guidelines and related documents produced by the Agency for Healthcare Research and Quality in partnership with the American Medical Association and the American Association of Health Plans

Evidence Published in Peer-Reviewed Journals

- Association Guidelines and Position Papers

Where evidence exists that has not yet been critically reviewed by one of the sources listed above, for example randomized controlled trials and clinical cohort studies, the evidence is summarized briefly, categorized, and fully referenced.

Clinical Experience

While recognizing the importance of these evidence-based resources, PDxMD also highlights the importance of experience in clinical practice. Therefore, our Editorial Advisory Board also provide advice from their own clinical experience, within Clinical Pearl sections of the MediFiles and elsewhere. Contributing expert physicians are identified in the Resources section of every MediFile.

Evaluation of Evidence

PDxMD evaluates all cited evidence according to the AAFP Recommended Basic Model for Evaluating and Categorizing the Clinical Content of CME, based on the model used by the University of Michigan:

Level M — Evidence from either:
Meta-analysis or
Multiple randomized controlled trials

Level P — Evidence from either:
A well-designed prospective clinical trial or
Several prospective clinical cohort studies with consistent findings (without randomization)

Level S — Evidence from studies other than clinical trials, such as:
Epidemiological studies
Physiological studies

References

The information provided by PDxMD is concise and action-oriented. As a result, our editorial policy is to cite only essential reference sources. References and evidence summaries are provided in four areas:

1. In the Diagnostic Decision section under Diagnosis
2. In the Guidelines and Evidence sections under Treatment
3. In the Outcomes section under Evidence
4. In the Key Reference Section under Resources

Where on-line references to the Cochrane Abstracts, BMJ Clinical Evidence and National Guideline Clearinghouse are cited in the text, the internet addresses of the home pages are given. The internet addresses of individual reports are not given.

When references are to association guidelines and position papers, the internet address of the association home page is generally provided. When possible, the internet address of the specific report is provided.

Editorial Faculty and Staff

Executive Committee

Editorial Board

Editorial Faculty and Staff

Editorial Faculty and Staff

Editorial Faculty and Staff

Clinical Reviewers

Editorial Faculty and Staff

Gail A Van Norman, MD
Cardiology
Clinical Associate Professor of Anesthesiology
Faculty Associate, Department of Biomedical
History and Ethics
University of Washington
Seattle, WA

Writers

Pim I Allen, MD
Solomon Almond, MB ChB, MRCP, DTM&H
Kim S Berman
Liza C Brettingham, MD, JCTGP
Patricia M Clark, MSN, RN, CS
Andrea L Clatworthy, PhD
Neil D Fisher, BSc PhD
Jay A Glasel, PhD
Norma-Jeanne Hennis
Adam Jacobs, MD
Tina Kohnstam, MB, BS
Shelley Minden
Saket Priyadarshi, BSc, MB ChB
Vicki L Rackner, MD, FACS
Ola N Soyinka, MB BS, MBA
Chris J Taylor, FRCS
Gail A van Norman, MD
Donald Venes, MD
Robert Whittle, MB BS (NSW)

Staff

Management Team
Fiona Foley, Steven Merahn, MD, Daniel Pollock, Zak Knowles, Howard Croft, Tanya Thomas, Lucy Hamilton, Julie Volck, Bill Bruggemeyer, Andrea Ford

Editorial Team
Anne Dyson, Sadaf Hashmi, Debbie Goring, Louise Morrison, Ellen Haigh, Robert Whittle, Claire Champion, Caroline Barnett, Laurie Smith, Li Wan, Paul Mayhew, Carmen Jones, Fi Ward

Technical Team
Martin Miller, Narinder Chandi, Roy Patterson, Aaron McGrath, John Wylie, Sarah Craze, Cameron Sangster

We would also like to acknowledge the extraordinary contributions of the following individuals to the conceptualization and realization of PDxMD over the initial years of its growth and development:

Tim Hailstone, Jonathan Black, Alison Whitehouse, Jayne Harris, Angela Baggi, Sharon Bambaji, Sam Bedser, Layla van den Bergh, Stuart Boffey, Siobhan Egan, Helen Elder, Mark Mitchenall, Chris Moodie, Tony Pollard, Simon Seljeflot, Liz Southey, Tim Stentiford, Matthew Whyte

ANGINA

SUMMARY INFORMATION

DESCRIPTION

- Angina is a symptom complex that results from myocardial ischemia; most commonly caused by narrowing of the coronary arteries
- Classic angina characterized by discomfort in the retrosternal area, which may radiate to the left shoulder and arm, the jaw, the neck, and – less frequently – to the back or to both arms
- Symptoms may also be associated with dyspnea, nausea, vomiting, light-headedness, and diaphoresis
- Usually precipitated by exertion; however, anginal variants may also occur at rest
- Symptoms typically resolve within minutes with rest or after taking prescribed antianginal medications
- Angina described as 'crescendo' in nature if symptoms occur increasingly frequently (and/or severely) with progressively less activity
- Unstable angina characterized by symptoms at rest which may persist despite antianginal therapy; refractory episodes may result in myocardial injury or infarction

URGENT ACTION

If there is a possibility of a myocardial infarction or ischemic event:

- Assess vital signs and establish means for rigorous monitoring of patient (heart rate, blood pressure, and oxygen saturation)
- Administer aspirin (325mg tablet, chewed) unless absolutely contraindicated
- Administer supplemental oxygen
- Administer nitroglycerin (sublingual tablet 0.3–0.4mg every 5min (three times) and/or topical ointment) as tolerated by blood pressure
- Place an intravenous line
- Consider administration of beta-blocker (intravenously or orally) as tolerated by blood pressure and heart rate
- Refer the patient urgently to a cardiologist or nearest emergency room for intensive investigation and management
- Obtain 12-lead ECG

ICD9 CODE

411.1 Unstable angina, preinfarction angina; 413 Angina pectoris; 413.0 Decubitus angina; 413.1 Prinzmetal's angina, variant angina; 413.9 Angina, unspecified; 528.3 Ludwig's angina

SYNONYMS

Angina pectoris, breast pang, coronarism, heart stroke, Heberden's angina, Rougnon–Heberden disease, stenocardia. Prinzmetal's (or variant) and 'microvascular' angina describe other rare forms of angina pectoris.

CARDINAL FEATURES

- Discomfort is often described as a heaviness, squeezing tightness, dull ache, or pressure in the chest
- Discomfort may radiate to the left arm, neck, jaw, or – less commonly – to the back or to both arms
- Symptoms are NOT ordinarily described as brief, sharp, pleuritic, stabbing, localized, throbbing, or migratory

Classic angina:

- Chest discomfort most commonly begins gradually and reaches maximal intensity over several minutes before resolving
- Discomfort usually resolves after rest or 2–3min after nitroglycerin is taken

Variant (Prinzmetal's) angina:

- Chest discomfort occurs at rest secondary to coronary vasospasm associated with ST-segment elevation on ECG
- Attacks usually occur in the early morning and most frequently resolve spontaneously, although they may be severe

Unstable angina:

- Chest discomfort occurs with increasing frequency and severity with progressively less activity or at rest

Syndrome X:

- Classic symptoms of angina pectoris are present along with evidence of myocardial ischemia
- Normal epicardial coronary arteries are seen on angiography

CAUSES

Common causes

Etiologies of myocardial ischemia:

- Coronary artery disease (CAD)
- Coronary vasospasm
- Aortic stenosis
- Mitral valve prolapse
- Hypertrophic cardiomyopathy
- Hypertensive heart disease
- Pulmonary hypertension

Rare causes

Syndrome X

Serious causes

Etiologies of myocardial ischemia:

- Coronary artery disease
- Coronary vasospasm
- Aortic stenosis
- Mitral valve prolapse
- Hypertrophic cardiomyopathy
- Hypertensive heart disease
- Pulmonary hypertension

Contributory or predisposing factors

- Inadequately controlled hypertension
- Cigarette smoking
- Hyperlipidemia
- Insulin resistance
- Family history of CAD
- Age (>65 years)
- Gender (male)
- Estrogen deficiency
- Obesity
- Sedentary lifestyle
- Other systemic issues that increase myocardial oxygen demand or decrease myocardial oxygen supply (e.g. infection, fever, anemia, hyperthyroidism)

EPIDEMIOLOGY

Incidence and prevalence

INCIDENCE

Males 26–56 per 1000, females 15–38 per 1000.

PREVALENCE

Over 30 per 1000 in those aged over 30 years.

Demographics

AGE

Relatively rare in adults under the age of 35 years, but the prevalence increases after age 35.

GENDER

More commonly affects men.

RACE

- Mortality from coronary heart disease (CHD) highest in African-Americans until late in life when it becomes higher in non-Hispanic Caucasians
- Overall, CHD incidence is lower in Hispanics than in Caucasians, but may be higher in long-term resident Hispanic populations than in recent immigrant populations

SOCIOECONOMIC STATUS

More prevalent in lower socioeconomic classes.

DIFFERENTIAL DIAGNOSIS

Myocardial infarction

FEATURES

- Symptoms may be similar to those of angina, but often are more severe and last longer (greater than 30min), more commonly with diaphoresis and shortness of breath
- Symptoms do not ordinarily resolve with rest or after taking sublingual nitroglycerin

Aortic dissection

FEATURES

- Pain usually described as a 'tearing' quality, located in the center of the chest with radiation between the scapulae or to the legs
- Precipitous onset of severe discomfort which may last for hours
- Absent pulses or inequality of blood pressure of the arms or legs
- Aortic regurgitation or enlarging pleural effusion present

Pulmonary embolism

FEATURES

- Pain may have precipitous onset and may be pleuritic in nature
- May be associated with hemoptysis
- May be associated with tachycardia, hypoxemia, and evidence of right ventricular strain by physical examination and ECG

Pleural inflammation

FEATURES

- Pain is typically 'sharp' or 'stabbing' in nature, and is exacerbated by deep breath, cough or change in position
- Symptoms are typically focal, localized to one side of the chest

Pericarditis

FEATURES

- Pain may be exacerbated by deep breath, cough, or change of position
- Symptoms may be alleviated by leaning forward
- Pain that radiates to the trapezius is common in pericarditis, but not characteristic of angina or myocardial infarction
- Characteristic ECG findings

Chest wall conditions and musculoskeletal conditions

FEATURES

- Conditions include fractured rib, costochondritis, intercostal neuritis, sprains and strains
- Pain is often sharp, fleeting and exacerbated by deep breath, cough, or movement of the arms, chest, or torso
- Pain can be worsened or reproduced by local palpation
- Site of discomfort may be red or swollen

Gastrointestinal disorders

FEATURES

- Pain relieved by food or antacids
- Non specific changes in T waves and ST segments have been reported in esophagitis, peptic ulcer disease, and cholecystitis. In addition, sublingual nitroglycerin and certain calcium channel blockers used to treat angina can occasionally alleviate pain due to esophageal reflux or spasm

SIGNS & SYMPTOMS

Signs

Examination of a patient who is actively suffering from angina may reveal:

- A third or fourth heart sound/gallop (due to myocardial ischemia and impaired diastolic relaxation)
- A reverse splitting of the second heart sound (due to dyssynergy of left ventricular systolic contraction and consequent delayed aortic valve closure)
- A systolic murmur at the apex (due to papillary muscle ischemia and consequent mitral regurgitation)

Symptoms

- Discomfort is often described as a heaviness, squeezing tightness, dull ache, or pressure in the chest
- The discomfort may radiate to the left arm, neck, jaw, or – less commonly – to the back or to both arms
- The symptoms are NOT ordinarily described as brief, sharp, pleuritic, stabbing, localized, throbbing, or migratory

Classic angina:

- Chest discomfort most commonly begins gradually and reaches maximal intensity over several minutes before resolving
- The discomfort usually resolves after rest or 2–3min after nitroglycerin is taken

Variant (Prinzmetal's) angina:

- Chest discomfort occurs at rest secondary to coronary vasospasm associated with ST-segment elevation on ECG
- Attacks usually occur in the early morning and most frequently resolve spontaneously, although they may be severe

In unstable angina:

- Chest discomfort occurs with increasing frequency and severity with progressively less activity or at rest

Syndrome X:

- The classic symptoms of angina pectoris are present along with evidence of myocardial ischemia on ECG
- Normal epicardial coronary arteries are seen on angiography
- Discomfort commonly located in the retrosternal area
- Radiation to the neck, shoulders, arms, jaws, epigastric region, or back
- Many patients DO NOT perceive angina as pain
- Some patients have dyspnea, profound fatigue, weakness, light-headedness, nausea, sweating, altered mental senses, or syncope in the absence of chest discomfort
- Symptoms typically triggered by physical activity, emotional stress, exposure to cold, consuming a heavy meal, or smoking
- Symptoms typically last 3–5min
- 'Second-wind' or 'walk-through' angina occurs when the second episode of anginal discomfort occurs 2–5min after the first episode; it is predictably longer in duration (lasting up to 30min)
- Decubitus angina occurs with change in posture
- Nocturnal angina is frequently associated with nightmares

ASSOCIATED DISORDERS

- Valvular heart disease
- Hypertrophic cardiomyopathy

CONSIDER CONSULT

Manifestations of ischemic heart disease that warrant immediate referral to the nearest emergency department:

- Chest pain lasting more than 30min or refractory to treatment with three sublingual nitroglycerin tablets (less likely classic angina; more likely unstable angina or myocardial infarction)
- Chest pain with new left bundle branch block or ST elevation on ECG (diagnostic of acute myocardial infarction)
- Chest pain associated with hemodynamic instability or clinical evidence of congestive heart failure (suggests significant left ventricular dysfunction)

Manifestations of ischemic heart disease that warrant referral to a cardiologist for further assessment:

- Episodic exertional chest discomfort which has persisted or gradually worsened despite medical therapy
- Symptoms of classic angina with a strongly positive exercise tolerance test
- Continued chest discomfort with nondiagnostic testing, leaving a diagnostic dilemma
- Intolerance to medications, creating treatment difficulties in patients with established angina

INVESTIGATION OF THE PATIENT

Direct questions to patient

Q What was the pain like? (describe it). Determine whether the pain is typical or atypical in quality, location, duration

Q Have you had any episodes like this before? If the patient has had episodes before, determine whether there are any differences in the onset, activity that triggered it, time to pain resolution, and response to medication or rest

Q What were you doing just before the onset of the pain or symptoms? The relationship to a triggering event may aid in defining the condition

Q How quickly did the pain subside? Symptoms typically last 3–5min, but chest pain triggered by emotional distress often lasts longer than that triggered by exercise. When pain lasts more than 15min, investigate possibility of myocardial infarction

Q How would you characterize the pain? Some patients describe angina as vague chest discomfort, not perceiving it as pain. Some patients have anginal equivalents, such as shortness of breath, in the absence of any chest discomfort

Q Did medication relieve or reduce the chest pain? If patient has been using nitroglycerin, determine whether treatment was ineffective in resolving the pain. If so, this may be indicative of unstable angina and will require further evaluation and treatment

Contributory or predisposing factors

Is there a history of predisposing factors? Etiologies of myocardial ischemia include:

- Coronary artery disease
- Coronary vasospasm
- Aortic stenosis
- Mitral valve prolapse (may cause atypical chest pain, not clearly ischemia)
- Hypertrophic cardiomyopathy
- Hypertensive heart disease
- Pulmonary hypertension

Family history

Because diabetes, hyperlipidemia, and hypertension may have genetic ties to predispose patients to CHD, the following questions are appropriate.

Q Is there a family history of angina, myocardial infarction, or other stigmata of coronary artery disease, particularly at an early age?

Q Any other heart disease in the family?

- Q Is there a family history of diabetes?
- Q Is there a family history of high blood pressure?
- Q Is there a family history of high cholesterol levels?

Examination

If the patient is experiencing chest discomfort at the time, evaluate the patient for:

- Rales, S3, S4, and systolic murmur (due to ischemic mitral regurgitation)
- Decreased S1 intensity or paradoxic splitting of S2 (due to delayed left ventricular emptying)

Look for evidence of carotid or peripheral vascular disease:

- Check eyes for corneal arcus, xanthelasma, and retinal arteriolar changes
- Decreased distal pulses, bruits, cutaneous signs of arterial insufficiency
- Look for diagonal earlobe crease

All of the above signs generally disappear when symptoms resolve.

Summary of investigative tests

- Resting 12-lead ECG: an essential test in evaluating the patient with chest pain
- Exercise tolerance test diagnoses ischemia in patients with exertional chest discomfort; pharmacologic stress modalities should be considered if patient is not physically capable of walking. Consider referral to cardiologist prior to test if there is concern of 'unstable' or rapidly escalating symptoms
- Echocardiography: warranted in patients in whom the history or physical examination suggest valvular or other structural heart disease, congestive heart failure, or left ventricular enlargement/dysfunction. When combined with a stress test, a stress echocardiogram can diagnose angina by finding exercise-induced wall motion abnormalities
- A fasting lipid panel (including total cholesterol, HDL cholesterol, triglycerides, and calculated LDL cholesterol) should be obtained to evaluate for hyperlipidemia – a modifiable risk factor for CAD
- Cardiac catheterization: the 'gold-standard' test for identifying coronary artery disease – the substrate for angina. Catheterization also provides the opportunity for (percutaneous) coronary intervention (see Choices). Decisions regarding when to refer a patient for catheterization require referral to a cardiologist
- A chest X-ray should be obtained for patients with signs or symptoms suggesting congestive heart failure, valvular heart disease, pericardial disease, or aortic dissection or aneurysm. Patients with signs or symptoms of pulmonary disease should also undergo this evaluation
- A blood glucose level should be obtained to assess for diabetes, if suspected from clinical history
- A hemoglobin level should be obtained to address contribution of anemia to manifestation of angina

DIAGNOSTIC DECISION

The American College of Cardiology, the American Heart Association, and the American College of Physicians–American Society of Internal Medicine have produced guidelines that give recommendations on the diagnosis of chronic stable angina:

- Guidelines for the management of patients with chronic stable angina. [1]

The European Society of Cardiology has also developed guidelines that cover the diagnosis of stable angina:

- Management of stable angina pectoris. Recommendations of the Task Force of the European Society of Cardiology. [2]

CLINICAL PEARL(S)

- In classic angina, many patients describe their angina as being more frequent in the morning, such as while walking to work, even though they are more energetic at that time of day
- The diagnosis of angina usually proceeds along a stepwise plan, becoming more complex and invasive if needed. Most angina is diagnosed on the basis of history and an exercise test, using more expensive imaging studies (such as nuclear stress test or stress echocardiogram) if needed. Finally, a cardiac catheterization is considered either because of concern for accelerating or severe angina, or because of a continued diagnostic dilemma
- A cardiac catheterization will provide the anatomic information about coronary artery disease, locating coronary artery stenoses. The functional significance of these stenoses, as shown on an exercise or pharmacologic stress test, will often provide the critical information in deciding whether or not to proceed with catheter intervention of the coronary stenoses. There is not always a reason to open a coronary artery stenosis 'just because it is there'

THE TESTS

Body fluids

BLOOD HEMOGLOBIN

Description

Cuffed venous blood sample.

Advantages/Disadvantages

- Advantage: Confirms or rules out anemia
- Disadvantage: Has no other diagnostic or monitoring role in angina

Normal

- Women: 12.0–16.0g/dL
- Men: 13.5–17.5g/dL

Abnormal

As an indication of anemia:

- An arbitrary level of <12g/dL is acceptable, but the erythrocyte count should also be evaluated
- Keep in mind the possibility of a false-positive result

Cause of abnormal result

Any cause of anemia.

Drugs, disorders, and other factors that may alter results

- Excessive fluid intake will cause decreased hemoglobin values
- Hemoglobin levels are normally decreased in pregnancy
- Many drugs are associated with anemia

BLOOD GLUCOSE

Description

Cuffed venous blood sample.

Advantages/Disadvantages

- Advantage: Confirms or rules out diabetes
- Disadvantage: Has no other diagnostic or monitoring role in angina

Normal

- Fasting serum: 70–110mg/dL
- Fasting whole blood: 60–100mg/dL
- Random: 85–125mg/dL for patients >50 years of age, 70–115mg/dL for patients <50 years of age

Abnormal

- If random glucose >200mg/dL (and classic symptoms of polyuria, polydipsia, and weight loss are present), the diagnosis of diabetes is made
- If fasting glucose is >140mg/dL on two occasions, the diagnosis of diabetes is made
- Keep in mind the possibility of a false-positive result

Cause of abnormal result

Common causes include:

- Cushing's disease
- Pheochromocytoma
- Pituitary adenoma or pancreatic adenoma
- Pancreatitis
- Hyperthyroidism
- Brain damage or trauma
- Chronic liver disease
- Chronic illness or malnutrition
- Potassium deficiency

Drugs, disorders, and other factors that may alter results

- Steroids, diuretics, and many other drugs will interfere with the test
- Pregnancy may normally cause a slight elevation in glucose
- Obesity
- Infection of the adrenals
- Stress
- Prolonged physical inactivity

LIPID PROFILE

Description

Cuffed venous blood sample (fasting).

Advantages/Disadvantages

- Advantage: identifies the presence of hyperlipidemia, a risk factor for CAD and consequent angina and myocardial infarction
- Disadvantage: has no other diagnostic or monitoring role in angina; not immediately modifiable

Normal

- **Total cholesterol:** 140–250mg/dL (<200 recommended)
- **HDL cholesterol:** women: 30–80mg/dL, men: 30–70mg/dL
- **Triglycerides:** 40–150mg/dL
- **LDL cholesterol** (calculated): 62–185mg/dL (<130 recommended)

Abnormal

- **Total cholesterol:** an upper limit of 220mg/dL for total cholesterol value is desirable; as the blood level rises, the risk of atherosclerosis and heart disease increases
- **HDL cholesterol:** low levels of HDL cholesterol are associated with a risk of coronary artery disease in men and women aged over 50 years
- **Triglycerides:** elevated triglycerides along with elevated cholesterol are risk factors in atherosclerotic disease
- **LDL cholesterol:** high levels of LDLs are closely correlated with an increased incidence of atherosclerosis and CHD
- Keep in mind the possibility of a false-positive result

Cause of abnormal result

- **Cholesterol:** obstructive jaundice, hypothyroidism, nephrosis, xanthomatosis, uncontrolled diabetes, nephrotic syndrome, diet
- **HDL cholesterol:** chronic physical inactivity, inheritance
- **Triglycerides:** liver disease, nephrotic syndrome, hypothyroidism, poorly controlled diabetes, pancreatitis, glycogen storage disease, myocardial infarction (elevations may last up to 1 year after infarct event), toxemia, inactivity, diet, obesity
- **LDL cholesterol:** as this is a calculated value based on total cholesterol, HDL cholesterol, and triglyceride results, factors that can cause abnormal results for each of these tests are applicable here

Drugs, disorders, and other factors that may alter results

Total cholesterol levels are:

- Slightly increased in pregnancy
- Decreased by elevated estrogen levels
- Increased by oophorectomy

HDL cholesterol levels are:

- Frequently elevated in long-distance runners
- Either elevated or decreased in primary biliary cirrhosis, chronic hepatitis, and alcoholism
- Decreased in smokers

Iodine contrast media and recent weight gains or losses can interfere with test results.

Triglyceride levels are:

- Transiently increased after a heavy meal or alcohol ingestion
- Increased by pregnancy and oral contraceptives

Imaging

CHEST X-RAY

Advantages/Disadvantages

Advantages:

- Helps to confirm or rule out congestive heart failure (a patient can have congestive heart failure without pulmonary edema visible on a chest X-ray), valvular heart disease, pericardial disease, aortic dissection/aneurysm, pulmonary disease
- May assist with the identification of pulmonary edema (a manifestation of congestive heart failure), cardiomegaly, calcification of coronary arteries (in severe CAD), valvular heart disease, pericardial disease, aortic dissection/aneurysm, and pulmonary disease

Disadvantage: Usefulness as a routine test is not well established; has no other diagnostic or monitoring role in angina

Abnormal

- More likely to be abnormal in patients with previous myocardial infarction (and consequent left ventricular dilatation), those with a non coronary artery cause of chest pain, and those with non cardiac chest discomfort
- Keep in mind the possibility of imaging artifacts

Other tests

RESTING 12-LEAD ECG

Advantages/Disadvantages

Advantages:

- In the absence of symptoms, the ECG may reveal Q waves, poor R-wave progression, or ST/T-wave changes that indicate prior myocardial infarction
- When obtained during symptoms of chest pain, the ECG may indicate whether or not there is active ischemia or acute myocardial infarction (also, it may identify stigmata of acute pericarditis, pulmonary embolus, or left ventricular hypertrophy found in other disease processes causing chest pain)
- Non invasive procedure

Disadvantage:

- Rest 12-lead ECG is normal in approx. 50% of patients with chronic stable angina
- Normal result does not exclude ischemia as the cause of chest pain

Abnormal

- Presence of Q waves, chronic ST-segment depression (or other ST/T-wave abnormalities), and poor R-wave progression may reflect prior myocardial infarction and indicate the substrate for myocardial ischemia in a patient with chest pain
- Evidence of left ventricular hypertrophy increases the probability that the chest discomfort is due to angina
- In an ECG recorded during an episode of chest pain, transient changes in T wave, ST segment, or conduction strongly suggest coronary ischemia or another cardiac source of pain

Cause of abnormal result

- Myocardial ischemia (ongoing)
- Myocardial infarction (old or acute)
- Left ventricular hypertrophy
- Pericardial disease
- Electrolyte abnormalities
- Drug interaction
- Metabolic disturbances
- Pulmonary disease
- Gastrointestinal causes
- Intracerebral insult

EXERCISE TOLERANCE TEST

Advantages/Disadvantages

Advantages:

- Diagnoses ischemia in patients with exertional chest discomfort (pharmacologic stress modalities should be considered if patient is not physically capable of walking)
- Adjunctive nuclear or echocardiographic imaging may increase sensitivity and specificity of test, and is essential in patients with a baseline ECG that is uninterpretable for ischemia (i.e. left bundle branch block, severe left ventricular hypertrophy, use of digitalis)

Disadvantage: clinical utility of test is diminished in patients with atypical symptoms

CONSIDER CONSULT

If there is evidence of an accelerating pattern of angina (i.e. more frequent episodes at lower activity levels), referral for cardiology intervention (usually cardiac catheterization) is indicated.

IMMEDIATE ACTION

If there is the possibility of a myocardial infarction or an ischemic event:

- Administer aspirin (325mg tablet, chewed) unless absolutely contraindicated
- Administer supplemental oxygen
- Administer nitroglycerin (sublingual tablet 0.3–0.4mg every 5min (three times) and/or topical ointment) as tolerated by blood pressure
- Place an intravenous line
- Consider administration of beta-blocker (intravenously or orally) as tolerated by blood pressure and heart rate
- Refer the patient emergently to a cardiologist or nearest emergency room for intensive management

PATIENT AND CAREGIVER ISSUES

Health-seeking behavior

- Self-medications? The patient may have been self-medicating with low-dose aspirin (due to high media coverage) or with nonsteroidal anti-inflammatory drugs (NSAIDs) for pain
- **Has the patient altered his/her lifestyle?** A patient who has reduced or modified activities that led to anginal episodes may be more compliant when other lifestyle changes are recommended

MANAGEMENT ISSUES

Goals

The aims are:

- To minimize symptoms of angina
- To modify risk factors and improve prognosis by preventing myocardial infarction

Management in special circumstances

Women:

- Anginal symptoms may be more likely to present in an atypical manner in women than in men. These symptoms, particularly in young women, are often dismissed as 'non cardiac' in origin
- As coronary artery disease is less prevalent in younger women, the exercise test is more likely to be falsely positive, but women with typical symptoms of exertional angina and a positive exercise tolerance test should be referred to a cardiologist for consideration of cardiac catheterization

The elderly:

- It may be difficult to obtain a history of exertionally induced chest discomfort if the patient leads a sedentary lifestyle
- Inactive patients may have difficulty performing an exercise tolerance test; pharmacologic stress modalities may need to be considered if clinically appropriate
- Alterations of drug metabolism and pharmacology in the elderly warrant vigilant clinical and laboratory surveillance
- The risk of drug interactions, multiple pharmacy use, and compliance problems must also be borne in mind when planning a treatment regimen

COEXISTING DISEASE

Aortic valve stenosis, hypertrophic obstructive cardiomyopathy:

- Nitrates should be used only with great caution, since the resultant drop in preload may result in progressively worsening left ventricular output and hypotension

Heart failure:

- Beta-blockers may simultaneously confer a symptomatic benefit for patients with angina and a mortality benefit for patients with heart failure
- Beta-blockers should be used judiciously in patients with impaired ventricular function due to their negative inotropic effect, and should be instituted only in patients who are in a 'compensated' state

Ischemic dilated cardiomyopathy:

- Calcium antagonists may certainly relieve angina in patients with ischemic dilated cardiomyopathy, although they may not confer a mortality benefit in this population. They should be used with caution in such patients due to the negative inotropic effect

Asthma:

- Beta-blockers should be avoided due to the potential exacerbation of bronchospasm

Peripheral vascular disease:

- Beta-blockers may worsen symptoms

Migraine:

- Beta-blockers and calcium antagonists may be beneficial, but nitrates may worsen headaches

COEXISTING MEDICATION

Beta-blockers and heart rate limiting calcium antagonists (diltiazem and verapamil) should be used with caution together due to their combined effects impairing conduction across the atrioventricular node.

PATIENT SATISFACTION/LIFESTYLE PRIORITIES

Quality of life issues are very important in drug therapy for CAD, and should be specifically addressed. For example, many patients will have side-effects such as lethargy, sexual dysfunction, or forgetfulness from one beta-blocker but not from another. In general experience, there are no predictable rules, so it should be kept in mind that it is common practice to switch from one drug to another in the same category, or in another category, if side-effects are limiting treatment or creating intolerable side-effects.

SUMMARY OF THERAPEUTIC OPTIONS

Choices

- Medical management is the mainstay of treatment, often controlling angina satisfactorily for many years
- Catheter interventions and coronary bypass surgery are treatments, not cures, and underlying issues of risk factor management must still be addressed
- The use of nitroglycerin prior to physical activity can often prevent angina, and should be recommended to active patients with predictable angina

In treatment of patients with angina, the following four strategies should be kept in mind:

1. Management of concomitant systemic illnesses that may exacerbate angina

- Transfuse if anemic
- Correct hyperthyroidism
- Treat systemic infection

2. Risk reduction and lifestyle modification

- Smoking cessation
- Management of hypertension
- Control of diabetes
- Weight loss, regular exercise regimen
- Dietary changes for weight loss and lipid reduction
- Limit alcohol ingestion
- Stress reduction
- Mind–body practices may be efficacious as complementary therapies for cardiovascular disease-related conditions

3. Pharmacologic management

- Lipid lowering: Lipid-lowering therapy has been demonstrated to confer a mortality benefit through reduction of primary and secondary cardiovascular events – see the NCEP guidelines [JAMA 1993; 269:3015-23]. Lipid-lowering medications used include simvastatin and pravastatin
- Aspirin therapy reduces mortality. Aspirin should be used in all patients with angina or suspected coronary artery disease (unless absolutely contraindicated) since it confers a marked reduction in mortality from myocardial infarction
- Beta-blockers (e.g. atenolol, metoprolol) may reduce symptoms in patients with chronic stable angina and improve survival in those who have suffered a prior myocardial infarction
- Calcium channel blockers (e.g. nifedipine, nicardipine) and/or long-acting nitrates (isosorbide mononitrate) should be considered if initial treatment with beta-blockers is ineffective. Short-acting dihydropyridine calcium antagonists should not be used as solo therapy (i.e. without concomitant use of a beta-blocker), as the resultant reflex tachycardia may precipitate sudden cardiac death in patients with coronary disease
- Nitrates (e.g. amyl nitrate): sublingual nitrates work rapidly with lasting effect. Effectiveness with frequent use may be limited due to tachyphylaxis
- Beta-blockers and angiotensin-converting enzyme (ACE) inhibitors confer survival benefit in management of patients who have previously suffered myocardial infarction
- For patients with vasospastic angina (Prinzmetal's angina), consider a combination of calcium channel blockers and long-acting nitrate therapy
- ACE inhibitors (e.g. ramipril) have been demonstrated to have a reduction in ischemic events following myocardial infarction and heart failure, but no studies have evaluated the outcome benefit of ACE inhibitors in chronic stable angina
- The use of hormone replacement therapy (HRT) for primary risk reduction in postmenopausal women is currently under debate. It appears that there is a higher incidence of cardiovascular events in the first year following initiation of therapy; but there is a reduction in events after 4–5 years. A tentative recommendation is to maintain HRT in those who are already taking it, but not to initiate it in those who are not
- Supplementation with selenium, B vitamins, L-carnitine, and coenzyme Q10 may be of benefit

4. Revascularization

- Consideration of percutaneous coronary intervention (angioplasty or stent) if symptoms are refractory to medical therapy or are 'unstable'
- Coronary artery bypass grafting surgery particularly beneficial in patients with multi vessel disease and reduced left ventricular systolic function, diabetes, or other coronary anatomy not amenable to percutaneous intervention

Guidelines

The American College of Cardiology, the American Heart Association, and the American College of Physicians–American Society of Internal Medicine have produced guidelines that give recommendations on the management of chronic stable angina:

- Guidelines for the management of patients with chronic stable angina. [1]

The European Society of Cardiology has also developed guidelines that cover the management of stable angina:

- Management of stable angina pectoris. [2]

The American College of Cardiology and the American Heart Association have developed guidelines for the management of unstable angina:

- Braunwald E, Antman EM, Beasley JW, et al. ACC/AHA guidelines for the management of patients with unstable angina and non-ST-segment elevation myocardial infarction. [3]

Clinical pearl(s)

The issue of HRT for women is unsettled. Given the conflicting data, the decision is generally made for other reasons, such as osteoporosis prevention or menopausal symptom control.

Never

- Beta-blockers should be used with great caution in patients who have significant bradyarrhythmias, asthma, congestive heart failure, or hypotension. They must also be used prudently in patients with diabetes mellitus and peripheral vascular disease
- ACE inhibitors should not be used to treat patients with hereditary angioedema or bilateral renal artery stenosis
- Diltiazem and verapamil (calcium channel blockers) should be used cautiously in patients with bradyarrhythmias. Verapamil is not recommended in patients with poor left ventricular systolic function. When used alone, short-acting dihydropyridine calcium antagonists may induce reflex tachycardia and thereby increase the risk of sudden cardiac death; concomitant use with beta-blockers may reduce this risk.

FOLLOW UP

Plan for review

Comparison of anginal episodes before and after initiating therapy/intervention:

- Frequency: more or less often?
- Intensity and duration: are episodes more or less severe?
- Precipitating factors: is more or less activity required to bring on symptoms?
- If episodes occur more frequently, are more severe, or are precipitated with less activity, then consider upward titration of medical regimen (increase dose of one agent or add second anti anginal agent); if conservative maneuvers are ineffective, discuss referral to cardiologist for consideration of catheterization/revascularization

Tolerance of medication:

- Drug side-effects
- Blood pressure response: titrate doses up or down to attain desired effect
- Impact on other organ system function
- Assure appropriate serum drug levels when indicated

Functional capacity:

- Activity level: improvement on therapy?
- Consider exercise tolerance testing for measurement of exercise capacity relative to threshold for developing ischemia (and consideration of need for revascularization)

General:

- Follow up by phone or in the office for a blood pressure check within a few days if medication changes are likely to cause hypotension or orthostasis
- Evaluation of the effect of medication changes on anginal symptoms may take several days or weeks

- Follow up should be determined by the patient's medical stability, reliability, the possibility of significant drug interactions or comorbidities, and understanding of his/her disease and medications

Information for patient or caregiver

Adjustment of lifestyle issues (cholesterol level, exercise, smoking, diet) can decrease attacks of angina.

DRUGS AND OTHER THERAPIES: DETAILS

Drugs

SIMVASTATIN

Dose

Adult: 5–40mg daily, gradually increasing dose

Efficacy

Effective in reducing hyperlipidemia, hypercholesterolemia, and hypertriglyceridemia.

Risks/Benefits

- Benefits: marked response seen within 2 weeks of initiation, maximum therapeutic response occurring within 4–6 weeks. Response is maintained during chronic therapy
- Use caution with past liver disease, alcoholism
- Use caution with severe acute infections, trauma, hypotension
- Use caution with uncontrolled seizure disorders, severe metabolic disorders, and electrolyte disorders

Side-effects and adverse reactions

- CNS: Dizziness, headache, insomnia, peripheral neuropathy
- Gastrointestinal: abdominal pain, nausea, vomiting, dyspepsia, pancreatitis, liver dysfunction
- Genitourinary: erectile dysfunction
- Hematologic: eosinophilia, hemolytic anemia, leukopenia
- Musculoskeletal: myalgia, myositis, rhabdomyolysis
- Skin: alopecia, pruritus, rash, Stevens–Johnson syndrome

Interactions (other drugs)

- Azole antifungals
- Cholestyramine
- Colestipol
- Danazol
- Fluoxetine
- Gemfibrozil
- Isradipine
- Macrolide antibiotics
- Nefazodone
- Warfarin

Contraindications

- Acute liver disease
- Pregnancy
- Nursing

Evidence

The 4S study, a large randomized, controlled trial, has demonstrated that lipid reduction with simvastatin reduced mortality, rate of major coronary events, and need for coronary revascularization in all patients; similar reductions in the rate of major coronary events were seen in women compared with men and in elderly patients (aged 65 years or more) compared with younger patients. There were too few female deaths to assess the effects on mortality in women, but the effect was significant in elderly patients [4, 5] *Level P*

Follow up plan

- Monitor patients for changes in liver function test results for the first year of treatment or until 1 year after the last elevation in dose
- Monitor patients for myopathy during the initial months of therapy and during any periods of upward drug dosage titration

Patient and caregiver information

The statin drugs should be taken at night, since the liver manufactures cholesterol during these hours.

PRAVASTATIN

Dose

Adult: 10–40mg/day (in the evening) by mouth, in gradually increasing doses

Risks/Benefits

- Benefits: marked response seen within 2 weeks of initiation, maximum therapeutic response occurring within 4–6 weeks. Response is maintained during chronic therapy
- Use caution with past liver disease, alcoholism
- Use caution with severe acute infections, trauma, hypotension
- Use caution with uncontrolled seizure disorders, severe metabolic disorders, and electrolyte disorders
- Use caution with children less than 18 years

Side-effects and adverse reactions

- CNS: dizziness, headache
- Cardiovascular: chest pain
- Gastrointestinal: abdominal pain, nausea, vomiting, dyspepsia, pancreatitis, liver dysfunction
- Genitourinary: erectile dysfunction
- Hematological: eosinophilia, hemolytic anemia, leukopenia
- Musculoskeletal: arthralgia, myalgia, myositis, rhabdomyolysis
- Skin: alopecia, pruritus, rash, Stevens–Johnson syndrome

Interactions (other drugs)

■ Azole antifungals ■ Cholestyramine ■ Clofibrate ■ Colestipol ■ Danazol ■ Fluoxetine ■ Gemfibrozil ■ Isradipine ■ Macrolide antibiotics ■ Nefazodone ■ Troleandomycin ■ Warfarin

Contraindications

■ Acute liver disease ■ Pregnancy ■ Nursing mothers

Evidence

- LIPID is a large multicenter, double-blind, randomized, placebo-controlled trial of secondary prevention of coronary events. It is comparing the effects of pravastatin (40mg/day), with placebo, given for 5 years or more, in patients aged 31–75 years with a total cholesterol level at baseline of 155–270mg/dL and a history of acute myocardial infarction or hospitalization for unstable angina pectoris. In the 3620 patients with unstable angina, mortality from coronary heart disease, total mortality, rate of myocardial infarction, need for coronary revascularization, the number of admissions to hospital, and the number of in-hospital days were significantly lower in pravastatin group [6,7] *Level P*
- A prospective, randomized, controlled trial in men with unstable angina on optimal antianginal treatment found pravastatin therapy significantly reduced the number of episodes of transient myocardial ischemia as measured by 48-hr ambulatory electrocardiography [8] *Level P*

ISOSORBIDE MONONITRATE

Dose

Adult oral: 30–60mg twice daily sustained release gradually increasing dose

Efficacy

Decreases exercise-induced myocardial ischemia, alleviates symptoms, and increases exercise tolerance.

Risks/Benefits

- Use with caution in hypertrophic cardiomyopathy
- Use with caution in hypotension, glaucoma
- Use with caution in nursing mothers
- Avoid continuous delivery without nitrate-free interval (tolerance will develop)

Side-effects and adverse reactions

- CNS: agitation, anxiety, confusion, dizziness, headache, insomnia, nightmares
- Cardiovascular: atrial fibrillation, cardiovascular collapse, crescendo angina, edema, hypotension, palpitations
- Gastrointestinal: abdominal pain, diarrhea,nausea, dyspepsia
- Genitourinary: dysuria, erectile dysfunction
- Hematologic: hemolytic anemia
- Musculoskeletal: arthralgia, muscle twitching
- Skin: dermatitis, flushing, pruritus, rash

Interactions (other drugs)

Viagra

Contraindications

- Hypersensitivity to nitrates
- Closed-angle glaucoma
- Severe anemia
- Increased intracranial pressure
- Hypotension
- Acute myocardial infarction and congestive heart failure
- Cerebral hemorrhage

Evidence

A controlled 6-month trial of sustained-release isosorbide mononitrate in patients with stable angina showed significant improvement in anginal indices and quality of life, and those who received 100mg/day showed significantly more improvement than those who received 50mg/day [9] *Level P*

Acceptability to patient

High.

Follow up plan

Monitor patients frequently for tolerance to prescribed dose of medication.

Patient and caregiver information

- Patients should be instructed to contact primary care physician if the anti anginal effect of the prescribed drug dose appears to be weakening

AMYL NITRITE

Dose

Adult inhalation: 0.18–0.3 mL cap as needed, may repeat 3min

Side-effects and adverse reactions
- CNS: dizziness, headache, syncope
- Cardiovascular: collapse, hypotension, palpitations
- Gastrointestinal: abdominal pain, nausea
- Hematologic: hemolytic anemia
- Musculoskeletal: muscle twitching
- Skin: flushing

Interactions (other drugs)
Viagra

Contraindications
- Hypersensitivity to nitrates ▪ Closed-angle glaucoma ▪ Severe anemia
- Increased intracranial pressure ▪ Hypotension
- Acute myocardial infarction and congestive heart failure ▪ Cerebral hemorrhage

ASPIRIN
Dose
Adult oral dose:165–325mg daily
Child oral dose: 60–90mg/kg daily

Efficacy
Effective in reducing potential for vascular events (myocardial infarction, first heart attack) in patients with chronic stable angina.

Risks/Benefits
- Benefits: simple dosing regimen allows for better patient compliance
- Use caution in anemia, Hodgkin's disease, bleeding disorders
- Use caution with gout, hepatic and renal disease
- Use caution with asthma, nasal polyps, nasal allergies
- Use caution with children and teenagers (Reye's syndrome)

Side-effects and adverse reactions
- CNS: dizziness, headache
- EENT: hearing loss and tinnitus
- Gastrointestinal: abdominal pain, nausea, dyspepsia, hepatotoxicity
- Hematological: bleeding disorders, thrombocytopenia
- Respiratory:hyperpnea, asthma
- Skin: angioedema, bruising, rash, urticaria

Interactions (other drugs)
- ACE inhibitors ▪ Acetazolamide ▪ Antacids ▪ Corticosteroids ▪ Diltiazem ▪ Ethanol
- Griseofulvin ▪ Methotrexate ▪ Oral anticoagulants ▪ Probenecid ▪ Sulfinpyrazone
- Sulfonylureas ▪ Warfarin

Contraindications
- Hypersensitivity to salicylates, NSAIDs or tartrazine ▪ Gastrointestinal bleeding
- Hemophilia ▪ Hemorrhagic states

Evidence
- An overview of randomized controlled trials of found that treatment with aspirin for 1 month or longer significantly reduced the risk of a vascular event. Most of the 70,000 patients were at

high risk of coronary events, although not all had a diagnosis of angina. Low-dose aspirin (75mg/day) was found to be as effective as higher-dose aspirin [10] *Level M*

- Aspirin (75mg/day) was compared with placebo in a randomized controlled trial involving 2000 people with stable angina. Aspirin reduced the rate of myocardial infarction or sudden death [11] *Level P*

Acceptability to patient

High.

Patient and caregiver information

Patients subject to aspirin sensitivity should be instructed to consult physician about alternative treatment.

ATENOLOL

$Beta_1$-selective adrenoreceptor blocking agent

Dose

Adult oral dose: 50–200mg daily in gradually increasing dose

Efficacy

Effective in reducing or eliminating angina as well as post infarction mortality.

Risks/Benefits

- Benefits: beta-blockers, when given in adequate dosage, help to prevent anginal attacks by reducing myocardial oxygen demand and the severity of ischemia
- Use with caution in diabetes mellitus, thyroid disease, renal disease
- Use with caution in chronic obstructive pulmonary disease
- Use with caution in peripheral vascular disease

Side-effects and adverse reactions

- CNS: Lethargy, depression, and vivid dreams.
- Cardiovascular: bradycardia, congestive heart failure, heart block, peripheral vascular disease
- EENT: dry eyes, sore throat
- Respiratory: bronchospasm, dyspnea, wheezing
- Gastrointestinal: ischemic colitis, nausea, dry mouth
- Hematologic: agranulocytosis, thrombocytopenia
- Metabolism: hyperglycemia, hyperlipidemia, masked hypoglycemia
- Skin: Alopecia, bruising, rash

Interactions (other drugs)

- Adenosine - Amoxicillin, ampicillin - Antacids - Calcium channel blockers
- Clonidine - Dipyridamole - Lidocaine - Neostigmine - NSAIDs - Physostigmine
- Prazosin - Tacrine - Theophylline - Verapamil

Contraindications

- Asthma - Cardiogenic shock - Congestive heart failure - Heart block
- Sinus bradycardia

Evidence

- A pooled study from nine randomized controlled trials reported a significant reduction in mortality after myocardial infarction in patients (including patients with angina) who were treated with beta-blockers [12] *Level M*

- A multicenter, double-blind, randomized, controlled study of the effects of atenolol on patients with asymptomatic or mildly symptomatic coronary artery disease found that atenolol significantly reduced the risk of cardiac events (including hospitalization for unstable angina and aggravation of angina) and also significantly reduced the average duration of ischemic events during 48-hr ambulatory monitoring [13] *Level P*

Acceptability to patient

High, but some patients may wish to discontinue treatment due to drug side-effects.

Follow up plan

Monitor patients frequently for tolerance to prescribed medication, lipid profile changes, and for significant side-effects that may require dosage or drug change.

Patient and caregiver information

Many patients who experience side-effects such as lethargy notice an improvement after several days on the drug and should be instructed to wait for improvement. Also, beta-blockers taken at bedtime can avoid some of the daytime beta-blocker side-effects. Many patients who experience side-effects such as lethargy notice an improvement after several days on the drug and should be instructed to wait for improvement. Also, beta-blockers taken at bedtime can avoid some of the daytime beta-blocker side-effects.

METOPROLOL

$Beta_1$-selective adrenoreceptor

Dose

Adult oral dose: 100–400mg daily in gradually increasing doses

Risks/Benefits

- Benefits: beta-blockers, when given in adequate dosage, help to prevent anginal attacks by reducing myocardial oxygen demand and the severity of ischemia
- Use with caution in diabetes mellitus, thyroid disease, renal disease
- Use with caution in chronic obstructive pulmonary disease
- Use with caution in peripheral vascular disease
- Use with caution in pregnancy

Side-effects and adverse reactions

- CNS: lethargy, depression, and vivid dreams.
- Cardiovascular: bradycardia, congestive heart failure, heart block, peripheral vascular disease
- EENT: tinnitus
- Respiratory: bronchospasm, dyspnea, wheezing
- Gastrointestinal: constipation, nausea, dry mouth, dyspepsia
- Genitourinary: impotence, sexual dysfunction
- Hematological: agranulocytosis
- Metabolism: hyperglycemia, hyperlipidemia, masked hypoglycemia
- Skin: alopecia, bruising, rash

Interactions (other drugs)

▪ Amiodarone ▪ Antidiabetics ▪ Antipyrine ▪ Barbiturates ▪ Benzodiazepines ▪ Calcium channel blockers ▪ Cimetidine ▪ Clonidine ▪ Dipyridamole ▪ Lidocaine ▪ NSAIDs ▪ Phenylephrine ▪ Physostigmine ▪ Prazosin ▪ Quinolones ▪ Rifampin ▪ Theophylline ▪ Verapamil

Contraindications

- Asthma
- Cardiogenic shock
- Congestive heart failure
- Heart block
- Sinus bradycardia

Evidence

- A pooled study from nine randomized controlled trials reported a significant reduction in mortality after myocardial infarction in patients (including patients with angina) who were treated with beta-blockers [14] *Level M*
- A randomized controlled trial of hospitalized patients with angina at rest compared the effects on recurrent angina and myocardial infarction of treatment with metoprolol, nifedipine, both, or placebo. Metoprolol was found to be significantly more effective than nifedipine [15] *Level P*

NIFEDIPINE

Dose

Adult oral dose: 10–120mg daily usually via sustained release

Efficacy

Calcium channel blockers decrease the number of anginal attacks.

Risks/Benefits

- Benefits: effective antianginal and antihypertensive medications
- Use caution in congestive heart failure, hypotension, and aortic stenosis
- Use caution in hepatic and renal disease
- Use caution in the elderly

Side-effects and adverse reactions

- CNS: dizziness, headache, paresthesia.
- Cardiovascular: bradycardia, peripheral edema, palpitations
- Gastrointestinal: constipation, nausea, dry mouth, dyspepsia
- Respiratory: cough, dyspnea
- Genitourinary: nocturia, polyuria, sexual dysfunction
- Skin: alopecia, pruritus, rash

Interactions (other drugs)

- Barbiturates
- Beta-blockers
- Calcium
- Grapefruit juice
- H_2 antagonists
- Lansoprazole
- Magnesium
- Phenytoin
- Quinidine
- Vincristine

Contraindications

- Severe coronary artery disease
- Recent myocardial infarction
- Hypertensive emergencies

Evidence

Calcium channel blockers reduce the symptoms of angina, although there is some question that some formulations of nifedipine (and other calcium channel blockers) have an adverse effect on mortality in some patients with CAD:

- A systematic review of trials of calcium channel blockers in patients with angina found that they reduced anginal symptoms and ischemia but had no effect on mortality or rate of myocardial infarction [14] *Level M*
- A meta-analysis of 16 randomized secondary prevention trials of nifedipine showed that short-acting nifedipine in moderate and high doses has an adverse effect on mortality in patients with coronary artery disease (not confined to angina) [15] *Level M*
- This same study separately reviewed studies of any calcium channel blocker, and it suggests that other calcium channel blockers, especially those of the dihydropyridine type, may have similar adverse effects on mortality in patients with coronary disease [15] *Level S*

Acceptability to patient
High.

Follow up plan
- If patient is taking bepridil, physician should perform periodic QT monitoring
- Use dependence occurs with verapamil, and the physician should monitor drug use

Patient and caregiver information
Patients may be reassured the calcium channel blockers do not affect bone calcium absorption.

NICARDIPINE
Calcium channel blocker

Dose
Adult oral dose: 20–40mg three times daily

Risks/Benefits
- Benefits: effective antianginal and antihypertensive medications
- Use caution in congestive heart failure, hypotension, and aortic stenosis
- Use caution in hepatic and renal disease
- Use caution in the elderly

Side-effects and adverse reactions
- CNS: depression, dizziness, headache, paresthesia
- Cardiovascular: angina, bradycardia, peripheral edema, palpitations
- Gastrointestinal: constipation, nausea, dry mouth, dyspepsia
- Respiratory: cough, dyspnea
- Genitourinary: nocturia, polyuria, sexual dysfunction
- Skin: alopecia, pruritus, rash

Interactions (other drugs)
- Beta-blockers
- Calcium
- Cyclosporin
- Neuromuscular blocking agents

Contraindications
Advanced aortic stenosis

Evidence
Calcium channel blockers reduce the symptoms of angina, although there is some question that some formulations may have an adverse effect on mortality in some patients with CAD:
- A systematic review of trials of calcium channel blockers in patients with angina found that they reduced anginal symptoms and ischemia but had no effect on mortality or rate of myocardial infarction [14] *Level M*
- A review of studies of calcium channel blockers in patients with coronary artery disease found that these agents, especially those of the dihydropyridine type, may have adverse effects on mortality [15] *Level S*

RAMIPRIL
ACE inhibitor

Dose
Adult oral dose: 2.5–50mg daily in gradual increasing doses
Adult oral dose in renal disease: 1.25–5mg daily

Efficacy

ACE inhibitors may act to decrease myocardial oxygen demand, and have been shown to reduce ischemic events in post revascularization patients and in those with congestive heart failure.

Risks/Benefits

- Benefits: in post-revascularization patients, ACE inhibitors may act to reduce the incidence of acute myocardial infarction or clinical heart failure
- Use caution with bilateral renal artery stenosis, renal and liver disease
- Use caution with diuretic therapy, congestive heart failure, and hypovolemia
- Use caution with collagen vascular diseases
- Use caution with the elderly

Side-effects and adverse reactions

- CNS: anxiety, dizziness, headache, paresthesia.
- Cardiovascular: angina, hypotension, postural hypotension, palpitations
- Gastrointestinal: constipation, nausea, dry mouth, pancreatitis
- Respiratory: cough, asthma, dyspnea
- Genitourinary: sexual dysfunction
- Hematologic: agranulocytosis, neutropenia, thrombocytopenia
- Metabolic: hyperkalemia, hyponatremia, hypoglycemia
- Musculoskeletal: arthralgia, arthritis, myalgia
- Skin: alopecia, pruritis, rash

Interactions (other drugs)

- Allopurinol
- Alpha-adrenergic blockers
- Aspirin
- Cyclosporin
- Insulin
- Iron
- Lithium
- Loop diuretics
- NSAIDs
- Potassium/potassium-sparing diuretics

Contraindications

- Bilateral renal artery stenosis
- Pregnancy

Evidence

ACE inhibitors have been shown to be effective in reducing ischemic events in post-myocardial infarction and heart failure patients:

- APRES, a long-term randomized controlled trial of patients with angina and left ventricular dysfunction, followed the effects of ramipril after the patients had undergone invasive revascularization procedures. The drug significantly reduced the incidence of cardiac death, acute myocardial infarction, and clinical heart failure [16] *Level P*

Acceptability to patient

High.

Follow up plan

- Patients should monitor blood pressure daily at home or in the office when an ACE inhibitor is initially added or increased, particularly if they are taking other medications that potentiate the antihypertensive effect of the ACE inhibitor
- Patients should have telephone or office contact with the physician within the first week to monitor for orthostasis, other side-effects

Patient and caregiver information

- Patients should be instructed to watch for a chronic, dry cough, which may necessitate switching to a different medication
- Patients should be instructed to monitor blood pressure carefully with addition or change in ACE inhibitor, and to report any weakness or orthostatic symptoms, particularly if they are taking other medications that potentiate the antihypertensive effect of the ACE inhibitor

Surgical therapy

PERCUTANEOUS TRANSLUMINAL CORONARY ANGIOPLASTY (PTCA)

Efficacy

Inflation of a balloon-tipped catheter within a diseased segment of coronary artery causes disruption of atherosclerotic plaque and consequent reduction in luminal stenosis.

Risks/Benefits

- Risks: risk of myocardial infarction or need for emergency coronary artery bypass grafting (CABG) surgery as a result of unsuccessful procedure (approx. 2%). Risk of embolic stroke (less than 0.5%), death (less than 0.5%) or vascular complication requiring transfusion and/or vascular surgical repair. Six-month rate of restenosis is 20–50%
- Benefits: procedural success is high (greater than 95%). Only a short period of hospitalization needed following the procedure. Return to work is rapid

Evidence

In patients with moderate to severe stable angina, PTCA appears to reduce the angina symptoms more effectively than medical therapy but is associated with a higher rate of subsequent need for coronary artery bypass grafting. It does not reduce the rate of subsequent myocardial infarction, the need for later PTCA, or death:

- One systematic review of trials involving a total of over 1900 patients with stable coronary artery disease found that PTCA reduced the rate of angina significantly but increased the rate of subsequent need for coronary artery bypass grafting compared with medical treatment [17] *Level M*
- The same review found no difference between PTCA and medical treatment in terms of subsequent myocardial infarction, the need for later PTCA, or death [17] *Level M*
- RITA-2, a randomized, controlled trial of over 1000 people (which was included in the review above), found that PTCA improved angina symptoms, breathlessness, and treadmill tolerance compared with medical treatment at 3 months and 1 year; however, there was no significant difference between the two types of therapy at 3 years [18] *Level P*
- Another study of the RITA-2 trial participants (also included in the review above) concluded that the benefits of PTCA were confined to people with moderate or severe angina and that people whose anginal symptoms were mild at the time of enrollment in the trial did not benefit from PTCA [19] *Level P*

PTCA is less effective than CABG at reducing the rate of angina and the need for repeat procedures, but there appears to be no difference between the two therapies in terms of mortality or quality of life measures:

- A systematic review compared PTCA with CABG and found that the rate of moderate or severe angina at 1 year was significantly lower after CABG, although there was no significant difference in mortality [20] *Level M*
- The BARI trial found that the rate of repeat procedures was significantly higher in patients with mutlivessel disease who underwent PTCA than it was in those who underwent CABG [21] *Level P*
- Two randomized studies have found that both PTCA and CABG appear to improve quality of life measures but that there appears to be no significant difference between the two [22, 23] *Level P*

Acceptability to patient

High.

Follow up plan

- Following angioplasty, all patients should be maintained on aspirin therapy for life
- Following stent implantation, all patients should be maintained on aspirin therapy for life and on additional antiplatelet therapy (clopidogrel or ticlopidine) as directed – typically for 4 weeks following the intervention

- Abrupt onset of chest pain following percutaneous intervention requires immediate evaluation to exclude the possibility of acute stent thrombosis (typically within the first days to weeks following the procedure)
- Recurrence of exertionally induced chest pain should be evaluated by exercise testing or angiography as clinically warranted to exclude restenosis; such symptoms typically occur within 6 months of the intervention

Patient and caregiver information

Adjustment of patient lifestyle (diet, smoking, other risk factors) can help to minimize possible recurrence.

CORONARY ARTERY BYPASS GRAFT (CABG)

Efficacy

Venous or arterial conduits are interposed from the aorta (or other arterial source) to the affected coronary artery, permitting perfusion distal to the point of obstruction.

Risks/Benefits

- Risk: inhospital risk of complications reflects severity of native coronary disease (number of vessels bypassed), degree of left ventricular systolic dysfunction, and presence of comorbid illnesses (diabetes, renal insufficiency, pulmonary disease). Recovery typically requires several days of hospitalization
- Benefit: procedural success is high

Evidence

CABG is more effective than medical therapy at reducing mortality, particularly in patients with more severe coronary heart disease:

- A systematic review of seven randomized, controlled trials involving a total of over 2649 patients with coronary heart disease compared CABG with medical therapy found that CABG reduced mortality at 5, 7, and 10 years but that CABG did not affect the rate of subsequent myocardial infarction; in the trials reviewed, the oldest patient was aged 65 years and almost all the patients (97%) were male [24] *Level M*
- The benefits of CABG were most pronounced in patients with an abnormal left ventricular ejection fraction, those with larger numbers of involved coronary arteries, and those with inovlement of the left anterior descending artery (regardless of the involvement of other vessels) [24] *Level M*

CABG is more effective than percutaneous transluminal coronary angioplasty (PTCA) at reducing the rate of angina and the need for repeat procedures, but there appears to be no difference between the two therapies in terms of mortality or quality of life measures:

- Another systematic review compared CABG with PTCA and found that the rate of moderate or severe angina at 1 year was significantly lower after CABG, although there was no significant difference in mortality [20] *Level M*
- The BARI trial found that the rate of repeat procedures was significantly lower in patients with mutlivessel disease who underwent CABG than it was in those who underwent PTCA [21] *Level P*
- Two randomized studies have found that both CABG and PTCA appear to improve quality of life measures but that there appears to be no significant difference between the two [22, 23] *Level P*

Acceptability to patient

Acceptability varies from patient to patient. The short-term drawbacks of post operative pain and need for several days of hospitalization are outweighed by the high success rate in treatment of angina and – in some patient populations – reduction of mortality.

Follow up plan
- Patient should return for evaluation when experiencing any episodes of chest pain after CABG for assessment of acute graft closure
- Consultation should be arranged with the responsible surgeon if any evidence of infection is noted at the sternotomy site or the saphenous vein graft harvest site
- Plans for physical therapy/cardiac rehabilitation should be arranged in conjunction with the surgeon and cardiologist
- Cardiovascular medications should be continued following hospital discharge
- All patients should remain on daily aspirin therapy for life unless absolutely contraindicated

Patient and caregiver information
Adjustment of patient lifestyle (smoking cessation, dietary modification, regular exercise) and optimization of other modifiable risk factors (control of hypertension, lipid reduction therapy, use of daily aspirin) can help to minimize recurrent CAD and rate of cardiovascular morbidity and mortality

Complementary therapy
SELENIUM
Efficacy
- Lower selenium levels correlate with a higher risk of CAD
- Selenium acts as an antioxidant and anti-inflammatory. It may prevent oxidation of lipids and it reduces platelet aggregation
- Epidemiologic studies have produced mixed results
- Dose is 100–200mcg/day

Risks/Benefits
- Use caution in gastrointestinal disease, renal impairment, and pregnancy
- Side-effects should not occur at the recommended doses
- Selenium toxicity includes: alopecia, dermatitis, diarrhea, fatigue, halitosis, irritability, metallic taste in mouth, nausea, vomiting
- Selenium is contraindicated in neonatal prematurity and benzyl alcohol hypersensitivity

Interactions:
- No known drug interactions

Acceptability to patient
Quite acceptable. Cost is an issue, because insurance does not usually pay for non prescription items.

Follow up plan
Regular care for angina; selenium should be used as a supplement to conventional therapy.

B VITAMINS
Efficacy
Hyperhomocysteinemia is a significant independent risk factor for CAD. Vitamin B6, folate and B12 are required as coenzymes in biochemical pathways in which a sulfur molecule moves between homocysteine and methionine.

Risks/Benefits
Vitamin B6:
- High doses of B6 can cause peripheral neuropathy
- CNS side-effects include paresthesia and sensory neuropathic syndromes
- Gastrointestinal side-effects include nausea, and altered liver function test results

Vitamin B12:
- Should not be used in patients with Leber's optic atrophy
- No known toxicity

Folate:
- Use caution in patients with undiagnosed anemia
- Respiratory side-effects include bronchospasm (rare)
- Skin side-effects include itching and rash

Vitamin B6 interactions:
■ **Amiodarone** ■ **Carbamazepine** ■ **Cycloserine** ■ **Ethionamide** ■ **Fosphenytoin** ■ **Hydralazine** ■ **Isoniazid** ■ **Levodopa** ■ **Oral contraceptives** ■ **Penicillamine** ■ **Phenelzine** ■ **Phenobarbital** ■ **Phenytoin** ■ **Theophylline** ■ **Valproic acid** ■ **Alcohol**

Vitamin B12 interactions:
■ **Antibiotics** ■ **Cholestyramine** ■ **Colchicine** ■ **Colestipol** ■ **H_2 blockers** ■ **Metformin** ■ **Nitrous oxide** ■ **Para-aminosalicylic acid** ■ **Potassium chloride** ■ **Proton pump inhibitors**

Folate interactions:
■ **Anticonvulsants** ■ **Cholestyramine** ■ **Colestipol** ■ **Colchicine** ■ **Fluoxetine** ■ **Lithium** ■ **Lometrexol** ■ **Metformin** ■ **Methotrexate** ■ **NSAIDs** ■ **Phenobarbital** ■ **Phenytoin** ■ **Pyrimethamine** ■ **Sulfasalazine**

Evidence
- An association between blood homocysteine levels and cardiovascular disease has been demonstrated. The causality has not been proven, and neither has the benefit of lowering the homocysteine level. Homocysteine-lowering therapy (folic acid, vitamin B6) is unlikely to cause harm [25] *Level C*
- Patients with elevated homocysteine levels should be considered for treatment with folate therapy [1] *Level C*
- A meta-analysis found that folic acid based supplements significantly reduced blood homocysteine levels. The addition of vitamin B12 produced a further reduction in homocysteine, but vitamin B6 did not have a significant additional effect [26] *Level M*

Acceptability to patient
Highly acceptable. Doses needed for reducing homocysteine (folic acid 400mcg/day, vitamin B6 5–50mg/day, vitamin B12 50–100mcg/day) are available in many multiple vitamin supplements at reasonable cost.

Follow up plan
Regular care is essential. The B vitamins are supplementary. Homocysteine levels should be evaluated at intervals.

L-CARNITINE
L-carnitine is a cofactor for the transformation of free long-chain fatty acids into acyl-carnitines for mitochondrial oxidation. Acyl-carnitines are the primary fuel source for heart and skeletal muscle. Carnitine improves oxygen utilization and energy metabolism in heart muscle.

Efficacy
- Older placebo-controlled trials show lower use of nitroglycerin, improved exercise tolerance, and improved stress test responses, but there are no recent studies (Watanabe S, Ajisaa R, Masuoka T, et al. Effects of L- and DL-carnitine on patients with impaired exercise tolerance. Jpn Heart J 1995;36:319–31. Medline)
- Dose range is 900–4000mg/day, typically 2000mg/day

Risks/Benefits

- There is no toxicity with use of the L-form alone
- The D-form has been known to cause muscle pain and weakness
- The D,L-carnitine product competitively inhibits L-carnitine
- Gastrointestinal side-effects include nausea, vomiting, abdominal pain, diarrhea
- Skin side-effects include drug-related body odor

Interactions:

- Choline
- D,L-carnitine

Acceptability to patient

No major problems.

Follow up plan

L-carnitine should be used in conjunction with conventional medical therapy.

MIND–BODY PRACTICES

Efficacy

Mind–body approaches including social support, cognitive–behavioral treatment, meditation, yoga, hope, faith, imagery, spiritual healing, hypnosis, music therapy, t'ai chi, qigong, and aikido may be efficacious as complementary therapies for cardiovascular disease-related conditions. The need for further research is evident.

Risks/Benefits

Benefits:

- An essentially risk-free approach
- Inexpensive/cost-effective

Acceptability to patient

Requires new learning and behavioral change/practice on the part of patient. Compliance challenging at times.

Follow up plan

Usual medical care should be ongoing. Support and encouragement to continue the mind–body practices is important.

COENZYME Q10

Efficacy

A small, double-blind, placebo-controlled, crossover trial of patients with stable angina showed a 50% reduction in anginal episodes per week, and lower nitroglycerine use, and longer treadmill tolerance time in those given coenzyme Q10.

Risks/Benefits

- Essentially no risks reported at 100mg/day for up to 6 years
- Use caution in young children
- Contraindicated in pregnancy and breast-feeding (no clinical trial data yet available yet in these patient populations)
- CNS side-effect of insomnia
- Gastrointestinal side-effects include nausea, diarrhea, dyspepsia, elevated hepatic enzymes, loss of appetite

Interactions:
- Antidiabetic drugs (coenzyme Q10 may improve glycemic control in some type II diabetics)
- Beta-blockers (propranolol may inhibit some coenzyme Q10-dependent enzymes)
- Doxorubicin (coenzyme Q10 may help ameliorate the cardiotoxicity of doxorubicin)
- Insulin
- Piperazine (may increase plasma coenzyme Q10)
- Statins (decrease coenzyme Q10 levels)
- Warfarin (effect of warfarin decreased)

Evidence

A small RCT compared coenzyme Q10 (Co Q10) with placebo in patients with stable angina pectoris. Co Q10 reduced anginal frequency and nitroglycerin consumption compared with placebo, although the reduction was not statistically significant. In terms of exercise testing, a significant increase in the duration of exercise before ST-segment depression occurred was noted in patients treated with Co Q10. An increase in CoQ10 plasma concentration was significantly related to the increase in exercise duration [27] *Level P*

Acceptability to patient

Apart from the expense, Coenzyme Q10 appears well tolerated by patients.

Follow up plan

Regular medical care to follow symptoms and objective parameters.

LIFESTYLE

Smoking cessation, weight reduction, stress reduction program, increased activity/regular exercise.

RISKS/BENEFITS

No risks except for a risk of exacerbation of anginal symptoms and of injury in the poorly conditioned patient. Benefits are:
- **Smoking cessation**: Greatly improves symptoms and patient prognosis
- **Weight reduction**: Maintaining a diet high in vegetables, fruit, fish, and poultry may help promote a more favorable lipid profile and thereby reduce risk of adverse cardiovascular events. Weight reduction may reduce strain on the heart
- **Stress reduction**: Reduction in anxiety and stress may reduce the need for medical intervention by decreasing the frequency of episodes/situations that precipitate angina, and by reducing blood pressure
- **Exercise**: Increases exercise tolerance, decreases angina, reduces blood pressure, lipids, stress, and weight

ACCEPTABILITY TO PATIENT
- **Smoking cessation**: Some patients may require pharmacologic support in order to quit smoking successfully. The use of transdermal nicotine is a safe and effective potential strategy. Multiple strategies are more likely to be successful. They may include group sessions, counseling with the physician, as well as pharmacologic intervention
- **Weight reduction**: Some patients may require nutritional consultation and supervision in order to achieve the goals with respect to diet. In some cases, enrollment in a weight reduction program may be indicated
- **Stress reduction**: Patients may need help in dealing with their stress and may benefit from relaxation techniques and other methods of stress control
- **Exercise**: Patients may be fearful of increasing exercise level with angina and may be resistant to a regimen that may require significant change in lifestyle and must be long-term to be effective

FOLLOW UP PLAN

- **Smoking cessation**: Monitor patient's success with goals and prescribe transdermal nicotine if needed. Bupropion nicotine chewing gum may assist
- **Weight reduction**: Monitor patient's success with diet goals and prescribe medical treatment if needed
- **Stress reduction**: Monitor patient's success with stress reduction goals, prescribe further therapy if needed
- **Exercise**: Regular monitoring of patient participation, weight reduction, tolerance, and reminders of the importance of activity are important components in maintaining compliance. Working with physical therapy or cardiac rehabilitation services if available is probably more effective than individual programs. Monitor for musculoskeletal injury, particularly in the obese patient

PATIENT AND CAREGIVER INFORMATION

Remind patient of the positive effects on prognosis and general health.

OUTCOMES

EFFICACY OF THERAPIES

Response to treatment varies between patients and depends greatly on the treatment involved:

- Although catheter revascularization can dramatically alleviate anginal symptoms, restenosis and the need for repeat procedures tempers its use
- Although coronary bypass surgery is very effective for relieving angina, the risks of surgery are significant and, if angina returns in the future, it is often more difficult to treat in a patient who has had bypass surgery previously

Patient satisfaction is thus an important measure of treatment efficacy. Negotiating an acceptable quality of life is important and must be individualized.

The follow-up exercise test or imaging study is the standard objective measurement of treatment efficacy.

Evidence

- Lipid reduction with statins reduces mortality and the rate of coronary events [4–8] *Level P*
- Isosorbide mononitrate is effective in reducing anginal symptoms and improving quality of life [9] *Level P*
- Aspirin in high-risk patients can reduce the risk of vascular events, including myocardial infarction, and sudden death [10, 11] *Level P*
- Beta-blockers can reduce mortality and the risk of cardiac events in patients with coronary artery disease and may be more effective than calcium channel blockers in reducing the symptoms of angina and the rate of myocardial infarction in patients with angina at rest [12] *Level M* [13, 28] *Level P*
- Calcium channel blockers reduce the symptoms of angina, although there is some question that some may have an adverse effect on mortality in some patients with coronary artery disease [14] *Level M*, [15] *Levels M and S*
- Angiotensin-converting enzyme (ACE) inhibitors reduce ischemic events in post myocardial infarction and heart failure patients [16] *Level P*
- Percutaneous transluminal coronary angiography (PTCA) appears to reduce the angina symptoms of patients with moderate to severe stable angina more effectively than medical therapy, but it is associated with a higher rate of subsequent need for coronary artery bypass grafting (CABG). It does not reduce the rate of subsequent myocardial infarction, the need for later PTCA, or death [17] *Level M*, [18, 19] *Level P*
- CABG is more effective than medical therapy at reducing mortality, particularly in patients with more severe coronary heart disease [24] *Level M*
- CABG is more effective than PTCA at reducing the rate of angina and the need for repeat procedures, but there appears to be no difference between the two procedures in terms of mortality or quality of life measures [20] *Level M*, [21–23] *Level P*

Review period

- Follow up by phone or in the office for a blood pressure check within a few days if medication changes are likely to cause hypotension or orthostasis
- Evaluation of the effect of medication changes on anginal symptoms may take several days or weeks

PROGNOSIS

The prognosis can be determined by the patient history, physical examination, non invasive data, and coronary angiographic results.

- Clinical findings suggestive of poor left ventricular function are associated with a worse prognosis

- Patients with poor exercise capacity and those with evidence of severe ischemia at low workload are at high risk
- Prognosis is worse in patients with severe proximal left anterior descending artery disease and two-vessel disease, left main disease, and three-vessel disease who have reduced left ventricular function and/or diabetes

Therapeutic failure

Percutaneous and intraoperative transmyocardial revascularization has application for those patients with coronary disease not amenable to PTCA or CABG. However, this laser procedure should be reserved for patients with medically refractive angina and no other revascularization option.

Trials are ongoing studying methods to induce vascular proliferation (angiogenesis) to improve myocardial perfusion in patients who are not candidates for percutaneous or surgical coronary revascularization.

Recurrence

With relapse of symptoms despite maximal medical therapy, consider methods for coronary revascularization (i.e. percutaneous coronary revascularization or CABG surgery).

Although present methods for percutaneous revascularization have at least a 95% procedural success rate, there still exists a 20–50% rate of restenosis within 6 months following the procedure.

There are many strategies for percutaneous revascularization of coronary arteries, which have developed restenosis:

- Repeat angioplasty or stent of diseased segment
- Directional atherectomy
- Rotablator
- Intravascular radiation therapy
- Referral for consideration of CABG surgery

If restenosis occurs, PTCA or CABG procedures can be performed.

COMPLICATIONS

Coronary artery disease (the substrate for angina), if left untreated, leads to myocardial infarction, left ventricular failure, arrhythmias, heart failure, and, ultimately, death.

PREVENTION

RISK FACTORS

- **Smoking**: Clinical trials have shown that smoking cessation is associated with a reduction in cardiac event rates. Other effects of smoking cessation include decreased blood carboxyhemoglobin levels, elevated HDL cholesterol, and reversal of coronary artery vasoconstriction
- **Hypertension**: Control of hypertension may dramatically reduce the risk of cardiovascular morbidity and mortality, particularly in those patients known to have symptomatic CAD.
- **Diabetes mellitus**: Type 1 diabetics show decreased risk of microvascular complications with better metabolic control
- **Obesity**: In obese patients, weight reduction and maintenance of a healthy diet and regular exercise regimen may reduce cardiovascular stress, improve lipid profile, and reduce risk of morbidity and mortality from cardiovascular causes
- **Inactive lifestyle**: Considering the effects of exercise on lipid levels and disease progression, an exercise training program may reduce cardiovascular stress, improve lipid profile, and reduce risk of morbidity and mortality from cardiovascular causes

MODIFY RISK FACTORS

- Hypertension should be monitored and managed as appropriate
- Cholesterol should be measured and managed
- Smoking cessation should be encouraged
- Regular exercise regimen and a healthy diet (low in fat) should be espoused

Lifestyle and wellness

Maintaining a regular exercise regimen, a healthy diet, and achieving target body weight for age/gender/height is recommended for all patients.

TOBACCO

Discontinuation of smoking is considered beneficial, even without diagnosed disease states.

ALCOHOL AND DRUGS

Limiting alcohol use and discontinuing the use of drugs is considered beneficial.

DIET

A low-fat diet, with emphasis on maintaining ideal body weight and optimizing lipid profile, will reduce the likelihood of cardiovascular morbidity and mortality.

PHYSICAL ACTIVITY

Maintaining a regular exercise regimen is recommended for all; those who lead a sedentary lifestyle may require more structured supervision in an exercise training program.

FAMILY HISTORY

If there is a history of cardiovascular disease in the family, an education program should make the patient aware of all risk factors for disease and preventive measures.

SCREENING

Most effective screen is careful history from patient.

PREVENT RECURRENCE

Patients should be instructed that changes in lifestyle (including altered diet, stress reduction, discontinuation of smoking) can help reduce recurrence. However, these changes may not totally prevent recurrence of anginal events, as angina is a symptom of an underlying condition.

Reassess coexisting disease

Attention should be paid to reducing all modifiable risk factors for CAD, including smoking cessation, management of hypertension, use of aspirin in all patients suspected of having CAD, optimization of lipid profile.

ASSOCIATIONS

National Heart, Lung, and Blood Institute
Information Office
P.O. Box 30105
Bethesda, MD 20892-0105
Telephone: (301) 592-8573
http://www.nhlbi.nih.gov

American Heart Association
National Center
7272 Greenville Avenue
Dallas, TX 7523
Heart and Stroke Information: (800) AHA-USA1
Stroke Information: (888) 4-STROKE, Women's Health Information: (888) MY HEART
http://www.americanheart.org

The Mended Hearts, Inc
Home Office, 7272 Greenville Avenue
Dallas, TX 7523
Telephone: (800) AHAUSA1
http://www.mendedhearts.org

KEY REFERENCES

- Agency for Health Care Policy and Research, National Heart, Lung and Blood Institute. Unstable angina: diagnosis and management, clinical practice guideline no. 10. Rockville, MD: US Department of Health and Human Services, Public Health Service, AHCPR Publication No. 94-0602, March 1994
- Braunwald E, ed. Heart disease: A textbook of cardiovascular medicine, 5th edn. Philadelphia, PA: WB Saunders, 1997
- Gibbons RJ, Chatterjee K, Daley J, et al. ACC/AHA/ACP-ASIM guidelines for the management of patients with chronic stable angina: a report of the American College of Cardiology/American Heart Association Task Force on Practice Guidelines. J Am Coll Cardiol 1999;33(7):2092–7.
- Simandl S, Cohn PF. Chronic ischemic heart disease. In: Alpert JS, ed. Cardiology for the primary care physician. St. Louis, MO: Mosby; 1996; chapter 17

Guidelines and evidence references:

1 Guidelines for the management of patients with chronic stable angina. J Am Coll Cardiol 1999;33:2092–197; available online from the National Guideline Clearinghouse
2 Anonymous. Management of stable angina pectoris. Recommendations of the Task Force of the European Society of Cardiology. Eur Heart J 1997;18:394–413; available online from the National Guideline Clearinghouse
3 Braunwald E, Antman EM, Beasley JW, et al. ACC/AHA guidelines for the management of patients with unstable angina and non-ST-segment elevation myocardial infarction. A report of the American College of Cardiology/American Heart Association Task Force on Practice Guidelines (Committee on the Management of Patients with Unstable Angina). J Am Coll Cardiol 2000;36:970–1062; Cathet Cardiovasc Intervent 2000;51:505–21; available online from the National Guideline Clearinghouse
4 Anonymous. Randomised trial of cholesterol lowering in 4444 patients with coronary heart disease: the Scandinavian Simvastatin Survival Study (4S). Lancet 1994;344:1383–9
5 Miettinen TA, Pyörölä K, Olsson AG, et al. Cholesterol-lowering therapy in women and elderly patients with myocardial infarction or angina pectoris: findings from the Scandinavian Simvastatin Survival Study (4S). Circulation 1997;96:4211–8
6 Anonymous. Design features and baseline characteristics of the LIPID (Long-Term Intervention with Pravastatin in Ischemic Disease) Study: a randomized trial in patients with previous acute myocardial infarction and/or unstable angina pectoris. Am J Cardiol 1995;76:474–9
7 Tonkin AM, Colquhoun D, Emberson J, et al. Effects of pravastatin in 3260 patients with unstable angina: results from the LIPID study. Lancet 2000;356:1871–5

8 van Boven AJ, Jukema JW, Zwinderman AH, et al. Reduction of transient myocardial ischemia with pravastatin in addition to the conventional treatment in patients with angina pectoris. REGRESS Study Group. Circulation 1996;94:1503–5

9 Zwinderman AH, Cleophas TJ, van der Sluijs H, et al. Comparison of 50-mg and 100-mg sustained-release isosorbide mononitrate in the treatment of stable angina pectoris: effects on quality of life indices. Dutch Mononitrate Quality of Life (DUMQOL) Study Group. Angiology 1999;50:963–9

10 Antiplatelet Trialists' Collaboration. Collaborative overview of randomised trials of antiplatelet therapy. I: prevention of death, myocardial infarction, and stroke by prolonged antiplatelet therapy in various categories of patients. BMJ 1994;308:81–106; reviewed in Clinical Evidence 2001;5:95–124

11 Juul-Möller S, Edvardsson N, Jahnmatz B, et al, for the Swedish Angina Pectoris Aspirin Trial (SAPAT) Group. Double-blind trial of aspirin in primary prevention of myocardial infarction in patients with stable chronic angina pectoris. Lancet 1992;340:1421–5; reviewed in Clinical Evidence 2001;5:95–12417

12 Beta-Blocker Pooling Project Research Group. The Beta-Blocker Pooling Project (BBPP): subgroup findings from randomized trials in post-infarct patients. Eur Heart J 1988; 9:8–16; reviewed in Clinical Evidence 2001;5:95–124

13 HINT Research Group. Early treatment of unstable angina in the coronary care unit: a randomized, double blind, placebo controlled comparison of recurrent ischaemia in patients treated with nifedipine or metoprolol or both. Br Heart J 1986;56:400–13; reviewed in Clinical Evidence 2001;5:95–124

14 Held PH, Yusuf S, Furberg CD. Calcium channel blockers in acute myocardial infarction and unstable angina: an overview. BMJ 1989; 299:1187–92; reviewed in Clinical Evidence 2001;5:95–124

15 Furberg CD, Psaty BM, Meyer JV. Nifedipine. Dose-related increase in mortality in patients with coronary heart disease.Circulation 1995;92:1326–31

16 Kjoller-Hansen L, Steffensen R, Grande P. The angiotensin-converting enzyme inhibition post revascularization study (APRES). J Am Coll Cardiol 2000;35:881–8

17 Bucher HC, Hengstler P, Schindler C, Guyatt GH. Percutaneous transluminal coronary angioplasty versus medical treatment for non-acute coronary heart disease: meta-analysis of randomised controlled trials. BMJ 2000;321:73–7; reviewed in Clinical Evidence 2001;5:95–12418

18 Pocock SJ, Henderson RA, Clayton T, et al. Quality of life after coronary angioplasty or continued medical treatment for angina: three-year follow-up in the RITA-2 trial. Randomized Intervention Treatment of Angina. J Am Coll Cardiol 2000;35:907–14; reviewed in Clinical Evidence 2001;5:95–124

19 Anonymous. Coronary angioplasty versus medical therapy for angina: the second Randomised Intervention Treatment of Angina (RITA-2) trial. RITA-2 trial participants. Lancet 1997;350:461–8

20 Pocock SJ, Henderson RA, Rickards AF, et al. Meta-analysis of randomised trials comparing coronary angioplasty with bypass surgery. Lancet 1995;346:1184–9; reviewed in Clinical Evidence 2001;5:95–124

21 Bypass Angioplasty Revascularization Investigation (BARI) Investigators. Comparison of coronary bypass surgery with angioplasty in patients with multivessel disease. N Engl J Med 1996;335:7–225; reviewed in Clinical Evidence 2001;5:95–124

22 Hlatky MA, Rogers WJ, Johnstone I, et al. Medical care costs and quality of life after randomization to coronary angioplasty or coronary bypass surgery. Bypass Angioplasty Revascularization Investigation (BARI) Investigators. N Engl J Med 1997;336:92–9; reviewed in Clinical Evidence 2001;5:95–124

23 Währborg P. Quality of life after coronary angioplasty or bypass surgery. 1-year follow-up in the Coronary Angioplasty versus Bypass Revascularization Investigation (CABRI) trial. Eur Heart J 1999;20:653–8; reviewed in Clinical Evidence 2001;5:95–124

24 Yusuf S, Zucker D, Peduzzi P, et al. Effect of coronary artery bypass graft surgery on survival: overview of 10-year results from randomized trials by the coronary artery bypass surgery trialists collaboration. Lancet 1994;244:565–70; reviewed in Clinical Evidence 2001;5:95–124

25 Institute for Clinical Systems Improvement. Stable coronary artery disease. Bloomington, MN: ICSI, 2002.

26 Homocysteine Lowering Trialists Collaboration. Lowering blood homocysteine with folic acid based supplements: meta-analysis of randomized trials. BMJ 1998; 316:894–8

27 Kamikawa T, Kobayashi A, Yamashita T, et al. Effects of coenzyme Q10 on exercise tolerance in chronic stable angina pectoris. Am J Cardiol 1985; 56: 247–51

28 Pepine CJ, Cohn PF, Deedwania PC, et al, for the the ASIST Study Group. Effects of treatment on outcome in mildly symptomatic patients with ischemia during daily life: the atenolol silent ischemia study (ASIST). Circulation 1994; 90:762–8; reviewed in Clinical Evidence 2001;5:95–124

CONTRIBUTORS

Russell C Jones, MD, MPH
Mark B Stockman, MD
Jane L Murray, MD
Doug Drachman, MD

ABDOMINAL AORTIC ANEURYSM

SUMMARY INFORMATION

DESCRIPTION

- Defined as a localized dilation of the abdominal aorta with an increase in diameter of at least 50%. In most instances, an aortic diameter above 3cm indicates an aneurysm
- Abdominal aortic aneurysm is seen in 5–7% of people above age 60 in the US. Incidence rises sharply after 55 years of age in men and 70 years of age in women. Cigarette smoking and hypertension are significant risk factors
- Due to the high death rate from rupture (70–80%), elective surgical repair or implantation of an endovascular stent graft is advisable in appropriate patients. In general, patients with aneurysms larger than 5cm in diameter, symptomatic aneurysms, or rapidly enlarging aneurysms should be considered for repair. Treatment for aneurysms between 4 and 5cm is controversial
- Most abdominal aortic aneurysms encountered by primary care physicians are intact and asymptomatic. These are often found incidentally on routine physical examination or in radiographic studies performed for other indications
- The possibility of a ruptured abdominal aortic aneurysm should be considered in middle-aged or elderly patients with any of the following: pain in abdomen, back, or flank; pulsatile abdominal mass; or hypotension. Diagnosis is clear-cut when all three signs coincide

URGENT ACTION

- Arrange urgent surgery for patients with the three classic signs of rupture: pain in abdomen, back, or flank; pulsatile abdominal mass; and hypotension
- Urgent evaluation is also appropriate for patients who are strongly suspected of having a ruptured aneurysm, typically due to presentation with pain in abdomen, back, or flank, and/or a pulsatile abdominal mass

KEY! DON'T MISS!

'Blue toe syndrome' or livedo reticularis should prompt an immediate evaluation for abdominal aortic aneurysm.

ICD9 CODE
- 441.4 Aneurysm, abdominal (aorta)
- 441.3 Ruptured abdominal aortic aneurysm

SYNONYMS
AAA.

CARDINAL FEATURES
Localized dilation of the abdominal aorta with an increase in diameter of at least 50% (1.5 times normal size). Most abdominal aortic aneurysms are infrarenal. The normal diameter in this region is approximately 2cm. A small percentage of abdominal aortic aneurysms are suprarenal; these are generally extensions of thoracic aneurysms.

Rupture of an abdominal aortic aneurysm may have the following characteristics:
- Free intraperitoneal rupture, marked by acute pain rapidly followed by cardiovascular collapse and death
- Bleeding through a small posterolateral tear in the aortic wall, with bleeding temporarily contained in the retroperitoneum. In such instances, patients may have time to obtain medical care before frank intraperitoneal rupture ensues
- Most aneurysms (75%) are asymptomatic and discovered on routine physical examination or incidental imaging studies

CAUSES
Common causes
Atherosclerotic disease of the aorta.

Rare causes
- Marfan's syndrome
- Ehlers–Danlos syndrome
- Collagen vascular disease
- Mycotic aneurysm
- Trauma to abdomen

Contributory or predisposing factors
Contributory factors for aneurysm development:
- Hypertension
- Cigarette smoking
- Chronic obstructive pulmonary disease
- Peripheral vascular disease
- Carotid artery disease
- Hernia

Contributory factors for aneurysm rupture:
- Large size of aneurysm
- Hypertension
- Chronic obstructive pulmonary disease

EPIDEMIOLOGY
Incidence and prevalence
INCIDENCE
Over 16,000 deaths per year (1996 data) due to rupture.

PREVALENCE

- Among people above age 60 in the US, present in 50–70/1000
- Of patients suspected of having abdominal aortic aneurysm by physical examination, only 15% are shown to have it by imaging studies

Demographics

AGE

- Present in 5–7% of people above age 60 in the US
- Extremely rare in children, although possible in those with Marfan's syndrome or blunt injury to the abdomen

GENDER

- Male:female ratio is 11:1 for ages 60–64; lowers to 3:1 for ages 85–90
- Women typically have smaller aneurysms than men
- Rate of aneurysm rupture in one study was 3-fold higher in women than in men

RACE

More prevalent among caucasians than African-Americans.

GENETICS

- First-degree relatives of individuals with abdominal aortic aneurysm at higher risk (12-fold increase). Male siblings at highest risk
- Marfan's syndrome a possible cause
- Ehlers–Danlos syndrome a possible cause

DIFFERENTIAL DIAGNOSIS

Renal colic

Leading misdiagnosis for abdominal aortic aneurysm. Some clinicians recommend obtaining an ultrasound or computed tomography (CT) scan to look for abdominal aortic aneurysm in patients above age 50 who present with an apparent kidney stone.

FEATURES

- Severe, possibly intermittent, flank pain that radiates to groin, scrotum, or labia
- Hematuria often present
- No abdominal tenderness
- Possible previous stone formation
- Diaphoresis
- Possible nausea and vomiting
- Possible fever

Abdominal tumor

FEATURES

- Patient may have palpable abdominal mass (nonpulsatile)
- Abdominal distention and pain may also be present
- Patients may show signs of obstruction

Pancreatitis

The main features of pancreatitis are as follows:

FEATURES

- Often associated with excessive alcohol ingestion or gallstones
- Symptoms range from mild abdominal pain to shock
- Steady midepigastric pain that radiates to back; pain often increases in the supine position
- Possible erythematous skin nodules
- Possible basilar rales with pleural effusion

Intestinal ischemia

FEATURES

- Severe abdominal pain, possibly with low back pain
- Possible diarrhea
- Possible blood in stool
- Edema is common
- Possible history of peripheral vascular disease

Diverticulitis

FEATURES

- Persistent abdominal pain, at first nonlocalized and then worst in left lower abdomen
- Anorexia common
- Possible nausea, vomiting
- Abdominal distention
- Possible increased urinary frequency

Cholecystitis

The main features of cholecystitis are as follows:

FEATURES

- Dull and aching pain at onset; later becomes sharp and localized
- Pain may radiate to tip of right scapula, acromion, or thoracic spine
- Murphy's sign present in most instances (inspiratory arrest due to pain on palpation of right upper quadrant)
- Possible history of biliary colic or known gallstones

Appendicitis

The main features of appendicitis are as follows:

FEATURES

- Abdominal pain is the leading symptom
- Pain is initially poorly localized; after 1–12h it localizes in the lower right quadrant
- With retrocecal appendix, pain may be in the back, flank, or testicles
- Anorexia nearly always present
- Vomiting is common
- Possible diarrhea or constipation

Perforated viscus

FEATURES

- Severe abdominal pain with abrupt onset
- Pain changes over time from localized to diffuse
- Abdomen rigid, guarded
- Lack of bowel sounds
- Possible hypovolemic shock

Bowel obstruction

FEATURES

- May follow progressive change in bowel habits
- Abdominal pain: typically begins intermittently and becomes constant
- Vomiting: bile-stained or feculent emesis
- Tachycardia
- Hypotension
- Examination reveals peritoneal signs of rebound/guarding

Musculoskeletal back pain

Musculoskeletal back pain is the most dangerous misdiagnosis for ruptured abdominal aortic abdomen because patients are often released from care.

FEATURES

- Possibly associated with injury or muscular strain
- In contrast to abdominal aortic aneurysm, pain usually improves in supine position and worsens with motion
- Spasm may be evident on examination

SIGNS & SYMPTOMS

Signs

Stable, intact aneurysm:

- Without signs in most instances
- Possible vague, dull pain with gradual onset
- Possible 'blue toe syndrome' resulting from embolization

Expanding aneurysm:
- Without signs in most instances
- Possible abdominal or back pain with abrupt onset; pain is unaffected by movement
- Possible gastrointestinal signs (early satiety, nausea, weight loss), reflecting intestinal compression
- Possible flank pain and pyelonephritis, reflecting ureteral obstruction
- Possible awareness of pulsation in abdomen (a 'second heart')
- Possible 'blue toe syndrome' resulting from embolization

Ruptured aneurysm:
- Severe abdominal pain that may radiate to groin, back, or legs; pain is unaffected by position
- Possible awareness of pulsation in abdomen
- Possible nausea and vomiting
- Possible hypotension
- Possible syncope
- Possible anxiety
- Possible shock

Symptoms

Stable, intact aneurysm:
- Asymptomatic in most instances
- Possible pain – vague, dull, or throbbing – with gradual onset
- Possible blue, painful toes
- Possible livedo reticularis

Expanding aneurysm:
- Asymptomatic in most instances
- Possible abdominal or back pain with abrupt onset
- Possible feeling of fullness after eating small amounts of food
- Possible sense of pulsation in abdomen
- Possible nausea/vomiting
- Possible blue, painful toes
- Possible livedo reticularis

Ruptured aneurysm:
- Severe abdominal pain that may radiate to groin, back, or legs; pain is unaffected by position
- Fast pulse
- Possible awareness of pulsation in abdomen
- Possible nausea and vomiting
- Possible light-headedness
- Possible fainting
- Possible anxiety
- Possible shock
- Possible livedo reticularis

The sensitivity of palpation for detection of abdominal aortic aneurysm varies with the size: 29% for abdominal aortic aneurysm 3–3.9cm, 50% for 4–4.9cm, 76% for >5cm.

ASSOCIATED DISORDERS

- 25% of people with abdominal aortic aneurysm have atherosclerotic occlusive disease
- Prevalence of coronary, renal, and cerebrovascular arterial disease is increased in those with abdominal aortic aneurysm. All patients who undergo surgical repair or stent graft implantation should be preoperatively evaluated with stress sestamibi and/or coronary angiography

KEY! DON'T MISS!

'Blue toe syndrome' or livedo reticularis should prompt an immediate evaluation for abdominal aortic aneurysm.

CONSIDER CONSULT

- All patients with symptomatic abdominal aortic aneurysms should receive urgent surgery
- Patients with an aneurysm larger than 4cm should be referred for consultation with a vascular specialist
- Patients with an aneurysm that has undergone documented enlargement beyond 0.5cm in <12 months should be referred for consultation with a vascular specialist

INVESTIGATION OF THE PATIENT

Direct questions to patient

- Q **Do you have severe pain (abdomen, back, flank, or groin)?** Pain consistent with rupture, particularly in male patients above age 50, provides cause to consider this diagnosis. Flank pain may also be caused by ureteral obstruction by an aneurysm; in such instances patient may have bouts of pyelonephritis
- Q **Are you aware of abnormal abdominal sensations, such as a pulsating feeling?** Affirmative answer requires immediate assessment for ruptured or expanding abdominal aortic aneurysm
- Q **If pain is present, when did it begin?** Abrupt onset is characteristic of rupture. Gradual onset may reflect expansion of aneurysm. In rare instances, patients survive with a ruptured aneurysm for days or weeks before seeking medical care
- Q **Have your symptoms worsened over time?** Rapidly progressive symptoms are characteristic of rupture
- Q **Do you feel light-headed or in danger of fainting when standing up?** Hypotension is the least consistent of the symptoms characterizing rupture. Nevertheless, syncope is sometimes the chief complaint of people with a ruptured aneurysm
- Q **Have you experienced trauma to your abdomen?** Blunt injury is a rare but possible cause of abdominal aortic aneurysm

Contributory or predisposing factors

- Q **Do you smoke cigarettes?** Smoking is a leading risk factor for abdominal aortic aneurysms
- Q **Do you have any of the following disorders: hypertension, atherosclerosis, chronic obstructive pulmonary disease, peripheral vascular disease, carotid artery disease, bronchiectasis, Marfan's syndrome, or Ehlers–Danlos syndrome?** Any of these conditions provides increased cause to suspect abdominal aortic aneurysm

Family history

- Q **Do you have any relatives, living or dead, with an abdominal aortic aneurysm?** First-degree relatives of an individual with an abdominal aortic aneurysm are at increased risk of this condition. Male siblings are at highest risk

Examination

- **Does the patient have a pulsatile abdominal mass?** Have the patient lie with knees slightly flexed. Palpate abdominal aorta during exhalation. Affected patients may have a pulsatile mass left of midline between the xyloid process and umbilicus. Palpation is most likely to detect large masses and masses present in nonobese patients
- **Does the patient have an abdominal bruit?** Perform auscultation. A bruit is a nonspecific finding evident in a small percentage of patients with an abdominal aortic aneurysm
- **Does the patient have embolization?** Check for 'blue toe syndrome,' manifested by one or more cyanotic toes and palpable pedal pulses. This syndrome suggests a proximal source of emboli. Livedo reticularis is a mottled skin appearance of the lower extremities due to showers of cholesterol emboli

Summary of investigative tests

- B-mode ultrasound: preferred diagnostic procedure in most instances. Used to screen patients at risk of abdominal aortic aneurysm and monitor aneurysms over time
- CT: preferred for suspected rupture. Also used following ultrasound identification of an aneurysm to provide detailed characteristics of the arterial wall
- Spiral CT: commonly used for planning stent graft placement
- Magnetic resonance angiography: used for preoperative assessment of aortic aneurysms

DIAGNOSTIC DECISION

According to the *Guide to clinical preventive services: screening for abdominal aortic aneurysms*, an abdominal aortic aneurysm is a focal dilation of the aorta that is at least 150% of normal aortic diameter.

CLINICAL PEARL(S)

- The majority of abdominal aortic aneurysms are found incidentally. A good abdominal examination should be part of every patient evaluation
- Patients complaining of suspicious abdominal pain should be screened with a thorough physical examination and abdominal ultrasonography
- Any patient with distal emboli should be screened for abdominal aortic aneurysm

THE TESTS

Imaging

B-MODE ULTRASOUND

Advantages/Disadvantages

Advantages:

- Readily available
- May be performed at bedside
- Inexpensive
- Accuracy of 82–99%
- Noninvasive

Disadvantages:

- Does not reveal leakage or rupture
- Quality of study may be decreased with obesity or with bowel gas
- Quality of study is dependent on skill of examiner

Abnormal

Focal dilation of aorta that is at least 50% above normal diameter.

Drugs, disorders, and other factors that may alter results

Bowel gas or obesity may impair image of the aorta.

CT

Advantages/Disadvantages

Advantages:

- Highest accuracy for determining size and location of abdominal aortic aneurysm
- Readily available
- Reveals anatomic abnormalities
- Noninvasive

Disadvantages:

- Expensive
- Involves ionizing radiation
- Poor delineation of renal and visceral arteries

Abnormal
Focal dilation of aorta that is at least 50% above normal diameter.

Drugs, disorders, and other factors that may alter results
Movement of patient degrades image.

SPIRAL CT
Advantages/Disadvantages
- Advantage: provides three-dimensional images of aorta and surrounding structures
- Disadvantage: expensive

Abnormal
Focal dilation of aorta that is at least 50% above normal diameter.

Drugs, disorders, and other factors that may alter results
Accurate reconstruction of image requires a technician with highly specialized training.

MAGNETIC RESONANCE ANGIOGRAPHY
Description
Computer-assisted magnetic resonance imaging (MRI) of arteries.

Advantages/Disadvantages
Advantages:
- Highly accurate in determining aneurysm size
- Depiction of blood vessels is similar to traditional angiography
- Identifies the proximal extent of disease and iliofemoral involvement in most cases

Disadvantages:
- Expensive
- Limited potential to define renal and mesenteric arterial occlusive disease

Abnormal
Focal dilation of aorta that is at least 50% above normal diameter.

TREATMENT

CONSIDER CONSULT

- Any patient in whom dissection or rupture is suspected should be referred urgently to a vascular specialist

IMMEDIATE ACTION

Any patient in whom dissection or rupture is suspected should be referred urgently to a vascular specialist.

PATIENT AND CAREGIVER ISSUES

Forensic and legal issues

Lawsuits may result from failure to diagnose ruptured abdominal aortic aneurysm.

Health-seeking behavior

Have you started or stopped smoking? Cigarette smoking is a significant risk factor for the development of abdominal aortic aneurysms. If surgery becomes necessary, smoking cessation can improve perioperative mortality rates.

MANAGEMENT ISSUES

Goals

- Prevent death from rupture
- Address symptoms caused by the aneurysm

Management in special circumstances

COEXISTING DISEASE

- Some physicians advise against aneurysm repair in patients with coexisting diseases that reduce life expectancy to less than 2 years
- Patients at high risk with regard to surgical repair (unstable angina, cardiac ejection fraction below 30%, congestive heart failure, serum creatinine above 3mg/dL, or chronic obstructive pulmonary disease) should receive intense perioperative monitoring if surgery becomes necessary
- Because coronary artery disease greatly increases the risk of surgery, all patients about to undergo nonemergency surgery or stent graft placement for an abdominal aortic aneurysm should receive preoperative stress sestamibi or coronary angiography

COEXISTING MEDICATION

Beta-blocking agents should be considered to reduce the risk of rupture.

SPECIAL PATIENT GROUPS

Screening and treatment for abdominal aortic aneurysm are sometimes considered inappropriate for people with a life expectancy of <2 years due to another disorder.

PATIENT SATISFACTION/LIFESTYLE PRIORITIES

Smoking cessation may be difficult for some patients.

SUMMARY OF THERAPEUTIC OPTIONS

Choices

- Nonoperative management: periodic monitoring, risk factor reduction, and treatment with a beta-blocker; appropriate for patients with a small aneurysm (<4cm), with a moderate aneurysm (4–6cm) and limited life expectancy, and with high operative mortality risk
- Open surgical repair: the traditional method for aneurysm repair

- Endovascular grafting: newer method for repair used typically for older patients and those at high operative risk
- Smoking cessation

Clinical pearl(s)

- The diagnosis is often missed; a high index of suspicion is necessary
- Screening of high-risk patients with multiple risk factors may provide the opportunity to perform elective surgery at low operative mortality risk

Never

Never delay surgery (e.g. by ordering a CT scan) in a patient with suspected rupture.

FOLLOW UP

For patients who have undergone surgical repair, follow up should be supervised by the surgeon.

Plan for review

- Patients with an intact aneurysm should receive periodic monitoring (ultrasound or CT): annual monitoring for aneurysms smaller than 3.5cm; monitor once every 6 months for aneurysms larger than 3.5cm
- Follow up should address hypertension and cigarette smoking
- Patients who have undergone surgery should be monitored for coronary artery disease, the primary cause of mortality following repair of an abdominal aortic aneurysm

Information for patient or caregiver

Patients with intact aneurysms should understand the need for periodic monitoring and the benefits of reducing blood pressure (if high) and smoking cessation. They should be alerted to the possible initial signs of rupture, expansion, and embolization.

DRUGS AND OTHER THERAPIES: DETAILS

Drugs

BETA-BLOCKER

Dose

Propranolol: dosage should be individualized.

Efficacy

- Reduces blood pressure
- Possibly causes beneficial changes in the arterial wall

Risks/Benefits

Risks:

- Use with caution in diabetes mellitus, thyroid disease, renal disease
- Use with caution in peripheral vascular disease, Raynaud's syndrome
- Use with caution prior to surgery or anesthesia
- Use caution in pregnancy and breast-feeding
- Do not withdraw abruptly

Benefits:

- Reduces blood pressure
- Possibly causes beneficial changes in the arterial wall

Side-effects and adverse reactions

- Cardiovascular: bradycardia, congestive heart failure, heart block, peripheral vascular disease

- CNS: lethargy, depression, and vivid dreams
- EENT: dry eyes, sore throat
- Gastrointestinal: nausea, vomiting, diarrhea, dry mouth, ischemic colitis
- Hematologic: agranulocytosis, thrombocytopenia
- Metabolism: hyperglycemia, hyperlipidemia, masked hypoglycemia
- Respiratory: bronchospasm, dyspnea, wheezing
- Skin: alopecia, bruising, rash

Interactions (other drugs)

- Adenosine - Alpha-adrenergic blockers - Amiodarone - Amoxicillin, ampicillin - Antacids - Antidiabetics - Beta-agonists - Calcium channel blockers - Clonidine - Cocaine - Digoxin - Dipyridamole - Lidocaine - Neostigmine - Neuroleptics - Nonsteroidal anti-inflammatory drugs (NSAIDs) - Physostigmine - Prazosin - Tacrine - Theophylline - Verapamil

Contraindications

- Bronchospastic diseases, asthma - Cardiogenic shock - Congestive heart failure - Advanced AV heart block - Severe bradycardia - Hepatic disease

Acceptability to patient

High.

Follow up plan

Monitor blood pressure near end of dosage interval.

Patient and caregiver information

Patient should adhere to established regimen and take radial pulse before each dose.

Surgical therapy

OPEN SURGICAL REPAIR

Excision of the aneurysm and insertion of a synthetic prosthesis.

Efficacy

Repair of aneurysm.

Risks/Benefits

- Risk: operative mortality rate is 4–6% (2% in low-risk patients)
- Benefit: averts risk of rupture

Acceptability to patient

Procedure has a long recovery and significant risk of mortality (4–6%). Patients with intact aneurysms should assess the risks and benefits of surgery.

Follow up plan

Should be supervised by surgeon.

Patient and caregiver information

Patients should understand the risks of surgery.

ENDOVASCULAR GRAFTING

A prosthetic tube graft is inserted through the femoral artery.

Efficacy

Graft bridges the aneurysm and allows aortic blood flow to continue.

Risks/Benefits

Risks:

- Not suitable for all abdominal aortic aneurysms
- Frequent occurrence of endoleaks, which may present a continuing risk for aneurysm expansion or rupture

Benefits:

- Faster surgical recovery
- Tolerable for some patients who would have a high risk of mortality from traditional surgery

Acceptability to patient

Patients should consider the risks and benefits of both types of surgical repair.

Follow up plan

Supervised by vascular specialist.

Patient and caregiver information

Patient should understand the risks and benefits of the procedure.

Other therapies

PERIODIC MONITORING

Monitor with ultrasound or CT to track possible changes in the size of the aneurysm:

- Monitor annually for aneurysms smaller than 3.5cm
- Monitor every 6 months for aneurysms larger than 3.5cm

Efficacy

Identifies patients for whom a surgical consult is appropriate due to increased risk for rupture.

Risks/Benefits

- Risk: without surgical repair, the aneurysm has the potential to rupture
- Benefit: spares patients with small aneurysms the risks involved in surgery, which has a mortality rate of 5–6%

Acceptability to patient

Patient may prefer to avoid or delay surgery.

Follow up plan

- For patients with aneurysms smaller than 3.5cm, monitor annually
- For patients with aneurysms larger than 3.5cm, monitor once every 6 months

Patient and caregiver information

Patients should understand the potential risks of aneurysm and the reason for monitoring.

LIFESTYLE

Smoking cessation.

RISKS/BENEFITS

Benefits:

- Reduces risk of aneurysm formation
- If surgery proves necessary, smoking cessation will increase chances of perioperative survival

ACCEPTABILITY TO PATIENT
May be difficult for some patients.

FOLLOW UP PLAN
Frequent reinforcement necessary.

PATIENT AND CAREGIVER INFORMATION
Patient should understand the importance of smoking cessation.

OUTCOMES

EFFICACY OF THERAPIES

Five-year survival rates after aneurysm repair range from 49–84%.

Review period

- For aneurysms below 3.5cm, monitor yearly
- For aneurysms above 3.5cm, monitor every 6 months
- For patients who have received surgery, review should be supervised by the surgeon

PROGNOSIS

- Mortality rate with elective repair of an abdominal aortic aneurysm ranges from 0.9–5% at university medical centers
- Emergency repair of a ruptured aneurysm has a mortality rate of about 75%
- Five-year survival rates after aneurysm repair range from 49–84%

Clinical pearl(s)

- Risk of rupture rises exponentially when diameter is >5cm
- Aneurysms <4cm rarely rupture
- Patients with diagnosed coronary disease should have coronary revascularization prior to abdominal aortic aneurysm repair

Therapeutic failure

- Surgical consultation for intact but large or rapidly growing aneurysm
- Surgery for ruptured or symptomatic aneurysm

Deterioration

Signs of rapid aneurysm expansion (>0.5cm/year) or expansion beyond 4cm warrants surgical consult.

Terminal illness

Facilitate emergency surgery.

COMPLICATIONS

- Rupture, usually resulting in death
- Pressure on intestines, causing gastrointestinal symptoms such as early satiety, nausea, and weight loss
- Ureteral obstruction, causing flank pain and periodic pyelonephritis
- Embolization, causing lower-extremity ischemia, including 'blue toe syndrome' and livedo reticularis

CONSIDER CONSULT

- Refer for postsurgical complications – coronary artery disease is the most likely threat following surgical repair of an abdominal aortic aneurysm

RISK FACTORS

- Cigarette smoking: adds significantly to risk of aneurysm development
- Hypertension: important risk factor for aneurysm development
- Diabetes: negatively associated with abdominal aortic aneurysm. This is a variance from other forms of peripheral artery disease

MODIFY RISK FACTORS

Lifestyle and wellness

TOBACCO

Cigarette smoking is a major risk factor for development of abdominal aortic aneurysm.

FAMILY HISTORY

- An individual with a first-degree relative who had an abdominal aortic aneurysm is at a higher than average risk of developing this condition
- Male siblings are at highest risk

SCREENING

ULTRASOUND OR PALPATION

According to the United States Preventive Services Task Force, there is insufficient evidence to recommend for or against routine screening for abdominal aortic aneurysm. Although there is no evidence that morbidity and mortality rates may be reduced with screening, selected high-risk patients may be screened. Whether abdominal palpation or ultrasound is the preferred test remains unclear – palpation is less expensive but not as sensitive as ultrasound. Repeat examination of patients with a previous normal ultrasound may not be indicated.

Reference

United States Preventive Services Task Force. Screening for abdominal aortic aneurysm. Guide to clinical preventive services, 2nd edn. Baltimore, MD: Williams & Wilkins, 1996, 67–72. Available at National Guideline Clearinghouse.

Cost/efficacy

'Cost-effective analysis suggests that repeat examination of individuals with a previous normal ultrasound [with regard to abdominal aortic aneurysm] is not indicated.'

Reference

United States Preventive Services Task Force. Guide to clinical preventive services, 2nd edn. Baltimore, MD: Williams & Wilkins, 1996, 67–72

RESOURCES

ASSOCIATIONS

American College of Cardiology
Heart House
9111 Old Georgetown Road
Bethesda, MD 20814-1699
Tel: (800) 253-4636
Fax: (301) 897-9745
http://www.acc.org

American College of Emergency Physicians
1125 Executive Circle
Irving, TX 75038-2522
Tel: (800) 798-1822
Fax: (972) 580-2816
http://www.acep.org

KEY REFERENCES

- Santilli JD, Santilli SM. Diagnosis and treatment of abdominal aortic aneurysms. Am Fam Physician 1997; 56(4):1081–90
- Gorski Y, Ricotta JJ. Weighing risks in abdominal aortic aneurysm. Postgrad Med 1999;106:69–80
- Braunwald E, Zipes DP, Libby P, Heart disease: a text book of cardiovascular medicine, 6th edn. Philadelphia: WB Saunders, 2001
- Deaton DH, Lederle FA. Abdominal aortic aneurysm: screening for a silent threat. Primary Care Treatment Update, Medical Education Collaborative, 2000.
- The UK Small Aneurysm Trial Participants. Mortality results for randomised controlled trial of early elective surgery or ultrasonographic surveillance for small abdominal aortic aneurysms. Lancet 1998;352:1649–55
- Brown LC, Powell JT. Risk factors for aneurysm rupture in patients kept under ultrasound surveillance. The UK Small Aneurysm Trial Participants. Ann Surg 1999;230:289–97
- Gadowski GR, Pilcher DB, Ricci MA. Abdominal aortic aneurysm expansion rate: effect of size and beta-adrenergic blockade. J Vasc Surg 1994;19:727–31
- US Preventive Services Task Force. Screening for abdominal aortic aneurysms, 1998. Available at the National Guideline Clearinghouse
- Moore WS, Kashyap VS, Vescera CL, et al. Abdominal aortic aneurysm: a 6-year comparison of endovascular versus transabdominal repair. Ann Surg 1999;230:298–306
- Hirsch AT, Jaff MR, eds. An office based approach to the diagnosis and treatment of peripheral arterial disease. Part VI: A primer to the vascular laboratory for the primary care physician. Belle Mead, NJ: Excerpta Medica, 2000, p23–8
- Townsend CM, Jr. Sabiston textbook of surgery, 16th edn. Philadelphia: WB Saunders, 2001
- Lederle FA, Simel DL. Does this patient have abdominal aortic aneurysm? JAMA 1999;281:77–82

FAQS

Question 1

When should I refer a patient with suspected aneurysm?

ANSWER 1

All patients should be referred to a vascular specialist. Even if the risk of rupture is low, emboli may occur or additional disease may be present.

Question 2
Which patient should have a cardiac work up prior to vascular surgery for abdominal aortic aneurysm?

ANSWER 2
Any patient with possible risk factors (age >50, diabetes, angina, Q-waves, ectopy, hypertension, other peripheral disease) should have at least a screening imaging stress test (e.g. adenosine sestamibi).

Question 3
What are the most common misdiagnoses?

ANSWER 3
Urinary tract infection or obstruction and spine pain are the most common missed diagnoses.

Question 4
What is the best way to follow abdominal aortic aneurysm size?

ANSWER 4
Ultrasound is the most cost-effective method for following asymptomatic abdominal aortic aneurysm to monitor size.

Question 5
When should aortic stent grafting be used instead of surgery?

ANSWER 5
Currently, aortic stent grafting is an emerging technology with few long-term data. It is generally reserved for patients who are poor operative candidates. Newer techniques and devices have the potential to change this trend in the future. Additional studies are needed.

CONTRIBUTORS
Russell C Jones, MD, MPH
John McB Hodgson, MD, FACC, FSCAI

AORTIC DISSECTION

SUMMARY INFORMATION

DESCRIPTION

- Entry of blood into intima–media space of thoracic aorta, with an intimal tear resulting in creation of a false lumen
- False lumen may extend in an anterograde or retrograde direction
- Range of symptoms and signs depends on location of dissection, degree of extension, presence of vascular branch (and end-organ) involvement, and presence of rupture
- Medical emergency that requires urgent assessment in the hospital
- Often requires emergent surgical repair

URGENT ACTION

- Arrange immediate transfer to the hospital if aortic dissection is suspected
- Admit to ICU for hemodynamic monitoring, preferably in cardiothoracic surgery center
- Administer intravenous fluid if cardiovascular collapse occurs
- Decrease contractility and blood pressure

KEY! DON'T MISS!

- New onset of an aortic murmur or change in character of a pre-existing aortic murmur
- Unequal pulses in major arterial sites (e.g. brachial, femoral)
- Discrepant limb blood pressure

ICD9 CODE
441.0 Dissection of aorta (ruptured)

SYNONYMS
Dissecting aortic aneurysm.

CARDINAL FEATURES
- Blood leaves aorta via transverse intimal tear
- Propagation of dissection anterogradely or retrogradely
- Location of dissection: ascending aorta 65%, descending aorta 20%, aortic arch 10%, abdominal aorta 5%
- Wide range of presentations depending on areas affected and aortic branches involved
- May present as acute myocardial infarction, acute aortic regurgitation, cardiac tamponade, cardiovascular collapse, limb ischemia, syncope, stroke, or spinal cord syndrome
- Usual presentation is with sudden, severe, central, tearing chest pain
- Cardinal signs are pulse deficits, asymmetric blood pressures, and an evolving aortic regurgitation murmur
- Management usually involves surgical repair
- Measures to reduce blood pressure important before surgery or when patient unsuitable for surgery

CAUSES
Common causes
- Hypertension (80%)
- Bicuspid aortic valve (congenital) (7–14%)
- Connective tissue diseases – Marfan syndrome (6–9%); Ehlers–Danlos syndrome

Rare causes
- Rare congenital abnormalities – unicuspid aortic valve, coarctation of the aorta
- Pregnancy, especially in the third trimester
- Giant cell arteritis (cranial arteritis)
- Cocaine use, especially in males
- Chest trauma
- Systemic lupus erythematosus, polycystic kidneys, hypertension associated with Cushing's syndrome
- Weight lifting

Serious causes
Marfan's syndrome and Ehlers–Danlos syndrome associated with cystic medial necrosis of the aorta which predisposes to dissection.

Contributory or predisposing factors
Iatrogenic:
- Aortic surgery (dissection may occur at the site of aortic incisions or cross-clamping)
- Following use of intra-aortic balloon pump

EPIDEMIOLOGY
Incidence and prevalence
INCIDENCE
- 0.05–0.10/1000 per year
- 2000 new cases per year in US

- 1 in 350 autopsies
- 6–9% have Marfan's syndrome

PREVALENCE
Since mortality is so high in untreated patients, no prevalence data are available.

Demographics
AGE
- Peak incidence 60–70 years
- 30–40 years in Marfan's syndrome

GENDER
Males are affected twice as commonly as females.

RACE
No racial predisposition has been established.

GENETICS
Marfan's syndrome and Ehlers-Danlos syndrome predispose to aortic dissection.

DIFFERENTIAL DIAGNOSIS

- 30–60% of aortic dissections are initially thought to be other disorders
- 30% of aortic dissections are discovered at autopsy

Myocardial infarction

Myocardial infarction is a disorder in which necrosis of heart muscle occurs because of an inadequate supply of oxygen.

FEATURES

- Pain of dissection typically maximal at onset, myocardial infarction typically increases over several minutes
- Pain of myocardial infarction is typically a dull pressure, that of aortic dissection is usually tearing
- Dissection flap can involve a coronary artery in proximal dissection causing associated myocardial infarction
- Right coronary artery usually involved, leading to inferior myocardial infarction
- Important to consider aortic dissection in inferior myocardial infarction; thrombolytic therapy carries 70% mortality rate when dissection present

Pulmonary embolus

Pulmonary embolus is an abrupt blocking of a pulmonary artery or one of its branches by a thrombus or foreign material.

FEATURES

- Usually associated with respiratory phenomena – pain that varies with respiration, cough, hemoptysis, and dyspnea
- Hemoptysis is common in pulmonary embolus, rare in aortic dissection

Angina

Angina is a symptom complex that results from myocardial ischemia; most commonly caused by narrowing of the coronary arteries.

FEATURES

- Angina pain can be similar in quality and distribution to that of aortic dissection
- Angina typically dull pressure, whereas aortic dissection pain is usually tearing
- Angina tends to rise to crescendo, aortic dissection pain is most often maximal at onset
- Leg pain and neurologic abnormalities can be seen in aortic dissection but not in angina

Pericarditis

Pericarditis is inflammatory or infective disease of the pericardial sac, which may be acute or chronic.

FEATURES

- Causes pain that is usually relieved by sitting forward
- Pericarditis is associated with characteristic ECG abnormalities, including diffuse ST-segment elevation (with concave-upward sloping), PR depression, and PR elevation in avR

Pneumothorax

Pneumothorax is the presence of air in the space between the visceral pleura and parietal pleura.

FEATURES

- Characterized by breathlessness and pain that is usually pleuritic
- Patients often have a history of previous pneumothorax, chronic respiratory disease, connective tissue disease, or lung neoplasm
- Clinical findings are resonance to percussion and diminished breath sounds on the affected side
- Chest X-ray is diagnostic

Pneumonia

FEATURES

- Characterized by dyspnea, productive cough, pleuritic pain, and signs of systemic infection
- Examination commonly reveals bronchial or diminished breath sounds, egophony, crepitations, and pleural rub, and dullness to percussion in the affected lung field
- Although fever is characteristic of pneumonia, low-grade fever is occasionally found in aortic dissection

Perforation of peptic ulcer

Aortic dissection may cause abdominal pain and rigidity similar to that found with perforated peptic ulcer.

FEATURES

- Pain is typically limited to the abdomen
- Whereas patients with perforated peptic ulcer commonly remain motionless with pain, those with aortic dissection often writhe in pain
- Erect chest X-ray shows subdiaphragmatic air in perforated peptic ulcer

Acute pancreatitis

Inflammation of the pancreas. Symptomatology and complications of pancreatitis are caused by autodigestion of the pancreas and surrounding tissue due to leaking pancreatic enzymes.

FEATURES

- Characterized by epigastric pain that radiates to the back
- Cardiovascular collapse and upper abdominal pain may occur in both aortic dissection and acute pancreatitis
- Acute pancreatitis does not give rise to pulse deficits, leg pain, or focal neurologic deficits
- In addition to clinical judgment and appropriate radiographic studies, assessment of serum amylase and lipase may assist in the differentiation of aortic dissection and pancreatitis

Acute aortic regurgitation

Aortic regurgitation is the retrograde flow of blood into the left ventricle from the aorta, due to incompetence of the aortic valve.

FEATURES

- In addition to aortic dissection, aortic valve endocarditis and blunt chest wall trauma may cause acute aortic regurgitation
- The presence of acute aortic regurgitation represents a medical emergency that requires immediate and rigorous assessment. Imaging modalities such as computed tomography scanning, transesophageal echocardiography, and/or magnetic resonance imaging should be undertaken to assist with diagnosis and direction of subsequent therapeutic intervention

SIGNS & SYMPTOMS

Signs

- Reflect location of the aortic dissection and associated aortic branch vessel involvement
- Hypertension in 90% of distal aortic dissections

- Hypotension in proximal aortic dissection is common; most often due to rupture into pericardium and subsequent cardiac tamponade
- Aortic dissection involving a brachiocephalic artery may reduce perfusion to the ipsilateral arm, with consequent reduction in blood pressure (pseudohypotension)
- Pulse deficit in 50% of proximal dissections and 15% of distal aortic dissections
- Blood pressure difference between the left and right arms
- Murmur of aortic regurgitation in up to 65% of proximal dissections; this is usually caused by a dissection dilating the aortic root
- Neurologic deficits in up to 20% of aortic dissections, with stroke in 3–6% and (less commonly) spinal artery involvement resulting in paraplegia
- Involvement of iliac arteries may result in acute ischemia of the lower limb (pallor, pain, paresthesia, pulselessness, coldness)
- Pleural effusion, typically on the left, is characterized by dullness to percussion at the lung base and decreased breath sounds; this may be due to inflammation around the aorta or contained rupture with hemothorax
- Acute cardiovascular collapse
- Rare signs include those of superior vena cava syndrome, upper airway obstruction and Horner's syndrome, and hoarseness and a pulsating neck mass

Symptoms

Pain:
- Present in 75–90% of cases
- Described as 'tearing'
- Radiation includes back, abdomen, neck, jaw
- Commonly located in extrathoracic sites, owing to involvement of branch vessels and subsequent regional ischemia
- Pain is frequently absent in patients with Marfan's syndrome

Less common symptoms include:
- Syncope
- Symptoms of congestive heart failure
- Paraparesis
- Dysphagia
- Hemoptysis caused by rupture into tracheobronchial tree
- Hematemesis caused by rupture into tracheobronchial tree or esophagus

ASSOCIATED DISORDERS

Myocardial infarction may result from dissection involving the coronary arterial circulation, most commonly the right coronary artery with inferior myocardial infarction.

KEY! DON'T MISS!

- New onset of an aortic murmur or change in character of a pre-existing aortic murmur
- Unequal pulses in major arterial sites (e.g. brachial, femoral)
- Discrepant limb blood pressure

CONSIDER CONSULT

- If aortic dissection is suspected, referral should be initiated immediately
- If possible, refer to a center with cardiothoracic surgery facilities

INVESTIGATION OF THE PATIENT

Direct questions to patient

Q **How would you describe the pain?** Typically 'tearing,' 'ripping,' 'searing'

Q **Where is the pain?** Usually central chest, may radiate to jaw, abdomen, leg, back

Q **Was the onset of the pain sudden or gradual?** Usually sudden and maximal at onset

Q **Have you previously experienced pain of this nature and severity?** This is unlikely in aortic dissection

Contributory or predisposing factors

Q **Do you have high blood pressure?** About 80% of patients with aortic dissection have hypertension

Q **Do you have any connective tissue diseases such as Marfan's syndrome or Ehlers–Danlos syndrome?** These are common causes of aortic dissection

Family history

Have any of your family members had diseases affecting the aorta? Note, however, that Marfan's syndrome and Ehlers–Danlos syndrome may elude diagnosis for generations.

Examination

- Measurement of blood pressure in both arms: hypertension requires acute treatment, and hypotension requires urgent stabilization, including volume replacement. Beware pseudohypertension in which the dissection involves one of the brachiocephalic arteries, resulting in low blood pressure measured in that arm. Involvement of one or both of the renal arteries may result in renal ischemia or infarction with consequent hypertension and possible acute renal failure
- Cautious evaluation of all peripheral pulses: a discrepancy or asymmetry in pulses (particularly between the two brachial, carotid, or femoral pulses) may indicate interruption of flow as a result of dissection
- Heart sounds: a new murmur of aortic regurgitation or a change in a pre-existing murmur is concerning for aortic dissection. A continuous murmur may reflect dissection with rupture via a false lumen into a cardiac chamber
- Breath sounds: pleural effusion may be present, more frequently on the left. Signs of left ventricular failure possible, especially with rupture into left atrium
- Neurologic examination: involvement of the carotid and spinal arteries may create a wide variety of focal neurologic deficits

Summary of investigative tests

If there is any suspicion of aortic dissection, the patient should be referred immediately to the hospital for evaluation.

- An ECG is useful to exclude myocardial infarction, which may exist alone or in association with an acute aortic dissection
- Blood should be drawn for electrolytes, urea and creatinine, complete blood count (CBC), and serum cardiac enzymes and cardiac troponins
- A chest X-ray may show widened mediastinum and/or displacement of aortic intimal calcium. It is a useful screening investigation in the hospital. Normal appearance does not exclude diagnosis
- Aortography used to be the main diagnostic imaging method for aortic dissection, but it has now been superseded
- Transesophageal echocardiography is very sensitive and specific but requires specialist equipment and skill
- Transthoracic echocardiography does not show the arch of the aorta and the descending aorta sufficiently well to be used as a reliable diagnostic technique; transesophageal echocardiography is therefore preferred
- Contrast-enhanced computed tomography of the chest is often more available than transesophageal echocardiography
- Magnetic resonance imaging is noninvasive and allows assessment of aortic branch involvement. It cannot be used to monitor critically ill patients and is unsuitable in patients with a metal implant or a pacemaker

- Intravascular ultrasonography is not yet widely available; it allows accurate evaluation of anatomic involvement of the aortic dissection

DIAGNOSTIC DECISION

- Any question of an aortic dissection should prompt immediate referral to the hospital
- High-risk factors include hypertension, Marfan's syndrome, and Ehlers–Danlos syndrome
- Acute, tearing central chest pain with precipitous onset suggests aortic dissection
- Asymmetry of pulses and unequal blood pressure in the extremities are findings that are suspicious for aortic dissection

Guidelines

- Imaging guidelines have been developed by the American College of Radiology Appropriateness Criteria Committee, Expert Panel on Cardiovascular Imaging. [1]

CLINICAL PEARL(S)

- A high index of suspicion is key to minimizing morbidity and mortality
- Transesophageal echocardiography is the best diagnostic test for critically ill patients
- Emergent catheterization, not thrombolytics, is indicated for myocardial infarction suspected to be related to dissection
- A normal chest X-ray does not rule out dissection

THE TESTS

Body fluids

ELECTROLYTES, UREA, AND CREATININE

Description

- Venous blood sample
- Measurement of renal function may indicate renal arterial involvement with dissection

Advantages/Disadvantages

Advantages:

- Will indicate whether renal function is impaired
- Serial measurements may be used to monitor patient's progress

Normal

- Sodium: 135–147mEq/L (135–147mmol/L)
- Potassium: 3.5–5.0mEq/L (3.5–5.0mmol/L)
- Urea: 8–18mg/dL (2.8–6.4mmol/L)
- Creatinine: 0.6–1.2mg/dL (53–106mcmol/L)

Note that reference ranges can vary; check with local laboratory.

Abnormal

Results outside normal range.

Cause of abnormal result

- Diminished renal function
- Dehydration
- Diuretics, corticosteroids, nonsteroidal anti-inflammatory drugs (NSAIDs)

Drugs, disorders, and other factors that may alter results

- Hemolyzed blood sample
- Significant delay between taking and analyzing blood sample

COMPLETE BLOOD COUNT (CBC)

Description

Venous blood sample.

Advantages/Disadvantages

Advantage: simple, straightforward, and routine investigation that is universally available.

Normal

- Leukocytes: 4.5–10.5x10^9/L
- Hemoglobin: men 13–18g/dL (8.06–11.17mmol/L); women 12–16g/dL (7.45–9.93mmol/L)
- Platelets: 130–400x10^9/L
- Hematocrit: men 39–49%; women 33–43%

Abnormal

Results outside normal range.

Cause of abnormal result

- Hematocrit may be low if contained rupture has occurred and sufficient time has elapsed (or fluids administered) to allow hemodilution
- Other causes of a low hematocrit could include perforated ulcer, pancreatitis, and esophageal pathology
- A raised white cell count is suggestive of infection

SERUM CARDIAC ENZYMES AND CARDIAC TROPONINS

Description

Venous blood sample to measure:

- Cardiac enzymes – creatine kinase (CK) and creatine kinase methyl bromide (CK-MB)
- Cardiac troponins – cardiac troponin I (cTnI) and cardiac troponin T (cTnT)

Advantages/Disadvantages

Advantages:

- Cardiac enzymes: CK is sensitive but not specific; CK-MB is more specific than undifferentiated CK for myocardial infarction; allows late diagnosis or confirmation of infarction
- Cardiac troponins: very high specificity and sensitivity for cardiac muscle; becomes positive in 3–12h; prolonged time course of decay (does not return to normal for 5–10 days in the case of cTnI and for 5–14 days in the case of cTnT) allows late diagnosis or confirmation of myocardial infarction

Disadvantage: cardiac enzymes may be elevated with chronic skeletal muscle injury.

Normal

- CK: 0–130U/L
- CK-MB: <5% of total CK
- cTnT: 0–0.10ng/ml
- cTnI: 0–0.15ng/ml

Normal values may vary by laboratory.

Abnormal

- CK: >130U/L
- CK-MB: >5% of total CK
- cTnT: >0.10ng/ml
- cTnI: >0.15ng/ml

Cause of abnormal result
Necrosis of cardiac muscle in myocardial infarction causes release of cardiac enzymes and cardiac troponins into blood.

Drugs, disorders, and other factors that may alter results
CK:
- Skeletal muscle disease (myositis, muscular dystrophy)
- Skeletal muscle injury (including intramuscular injections, surgery)
- Recent moderate to severe exercise
- Alcohol intoxication (with or without delirium tremens or convulsions)
- Hypothyroidism
- Severe hypokalemia
- Statins may cause myositis and thus elevate CK, particularly when used in conjunction with niacin, fibrates, or cyclosporin
- Renal insufficiency

CK-MB:
- Severe skeletal muscle injury (skeletal muscle also has a small amount of CK-MB) and renal insufficiency

Cardiac troponins:
- cTnT may be affected by renal insufficiency

Imaging
CHEST X-RAY
Advantages/Disadvantages
Advantages:
- Widely available
- Requires little specialist skill to assess
- Relatively inexpensive
- Noninvasive
- Easily and quickly performed; may be advantageous with critically ill patients
- Minimal radiation dose

Disadvantage: findings nonspecific and not diagnostic alone.

Abnormal
- Widened aortic silhouette in 85% of aortic dissections
- Distinct localized swelling can be seen in dissection of limited dimensions
- Separation of calcified aortic intima from outer border >1cm very suggestive of aortic dissection – 'calcium sign'
- Left-sided pleural effusion sometimes seen
- Comparison with previous chest films helpful

Cause of abnormal result
Blood within false lumen of aorta causes widened aortic outline.

Drugs, disorders, and other factors that may alter results
Aortic unfolding in the elderly may produce a widened aortic silhouette, as may aortic aneurysm.

CONTRAST-ENHANCED COMPUTED TOMOGRAPHY

Advantages/Disadvantages

Advantages:

- Widely available
- Noninvasive
- More rapid to perform than magnetic resonance imaging (MRI)
- May often distinguish between aortic dissection and other causes of widening of the aorta

Disadvantages:

- Does not show aortic regurgitation, if present
- Not as good as MRI at localizing the site and extent of dissection

Abnormal

- Widening of the aorta
- Presence of false lumen/dissection flap
- Communications between true and false lumens
- Aortic wall hematoma

Cause of abnormal result

- Aortic dissection
- Periaortic hematoma
- Tumor

Drugs, disorders, and other factors that may alter results

Any cause of widening of the aorta may mimic the CT appearance of dissection of the aorta.

MAGNETIC RESONANCE IMAGING (MRI)

Advantages/Disadvantages

Advantages:

- Most accurate technique for detecting aortic dissection (specificity and sensitivity approaches 100%) and for showing its site and extent
- Noninvasive
- Allows assessment of aortic branch involvement
- Cine-MRI can be used to assess for aortic regurgitation

Disadvantages:

- Cannot be used to monitor critically ill patients
- Unsuitable in patients with a metal implant or a pacemaker

Abnormal

MRI in the presence of aortic dissection may show:

- Presence of false lumen
- Communications between true and false lumens
- Blood flow pattern
- Aortic insufficiency
- Thrombus

Drugs, disorders, and other factors that may alter results

- Chronic aortic dissection and chronic aortic insufficiency can have similar results
- Good for demonstrating dissection without intimal tear

TRANSESOPHAGEAL ECHOCARDIOGRAPHY

Advantages/Disadvantages

Advantages:

- Widely available
- Can be performed at the bedside
- Provides good visualization of the thoracic aorta
- Can show aortic regurgitation and involvement of the coronary arteries
- Color Doppler allows accurate definition of entry and exit sites
- Allows view of cardiac function and segmental wall motion
- Allows diagnosis of pericardial effusion/tamponade
- Allows diagnosis of minor intramural hematomas

Disadvantages:

- Invasive – requires esophageal intubation under sedation
- Poor at visualizing the top of the arch and great vessel origins in some patients

Abnormal

- Presence of false lumen
- Blood flow between true and false lumen (indicating entry site)
- Intramural hematoma

Other tests

ELECTROCARDIOGRAM (ECG)

Description

Standard 12-lead ECG.

Advantages/Disadvantages

Advantages:

- Quick, portable, noninvasive
- Requires little specialist knowledge

Disadvantages:

- ECG often not changed from baseline in aortic dissection
- Not specific or sensitive for the identification of aortic dissection but useful to rule out myocardial infarction

Abnormal

- As 80% of patients with aortic dissection have baseline hypertension, ECG may reflect stigmata of chronic hypertension, including left ventricular hypertrophy with repolarization abnormality
- Concomitant coronary artery disease may be reflected in baseline ECG abnormalities, including Q waves, ST-segment abnormalities, and poor R-wave progression
- If aortic dissection involves a coronary artery, the ECG may reveal evidence of consequent acute myocardial, most often in inferior (right coronary artery) distribution

Cause of abnormal result

Coexistent chronic ischemic heart disease or hypertension, or associated cardiac involvement in the acute dissection.

TREATMENT

CONSIDER CONSULT

- Full examination and blood pressure measurement in both arms should be done in the office assuming the patient is hemodynamically stable
- 12-lead ECG should be done if possible but should not delay transfer
- Specialist evaluation and appropriate diagnostic studies should be orchestrated on an urgent basis
- Transfer to the hospital should be under paramedic or physician supervision, with resuscitation equipment available

IMMEDIATE ACTION

- Venous access should be obtained
- Control of hypertension is important, and should be initiated as early as possible with careful attention to hemodynamic parameters

MANAGEMENT ISSUES

Goals

- Diagnosis of aortic dissection
- Communication with tertiary care physician advising of potential emergency
- Arrangement of early transfer to a hospital, preferably with critical care and cardiac surgical facilities

Management in special circumstances

- Importance of coexisting acute myocardial infarction must be borne in mind
- Aortic dissection with sudden onset of pain is possible in patients with hypertension or with Marfan's syndrome or Ehlers–Danlos syndrome
- Asymmetry in pulse deficits or blood pressure measurements is a critical indication that aortic dissection may be present
- Anticoagulant and thrombolytic therapy in the presence of aortic dissection can be catastrophic
- Patients with suspected aortic dissection should be considered unstable, and transfer to the hospital should be arranged as quickly as possible

COEXISTING DISEASE

- Coexisting severe cardiorespiratory disease that would render the patient unfit for major surgery would necessitate the use of conservative medical management
- Medical management consists of control of hypertension
- Assessment of surgical risk should be considered carefully by members of cardiology, surgery, and anesthesiology teams

SPECIAL PATIENT GROUPS

- Aortic dissection is a very rare complication of pregnancy, occurring most often in the third trimester
- Urgent specialist assessment is required if aortic dissection is suspected in pregnancy
- Half of all dissections occurring in women under 40 occur during pregnancy

SUMMARY OF THERAPEUTIC OPTIONS

Choices

A new diagnosis of aortic dissection represents an emergency that requires specialist attention in a hospital setting; it should not be managed in the outpatient setting.

The decision about surgical versus medical ('conservative') management reflects a variety of considerations including the location, chronicity, and severity (rupture, organ involvement, hemodynamic instability of patient) of the dissection and the presence of comorbid illnesses.

Generally, dissections involving the ascending aorta (type II) or the ascending and arch portions (type I) are corrected surgically as soon as possible. Those involving only the descending aorta (type III) are initially managed medically, with operation reserved for special situations.

Surgery to repair the aortic dissection may be the definitive therapy for selected patients. Indications for surgery include:
- Involvement of the ascending aorta and/or arch
- Involvement of the carotid artery presenting as neurologic abnormality
- Renal artery involvement presenting as accelerated hypertension or renal failure
- Signs of rupture of the dissection (e.g. signs of cardiac tamponade, cardiovascular collapse)
- Acute aortic insufficiency
- Acute myocardial infarction due to dissection of coronary ostium

Medical management is sometimes appropriate:
- For patients in whom comorbidity precludes surgery, 'conservative therapy,' with a focus on blood pressure reduction, may be the treatment of choice
- Some centers advocate medical therapy for clinically stable patients with distal aortic dissection and chronic aortic dissection (i.e. presentation beyond 2 weeks of onset of symptoms)
- In medically managed patients, chest pain, new neurologic signs, or limb pain should prompt urgent consideration of surgical repair

The focus of medical therapy is on control of hypertension and reduction of the 'shear force' (dP/dt) imparted to circulating blood during systolic contraction:
- Intravenous nitroprusside may be used for acute management of hypertension
- Intravenous and/or oral beta-blockers are effective for acute and long-term management of hypertension. Labetalol, which has both alpha- and beta-blocking properties, is thought to benefit both control of hypertension and reduction of inotropy, with resultant reduction of the 'shear forces' (dP/dt)
- Calcium channel blockers should be considered in patients who do not tolerate beta-blocker therapy
- Angiotensin-converting enzyme (ACE) inhibitors may be particularly effective in refractory hypertension due to renal artery compromise in aortic dissection

Clinical pearl(s)
- Do not delay treatment of hypertension and increased inotropic state with nitroprusside and beta-blockers
- Emergency transfer by ACLS ambulance or helicopter is required

Never
Never delay transfer to do CT or MRI locally – they almost always need to be redone at the referral center. Transfer is based on clinical suspicion and simple examinations.

FOLLOW UP
- Recurrent dissection (particularly in medically treated patients) and aortic aneurysm (particularly in surgically treated patients) are most likely to occur within the first 2 years after diagnosis
- Initial follow-up should be frequent and intensive (i.e. every 1–3 months); once clinical stability has been ascertained, less frequent follow up (i.e. every 6 months) is possible
- Serial evaluation of peripheral pulses, blood pressures, chest X-ray, and chest CT scanning, transesophageal echocardiography, or MRI scanning

Plan for review
Blood pressure measurement – careful control is essential. A beta-blocker should be part of the chronic medication plan.

Information for patient or caregiver

- Compliance with antihypertensive medication is critical
- Any symptoms suggestive of recurrence of dissection (usually similar to those of initial presentations) should prompt urgent reporting to the emergency room

DRUGS AND OTHER THERAPIES: DETAILS

Drugs

NITROPRUSSIDE

- Intravenous nitroprusside may be used for acute management of hypertension
- May be started in the outpatient setting
- Should be used in conjunction with beta-blocker to reduce dP/dt

Dose

0.3mcg/kg/min initially, increased up to a maximum dose of 10mcg/kg/min. Titrate to systolic blood pressure of 110mmHg. Use with a beta-blocker.

Efficacy

- Effective at lowering blood pressure in a hypertensive crisis
- Medical management is effective in managing patients with aortic dissection (especially type III)

Risks/Benefits

Risks:

- Potential cyanide toxicity with continued administration
- Use caution in hepatic disease, hypothyroidism, and hyponatremia

Benefit:

- Dose can be rapidly titrated against effect

Side-effects and adverse reactions

- Cardiovascular: hypotension, palpitations, tachycardia, bradycardia
- CNS: dizziness, headache
- Hematologic: methemoglobinemia
- Gastrointestinal: nausea
- Other: cyanide toxicity

Interactions (other drugs)

- Clonidine
- Diltiazem
- Guanabenz
- Guanfacine

Contraindications

- Compensatory hypertension (e.g. in coarctation of the aorta, arteriovenous shunt)
- Reduced cerebral perfusion
- Leber's (optic) atrophy

Follow up plan

- Close follow up under the supervision of a hospital specialist is necessary for aortic dissection patients treated medically
- Clinical examination and an imaging test, usually computed tomography or magnetic resonance imaging, should be done
- Significant progression of the dissection, or chest pain, new neurologic signs, or limb pain should prompt early consideration of surgical repair if possible

LABETALOL

$Alpha_1$- and beta-blocker. May be used as monotherapy for aortic dissection.

Dose

- Intravenous: 10mg over 2min; repeated as needed every 10–15min with escalating doses (20–80mg) to a total of 300mg; then continuous infusion (1–2mg/min)
- Oral: 100mg twice daily, increased every 2–3 days by 100mg/day up to a usual maintenance dose of 200–400mg twice daily (maximum 1200–2400mg twice daily)

Efficacy

Labetalol has both alpha- and beta-blocking properties and is felt to benefit both control of hypertension and reduction of inotropy, with resultant reduction of 'shear forces' (dP/dt).

Risks/Benefits

Risks:

- Caution in patients with chronic liver disease – need to decrease the dose by 50%
- Use caution in congestive heart failure, bronchospastic airways, diabetes mellitus, peripheral vascular disease, and renal disease

Side-effects and adverse reactions

- Cardiovascular: atrioventricular block, bradycardia, ventricular dysrhythmias
- CNS: anxiety, dizziness
- EENT: double vision, dry eyes, tinnitus
- Gastrointestinal: nausea, diarrhea, vomiting
- Hematologic: agranulocytosis, trombocytopenic purpura (with beta-blockers)
- Respiratory: bronchospasm
- Skin: rash

Interactions (other drugs)

- Alpha-adrenergic blockers
- Amiodarone
- Cimetidine
- Clonidine
- Digoxin
- Dihydropyridine calcium channel blockers
- Diltiazem
- Epinephrine
- Hypoglycemic agents
- Non steroidal anti-inflammatory drugs
- Theophylline
- Verapamil

Contraindications

- Hypersensitivity reaction
- Bronchial asthma
- Cardiogenic shock
- Second- or third-degree heart block

Follow up plan

- Close follow up under the supervision of a hospital specialist is necessary for aortic dissection patients treated medically
- Clinical examination and an imaging test, usually computed tomography or magnetic resonance imaging, should be carried out
- Significant progression of the dissection, or chest pain, new neurologic signs, or limb pain should prompt early consideration of surgical repair if possible

CALCIUM CHANNEL BLOCKERS

Dose

Depends on agent (e.g. verapamil 80mg twice daily initially, increased as needed up to 240mg twice daily).

Risks/Benefits

Risks:

- The vasodilatory effects of verapamil may cause hemodynamic complications in patients with a substantial outflow gradient or markedly elevated pulmonary pressure
- Use caution with congestive heart failure, hypotension, renal and hepatic disease, Duchenne's muscular dystrophy, and acute phase of myocardial infarction

- Use caution in children
- Use caution in concomitant beta-blocker therapy

Benefit: can be used as an alternative in those unable to tolerate beta-blocker therapy.

Side-effects and adverse reactions

- Cardiovascular: tachycardia, bradycardia, palpitations, congestive heart failure, atrioventricular block, hypotension, peripheral edema
- CNS: dizziness, flushing, headache, fatigue
- EENT: tinnitus
- Gastrointestinal: nausea, constipation, vomiting, abdominal pain
- Genitourinary: impotence, nocturia, polyuria, gynecomastia
- Skin: rash

Interactions (other drugs)

■ Antidysrhythmics (amiodarone, digoxin, disopyramide, dofetilide, encainide, flecainide, procainamide, quinidine) ■ Antihypertensives (particularly alpha- and beta-blockers) ■ Antivirals ■ Aspirin ■ Azole antifungals ■ Barbiturates ■ Benzodiazepines ■ Buspirone ■ Calcium ■ Carbamazepine ■ Cardiac glycosides ■ Cimetidine ■ Cisapride ■ Clarithromycin, erythromycin ■ Cyclosporine, tacrolimus ■ Dantrolene ■ Diclofenac ■ Doxorubicin ■ Ethanol ■ Fentanyl ■ General and local anesthetics ■ Grapefruit juice ■ Histamine H_2 antagonists ■ Imipramine ■ Lithium ■ Neuromuscular blockers ■ Phenytoin ■ Rifampin ■ SSRIs ■ Statins ■ Theophylline

Contraindications

- Sick sinus syndrome or second- or third-degree AV block except with a functioning pacemaker, hypotension <90mmHg systolic (diltiazem and verapamil).
- Acute myocardial infarction and pulmonary congestion (diltiazem)
- Severe left ventricular dysfunction; cardiogenic shock and severe congestive heart failure, unless secondary to a supraventricular tachycardia amenable to verapamil therapy and in patients with atrial flutter or atrial fibrillation and an accessory bypass tract (verapamil)
- Do not administer intravenous verapamil concomitantly with intravenous beta-adrenergic blocking agents (within a few hours)
- Ventricular tachycardia (verapamil)
- Advanced aortic stenosis (nicardipine)

Follow up plan

- Close follow-up under the supervision of a hospital specialist is necessary for aortic dissection patients treated medically
- Clinical examination and an imaging test, usually computed tomography or magnetic resonance imaging, should be carried out
- Significant progression of the dissection, or chest pain, new neurologic signs, or limb pain should prompt early consideration of surgical repair if possible

ANGIOTENSIN CONVERTING ENZYME (ACE) INHIBITORS

Dose

Depends on agent, e.g. captopril 25mg three times daily, increased if necessary every 1–2 weeks to 50mg three times daily; usual maintenance dose 25–150mg three times daily.

Efficacy

May be particularly effective in refractory hypertension due to renal artery compromise in aortic dissection.

Risks/Benefits

Risks: use caution in renal impairment, hypotension and aortic stenosis, hyperkalemia, and neutropenia

Side-effects and adverse reactions

- Cardiovascular: orthostatic hypotension and syncope, angina, palpitations, sinus tachycardia
- CNS: headache, dizziness, fatigue
- EENT: cough
- Gastrointestinal: nausea, vomiting, diarrhea, constipation, abdominal pain
- Genitourinary: renal damage, impotence
- Hematologic: neutropenia, agranulocytosis, aplastic and hemolytic anemia, pancytopenia, thrombocytopenia
- Metabolic: hyperkalemia, hyponatremia
- Skin: angioedema, maculopapular rash

Interactions (other drugs)

- Allopurinol
- Antihypertensives (loop and potassium-sparing diuretics, prazosin, terazosin, doxazosin)
- Azathioprine ▪ Heparin ▪ Insulin ▪ Iron ▪ Lithium ▪ NSAIDs ▪ Potassium ▪ Sodium
- Trimethoprim

Contraindications

- Pregnancy ▪ Angioedema ▪ Hypotension ▪ Children

Follow up plan

- Close follow up under the supervision of a hospital specialist is necessary for aortic dissection patients treated medically
- Clinical examination and an imaging test, usually computed tomography or magnetic resonance imaging, should be carried out
- Significant progression of the dissection, or chest pain, new neurologic signs, or limb pain should prompt early consideration of surgical repair if possible

Surgical therapy

- Surgery may be the definitive therapy for selected patients with aortic dissection
- Blood pressure reduction prior to surgery is important for hypertensive patients
- Acute blood pressure reduction may be accomplished with intravenous agents, such as nitroprusside (with beta-blockers) or labetalol, with access to intensive hemodynamic monitoring
- Conservative therapy,' with a focus on blood pressure reduction, may be the treatment of choice for patients in whom comorbidity precludes surgery
- Some centers advocate medical therapy for clinically stable patients with distal aortic dissection and chronic aortic dissection (i.e. presentation beyond 2 weeks of onset of symptoms)

REPAIR OF AORTIC DISSECTION

- Surgery aims to resect severely damaged aorta and to excise the intimal tear
- Interposition of prosthetic aortic sleeve graft is usually done to restore continuity of the aorta after surgery

Efficacy

- Early mortality of patients not treated surgically is 1% per h
- Survival rate to discharge following emergency repair of aortic dissection is 80%

Risks/Benefits

Risks:

- Surgical risks are largely dependent on dissection location and associated conditions including hemodynamic status, perforation, tamponade, aortic insufficiency, great vessel involvement, left ventricular function, myocardial infarction, pulmonary status, and renal status
- Therapy is life-saving for most patients; however, the magnitude of the operation means recovery is slow and may be complicated

Evidence

- A retrospective study examined the efficacy of surgery for patients with complications of aortic dissection from 1956 to 1988. The cumulative survival rate was 86% for all patients and 94% for patients treated in more recent years. Long-term survival after final reoperation was 66% at 5 years, and 44% at 10 years [2] *Level S*
- A prospective study (non randomized) compared the open resection technique with the graft inclusion technique in the management of acute ascending aortic dissection. The early mortality rate was 31% following graft inclusion, and 16% for the open technique group. The open technique also showed better late outcomes, with 8-year survival being significantly higher [3] *Level P*

Follow up plan

- Regular and indefinite follow up after surgical repair should involve clinical examination and computed tomography, transesophageal echocardiography, or magnetic resonance imaging of the aorta
- Follow up should be carried out under the guidance of those with cardiac surgical expertise

OUTCOMES

EFFICACY OF THERAPIES

- Mortality rate of untreated aortic dissection 1% per h in the first 48h
- Efficacy of early surgical resection established in several large series reported in the 1980s
- Early mortality high but good long-term survival following surgical repair
- Improvements in surgical techniques have led to better long-term outcome in recent series, but early mortality remains high

Evidence

PDxMD are unable to cite evidence that meets our criteria for evidence.

Review period

Review after surgery should be continued indefinitely.

PROGNOSIS

- Mortality rate of untreated aortic dissection is 1% per h in the first 48h
- Nearly all deaths occur within 1 month of diagnosis
- Survival rate after succesful medical or surgical therapy is 75–82% at 5 years

Clinical pearl(s)

- Patients with poorly controlled blood pressure after initial treatment are 10 times more likely to have recurrence or rupture
- Aneurysm formation occurs at a remote site in 17–25% of patients at a mean of 18 months; this should be treated aggressively as aneurysms are more prone to rupture
- Renal or visceral artery involvement carries a >50% acute mortality rate

Therapeutic failure

- Failure of medical therapy in a stable patient with distal dissection is an indication for surgery
- Any evidence of recurrence (e.g. pain, cardiovascular collapse, new neurologic abnormality) in a patient treated surgically is an indication for urgent assessment by a cardiothoracic surgeon

Recurrence

- Recurrence generally relates to advanced and diffuse atherosclerosis. Aneurysm formation at a remote site occurs in 17–25% of patients at a mean of 18 months; this should be treated aggressively as aneurysms are more prone to rupture
- Aortic insufficiency may progress over time if it was not repaired initially

Deterioration

- Surgical repair of the dissection may be the treatment of choice in the clinically unstable patient, whether previously treated surgically or not
- If other factors exist that preclude surgical intervention, medical management with antihypertensive therapy should be pursued

COMPLICATIONS

- Recurrent aneurysms often form in the distal portions of the original dissection plane and are, therefore, thin-walled and more prone to rupture
- Progressive aortic insufficiency if the valve was not repaired/replaced initially (in ascending dissections)

CONSIDER CONSULT

- In a patient known to have a chronic aortic dissection managed medically or a previously operated aortic dissection, any sign of deterioration should prompt urgent referral. Signs of recurrence are acute chest pain, new neurologic events, cardiovascular collapse

PREVENTION

- Control of hypertension is the cornerstone in prevention of aortic dissection
- Attention to other modifiable cardiac risk factors (i.e. cholesterol, smoking, obesity) is also recommended

RISK FACTORS

- The major modifiable risk factor for aortic dissection is hypertension
- Other risk factors include Marfan's syndrome and Ehlers–Danlos syndrome

MODIFY RISK FACTORS

Lifestyle and wellness

ALCOHOL AND DRUGS

- Excessive alcohol intake can contribute to hypertension
- Numerous prescription and over-the-counter drugs are associated with hypertension, including oral contraceptives and corticosteroids
- Several drugs of abuse are associated with hypertension, particularly cocaine and amphetamine
- Tobacco use may worsen hypertension

DIET

A low-salt diet should be advised to patients who are hypertensive.

PHYSICAL ACTIVITY

Exercise should be encouraged in hypertensive patients.

FAMILY HISTORY

- A family history of aortic dissection may occur with unrecognized Marfan's syndrome or Ehlers–Danlos syndrome
- First-degree relatives should be screened if multiple family members have aortic dissection, particularly at a young age

PREVENT RECURRENCE

Prevention of recurrence of aortic dissection involves careful control of hypertension. Patients with poorly controlled hypertension are 10 times more likely to have rupture or recurrence.

ASSOCIATIONS

American Heart Association
National Center
7272 Greenville Avenue
Dallas, Texas 75231
http://www.americanheart.org

American College of Cardiology
Heart House
9111 Old Georgetown Road
Bethesda, MD 20814-1699
Tel: (800) 253-4636 or (301) 897-5400
Fax: (301) 897-9745
http://www.acc.org

National Marfan Foundation
382 Main Street
Port Washington, NY 11050
Tel: (800) 8-MARFAN and (516) 883-8712
Fax: (516) 883-8040
http://home.talkcity.com/LOLWay/uncle_dan/marfan/pub/resourcebook/

Ehlers–Danlos National Foundation
6399 Wilshire Blvd, Ste 203
Los Angeles, CA 90048
Tel: (323) 651-3038
Fax: (323) 651-1366
http://www.ednf.org/

KEY REFERENCES

- Varon J, Marik PE. The diagnosis and management of hypertensive crises. Chest 2000;118:214–27
- Dmowski AT, Carey MJ. Aortic dissection [review]. Am J Emerg Med 1999;17:372–5
- Slater EE. The clinical recognition of dissecting aortic aneurysm. Am J Med 1976;60:625–33
- Rosman HS, Patel S, Borzak S, et al. Quality of history taking in patients with aortic dissection. Chest 1998;114(3):793–5
- Sullivan PR. Diagnosis of acute thoracic aortic dissection in the emergency department. Am J Emerg Med 2000;18:46–50
- Fann JI, Smith JA, Miller DC, et al. Surgical management of aortic dissection during a 30-year period. Circulation 1995;92:113–21
- Niederhauser U, Rudiger H, Kunzli A, et al. Surgery for acute type A aortic dissection: comparison of techniques. Eur J Cardiothorac Surg 2000;18:307–12

Evidence references and guidelines

1 Imaging guidelines have been developed by the American College of Radiology Appropriateness Criteria Committee, Expert Panel on Cardiovascular Imaging. ACR Appropriateness Criteria for acute chest pain – suspected aortic dissection. Radiology 2000;215:1–5
2 Crawford ES, Svensson LG, Coselli JS, et al. Aortic dissection and dissecting aortic aneurysms. Ann Surg 1988;208:254–73. Medline
3 Niederhauser U, Rudiger H, Kunzli A, et al. Surgery for acute type A aortic dissection: comparison of techniques. Eur J Cardiothorac Surg 2000;18:307–12. Medline

FAQS

Question 1

Which patients should be referred for emergency surgery?

ANSWER 1

Those with the 'proximal' type I and type II dissections (both involve the ascending aorta). Untreated patients have 25% mortality rate at 24 h, 50% at 1 week, 75% at 1 month, and 90% at 1 year.

Question 2

Do older patients at risk for coronary artery disease need coronary angiography prior to surgery?

ANSWER 2

Not generally. Recent studies suggest that surgical mortality is increased by the time delay to perform angiography.

Question 3

What should I do if a patient presents with suspected tamponade?

ANSWER 3

Emergency pericardiocentesis may actually cause the patient to worsen by allowing the blood pressure to increase. If the patient has an adequate blood pressure they should be taken emergently to the operating room for surgical repair and intraoperative drainage. If the patient is in cardiovascular collapse, pericardiocentesis should be performed, but only enough fluid should be removed to achieve a systolic blood pressure of approximately 110mmHg.

Question 4

I am at a small hospital without invasive monitoring capabilities. How can I initiate medical management while awaiting transfer?

ANSWER 4

Automated blood pressure cuffs can be placed on the extremity with the best pulse (may be one of the calves). If nitroprusside is not available, intravenous enalaprilate (0.625mg boluses) may be used with intravenous esmolol (standard titration) or intravenous lopressor. Alternatively, intravenous labetalol could be used. Treatment should not be delayed. Package inserts or tertiary center physician contact can assist with initiation of therapy.

Question 5

My patient complains of increasing pain and is becoming hypotensive. I want to start dopamine to keep the pressure up. Is this OK?

ANSWER 5

No, dopamine will increase contractility and systemic resistance, both of which will worsen the dissection. Most patients with dissection are hypertensive due to catechol surge and pain. If your patient is hypotensive, he or she either has acute aortic insufficiency, pericardial tamponade, or has ruptured and is exsanguinating. Treatment should include rapid fluid resuscitation, avoid nitrates, and transfuse blood emergently. In any case, emergency surgery is the only definitive therapy. Transfer should be arranged as soon as possible. While waiting, evaluation of the jugular venous pressure, cardiac auscultation, and an echocardiogram can assist with the diagnosis of tamponade or aortic insufficiency.

CONTRIBUTORS

Fred F Ferri, MD, FACP
John McB Hodgson, MD, FACC, FSCAI
Doug Drachman, MD

AORTIC REGURGITATION

SUMMARY INFORMATION

DESCRIPTION

Retrograde flow of blood into the left ventricle from the aorta, secondary to incompetent aortic valve.

URGENT ACTION

Urgent action is indicated in cases of:

- Acute aortic regurgitation complicated by left ventricular failure, cardiogenic shock, and/or pulmonary edema: emergency surgical intervention may be life-saving in such cases
- Acute aortic regurgitation as a presenting sign of aortic trauma or suspected aortic dissection: emergency surgery is indicated, and antihypertensive therapy for acute aortic dissection with nitroprusside in combination with beta-blockade should be instituted before imaging studies are completed
- Suspected aortic valvular endocarditis: a high index of suspicion for valvular endocarditis is an indication for obtaining at least three sets of blood cultures prior to institution of empiric antimicrobial therapy

KEY! DON'T MISS!

When many of the signs of severe aortic regurgitation are not present, diagnosis of aortic regurgitation is easy to miss.

ICD9 CODE
424.1 Aortic valve regurgitation/insufficiency

SYNONYMS
Aortic insufficiency, AI, AR.

CARDINAL FEATURES
- Retrograde blood flow into left ventricle from the aorta, due to incompetence of the aortic valve
- Left ventricular volume overload from regurgitant blood volume
- Initially, increased left ventricular ejection due to increased left ventricular volume
- Increased left ventricular end-diastolic pressure
- Eventually, left ventricular dilation and failure, with secondary pulmonary hypertension

CAUSES
Common causes
- Aortic root dilation
- Aortic root dissection (acute aortic regurgitation)
- Infectious endocarditis (acute aortic regurgitation)
- Rheumatic fever (two-thirds of patients with aortic regurgitation and mitral valvular disease)
- Trauma (acute aortic regurgitation)
- Marfan's syndrome (acute and chronic aortic regurgitation)

Rare causes
- Ehlers–Danlos syndrome
- Cystic medionecrosis of the aorta
- Myxomatous proliferation of the aortic valve
- Systemic lupus erythematosus
- Whipple's disease
- Congenital bicuspid valve with aortic regurgitation
- Syphilis
- Osteogenesis imperfecta
- Arthritis/collagen vascular disease: psoriatic arthritis, ankylosing spondylitis, relapsing polychondritis, Reiter's syndrome, giant cell arteritis
- Discrete membranous subaortic stenosis
- Ventricular septal defect with aortic valve prolapse (in children)
- Takayasu's disease
- Fenfluramine (fen-phen) use

Serious causes
- Trauma
- Aortic root dissection
- Infectious endocarditis
- Marfan's syndrome
- Ventricular septal defect with aortic valve prolapse (in children)

Contributory or predisposing factors
Hypertension.

EPIDEMIOLOGY

Incidence and prevalence

PREVALENCE

- Aortic regurgitation of more than trace severity is present in 13% of men and 8.5% of women
- In a study of native Americans, mild aortic regurgitation was present in 7.3%, moderate in 2.4%, and severe in 0.3% of adults

Demographics

AGE

- More common in adults; age of onset depends on underlying cause. In a study of native Americans, aortic regurgitation correlated with age >60 years (14.4% vs 5.8% under age 60 years)
- In one study, prevalence of aortic regurgitation in normal children and adolescents was 0.3%, suggesting that it should not be considered a normal finding in children and adolescents

GENDER

- Three-quarters of patients with pure or predominant aortic regurgitation are male
- Women predominate among patients with aortic regurgitation and associated mitral valvular disease
- Takayasu's disease occurs predominantly in women

GENETICS

- Marfan's syndrome: autosomal dominant
- Ehlers–Danlos syndrome: a group of heritable disorders, which includes autosomal-dominant, autosomal-recessive, and X-linked forms
- Takayasu's disease: some association with histologic tissue types
- Osteogenesis imperfecta: a group of heritable disorders with autosomal-dominant, autosomal-recessive, and sporadic inheritance
- Arthritis/collagen vascular disease: familial predisposition with complex inheritance

GEOGRAPHY

- Cases related to rheumatic fever are more common in developing countries
- Takayasu's disease is more common in Asian countries, but is not more common in Asian races

SOCIOECONOMIC STATUS

Cases resulting from rheumatic fever are more common in lower socioeconomic classes.

DIFFERENTIAL DIAGNOSIS

Aortic regurgitant murmur must be distinguished from other causes of diastolic murmur.

Pulmonic valve regurgitation

Can be congenital in origin. Most often results from dilation of the pulmonic valve ring secondary to pulmonary hypertension. Very uncommonly a seat of infectious endocarditis.

FEATURES

- Murmur: high-pitched diastolic decrescendo Graham Steell murmur heard best over the left sternal border and pulmonic area; loud P2; murmur increases with inspiration; rarely audible at the second right intercostal space (in contrast to aortic regurgitation)
- Signs of right ventricular volume and pressure overload; prominent right ventricular heave, elevated jugular venous pressure

Mitral stenosis

Mitral stenosis is narrowing of the outflow path from the left ventricle.

FEATURES

- Usually rheumatic in origin; two-thirds of patients with mitral stenosis are female
- Isolated valvular lesion in 40% of cases
- Presentation in pulmonary edema can occur with minor increases in cardiac output: exertion, fever, thyrotoxicosis, pregnancy, sexual intercourse
- Symptoms develop up to 20 years after rheumatic fever
- Once symptomatic, death usually occurs within 2–5 years, if not treated
- Hemoptysis occurs in patients with elevated left atrial pressure, most often in those without markedly elevated pulmonary vascular resistance
- Late disease can be complicated by pulmonary embolus or infarction, and systemic emboli can result from left atrial thrombus formation
- Pulmonary infections are common
- Murmur: low-pitched, mid-to-late diastolic rumble heard best with the bell of the stethoscope over the apex; loud S1; murmur begins after opening snap; presystolic accentuation with onset of atrial systole
- Peripheral and facial cyanosis; malar flush in advanced mitral stenosis
- Prominent jugular a-waves indicative of secondary pulmonary hypertension
- Atrial arrhythmia, particularly atrial fibrillation, is common

Tricuspid stenosis

Tricuspid stenois is an uncommon valvular lesion, usually rheumatic in origin.

FEATURES

- Predominantly occurs in women
- Rarely an isolated lesion – usually seen in combination with mitral stenosis or mitral regurgitation
- Because patients often have associated mitral stenosis, presentation is often with pulmonary congestion
- Signs of right-sided cardiac congestion: hepatomegaly, ascites, edema, elevated jugular venous pressure with giant a-waves
- Low-pitched diastolic murmur heard along left sternal border that increases with inspiration, and is reduced with expiration and Valsalva (Carvallo's sign)

SIGNS & SYMPTOMS

Signs

- In acute aortic regurgitation, patient may appear acutely ill, with tachycardia, peripheral vasoconstriction, and cyanosis. Murmur may be soft or inaudible
- Decrescendo high-pitched early diastolic murmur is heard along sternal border in second right intercostal space. It is best heard with patient sitting upright and forward, and breath held in deep expiration. It is accentuated by raising arterial blood pressure via vasopressive drugs, squatting, and isometric exercise, and is reduced by maneuvers that lower arterial blood pressure, such as amyl nitrate or Valsalva (second phase)
- Soft S1 (preclosure of mitral valve) and prolongation of PR interval
- Displacement of cardiac impulse downward and to the left
- Low-pitched apical diastolic rumble (Austin Flint murmur) caused by contact of aortic regurgitant jet with left ventricular wall or mitral valve, causing it to vibrate (origin debatable)
- Early systolic apical ejection murmur (related to increased ejection rate and stroke volume)
- Signs of congestive heart failure: tachypnea, tachycardia, edema, rales, pulmonary effusion, S3 gallop, elevated jugular venous pressure
- Signs of pulmonary edema: rales, wheezing, tachypnea, frothy pink or blood-tinged sputum, cyanosis, decreased arterial oxygen saturation (SaO_2)
- Myocardial ischemia
- Arrhythmias
- Widened pulse pressure, increased systolic arterial pressure with decreased diastolic arterial pressure
- Bounding pulses: head bobbing in systole (de Musset's sign); water-hammer, pistol-shot, or collapsing pulse (Corrigan's pulse); capillary pulsations (Quincke's pulse) in nail beds
- To and fro 'double Duroziez' murmur heard over femoral arteries with slight compression
- Popliteal systolic pressure is increased over brachial systolic pressure >40mmHg (Hill's sign)

Symptoms

- Fatigue
- Shortness of breath
- Edema
- Palpitations
- Chest pain
- Orthopnea

KEY! DON'T MISS!

When many of the signs of severe aortic regurgitation are not present, diagnosis of aortic regurgitation is easy to miss.

CONSIDER CONSULT

Refer to a specialist if:

- New onset of diastolic murmur associated with recent chest trauma or deceleration injury. Refer immediately for possible acute aortic dissection and emergency surgical intervention, whether or not there are signs or symptoms of heart failure
- New onset of diastolic murmur associated with signs and symptoms of congestive heart failure or pulmonary edema
- New onset of diastolic murmur associated with chest pain suggestive of angina. Refer immediately for work-up of coronary insufficiency secondary to acute rise in left ventricular diastolic pressure associated with acute aortic regurgitation, or possible coronary insufficiency seoncary to acute aortic dissection with involvement of the coronary ostium
- New onset of diastolic murmur in patients with signs and symptoms of infection or sepsis
- Patient with known chronic aortic regurgitation developing symptoms or signs of cardiac decompensation

INVESTIGATION OF THE PATIENT

Direct questions to patient

- **Q Have you ever been told you have a heart murmur?** This may indicate chronicity, the presence of a congenital bicuspid aortic valve
- **Q Have you ever had rheumatic fever or recurrent strep throat?** Cause of aortic valvular disease
- **Q Do you have shortness of breath at rest or in the middle of the night?** Signs of cardiac decompensation
- **Q Do you have chest pain or pressure, particularly during physical activity, that radiates to the jaw or down the left arm?** Signs of coronary insufficiency
- **Q Have you had palpitations or racing pulse?** Symptomatic of arrhythmias
- **Q Have you noticed swelling in your feet or legs?** Sign of cardiac decompensation
- **Q Have you been coughing up pink or blood-tinged sputum?** Sign of cardiac decompensation or pulmonary edema
- **Q Have you had fevers, chills, night sweats?** May indicate bacterial endocarditis

Contributory or predisposing factors

- **Q Have you had problems with high blood pressure? Are you on medication for high blood pressure?** Predisposing factor for aortic dissection
- **Q Have you recently been in an automobile accident, suffered a fall, or otherwise injured your chest?** Predisposing factor for aortic dissection
- **Q Do you use illicit intravenous drugs of any kind?** Predisposing factor for endocarditis
- **Q Have you had recent dental work?** Predisposing factor for endocarditis in patients with underlying valvular abnormalities
- **Q Have you ever used fen-phen or other prescription medications to lose weight?** Even a short course of therapy (<1 month) may predispose to valvular heart disease
- **Q Have you had any unusual problems with your eyes, such as retinal detachment or lens dislocation?** May indicate presence of Marfan's disease
- **Q Do you have a history of sexually transmitted disease? Do you use barrier protection for sexual intercourse?** May indicate risk for syphilis

Family history

- **Q Did anyone in your family die suddenly, particularly under age 65 years, or does anyone have long slender limbs?** May indicate Marfan's syndrome
- **Q Have you or anyone in your family had problems with aneurysms or lax joints?** May indicate Ehlers–Danlos syndrome, or other collagen vascular disease

Examination

Specific:

- **Widened pulse pressure** in cases of chronic regurgitation (pulse pressure may not be increased in acute aortic regurgitation)
- **Cardiac examination** and auscultation: presence of diastolic murmur along left sternal border, diastolic rumble at ventricular apex (Austin Flint murmur), S3 gallop, early systolic ejection murmur, displacement of apical impulse downward and to the left
- **Pulmonary auscultation:** wheezes, rales suggestive of pulmonary edema
- **Vascular**: pistol-shot pulses, Quincke's pulses, water-hammer pulses, head-bobbing in systole, Corrigan's pulse
- **Peripheral:** edema, cyanosis, vasoconstriction

General:

- Fever, tachycardia, tachypnea, general ill-appearance (infective endocarditis)
- Elevated jugular venous pressure, hepatomegaly, ascites, edema suggestive of right heart failure
- High, arched palate; tall; long fingers; blonde/blue-eyed (Marfan's syndrome)
- Excessive joint or skin laxity (Ehlers–Danlos)
- Arthritis, psoriasis

Summary of investigative tests

- Electrocardiography (ECG): may reveal findings that are suggestive of other associated disease, but is not diagnostic in itself for aortic regurgitation
- Chest X-ray: used to gauge secondary effects of aortic regurgitation, such as congestive heart failure, rather than as a test for the primary diagnosis of aortic regurgitation. However, signs such as aortic root dilation, when present, encourage further investigation. A widened mediastinum should prompt evaluation for dissection
- Echocardiogram, transthoracic (TTE) or transesophageal (TEE): used to identify presence and severity of aortic regurgitation, as well as associated cardiac abnormalities. Done by a specialist
- Blood cultures, and complete blood count (CBC) with differential, erythrocyte sedimentation rate, in suspected cases of endocarditis
- Cardiac catheterization: may be used to assess severity of aortic regurgitation when noninvasive tests are inconclusive or discordant with clinical findings, and is ordered, performed, and interpreted by a specialist
- Radionuclide angiography: may be used to determine left ventricular volume when echocardiographic data are inconclusive or absent, and is employed in routine assessment of exercise ejection fraction; done by a specialist
- Aortogram: intravenous contrast dye is injected into the aortic arch and radiographic images are examined for presence of aortic dilation, dissection flap, false lumen, dye extravasation, and aortic regurgitation. Indicated emergently when presenting trauma suggests possibility of aortic tear and dissection, or when signs and symptoms of aortic dissection (tearing chest pain radiating to back or down the arms, dyspnea, syncope) with or without aortic regurgitation are present. Done by a specialist
- Ascending aortic computed tomography (CT) scan: uses contrast dye and requires intravenous and/or arterial access. Indicated to diagnose aortic dissection or disruption (potential causes of aortic regurgitation) and not to diagnose aortic regurgitation. It requires a specialist for procedure and interpretation, and is 83–100% sensitive for aortic dissection. However, it is not portable, is relatively expensive, and moderately invasive, and involves moderate radiation exposure
- Ascending aortic magnetic resonance imaging (MRI) scan: uses contrast dye and requires intravenous and/or arterial access. Indicated to diagnose aortic dissection or disruption (potential causes of aortic regurgitation) and not aortic regurgitation. It requires a specialist for procedure and interpretation, and is 90–100% sensitive for aortic dissection. However, it is not portable or available everywhere, can be difficult to accomplish in intubated/ventilated patients, and is relatively expensive and moderately invasive
- Exercise testing, with or without dobutamine infusion, echocardiography, or radionuclide study: used in patients with known aortic regurgitation to assess functional capacity, symptomatic response, and left ventricular function, and is usually done by a specialist
- Tissue testing/DNA testing for genetic abnormalities: indicated for work-up of genetic causes of aortic root dissection and dilation resulting in aortic regurgitation, such as Marfan's syndrome and Ehlers–Danlos syndrome. Only ordered by a specialist

DIAGNOSTIC DECISION

Based on establishing the presence and severity of aortic regurgitation, whether aortic regurgitation is acute or chronic, and the presence of underlying causes that are either treatable (e.g. endocarditis, aortic trauma or dissection) or require long-term surveillance (e.g. Marfan's syndrome).

- Presence of aortic regurgitation is suspected on physical examination and its severity established by echocardiography, using either transthoracic (TTE) or transesophageal (TEE)
- Severity of aortic regurgitation is also established by cardiac catheterization in some cases, and other tests such as chest X-ray
- Acute aortic regurgitation is determined by acute clinical presentation of patient, history of trauma, dissection, endocarditis
- Chronic aortic regurgitation is determined by clinical presentation, history, and echocardiographic findings

- Underlying causes: established by history, physical examination, laboratory work-up, echocardiography, and CT, MRI, with or without aortography

Guidelines

Guidelines are available at the National Guideline Clearinghouse:

- The American College of Cardiology and the American Heart Association. [1]
- ACC/AHA Guidelines for the clinical application of echocardiography. [2]

CLINICAL PEARL(S)

- Left ventricular function can decline even when patient is asymptomatic. This must be followed closely using echocardiography
- Angina may occur in the absence of coronary disease. Patients with new angina should have a careful examination to listen for aortic regurgitation
- As the aortic regurgitation progresses and S1 diminishes, the timing of the cardiac cycle may be difficult, resulting in the murmur being misinterpreted as systolic

THE TESTS

Body fluids

BLOOD CULTURES

Description

- Obtain three to five sets of venous blood cultures over 24h. Each set should include one aerobic and one nonaerobic culture flask
- If patient is acutely ill, four or more cultures may be taken over a 1-h period, each with a separate venipuncture
- Inform laboratory that infective endocarditis is a possible diagnosis and request incubation for 3 weeks; also notify laboratory if unusual bacteria or other pathogens are suspected

Advantages/Disadvantages

Advantages:

- Routine laboratory procedure
- Critical to diagnosis of infective endocarditis
- With exception of highly fastidious microorganisms, reveals etiologic agent in >95% of cases

Disadvantages:

- In a small number of instances, etiologic agent is culture negative
- If antibiotic treatment was started before blood was drawn, cultures are likely to yield negative results

Normal

No microorganisms in blood.

Abnormal

Presence of infectious agent(s).

Cause of abnormal result

- Patient fulfils a major diagnostic criterion for infective endocarditis when culture results are consistent with either: two separate cultures yielding microorganisms that typically cause infective endocarditis (viridans streptococci, *Streptococcus bovis*, HACEK organisms, community-acquired *Staphylococcus aureus* or enterococci), in the absence of a primary focus of infection; or microorganisms consistent with infective endocarditis are identified from persistently positive cultures – at least two positive cultures of blood drawn more than 12h

apart, or all three of three cultures, or a majority of four or more separate cultures, with first and last drawn at least 1h apart
- Patient fulfils a minor diagnostic criterion if above criteria are not met, but has one or more positive blood culture

Drugs, disorders, and other factors that may alter results
- Recent antibiotic treatment is the most common reason for culture-negative infective endocarditis. In hemodynamically stable patients with subacute presentation who have received antibiotics during the past 2 weeks, treatment should be delayed for several days so that etiologic agent can be cultured and identified
- Length of culture may be a factor in growth of fastidious organisms, such as the HACEK group. Laboratory should incubate cultures for 3 or more weeks before cultures are confirmed negative
- Pathogen may not grow in culture media: fungi, *Brucella* spp., *Legionella* spp., *Coxiella burnetii*, *Chlamydia*, and *Bartonella* spp.

Imaging

CHEST X-RAY

Advantages/Disadvantages

Advantages:
- Safe, noninvasive, relatively inexpensive, very low radiation exposure
- May demonstrate cardiomegaly, pleural effusion, Kerly B lines, indicative of possible congestive heart failure
- May demonstrate widening of the mediastinum, consistent with ascending aortic aneurysm or dissection

Disadvantages:
- Insensitive and nonspecific
- Provides supportive evidence only; nondiagnostic

Normal
- Normal cardiac silhouette
- No widening of the mediastinum
- No pleural fluid or increased pulmonary vascularity

Abnormal
- Enlarged cardiac silhouette, apex displaced downward and to the left
- Widened mediastinum
- Ascending aorta and/or aortic knob may be dilated
- Pleural fluid, Kerly B lines, increased pulmonary vascularity, and signs of pulmonary edema

Cause of abnormal result
- Enlarged cardiac silhouette may indicate cardiac dilation, pericardial fluid
- Widened mediastinum may indicate aortic dissection from trauma or hypertension, or ascending aortic aneurysm
- Pleural fluid, Kerly B lines, increased pulmonary vascularity may indicate congestive heart failure with increased pressure in the pulmonary vascular system

Drugs, disorders, and other factors that may alter results
- Any cause of apparent cardiomegaly or congestive heart failure, such as pericardial fluid, myocardial infarction, myocarditis, cardiomyopathy, and valvular dysfunction, from causes other than aortic regurgitation, can cause signs of congestive heart failure on chest X-ray
- Any cause of pulmonary edema, including congestive heart failure, arrhythmia, aspiration, and drug reaction, may cause pulmonary vascular abnormalities on chest X-ray

ECHOCARDIOGRAPHY – TRANSTHORACIC (TTE) AND TRANSESOPHAGEAL (TEE)

Description

- TTE: an ultrasound transducer applied to the chest wall is used to produce two-dimensional and Doppler images of cardiac structures
- TEE: an ultrasound transducer is introduced into the esophagus, where ultrasound imaging of the mediastinal structures occurs. Procedure requires local anesthetic application to the oropharynx, with or without sedation or general anesthesia

The American College of Cardiology Guidelines for Management of Patients with Valvular Heart Disease (http://www.guidelines.gov) recommends an echocardiogram (TTE or TEE) to:

- Confirm presence of acute aortic regurgitation
- Diagnose chronic aortic regurgitation in patients with equivocal physical findings
- Assess etiology of regurgitation (including valve morphology and aortic root size and morphology)
- Assess left ventricular hypertrophy, size, and systolic function
- Perform semiquantitative estimate of severity of aortic regurgitation
- Re-evaluate patients with mild, moderate, or severe aortic regurgitation with new or changing symptoms
- Re-evaluate left ventricular size and function in asymptomatic patients with severe aortic regurgitation
- Re-evaluate asymptomatic patients with mild, moderate, or severe aortic regurgitation and enlarged aortic root

Advantages/Disadvantages

Advantages – TTE:

- Safe, sensitive, specific, noninvasive technique
- Does not require sedation
- Portable and can be done in ICU setting
- Can evaluate presence of structural as well as functional valvular abnormalities, and may also demonstrate associated structural causes of aortic regurgitation (i.e. presence of ventricular septal defect with aortic valve prolapse, increased diameter of ascending aorta suggesting ascending aortic aneurysm or dissection)
- Pulsed and continuous-wave Doppler evaluation can evaluate regurgitant orifice size, regurgitant volume, and left ventricular ejection fraction
- Can demonstrate extent of left ventricular dysfunction

Disadvantages – TTE:

- Aortic valvular anatomy may be less well defined than on TEE
- Less sensitive and specific than TEE for aortic dissection (sensitivity and specificity for dissection 59–83% and 63–93%, respectively)
- Less sensitive and specific than TEE for valvular vegetations (sensitivity 94–100%, specificity 100%)
- Requires expert interpretation
- Somewhat operator-dependent

Advantages – TEE:

- Relatively safe procedure
- Portable and can be done in ICU setting
- Color and continuous-wave Doppler allow for functional as well as structural evaluation of the aortic valve
- Allows examination of cardiac structures for other abnormalities of structure and function that may explain or contribute to patient's clinical picture

- More sensitive and specific for diagnosis of aortic dissection than TTE (sensitivity and specificity 99% and 98%, respectively)
- More sensitive and specific for diagnosis of aortic valve vegetations than TTE (sensitivity and specificity 94% and 100%, respectively)

Disadvantages – TEE:
- More invasive than TTE, and carries risk of oropharyngeal and esophageal damage
- Requires sedation or general anesthesia in a significant proportion of patients
- Can cause sudden hypertension in patients who are not properly sedated or anesthetized; in aortic dissection or trauma patients, risk of rupture due to uncontrolled hypertension may be increased
- Less effective at determining flow velocities across the aortic valve than TTE, and may tend to underestimate flow and degree of regurgitation
- Requires a specialist

Normal
- Normal aortic valve structure
- Normal anatomy of ascending aorta
- Normal left ventricular size and function
- Normal Doppler color flow studies of aortic valve (no regurgitant jet)
- Normal continuous-wave Doppler studies of aortic valve (normal ejection peak velocity suggestive of no stenosis and normal ejection volumes)
- No septal defects

Abnormal
Abnormalities directly related to aortic valve disease include:
- Abnormal aortic valve structure (e.g. bicuspid or stenotic valve), abnormal valve leaflets (myxomatous or redundant prolapsing leaflets), abnormal systolic opening, and abnormal diastolic coaptation of valve leaflets
- Doppler studies indicating regurgitant flow in diastole across aortic valve
- Fluttering of anterior leaflet of mitral valve during diastole from regurgitant aortic flow
- Presence of vegetations on valve leaflets
- Presence of ventricular septal defect with leaflet prolapse
- Abnormal structure of left ventricular outflow tract, such as subaortic web
- Dilated or poorly contractile left ventricle, or eccentric hypertrophy suggesting chronic aortic regurgitation
- Dilated ascending aorta
- Presence of dissection flap or false lumen of ascending aorta
- Presence of cardiac structural or functional abnormalities that might cause a diastolic murmur mistaken for aortic regurgitation (e.g. pulmonic regurgitation)

Cause of abnormal result
- Ultrasound artifacts mistaken for vegetations on aortic valvular apparatus, or for dissection in ascending aorta
- Causes other than aortic regurgitation for left ventricular dilation, hypertrophy, or abnormal contractility
- Poor alignment of the TEE probe may lead to underestimation of peak velocities across the aortic valve, tending to underestimate valve flows; may underestimate regurgitation

Drugs, disorders, and other factors that may alter results
- Hypovolemia or peripheral vascular dilation ('unloading' of ventricle) may cause a reduction in apparent valvular regurgitation and underestimate the severity of dysfunction
- Hypervolemia or severe peripheral vasoconstriction ('loading' of ventricle) may cause a temporary increase in apparent valvular regurgitation, and lead to overestimate of the severity of dysfunction

CARDIAC CATHETERIZATION

Description

- Contrast dye is introduced into the coronary arteries and left ventricle via arterial catheters placed through access in a peripheral artery, such as the femoral artery or brachial artery
- Radiographic images of contrast allow structural evaluation of coronary arteries and left ventricle
- Used in evaluation of aortic regurgitation presenting with angina for evaluation of coronary anatomy that may require concomitant surgical repair

The American College of Cardiology Guidelines for Management of Patients with Valvular Heart Disease (http://www.guidelines.gov/) recommends cardiac catheterization for aortic regurgitation in the following circumstances:

- Before aortic valve replacement in patients at risk for coronary artery disease
- To assess the severity of aortic regurgitation when noninvasive tests are inconclusive or discordant, with clinical findings regarding severity of aortic regurgitation or need for surgery
- To assess left ventricular function when noninvasive tests are inconclusive or discordant with clinical findings regarding left ventricular dysfunction and need for surgery in patients with severe aortic regurgitation
- To assess left ventricular function and severity of aortic regurgitation before valve replacement when noninvasive tests are adequate and concordant with clinical findings, and coronary angiography is not needed (may be questionable)

Cardiac catheterization is not recommended to assess left ventricular function and severity of regurgitation in asymptomatic patients when noninvasive tests are adequate.

RADIONUCLIDE ANGIOGRAPHY

Description

- Intravenous injection of radionuclide is followed by nuclear imaging to detail left ventricular volume and ejection fraction. Requires specialist interpretation

The American College of Cardiology Guidelines for Management of Patients with Valvular Heart Disease (http://www.guidelines.gov/) recommends radionuclide angiography for aortic regurgitation in the following circumstances:

- Initial and serial assessment of left ventricular volume and function at rest in patients with suboptimal echocardiograms or equivocal echocardiographic data
- Serial assessment of left ventricular volume and function at rest when serial echocardiograms are not used
- Assessment of left ventricular volume and function in asymptomatic patients with moderate-to-severe aortic regurgitation when echocardiographic evidence of declining left ventricular function is suggestive, but not definitive
- Confirmation of subnormal left ventricular ejection fraction before recommending surgery in an asymptomatic patient with borderline echocardiographic evidence of left ventricular dysfunction
- Assessment of left ventricular volume and function in patients with moderate to severe aortic regurgitation when clinical assessment and echocardiographic data are discordant
- Routine assessment of exercise ejection fraction (lower recommendation)
- Quantification of aortic regurgitation in patients with unsatisfactory echocardiograms (lower recommendation)

Special tests

EXERCISE TESTING

Description

Clinical symptoms and signs, hemodynamic parameters (pulse, blood pressure), and ECG are recorded during a graded treadmill exercise to evaluate cardiac performance during exercise. It is usually done by a specialist.

The American College of Cardiology Guidelines for Management of Patients with Valvular Heart Disease (http://www.guidelines.gov/) recommends exercise testing in the following circumstances:

- Assessment of functional capacity and symptomatic responses in patients with a history of equivocal symptoms
- Evaluation of symptoms and functional capacity before participating in athletic activities
- Prognostic assessment before valve replacement in patients with left ventricular dysfunction
- Exercise echocardiography or dobutamine stress echocardiography for assessing left ventricular function in asymptomatic or symptomatic patients
- To determine the effects of aortic regurgitation on left ventricular function

Advantages/Disadvantages

Advantages:

- Relatively safe, noninvasive
- Can be combined with radionuclide study for evaluation of left ventricular function
- Can be combined with dobutamine infusion/echocardiography to evaluate left ventricular function

Disadvantages:

- Usually done by a specialist
- Moderately expensive
- Results are nonspecific to aortic regurgitation

Normal

- Normal hemodynamic response to exercise (no syncope, dyspnea)
- No symptoms of cardiac ischemia (chest pain) or arrhythmia

Abnormal

- Abnormal hemodynamic response to exercise
- Signs, symptoms, or ECG changes of myocardial ischemia
- Syncope
- Arrhythmia
- Inability to complete test due to dyspnea, exaggerated fatigue, claudication

Cause of abnormal result

- Symptoms or signs of myocardial ischemia may be due to presence of coronary disease or abnormal coronary artery hemodynamics resulting from aortic regurgitation
- Abnormal hemodynamic response to exercise may be due to aortic regurgitation, any cause of left ventricular dysfunction, or other valvular disease
- Syncope may be due to any cause of decreased cardiac output
- Arrhythmia may be secondary to effects of exercise in the presence of aortic regurgitation, or due to any cause of arrhythmia, e.g. other valvular heart disease, primary arrhythmia, electrolyte disturbances, or myocardial ischemia

Drugs, disorders, and other factors that may alter results

- Antihypertensive medication may prevent normal increases in blood pressure with exercise and mimic left ventricular dysfunction
- Beta-blockade may prevent normal increases in heart rate with exercise
- Concomitant cardiac and noncardiac disorders causing cardiac failure or ischemia may alter results

Other tests

ELECTROCARDIOGRAPHY (ECG)

Advantages/Disadvantages

Advantages:

- Safe, inexpensive, noninvasive
- Used for evaluating patients with aortic regurgitation for myocardial ischemia, arrhythmias, atrioventricular or intraventricular conduction defects

Disadvantages:

- Not in itself diagnostic of aortic regurgitation
- Nonspecific test

Abnormal

- With aortic regurgitation, ECG findings may be normal
- With severe, chronic aortic regurgitation, left ventricular hypertrophy may be present
- Severe chronic aortic regurgitation may be associated with tall R waves over the left precordium, and deep S waves over the right precordium, ST-segment depression, and T-wave inversions in leads I, aVL, V5, and V6 (left ventricular strain pattern)
- Left axis deviation
- Prolonged QRS: intraventricular conduction disturbances; ST-T abnormalities
- Arrhythmias

Cause of abnormal result

- ECG findings of left ventricular hypertrophy and strain, left axis deviation, and prolongation of QRS can result from chronic pressure/volume overload to left ventricle
- ST-T segment changes are due to ischemia or secondary to left ventricular hypertrophy
- In advanced endocarditis, perivalvular abscess may cause heart block

Drugs, disorders, and other factors that may alter results

- Antihypertensive medications, calcium channel blockers, and beta-blockers can all cause prolongation of QRS
- Left ventricular hypertrophy of another origin may show similar patterns

TREATMENT

CONSIDER CONSULT

Refer to a specialist if:

- Aortic valve replacement or repair is recommended
- Symptoms or signs of aortic regurgitation worsen in the face of vasodilator therapy
- Symptoms and signs of aortic regurgitation appear or worsen on appropriately directed antibiotic therapy for aortic valve endocarditis

IMMEDIATE ACTION

- If signs and symptoms of endocarditis are present on presentation: after obtaining appropriate cultures, institution of empiric antibiotic therapy should not await culture results
- If acute ascending aortic dissection is suspected: vasodilator therapy with nitroprusside and beta-blockade should be instituted even before imaging studies are completed. (Note: vasodilator therapy should be used only with beta-blockade; vasodilator therapy alone can increase ejection 'shear force' and worsen dissection, if not accompanied by therapy to decrease cardiac contractility)
- New onset of signs or symptoms of aortic regurgitation during medical management of descending aortic dissection: referral for immediate cardiac surgical work-up is indicated

PATIENT AND CAREGIVER ISSUES

Forensic and legal issues

If emergency/urgent diagnosis and therapy is indicated in a patient who is not competent to make medical decisions (e.g. work-up of possible aortic trauma in a patient with altered consciousness), primary care practitioner may have to initiate tests and treatment without patient's consent.

Impact on career, dependants, family, friends

- Aortic regurgitation may limit patient's ability to participate in competitive sports and some strenuous physical activities, thus potentially impacting on career choices, lifestyle, and family activities
- Need for anticoagulation after some types of aortic valve replacement therapy may also impact on safety of certain physical activities, thus impacting on career choices, lifestyle, and family activities

Patient or caregiver request

- **Do I have to give up competitive sports?** Possibly. Depending on the severity of aortic regurgitation, some physical activities may negatively impact on natural course of disease. In the case of anticoagulation following some types of aortic valve surgery, some curtailment of physical activities may be necessary
- **Should I take antibiotics for dental work or other medical procedures?** Yes. Whether or not you have undergone aortic valve replacement, aortic valve regurgitation predisposes you to a serious cardiac infection, called 'endocarditis', if your bloodstream is exposed to bacteria during dental and some surgical procedures. You should consult your physician and dentist for specific recommendations
- **I took fen-phen for 1 month several years ago. Am I at risk for aortic regurgitation? If I have an abnormal heart valve, will it ever get better?** Even 1 month of therapy exposes you to risk for aortic regurgitation. In one series, 30% of patients who took fen-phen developed aortic regurgitation. Several patients have been discovered to have aortic regurgitation after taking fen-phen for only 23–30 days. Aortic regurgitation may regress when you have been off fen-phen for at least 1 year, but it is unknown whether this occurs with everyone, or even in the majority of patients
- **What is my likelihood of having aortic or aortic valve problems if one of my parents has Marfan's disease?** Marfan's syndrome is an autosomal-dominant disorder, i.e. you have a 50:50 chance of inheriting the disorder from your parent. In those who have Marfan's

disease, aortic and aortic valvular disease is common, so you should consult a physician about cardiac screening if you suspect you have Marfan's syndrome, or if you know of a relative who has been diagnosed with Marfan's syndrome. Up to 30% of Marfan's syndrome cases arise spontaneously, i.e. you do not have to have a parent with the disease to get it

MANAGEMENT ISSUES

Goals

Acute aortic regurgitation:

- To institute prompt treatment for acute, severe aortic regurgitation, which is usually a surgical emergency
- To consider aortic valve replacement in patients with acute aortic insufficiency who have evidence of even mild congestive cardiac failure or mitral valve preclosure
- To direct medical management at temporizing cardiovascular condition (e.g. treatment of congestive heart failure and pulmonary edema, institution of afterload reduction, and then immediate referral for surgical consultation and intervention)

Chronic aortic regurgitation – as symptoms may be absent until left ventricular dysfunction is advanced, chronic aortic regurgitation should be corrected when more than mild symptoms are present and probably before onset of permanent left ventricular damage, even in asymptomatic patients:

- To optimize cardiovascular condition
- To institute appropriate treatment of medical causes if surgery is not indicated or contraindicated (e.g. treatment of hypertension, endocarditis)
- To monitor for appropriate timing of surgical intervention
- To institute prophylaxis for bacterial endocarditis

Management in special circumstances

Acute aortic regurgitation is an indication for emergency work-up and therapy for underlying cause. Left ventricular volume and pressure overload occurs suddenly, without time for ventricular compensation. Acute pulmonary congestion and a precipitous fall in cardiac output may result unless prompt treatment is instituted. Emergency surgery for valve replacement is often indicated.

COEXISTING DISEASE

Infectious disease:

- Those that cause aortic regurgitation require appropriately directed antimicrobial therapy. Includes: endocarditis, bacterial or fungal; syphilis, long-term prophylaxis in patients with rheumatic fever

Hypertension:

- Strict control to prevent progression of aortic regurgitation, and in medical management of aortic dissection

COEXISTING MEDICATION

Medications that increase afterload to left ventricle have a deleterious effect on aortic regurgitation:

- Sympathomimetics present in many cough and cold remedies
- Appetite-suppressant medication
- Drugs used to treat attention-deficit disorders, such as methylphenidate, amphetamine
- Some over-the-counter herbal medications may have sympathomimetic effects, such as ephedrine, ephedra, ma huong, and others: pharmacology of herbal medications (http://www.fpnotebook.com/PHACh2.htm)

SPECIAL PATIENT GROUPS

Pregnancy:

- No large series of patients with aortic regurgitation and pregnancy have been studied
- Pregnant women with aortic stenosis may also have aortic regurgitation: in one series of pregnant women with aortic stenosis, 54% had aortic regurgitation, and all did well during pregnancy
- Pregnant women with Marfan's syndrome are at risk for aortic dissection, and aortic regurgitation with aortic dilation, although only a handful of cases has been described in the literature

Terminal illness:

- Medical management for aortic regurgitation is more likely to be chosen than surgical intervention in the terminally ill, due to mitigation of the primary benefit of surgical over medical management (i.e. long-term survival)

PATIENT SATISFACTION/LIFESTYLE PRIORITIES

Choice of specific medical or surgical management can have significant effects on patient lifestyle; e.g. young patients who face potentially prolonged anticoagulation, or patients with particularly active lifestyles or athletic careers may opt for a surgical procedure (Ross procedure) that is less likely to require postoperative anticoagulation.

SUMMARY OF THERAPEUTIC OPTIONS

Choices

Medical management:

- Acute therapy to correct congestive heart failure and initiate afterload reduction: angiotensin-converting enzyme (ACE) inhibitors (e.g. enalapril), calcium channel blockers (e.g. nifedipine), nitroprusside (for urgent afterload reduction in acute aortic regurgitation)
- Long-term vasodilator therapy for chronic aortic regurgitation: hydralazine, nifedipine, enalapril
- Antimicrobial prophylaxis for surgical and dental procedures

Surgical therapy:

- Aortic valve replacement or repair of aortic dissection is employed in patients with acute aortic regurgitation due to endocarditis, trauma, or dissection
- May also be used in patients with chronic severe aortic regurgitation

Lifestyle issues:

- Dietary sodium restriction may help to preserve left ventricular systolic function and heart failure in patients who have hemodynamic compromise from aortic regurgitation

Guidelines

- The American College of Cardiology and the American Heart Association have produced guidelines providing recommendations for vasodilator therapy and aortic valve replacement in patients with chronic aortic regurgitation. [1]
- The American Academy of Family Physicians has produced the following: Cheitlin MD. Surgery for chronic aortic regurgitation: when should it be considered? [3]

Clinical pearl(s)

- Avoid placement of central venous lines in the neck or subclavian regions. The excessive arterial pulsations seen with aortic regurgitation often lead to inadvertent arterial stick with possible uncontrollable bleeding

- Atrial arrhythmias are poorly tolerated in patients with aortic regurgitation. If they occur, urgent restoration of sinus rhythm is indicated, usually in concert with a cardiac specialist

Never

Never institute vasodilator (nitroprusside) therapy for acute aortic dissection without accompanying beta-blockade. Vasodilation alone can increase 'shear' force on the aorta and worsen dissection, if a concomitant beta-blocker is not also administered.

FOLLOW UP

- Degree of aortic regurgitation and ventricular response should be established on initial work-up
- If chronic nature of lesion is uncertain and patient does not present with indications for surgery, a follow-up, physical examination, and echocardiogram is recommended by the American College of Cardiology 2–3 months after initial evaluation
- Thereafter, frequency of clinical re-evaluation depends on severity of aortic regurgitation, degree of left ventricular dilation, level of systolic left ventricular function, and whether previous studies have demonstrated progressive changes in left ventricular size and function
- Follow up evaluations should in general include history, physical examination, and echocardiography. Serial chest X-ray and ECG may be helpful in selected patients
- Asymptomatic patients with mild aortic regurgitation, little or no left ventricular dilation, and normal left ventricular systolic function: follow up with history and physical examination annually, and echocardiography every 2–3 years
- Asymptomatic patients with normal systolic function but severe aortic regurgitation and significant left ventricular dilation (left ventricular end-diastolic dimension >60mm): repeat history and physical examination every 6 months, and echocardiogram every 6–12 months. In cases with advanced dilation (left ventricular end-diastolic dimension >70mm, left ventricular end-systolic dimension >50mm), echocardiogram every 4–6 months
- Serial echocardiograms are recommended in patients with aortic root dilation
- Repeat echocardiograms are indicated for onset of symptoms or clinical findings suggesting worsening aortic regurgitation or progressive left ventricular dilation

Information for patient or caregiver

Advise of importance of follow up at recommended intervals, and need to report worsening symptoms or decreased exercise tolerance to their physician immediately. Up to 20% of asymptomatic patients with aortic regurgitation who have echocardiographic evidence of left ventricular dilation will become symptomatic or develop left ventricular dysfunction each year. Prompt surgical intervention may be indicated to prevent deterioration in left ventricular function.

DRUGS AND OTHER THERAPIES: DETAILS

Drugs

HYDRALAZINE

Preferentially dilates arterioles, and decreases afterload by decreasing systemic vascular resistance.

Dose

- Oral dose: 10mg four times daily; increase by 10–25mg/dose every 2–5 days as needed to a maximum of 300mg/day
- Intramuscular/intravenous dose: 10–20mg every 4–6h; may increase to 40mg/dose

Efficacy

- Reduces left ventricular end-diastolic volume and left ventricular end-systolic volume
- Increases ejection fraction in aortic insufficiency

Risks/Benefits

Risks:

- Use caution in renal disease or 'slow acetylation' phenotype
- Use caution in systemic lupus erythematosus (patients should be instructed to report adverse symptoms of joint pain, angina, fever, or continued weakness to their physician)
- Use caution in pregnancy (however, it is widely used in pre-eclampsia), children, and elderly patients

Benefit: reduces afterload by reducing systemic vascular resistance, reducing regurgitant aortic flow, and increasing forward cardiac output.

Side-effects and adverse reactions

- Cardiovascular: angina, palpitations, sinus tachycardia, orthostatic hypotension, sodium and water retention, edema
- Genitourinary: glomerulonephritis
- CNS: headache, dizziness, peripheral neuritis, paresthesias
- Gastrointestinal: nausea, vomiting, diarrhea, anorexia, constipation, weight gain
- Hematologic: blood dyscrasias
- Skin: lupus-like symptoms, rash

Interactions (other drugs)

▪ Antihypertensive agents ▪ Estrogens ▪ Monoamine oxidase inhibitors ▪ NSAIDs ▪ Sympathomimetics

Contraindications

▪ Coronary artery disease ▪ Mitral valvular rheumatic heart disease ▪ Pregnancy category C ▪ Breast-feeding ▪ Safety and efficacy in pediatric patients have not been established in controlled clinical trials; however, there is experience with the use of hydralazine hydrochloride in these patients

Evidence

One RCT compared hydralazine with placebo in minimally symptomatic patients with moderate-to-severe aortic regurgitation. Hydralazine-treated patients demonstrated a significant reduction in left ventricular end-diastolic volume index. There was also a significant reduction in left ventricular end-systolic volume index, and a significant increase in ejection fraction compared with placebo [4] *Level P*

Acceptability to patient

Many patients do not tolerate long-term therapy with this drug because of its significant side-effects.

Follow up plan

Follow up with echocardiographic studies if patient's symptoms worsen, or according to the American College of Cardiology's Guidelines for Management of Patients with Valvular Heart Disease.

Patient and caregiver information

Withdrawal of medication without substitution of other vasodilator therapy may cause worsening of cardiac condition.

ENALAPRIL

Competitive inhibitor of angiotensin-converting enzyme (ACE).

Dose

- Oral dose: 2.5–5mg once daily; increase as needed. Usual dosing range 10–40mg/day in once daily or divided doses twice daily
- Intravenous dose: 0.625–1.25mg given over 5min, every 6h

Efficacy

- Reduces left ventricular end-diastolic and end-systolic volume indexes, and increases exercise duration (mild)
- In one series, enalapril achieved significant left ventricular mass regression

Risks/Benefits

Risks: use caution in renal impairment, hypotension, aortic stenosis, hyperkalemia, and neutropenia.

Benefits:

- Decreases plasma concentration of angiotensin II and aldosterone
- Decreases systemic vascular resistance, preload and afterload, without significant changes in heart rate

Side-effects and adverse reactions

- Gastrointestinal: nausea, vomiting, diarrhea, constipation, abdominal pain
- Cardiovascular: orthostatic hypotension and syncope, angina, palpitations, sinus tachycardia
- Hematologic: neutropenia, agranulocytosis, aplastic and hemolytic anemia, pancytopenia, thrombocytopenia
- CNS: headache, dizziness, fatigue
- Genitourinary: renal damage, impotence
- Metabolic: hyperkalemia, hyponatremia
- Respiratory: cough
- Skin: angioedema, maculopapular rash

Interactions (other drugs)

- Allopurinol
- Antihypertensives (loop and potassium sparing diuretics, prazosin, terazosin, doxazosin)
- Azathioprine
- Heparin
- Insulin
- Iron
- Lithium
- NSAIDs
- Potassium
- Sodium
- Trimethoprim

Contraindications

- Pregnancy
- Angioedema
- Renal artery stenosis
- Hypotension
- Children

Evidence

An RCT compared enalapril with hydralazine in patients with chronic, asymptomatic, nonrheumatic aortic regurgitation. After 1 year of treatment, patients receiving enalapril had significantly reduced left ventricular end-diastolic and end-systolic volume indices, and reduced mass index compared with hydralazine. Both medications reduced left ventricular mean wall stress [5] *Level P*

Acceptability to patient

Occasionally patients experience a dry cough (1.3–2.2%).

NIFEDIPINE

Calcium-channel blocking agent.

Dose

- Oral dose: 10mg three times per day initially; usual range 10–20mg three times per day. Doses >120mg/day rarely needed
- For XL form: 30–60mg daily; titrating to doses >120mg/day not recommended

Efficacy

Improves hemodynamics and reduces need for valve replacement.

Risks/Benefits

Risks:

- Nifedipine should be used during pregnancy only if the potential benefit justifies the potential risk to the fetus
- Use caution when administering to patients with congestive heart failure, hypotension, aortic stenosis, hepatic and renal disease
- Use caution when administering to the elderly and in recent beta-blocker withdrawal

Benefits:

- Produces relaxation of coronary and peripheral vascular smooth muscle
- Decreases peripheral vascular resistance, increases cardiac output
- Effective antianginal and antihypertensive medication

Side-effects and adverse reactions

- Cardiovascular: bradycardia, peripheral edema, palpitations
- CNS: dizziness, headache, paresthesias
- Gastrointestinal: constipation, nausea, dry mouth, dyspepsia
- Genitourinary: nocturia, polyuria, sexual dysfunction
- Respiratory: cough, dyspnea
- Skin: alopecia, pruritus, rash

Interactions (other drugs)

- Anticoagulants
- Barbiturates
- Beta-blockers
- Cimetidine, ranitidine
- Carbamazepine
- Cardiac glycosides
- Diltiazem
- Doxazosin
- Fentanyl
- Grapefruit juice
- H_2 antagonists
- Insulin
- Lansoprazole
- Magnesium
- Phenytoin
- Quinidine
- Theophylline
- Vincristine

Contraindications

- Severe coronary artery disease
- Recent myocardial infarction
- Hypertensive emergencies
- Pregnancy category C
- Safety and efficacy in pediatric patients have not been established

Evidence

- An RCT compared nifedipine with digoxin in patients with severe aortic regurgitation and normal left ventricular systolic function. Patients treated with nifedipine had reduced rates of aortic valve replacement at 6 years (15% vs 34% with digoxin) [6] *Level P*
- Another RCT compared nifedipine with placebo in patients with asymptomatic, severe aortic regurgitation. After one year, patients treated with nifedipine had a significantly reduced left ventricular end-diastolic volume index and mass, reduced left ventricular mean wall stress, and an increased ejection fraction [7] *Level P*

Acceptability to patient

XL form allows once-a-day dosing regimen, which may be more acceptable to patients.

Follow up plan

Follow up should be according to American College of Cardiology's Guidelines for management of patients with valvular heart disease.

NITROPRUSSIDE

- Relaxes peripheral vascular smooth muscle – veins somewhat more than arteries
- Useful for acutely lowering afterload in cases of acute aortic regurgitation
- Mainstay of therapy for hypertensive crisis and, in combination with beta-blockade, for emergency treatment of aortic dissection
- Should be used only in ICU setting

Dose

- Intravenously: 0.25–1mcg/kg per min initially, titrate to 10mcg/kg per min if needed
- Infusions >10mcg/kg per min can rapidly be associated with cyanide toxicity

Efficacy

Acutely reduces afterload and systemic vascular resistance, and increases forward cardiac output.

Risks/Benefits

Risks:

- Potential cyanide toxicity with continued administration
- Use caution in hepatic disease, hypothyroidism, hyponatremia

Benefit: Reduces systemic vascular resistance, systolic arterial pressure, and mean arterial pressure.

Side-effects and adverse reactions

- Cardiovascular: hypotension, palpitations, tachycardia, bradycardia
- CNS: dizziness, headache
- Hematologic: methemoglobinemia
- Gastrointestinal: nausea
- Other: cyanide toxicity

Interactions (other drugs)

- Clonidine ■ Diltiazem ■ Guanabenz ■ Guanfacine

Contraindications

- Compensatory hypertension (e.g. in coarctation of the aorta, arteriovenous shunt)
- Reduced cerebral perfusion ■ Leber's (optic) atrophy

Acceptability to patient

Requires intravenous access and invasive arterial blood pressure monitoring.

Follow up plan

Therapy is used only in ICU setting with continuous monitoring.

Patient and caregiver information

Patient must be informed that therapy for more than 1 day, at high dosage, or in patients with renal failure, may cause tinnitus, delirium, or blurred vision (thiocyanate accumulation).

Surgical therapy

AORTIC VALVE REPLACEMENT OR REPAIR

- In acute aortic regurgitation, while medical therapy may by instituted to temporize, surgical intervention with valve replacement and/or ascending aortic surgery is the definitive therapy
- In chronic aortic insufficiency, the vast majority of patients with significant hemodynamic regurgitation will require surgical intervention, and timing of surgical therapy is key
- The American College of Cardiology/American Heart Association guidelines (Management of patients with valvular heart disease. J Am Coll Cardiol 1998;32:1486–588. Available at the National Guideline Clearinghouse) recommend aortic valve replacement in selected patients with chronic severe aortic regurgitation. Patients with mild aortic regurgitation are not candidates for aortic valve replacement. Symptoms in such patients should stimulate a search for other causes such as coronary artery disease, hypertension, or cardiomyopathy

Surgical treatment options:

- Aortic valve replacement with mechanical valve – requires coagulation, may last longer; bioprosthetic homograft – higher incidence of structural failures, may not require coagulation; or autograft (Ross procedure) – patient's native pulmonic valve is transplanted to the aortic position, and a bioprosthetic valve is inserted in the pulmonic position
- Although uncommon, occasionally aortic valve repair is undertaken. This will often not require long-term anticoagulation therapy postoperatively
- Ascending aortic graft with or without valve repair in cases of ascending aortic aneurysm or dissection

Efficacy

- Operative mortality for aortic valve replacement is 3–5%. Historic data from the presurgical era indicate that symptomatic patients have a poor outcome with medical therapy: mortality rate >10% per year in patients with aortic regurgitation and angina, and >20% per year in patients with congestive heart failure
- Left ventricular dysfunction after aortic valve replacement may not return to normal; hence the importance of timing surgery in asymptomatic patients with aortic regurgitation before the onset of significant left ventricular dysfunction

Risks/Benefits

Benefits:

- Decreased long-term mortality
- Prevents progression of left ventricular dysfunction if timed early in course of disease

Acceptability to patient

- Patients may better accept surgical intervention than chronic medical therapy, particularly if left ventricular dysfunction is affecting symptoms and activity level
- Morbidity and mortality of surgery, period of postoperative recovery, and need for anticoagulation after surgery may all negatively impact on acceptability of aortic valve replacement

Follow up plan

After aortic valve replacement, early and long-term postoperative follow up is needed to assess prosthetic valve function and left ventricular function:

- After surgery, baseline echocardiogram
- If patient has persistent left ventricular dilation on initial postoperative echocardiogram, treat the same as patients with symptomatic or asymptomatic left ventricular dysfunction, including use of ACE inhibitors

Patient and caregiver information

Stress the importance of surgical follow up and rigorous adherence to medication regimens for anticoagulation and afterload reduction (where needed) to prevent thrombotic complications of surgery, and to preserve left ventricular systolic function.

LIFESTYLE

Low sodium diet.

RISKS/BENEFITS

May help preserve left ventricular systolic function and prevent heart failure in patients who have hemodynamic compromise from aortic regurgitation.

ACCEPTABILITY TO PATIENT

Some patients have difficulty adhering to sodium restriction.

OUTCOMES

EFFICACY OF THERAPIES

- Morbidity and mortality of patients with chronic aortic regurgitation and left ventricular systolic dysfunction is high, even in asymptomatic patients, whereas patients with mild-to-moderate aortic regurgitation and preserved left ventricular function may be able to postpone or avoid valve replacement surgery
- In patients with mild-to-moderate aortic regurgitation and preserved left ventricular function, chronic vasodilator therapy with ACE inhibitors or nifedipine can reduce need for aortic valve replacement
- In patients with severe aortic regurgitation, or aortic regurgitation with left ventricular systolic dysfunction, early valve replacement decreases overall mortality, and improves quality of life
- In patients with acute aortic regurgitation due to aortic aneurysm, dissection, or trauma, medical therapy is used only to temporize for definitive surgical therapy. Short-term mortality for ascending aortic dissection approaches 100%, whereas operative mortality rate is about 45%

Evidence

- Hydralazine has been shown significantly to reduce left ventricular end-diastolic and end-systolic volume index, and significantly increase ejection fraction compared with placebo in minimally symptomatic patients with moderate-to-severe aortic regurgitation [4] *Level P*
- Enalapril has been shown significantly to reduce left ventricular end-diastolic and end-systolic volume indices, and mass index compared with hydralazine in patients with chronic asymptomatic aortic regurgitation. Both medications reduced left ventricular mean wall stress in this RCT [5] *Level P*
- Nifedipine significantly reduced left ventricular end-diastolic volume index and mass, reduced left ventricular mean wall stress, and increased ejection fraction compared with placebo in patients with asymptomatic, severe aortic regurgitation [7] *Level P*
- There are no randomized, controlled studies comparing aortic valve replacement with medical therapy in patients with severe aortic regurgitation, because of ethical considerations

PROGNOSIS

Acute aortic regurgitation is usually an indication for surgery and valve replacement. Operative mortality rate is 3–5%.

Chronic aortic regurgitation, asymptomatic:

- 4.3% per year will develop symptoms of left ventricular dysfunction
- 0.2% per year overall mortality rate
- 1.3% per year will develop asymptomatic left ventricular dysfunction
- Vast majority are symptomatic within 2–3 years
- Average rate of symptom onset is >25% per year

Chronic aortic regurgitation, symptomatic:

- Mortality rate is >10% per year in medically treated patients
- Mortality rate is 20% per year in patients presenting with congestive heart failure

Clinical pearl(s)

- Outcome after aortic valve replacement depends on presence, severity, and duration of ventricular systolic dysfunction. Best results are seen if dysfunction was short-lived
- Even if ventricular function does not improve after valve replacement, symptomatic relief is often achieved

Therapeutic failure

- Patients who fail on medical therapy should be referred for surgical intervention
- Persistent left ventricular dysfunction (not unexpected) after aortic valve replacement should be managed medically with chronic vasodilator therapy, as per the American College of Cardiology guidelines. Referral for initial management is indicated

Recurrence

Patients with valvular leak, or failure of prosthesis, should be referred to a specialist.

Deterioration

Deterioration of patient being medically followed for aortic regurgitation with or without chronic vasodilator therapy, as evidenced by new onset of symptoms, worsening of existing symptoms or exercise capacity, or deteriorating left ventricular performance by imaging tests, should be referred for possible surgical intervention.

Terminal illness

Therapy in the terminally ill patient with aortic regurgitation is directed toward medical options (vasodilator therapy) to improve left ventricular performance, and to minimize symptoms.

COMPLICATIONS

- The natural history observed in patients with chronic severe aortic regurgitation who are managed conservatively includes congestive heart failure, thromboembolism, and aortic dissection
- Other complications include side-effects of vasodilator medications, bleeding complications in patients who are anticoagulated after surgery, morbidity and mortality of surgical valve replacement, and prosthetic valve failure

CONSIDER CONSULT

Referral to a specialist if:

- New onset of symptoms, including decline in normal exercise tolerance, develops in an asymptomatic patient being followed for aortic regurgitation
- Symptoms develop or worsen in a symptomatic patient being medically managed
- Imaging studies indicate worsening left ventricular performance on medical therapy

PREVENTION

RISK FACTORS

- **Use of diet pills:** fen-phen has been associated with new-onset aortic regurgitation
- **Hypertension**: associated with aortic aneurysm and dissection, especially in collagen-vascular disorders
- **Smoking** is a risk factor for hypertension and coronary heart disease, which worsens the long-term prognosis in patients with aortic regurgitation
- **Bacteremia from surgical/dental procedures**: increases risk of endocarditis in patients with underlying abnormal valve anatomy
- **Intravenous drug abuse:** increases likelihood of bacteremia/endocarditis from contaminated needles
- **Behavior predisposing to sexually transmitted disease**: syphilis is a known cause of aortitis, aortic aneurysm, and aortic regurgitation
- **Streptococcal infections**: rheumatic valvular heart disease remains a prominent cause of aortic regurgitation
- **Family predisposition** (e.g. Marfan's syndrome, Ehlers–Danlos syndrome) to aortic disease, ascending aortic aneurysm, and aortic regurgitation

MODIFY RISK FACTORS

Lifestyle and wellness

TOBACCO

Cessation of smoking, especially by patients prone to hypertensive aortic disease and aortic regurgitation, may decrease risk.

ALCOHOL AND DRUGS

Cessation of intravenous drug use may decrease risk, especially in patients who have underlying abnormalities of aortic valve anatomy, such as bicuspid aortic valve.

DIET

A low-sodium diet may reduce risk of hypertension.

SEXUAL BEHAVIOR

Reducing risky sexual behaviors can reduce risk of contracting syphilis. Measures primarily include use of barrier protection during intercourse to decrease risks of sexually transmitted disease.

FAMILY HISTORY

Patients with known familial history of Marfan's syndrome, Ehlers–Danlos syndrome, and other disorders known to be associated with aortic regurgitation should receive regular physician evaluation for the presence of aortic regurgitant murmur. Institution of antihypertensive therapy or vasodilator therapy can retard progression of aortic disease when present.

DRUG HISTORY

Discontinue anorexic medications shown to be associated with new onset of aortic regurgitation: up to 30% of patients who took the diet pills fen-phen later developed aortic regurgitation; some patients developed valvular heart disease after only 23 days of therapy. An initial echocardiogram is recommended in anyone with a history of fen-phen use, for the purpose of evaluating potential asymptomatic valvular heart disease and for determining need for antibiotic prophylaxis for dental work. (http://www.fda.gov/cder/news/phen/fenphenqa2.htm)

CHEMOPROPHYLAXIS

- For patients with known anatomic abnormalities of the aortic valve, antimicrobial prophylaxis is indicated for certain surgical and dental procedures to prevent valvular endocarditis and subsequent aortic regurgitation
- Appropriate screening and antimicrobial therapy for suspected streptococcal pharyngitis reduces incidence of rheumatic valvular heart disease

Cost/efficacy

Antimicrobial prophylaxis and treatment of streptococcal pharyngitis is inexpensive and widely available. A reduced incidence of rheumatic valvular disease in developed nations is largely due to antimicrobial therapy.

SCREENING

Patients with known Marfan's syndrome should be followed regularly with chest X-ray and echocardiography studies to detect early onset of aneurysmal dilation of the ascending aorta; this potentially may allow for life-saving early intervention.

CHEST X-RAY

May detect asymptomatic mediastinal enlargement before onset of symptoms.

Cost/efficacy

- Relatively inexpensive, noninvasive, low radiation exposure
- Relatively insensitive and nonspecific test: further testing needed if results are suggestive

ECHOCARDIOGRAPHY

- Can detect and quantify aortic root dilation and aortic valvular incompetence prior to onset of symptoms
- Screening of first-degree relatives of patients with Marfan's syndrome is recommended by the American College of Cardiology/American Heart Association

Guidelines

ACC/AHA Guidelines for the clinical application of echocardiography. A report of the American College of Cardiology/American Heart Association Task Force on Practice Guidelines (Committee on Clinical Application of Echocardiography). [2]

Cost/efficacy

- Moderately expensive, noninvasive
- Test is both sensitive and specific

RESOURCES

ASSOCIATIONS

American College of Physicians
ACP-ASIM Headquarters
190 N Independence Mall W
Philadelphia, PA 19106-1572
Tel: (800) 338-2746 / (202) 261-4500 / (215) 351-2600
http://www.acponline.org/

American Heart Association
National Center
7272 Greenville Ave
Dallas, TX 75231
Tel: (800) 242-8721
http://www.americanheart.org/presenter.jhtml?identifier=1200000

American College of Chest Physician
3300 Dundee Rd
Northbrook, IL 60062-2348
Tel: (847) 498-1400
http://www.chestnet.org/

American College of Cardiology
Heart House
9111 Georgetown Rd
Bethesda, MD 20814-1699
Tel: (800) 253-4636
http://www.acc.org

KEY REFERENCES

- Bolger A. Aortic dissection. In: Otto C, ed. The practice of clinical echocardiograpy. Philadelphia: WB Saunders, 1997, p547–63
- Bonow RO, Carabello B, de Leon AC Jr, et al. Management of patients with valvular heart disease. J Am Coll Cardiol 1998;32(5):1486–588
- Cheitin M. Finding 'just the right moment' for operative intervention in the asymptomatic patient with moderate to severe aortic regurgitation. Circulation 1998;97(6):518–20
- Cheitin M, Alpert JS, Armstrong WF, et al. ACC/AHA guidelines for the clinical application of echocardiography. Circulation 1997;95(6):1686–744
- Connally HM, Crary JL, McGoon MD, et al. Valvular heart disease associated with fenfluramine–phenteramine. N Engl J Med 1997;337(9):581–8
- Curfman GD. Diet pills Redux. N Engl J Med 1997;337(9):629–30
- Devereaux RB. Appetite suppressants and valvular heart disease. N Engl J Med 1998;339:756–66
- Dujardin KS, Enriquez-Sarano M, Schaff HV, et al. Mortality and morbidity of aortic regurgitation in clinical practice: a long-term follow-up study. Circulation 1999;99(14):1851–7
- Elkayam U, Ostrzega E, Shotan A, Mehra A. Cardiovascular problems in pregnant women with the Marfan syndrome. Ann Intern Med 1995;123(2):117–22
- Kvidal P, Bergstrom R, Horte LG, Stahle E. Observed and relative survival after aortic valve replacement. J Am Coll Cardiol 2000;35(3):747–56
- Lebowitz NE, Bella JN, Roman MJ, et al. Prevalence and correlates of aortic regurgitation in American Indians: the Strong Heart Study. J Am Coll Cardiol 2000;36(2):461–7
- O'Gara PT. Acute aortic dissection. Curr Treat Options Cardiovasc Med 1999;1(1):11–8
- Pretre R, Von Segesser LK. Aortic dissection. Lancet 1997;349(9063):1461–4
- Schiller NB. Clinical decision making in patients with endocarditis. In: Otto C, ed. The practice of clinical

echocardiography. Philadelphia: WB Saunders, 1997, p389–403

- Singh JP, Evans JC, Levy D, et al. Prevalence and clinical determinants of mitral, tricuspid, and aortic regurgitation (the Framingham Heart Study). Am J Cardiol 1999;84(9):1143
- Thomson JD, Gibbs AJ. Left sided valvular regurgitation in normal children and adolescents. Heart 2000;3(2):185–7
- Tronos M, Olona M, Permanyer-Miralda G, et al. Heart failure after aortic vavle replacement for aortic regurgitation: prospective 20-year study. Am Heart J 1998;36(4) (part 1):681–7
- Weissman NJ, Panza JA, Tighe JF, Gwynne JT. Natural history of valvular regurgitation 1 year after discontinuation of dexfenfluramine therapy. A randomized double-blind placebo controlled trial. Ann Intern Med 2001;34(4):267–73
- FDA site discussing fen-phen. Available online: http://www.fda.gov/cder/news/phen/fenphenqa2.htm
- Family Practice Notebook, web page on alternative pharmacology. Available online: http://www.fpnotebook.com/PHACh2.htm

Evidence references and guidelines

1 The American College of Cardiology and the American Heart Association. Management of patients with valvular heart disease. J Am Coll Cardiol 1998;32:1486–588. Available at the National Guideline Clearinghouse

2 Cheitin M, Alpert JS, Armstrong WF, et al. ACC/AHA guidelines for the clinical application of echocardiography. Circulation 1997;95(6):1686–744

3 The American Academy of Family Physicians has produced the following: Cheitlin MD. Surgery for chronic aortic regurgitation: when should it be considered? Am Fam Physician 2001;64:1709–14

4 Greenberg B, Massie B, Bristow JD, et al. Long-term vasodilator therapy of chronic aortic insufficiency. A randomized double-blinded, placebo-controlled clinical trial. Circulation 1988;78:92–103. Medline

5 Lin M, Chiang HT, Lin SL, et al. Vasodilator therapy in chronic asymptomatic aortic regurgitation: enalapril versus hydralazine therapy. J Am Coll Cardiol 1994;24:1046–53. Medline

6 Scognamiglio R, Rahimtoola SH, Fasoli G, et al. Nifedipine in asymptomatic patients with severe aortic regurgitation and normal left ventricular function. N Engl J Med 1994;331:689–94. Medline

7 Scognamiglio R, Fasoli G, Ponchia A, Dalla-Volta S. Long-term nifedipine unloading therapy in asymptomatic patients with chronic severe aortic regurgitation. J Am Coll Cardiol 1990;16:424–9. Medline

FAQS

Question 1

What should be my first step if I think I hear a diastolic murmur consistent with aortic regurgitation?

ANSWER 1

Diagnosis should be confirmed by echocardiography. This will also give information about ventricular function and size.

Question 2

How should I follow a patient with asymptomatic, but echo-proven, moderate-to-severe aortic regurgitation?

ANSWER 2

Echocardiography and physical examination should be repeated every 6 months. In very stable patients with little ventricular dilation, echocardiogram can be obtained every 12 months.

Question 3

My patient has aortic regurgitation, but is asymptomatic. What activity can they do?

ANSWER 3

These patients may participate in any normal daily activity. They may engage in mild forms of exercise, but should avoid isometric exercise (e.g. weight lifting). Competitive sports should not be undertaken unless approved by a specialist.

Question 4

When is a stress test indicated to evaluate patients with aortic regurgitation?

ANSWER 4

Exercise testing is rarely needed in patients with aortic regurgitation. Response to exercise may assist in decision-making about valve replacement in patients with normal global ventricular function but severe ventricular dilation. If pulmonary artery pressures rises, exercise tolerance is impaired, or ejection fraction falls with exertion, surgery is indicated.

Question 5

Which is the drug of first choice in treating a patient with severe chronic aortic regurgitation who has no symptoms?

ANSWER 5

Based on current evidence, nifedipine offers good long-term results and does not appear to mask the progression of disease. Patients treated with nifedipine who later have valve replacement have done very well.

CONTRIBUTORS

Russell C Jones, MD, MPH
John McB Hodgson, MD, FACC, FSCAI
Raul J Frances, MD, PhD

AORTIC VALVULAR STENOSIS

SUMMARY INFORMATION

DESCRIPTION

- Aortic valvular stenosis, the most common valvular heart disease, is characterized by a narrowing at the aortic valve
- It produces a significant obstruction to left ventricular outflow and compensatory concentric left ventricular hypertrophy
- It may be congenital in origin, secondary to rheumatic inflammation of the aortic valve, or due to degenerative calcification of the aortic cusps
- It is most commonly caused by progressive valvular calcification superimposed on a congenitally bicuspid valve or, in the elderly, on a previously normal valve
- The characteristic features of aortic valvular stenosis are exertional dyspnea, angina pectoris, syncope, and heart failure
- Patients with aortic valvular stenosis may be asymptomatic until the fifth to seventh decades. Once symptoms occur, the prognosis is poor if the obstruction is left untreated (3-year mortality rate 50%)

URGENT ACTION

It is critical to avoid administering vasodilators or diuretics to any patient with suspected critical aortic stenosis as these agents can precipitate hemodynamic collapse. If the patient presents with heart failure symptoms that require therapy, hospitalization is advisable until the severity of the valvular disease has been determined.

KEY! DON'T MISS!

- A left ventricular strain pattern (depression of the ST segment with inverted T waves) may be present in leads I, aVL, and the left precordial leads. This is consistent with severe aortic valvular stenosis and an enhanced probability of sudden death
- The harsh murmur of senile aortic sclerosis may be difficult to distinguish from that of aortic stenosis; however, it is typically harsh and mid-peaking, does not radiate to the carotids, and carotid upstrokes are brisk and early

ICD9 CODE

424.1 Aortic valve disorders.

SYNONYMS

Aortic stenosis.

CARDINAL FEATURES

- Critical aortic valvular stenosis is defined when the aortic valve area is less than $0.8cm^2$ (normal values are between 3.5 and $4.0cm^2$). At this point, the systolic gradient between the left ventricle and the aorta can exceed 150mmHg and most patients are symptomatic
- A characteristic harsh systolic murmur is present, occasionally with thrill along the left sternal border, often radiating to the neck
- The characteristic features are exertional dyspnea, angina pectoris, syncope, and heart failure, but patients may be asymptomatic until the fifth to seventh decades
- Left ventricular hypertrophy is usually present, owing to the increasingly higher left ventricular pressure required to drive blood across the obstructed valve
- Typically, the congenitally stenotic aortic valve is bicuspid or unicuspid, with inflexible leaflets that dome upwards in systole and may not close completely during diastole
- The valve in acquired aortic valvular stenosis has thickened, rigid, fibrotic or calcified leaflets with the addition of fusion of the commissures in rheumatic heart disease
- In rheumatic aortic stenosis both the aortic and mitral valves are usually abnormal

CAUSES

Common causes

- Progressive valvular calcification superimposed on a congenitally bicuspid valve or, in the elderly, a previously normal valve (most common cause)
- Congenital valvular abnormalities include unicuspid, bicuspid, or quadricuspid malformations

Rare causes

- Rheumatic fever: rheumatic aortic valvular stenosis is almost always associated with rheumatic involvement of the mitral valve
- Homozygous type II hyperlipoproteinemia, an extremely rare childhood condition
- Alkaptonuria: accumulation of metabolites in heart valves can lead to aortic valvular stenosis

Serious causes

Unicuspid valves produce severe obstruction in infancy and are the most frequent malformations found in fatal aortic valvular stenosis in children under the age of 1 year

Contributory or predisposing factors

- Rheumatic fever: the primary etiology of noncongenital, nonrheumatic aortic stenosis is thought to be degenerative changes resulting from decades of trauma to the valve leaflets exposed to high velocity flow

The following factors appear to play a role in accelerating progression of the disease:

- Atherosclerosis
- Hypercholesterolemia
- Diabetes mellitus type 1 and diabetes mellitus type 2
- Calcific aortic valvular stenosis is observed in Paget's disease of bone as well as in endstage renal disease
- Hypertension
- Cigarette smoking

EPIDEMIOLOGY

Incidence and prevalence

PREVALENCE

Approximately 25% of patients over 65 years of age and 35% of those over 70 years of age have echocardiographic evidence of sclerosis; 2–3% of these patients exhibit hemodynamic evidence of stenosis.

Demographics

AGE

- Congenital aortic valvular stenosis: patients usually develop symptoms before 30 years of age
- Rheumatic aortic valvular stenosis: symptoms usually develop between 30 and 70 years of age, or approximately 30 years after the attack of rheumatic fever
- Degenerative aortic valvular stenosis: rarely becomes symptomatic before 65 years of age and is the most likely cause of aortic valvular stenosis in patients 70 years of age and older

GENDER

Degenerative valve disease is three to four times more frequent in men than in women.

GENETICS

There is no clear strong genetic component.

DIFFERENTIAL DIAGNOSIS

Besides aortic valvular stenosis, three other lesions may be responsible for obstruction to left ventricular outflow:

Hypertrophic cardiomyopathy

The characterisitic features of hypertrophic cardiomyopathy are as follows.

FEATURES

- The hallmark is unexplained marked hypertrophy of the left ventricle
- In particular, the interventricular septum of the left ventricular outflow tract is involved
- The hypertrophied septum thickens during systole and obstructs left ventricular outflow, producing the murmur and symptoms
- Most patients are either asymptomatic or only mildly symptomatic and are identified during screening of relatives of patients with the disease
- Disease is identified most often in adults between 30 and 40 years of age
- Most common symptoms are primarily related to increased left ventricular stiffness and late systolic obstruction of ventricular outflow, and include: dyspnea, exertional angina pectoris, palpitations, syncope, and near-syncope
- A similar systolic murmur to that noted for aortic valvular stenosis is heard in hypertrophic cardiomyopathy. However, the murmur is often present only in mid to late systole
- Having the patient stand or perform Valsalva's maneuver causes the murmur of hypertrophic cardiomyopathy to increase. In aortic valvular stenosis, these maneuvers cause a decrease in the murmur due to a decrease in the absolute blood volume that will flow across the stenotic aortic valve

Discrete congenital subvalvular aortic stenosis

FEATURES

- A congenital abnormality produced either by a membranous diaphragm or by a fibrous ring encircling the left ventricular outflow tract just beneath the aortic valve
- Subvalvular rings may be associated with congenitally abnormal aortic valves
- The turbulent flow at the valvular level caused by the subvalvular membrane often causes damage to the valve leaflets, most commonly resulting in aortic insufficiency, but occasionally leading to valvular stenosis
- A discrete form of congenital subvalvular aortic stenosis resembles valvular aortic stenosis both clinically and physiologically
- Careful echocardiography demonstrates the subaortic obstruction
- Subvalvular rings may recur following surgical excision

Supravalvular aortic stenosis

FEATURES

- An uncommon congenital anomaly
- Consists of a localized or diffuse narrowing of the ascending aorta originating just above the level of the coronary arteries at the superior margin of the sinuses of Valsalva
- In contrast to the other forms of aortic stenosis, the coronary arteries are often dilated and tortuous as a result of being subjected to the elevated pressures that occur within the left ventricle
- In supravalvular aortic stenosis, there is often a pulse differential in the carotid arteries and arms, with the right carotid and right arm pulses remaining brisk with a wider pulse pressure, and the left carotid and left arm being diminished with decreased pulse pressure. This is due to the anatomic configuration of the ring leading to superiorly directed blood flow

SIGNS & SYMPTOMS

Signs

- A harsh systolic murmur, occasionally with thrill along left sternal border, often radiating to the neck. May be louder at the apex in older patients. The severity of the stenosis correlates with the lateness of the peak intensity of the murmur but not with its intensity
- Delayed and diminished carotid pulses
- As stenosis severity worsens, valve motion is reduced, resulting in soft, absent or (more rarely) paradoxically split second heart sound
- A fourth heart sound is often present
- The jugular venous pulse usually shows prominent a-waves, reflecting reduced right ventricular compliance
- Although ECG may be surprisingly normal in some patients (particularly females) with significant stenosis, tall R waves over the left precordium are usually present, and broad P waves, associated with atrial enlargement, are often present
- In congenital aortic stenosis, the ascending aorta is usually dilated (poststenotic dilation) late in the course of the disease
- Rheumatic aortic valvular stenosis is almost always associated with rheumatic involvement of the mitral valve

Symptoms

- In adults, usually asymptomatic until the fifth to seventh decades
- Exertional dyspnea
- Angina pectoris occurs in two-thirds of patients with critical aortic valvular stenosis. It is commonly precipitated by exertion and relieved by rest. Of these patients, 50% have associated significant coronary artery obstruction
- Syncope – typically exertional. May be due to arrhythmias, hypotension, or decreased cerebral perfusion
- Orthopnea and paroxysmal nocturnal dyspnea are relatively late symptoms in aortic valvular stenosis
- Marked fatigability, debilitation, and peripheral cyanosis become prominent late in the course of the disease
- Atrial fibrillation: severe pulmonary hypertension leading to right ventricular failure, systemic venous hypertension, hepatomegaly, and tricuspid regurgitation are often preterminal findings

ASSOCIATED DISORDERS

- Coronary artery disease: one-half of patients with calcific aortic stenosis and angina have significant associated coronary artery disease
- Mitral annulus calcification: degenerative aortic valvular stenosis is often accompanied by calcification of the mitral annulus
- Infective endocarditis may develop on any congenitally abnormal valve or aortic valves with rheumatic deformity. All patients with prosthetic aortic valves are also at increased risk of infective endocarditis. Antibiotics should be administered to all of these patients before dental procedures and some surgical procedures
- Mitral regurgitation: aortic valvular stenosis intensifies the severity of mitral regurgitation by increasing the pressure that drives blood from the left ventricle to the left atrium
- Gastrointestinal bleeding, either idiopathic or due to angiodysplasia or other vascular malformations, occurs more frequently in patients with calcific aortic valvular stenosis
- Calcific aortic valvular stenosis may cause embolization of calcium to a variety of organs, including the heart, kidney, and brain
- Stroke: it has recently been reported that the risk for stroke is three times higher among those who have aortic (or mitral) valve disease than it is for those without the condition

KEY! DON'T MISS!

- A left ventricular strain pattern (depression of the ST segment with inverted T waves) may be present in leads I, aVL, and the left precordial leads. This is consistent with severe aortic valvular stenosis and an enhanced probability of sudden death
- The harsh murmur of senile aortic sclerosis may be difficult to distinguish from that of aortic stenosis; however, it is typically harsh and mid-peaking, does not radiate to the carotids, and carotid upstrokes are brisk and early

CONSIDER CONSULT

- If a patient presents with any of the classic symptoms of aortic valvular stenosis (exertional dyspnea, angina pectoris, syncope, and heart failure), refer to cardiologist
- If a patient is asymptomatic but shows signs of significant aortic stenosis on echocardiographic examination, refer to cardiologist for further evaluation

INVESTIGATION OF THE PATIENT

Direct questions to patient

Q Have you been diagnosed with a heart murmur before?

Q Have you had rheumatic fever?

Q Do you experience shortness of breath or chest pain on exercise?

Q Do you experience dizziness or blackouts after physical exertion?

Q Have you had a heart attack?

Q Do you suffer from hypertension?

Q Do you smoke?

Contributory or predisposing factors

Q Is there a history of predisposing factors? Rheumatic fever, atherosclerosis, hypercholesterolemia, diabetes mellitus type 1 and diabetes mellitus type 2, and hypertension are predisposing factors, although all are weak

Family history

Q Is there a family history of valvular heart disease?

Q Is there a family history of coronary artery disease?

Q Is there a family history of hypertension?

Q Is there a family history of hypercholesterolemia?

Examination

- Location and intensity of the point of maximal impulse to evaluate for left ventricular hypertrophy
- Palpation of the carotid pulse: a slow rise of the impulse and poor volume of the carotid pulse is consistent with aortic valvular stenosis (pulsus parvus et tardus)
- Determination of the brachial–radial and apical–carotid delay. Brachial–radial delay is determined by simultaneously palpating the brachial and radial pulses – any delay is considered abnormal. Apical–carotid delay is determined by palpating the precordial apex pulsation and the carotid artery pulsation
- Careful auscultation of the heart for a mid- to late-peaking systolic crescendo–decrescendo murmur that is loudest in the second right interspace and that radiates to the clavicle and the carotid artery
- Evaluation of the second heart sound for decreased intensity, paradoxical splitting or absence
- Evaluate the murmur during Valsalva maneuver to note any decrease in intensity, which will rule out hypertrophic cardiomyopathy

Summary of investigative tests

- The echocardiogram is the preferred noninvasive test for the diagnosis of aortic valvular stenosis and for following the progression of the disease
- Cardiac catheterization with coronary angiography should be performed in patients suspected of having severe aortic valvular stenosis. It is useful to confirm the diagnosis of and assess the degree of severity of aortic valvular stenosis. The patient can also be assessed for concomitant coronary artery disease
- The ECG may reveal left ventricular hypertrophy or suggest repolarization changes
- Chest X-ray may show a normal or enlarged cardiac silhouette, calcification of the aortic valve, and calcification and/or dilation of the ascending aorta

DIAGNOSTIC DECISION

The presence of any of the following findings significantly increases the likelihood of a diagnosis of aortic valvular stenosis:

- Effort syncope
- Slow rate of rise of the carotid arterial impulse
- Timing of peak murmur intensity in mid or late systole
- Decreasing intensity of a previously loud murmur
- Apical–carotid or brachioradial delay
- The absence of any systolic murmur or murmur radiation to the right carotid artery significantly decreases the likelihood of aortic valvular stenosis. However, in extremely severe, undiagnosed aortic stenosis with resultant left ventricular dysfunction, the murmur may become nearly inaudible. Aortic stenosis may thus be the cause of severe heart failure in a patient who has not received regular medical care
- Absent second heart sound

CLINICAL PEARL(S)

- The intensity of the aortic valve closure sound (A2) can be used to distinguish aortic stenosis from aortic sclerosis: A2 may be soft, late, or absent in aortic stenosis; in aortic sclerosis, A2 is usually normal in intensity and timing
- A narrow pulse pressure is often seen in critical aortic stenosis
- The absence of ECG evidence of left ventricular hypertrophy does not rule out critical aortic stenosis

THE TESTS

Imaging

ECHOCARDIOGRAPHY

Advantages/Disadvantages

Advantages:

- Confirms diagnosis
- Quantifies degree of stenosis
- It is particularly useful for identifying valvular abnormalities such as mitral stenosis and aortic regurgitation, which sometimes accompany aortic valvular stenosis
- It also allows definition of valvular morphology in the case of congenitally abnormal valves
- It can assist with differentiation of valvular stenosis from obstructive hypertrophic cardiomyopathy, subvalvular abnormalities, and supravalvular abnormalities
- Ventricular ejection fraction and the extent of concentric left ventricular hypertrophy can also be assessed
- Doppler interrogation of the valve provides measurement of the peak instantaneous transvalvular gradient, as well as the mean transvalvular gradient
- Non invasive test

Disadvantages:

- Echocardiography may not provide adequate viewing of the aortic valves and assessment of ventricular function in obese patients
- Low flow velocities cannot exclude aortic valvular stenosis because both reduced stroke volume and an inability to position the Doppler beam parallel to the flow may appreciably reduce the measured velocity. The echocardiographic calculation of valve area will remain accurate even in the presence of reduced cardiac output, however, and this is the number that should be carefully obtained in these patients

Abnormal

- The characteristic echocardiographic appearance in aortic valvular stenosis is an increased echo density of the aortic valve with reduced systolic excursions of the leaflets. A bicuspid, unicuspid, or quadricuspid morphology may be visualized
- A high flow velocity across the valve corresponds to a high transvalvular gradient, which indicates the presence of aortic valvular stenosis; however, significant aortic stenosis may be present despite a low gradient if cardiac output is reduced. Calculation of valve area is accurate even in the presence of reduced cardiac output
- Keep in mind the possibility of imaging artifacts

Cause of abnormal result

The abnormal morphology of a stenosed valve leads to turbulent blood flow in the region of the valve leaflets. The turbulent flow causes the normally thin, pliable valve to thicken. This shows up on echocardiography as increased echo density.

CHEST X-RAY

Advantages/Disadvantages

Advantages:

- Inexpensive
- Noninvasive
- Can help distinguish cardiovascular and pulmonary causes of dyspnea

Disadvantages:

- Nonspecific for cardiovascular abnormalities; additional testing will always be necessary
- Chest X-ray may be normal in up to 10% of patients with aortic valvular stenosis
- Keep in mind the possibility of imaging artifacts

Abnormal

- Although the chest X-ray may be normal in up to 10% of patients, often an enlarged cardiac silhouette or a boot-shaped heart may be seen
- Occasionally, aortic valve calcification is seen on lateral view and/or dilation and calcification of the ascending aorta (poststenotic dilation)
- Keep in mind the possibility of false-positive results

Cause of abnormal result

Left ventricular hypertrophy due to the increasingly higher left ventricular pressure that is required to drive blood across the obstructed valve.

CARDIAC CATHETERIZATION

Advantages/Disadvantages

Advantages:

- Useful for evaluating coronary circulation and to confirm or clarify the diagnosis of aortic valvular stenosis

- Indicated for patients suspected of having coronary artery disease prior to aortic valve replacement. This is important since patients with aortic valvular stenosis often have concomitant coronary artery disease
- A complete left and right heart catheterization may be required to determine the hemodynamic severity of the aortic valvular stenosis if a discrepancy exists between clinical and echocardiographic findings, or if there is evidence of associated valvular disease or pulmonary hypertension
- Can accurately define the degree of stenosis, assess the status of left ventricular function, and determine the location of left ventricular outflow obstruction

Disadvantages:

- Expensive
- High-risk, invasive procedure
- Accurate determination of valve area requires careful measurement of oxygen consumption, which is difficult and rarely done. Therefore, most often the area is calculated using an assumed oxygen consumption, which may be inaccurate. This is a particular issue in patients with lower gradients and left ventricular dysfunction

Abnormal

- A valve area below $0.8 cm^2$ indicates severe stenosis
- A high flow velocity across the valve corresponds to a high transvalvular gradient, which indicates the presence of aortic valvular stenosis. The flow velocity across the valve may be low in the presence of severe left ventricular dysfunction and reduced cardiac output
- Using angiography the presence of coronary artery disease may be determined by visualization of arterial stenoses
- Keep in mind the possibility of false-positive results

Other tests

ECG

Advantages/Disadvantages

Advantages:

- Can aid in diagnosis of aortic valvular stenosis
- Useful to rule out acute coronary syndromes
- Noninvasive

Disadvantages:

- Nonspecific
- May be surprisingly normal in patients (particularly females) with significant stenosis

Abnormal

- Tall R waves over the precordium are usually present
- A left ventricular strain pattern (depression of the ST segment with inverted T waves) may be present in leads I, aVL, and the left precordial leads. This is consistent with severe aortic valvular stenosis and an enhanced probability of sudden death
- Broad P waves may be present due to atrial enlargement
- Left ventricular hypertrophy is seen in the majority of patients
- Keep in mind the possibility of false-positive results

Cause of abnormal result

Left ventricular hypertrophy and atrial enlargement induced by aortic valvular stenosis.

TREATMENT

CONSIDER CONSULT

- Drug therapy for symptoms requires the cardiologist's guidance

IMMEDIATE ACTION

- Hypotension in a patient with critical aortic stenosis is an emergency. Any patient with known or suspected aortic stenosis and symptomatic low blood pressure should immediately be transferred to an intensive care setting, preferably one with cardiac surgical availability
- Avoid any therapy, including diuretics, that may lower the blood pressure further

MANAGEMENT ISSUES

Goals

- Immediate valve replacement if the symptoms of dyspnea, angina, syncope, or heart failure have developed as a result of aortic valvular stenosis
- Valve replacement for asymptomatic patients who have progressive left ventricular dysfunction, very severe left ventricular hypertrophy, and very high gradients (>80mmHg) (rare)
- Prophylaxis of infective endocarditis
- In a patient with questionable symptoms or a patient who reports no symptoms but whom you suspect of having severely limiting activity, an exercise test can be very useful. Exercise testing has been shown to be safe in asymptomatic patients with aortic stenosis, although it should never be performed in patients with the classic symptoms of heart failure, angina, or syncope

Management in special circumstances

COEXISTING DISEASE

It is generally accepted that patients with moderate or severe aortic valvular stenosis (regardless of symptom status) presenting for coronary artery bypass grafting undergo concomitant aortic valve replacement.

SPECIAL PATIENT GROUPS

- In children, adolescents, and young adults with congenital noncalcific aortic valvular stenosis, balloon aortic valvuloplasty is the preferred therapy until fully grown or past childbearing years. Early valve replacement surgery will require subsequent operations to upgrade the valve to an adult size
- The Ross procedure (in which a patient's abnormal aortic valve is replaced with the patient's own pulmonary valve, and a bioprosthesis placed in the pulmonary position) has recently been recognized as an alternative therapy in children and adolescents in the absence of available homographs. This is a very long surgical procedure and cardiopreservation must be carefully monitored. Patients with severe left ventricular hypertrophy are not candidates for this procedure
- In severely symptomatic patients who are not candidates for aortic valve replacement (i.e. those with comorbid conditions such as malignancy, pregnant women with severe aortic valvular stenosis), balloon aortic valvotomy may provide temporary relief of symptoms (the risk of restenosis within 6 months is very high)
- Patients with moderate or severe aortic valvular stenosis (regardless of symptom status) presenting for coronary artery bypass grafting should undergo concomitant aortic valve replacement

PATIENT SATISFACTION/LIFESTYLE PRIORITIES

- Aortic valvular stenosis is a progressive disease for which surgical therapy is the only definitive treatment. It is appropriate to consider aortic valve replacement even in the very elderly presenting with symptomatic aortic stenosis. Octogenarians with aortic stenosis in the absence of coronary artery disease or left ventricular dysfunction have quite low operative risk

- Obviously the decision regarding surgery has to be individualized to each patient
- Aortic valve replacement can be done with mechanical prostheses, which require lifelong anticoagulation; or with bioprostheses, which avoid the need for anticoagulation but which degenerate. Pericardial valves have a mean lifetime of 10 years, whereas aortic homografts (not as readily available) probably extend that time to about 15 years. The decision about which type of valve to use should be made taking into account the needs and desires of the patient, as well as any relevant surgical issues

SUMMARY OF THERAPEUTIC OPTIONS

Choices

There are no standard drug regimens, and all drug therapy in this disease should be undertaken with extreme caution, as overmedication can precipitate hemodynamic instability and death. Drug therapy for symptoms should be undertaken only under the guidance of a cardiologist.

Successful aortic valve replacement results in substantial clinical and hemodynamic improvement in patients with symptomatic aortic valvular stenosis as well as improved survival.

Useful guidelines for therapy include:
Bonow et al. ACC/AHA guidelines for the management of patients with valvular heart disease. J Am Coll Cardiolol 1998;32(5):1486–588

Clinical pearl(s)

Don't forget endocarditis prophylaxis for all patients with aortic valvular stenosis!

Never

- Beta-blockers, calcium channel blockers, and other negatively inotropic medications may precipitate cardiovascular collapse and should be avoided in the treatment of angina in patients with aortic valvular stenosis
- Angiotensin-converting enzyme (ACE) inhibitors and other vasodilators, as well as diuretics used routinely in the treatment of heart failure, may precipitate syncope and even death in aortic valvular stenosis and are contraindicated, even in patients with symptomatic heart failure. These patients should be hospitalized for initiation of therapy, if surgery will be delayed

FOLLOW UP

Plan for review

- Asymptomatic patients with valvular velocities <3m/s may be followed yearly, possibly with yearly echocardiograms, since the disease may progress fairly rapidly. If there is any question about whether a patient is truly asymptomatic, exercise testing should be considered
- Patients with valvular velocities >3m/s should be seen every 6 months. Once the valvular velocity is >4m/s the likelihood of eventual symptom development is high and patients should be followed closely. Consecutive echocardiograms are likely not useful in this group

Information for patient or caregiver

- All asymptomatic patients should receive careful education, including written lists of the symptoms that require immediate attention – particularly heart failure, chest pain, and syncope
- In addition, all patients with abnormal aortic valves should receive information about endocarditis prophylaxis and prescriptions for appropriate antibiotics
- In asymptomatic patients with moderate to severe aortic stenosis, the likelihood of eventual progression and need for cardiac surgery is significant. It is useful to discuss this with the patient to determine the patient's thoughts and fears regarding surgery, preference for type of valve, etc

DRUGS AND OTHER THERAPIES: DETAILS

Surgical therapy

AORTIC VALVE REPLACEMENT

Efficacy

Successful replacement of the aortic valve results in substantial clinical and hemodynamic improvement in patients with symptomatic aortic valvular stenosis as well as improved survival.

Risks/Benefits

Risks:

- The surgical mortality rate for valve replacement is 2–5%, but for patients above 75 years of age, it rises to 10%
- Patients with prosthetic heart valves have an increased risk of thromboembolism, endocarditis, prosthetic valve failure, and, if anticoagulation therapy is required, hemorrhage

Benefits:

- Following the onset of symptoms (dyspnea, angina, syncope, heart failure), the prognosis without surgery is poor, with a >50% mortality rate at 3 years

Acceptability to patient

- The needs, fears, and wishes of any patient being considered for cardiac surgery must be addressed. Since there is no other therapy for aortic stenosis, most symptomatic patients will eventually agree to undergo the procedure
- The choice of mechanical or bioprosthesis will depend on patient preference and the dictates of concomitant medical conditions as well as surgical considerations

Follow up plan

- Any patient receiving a prosthetic aortic valve should receive a yearly history and physical examination
- Echocardiography should be performed when there is any symptom or sign that suggests alteration in valvular function
- When a patient has a bioprosthesis, yearly echocardiography should be performed, beginning approximately 7–8 years postoperatively, to monitor for valve degeneration

Patient and caregiver information

Patients should receive information about antibiotic prophylaxis for bacterial endocarditis, as well as a prescription for antibiotics. Patients with mechanical prostheses must be educated regarding warfarin therapy, its risks, benefits, and idiosyncrasies.

LIFESTYLE

- Patients with severe obstruction should be cautioned to avoid vigorous athletic and physical activity. If limiting activity is not a viable choice for a given patient, then valve replacement should be pursued
- The necessity for endocarditis prophylaxis should be explained

OUTCOMES

EFFICACY OF THERAPIES

Aortic valve replacement surgery is a very effective therapy for symptomatic aortic stenosis and results in dramatic symptomatic improvement and increased survival.

Although the perioperative morbidity and mortality of aortic valve surgery is low, there is long-term morbidity and mortality associated with both mechanical and bioprosthetic valves. It is therefore not the current recommendation that asymptomatic persons with severe aortic stenosis undergo surgical valve replacement.

There is disagreement about this, however. The surgical risk is different for each patient, and must be taken into account when making the decision regarding timing of surgery.

PROGNOSIS

- Successful replacement of the aortic valve results in substantial clinical and hemodynamic improvement in patients with aortic valvular stenosis. Survival is increased in patients undergoing surgical therapy compared to those not undergoing valve replacement
- Balloon valvuloplasty carries a very high risk of restenosis within 6 months

Clinical pearl(s)

Balloon valvuloplasty can be used as a 'bridging' procedure for patients with severe aortic stenosis who will eventually require valve replacement.

Terminal illness

- The patient with critical symptomatic aortic stenosis who refuses or is inappropriate for cardiac surgery has a reduced life expectancy
- Efforts should be made to emphasize comfort and dignity as death nears, including obtaining hospice care for the patient
- If an implantable defibrillator has been previously placed, it should be turned off

COMPLICATIONS

Sudden death can occur in patients with severe, symptomatic aortic valvular stenosis but has rarely been reported to occur in asymptomatic patients.

PREVENTION

RISK FACTORS

- **Coronary artery disease:** investigate and institute therapy
- **Hypercholesterolemia:** investigate and institute therapy
- **Hypertension:** investigate and institute therapy
- **Smoking:** recommend cessation

MODIFY RISK FACTORS

Lifestyle and wellness

There are no lifestyle changes that have been shown significantly to affect progression of aortic stenosis.

TOBACCO

All patients should be advised to stop smoking.

SCREENING

- When aortic valvular stenosis is detected on the physical examination of an asymptomatic patient, an echocardiogram should be performed to confirm diagnosis and quantify severity
- If a patient has questionable symptoms or is very sedentary, or you are suspicious that the patient is slowly and progressively limiting activity so as to remain asymptomatic, exercise testing is a safe and useful adjunct to assess clinical significance of the stenosis
- If the peak gradient is less than 50mmHg the patient should be followed yearly with a history and physical examination
- If the peak gradient exceeds 50mmHg, follow up should be performed every 6 months
- In a patient who is physically active, repeat echocardiography is indicated if the patient reports the onset of one or all of the classic symptoms: exertional dyspnea, angina, syncope, or heart failure
- In sedentary patients, more frequent echocardiograms are indicated to detect the onset of left ventricular dysfunction in the absence of symptoms

RESOURCES

ASSOCIATIONS

American Heart Association
National Center
7272 Greenville Avenue
Dallas, Texas 75231
http://www.americanheart.org/

KEY REFERENCES

- Bonow RO, Carabello B, de Leon AC Jr, et al. ACC/AHA guidelines for the management of patients with valvular heart disease. J Am Coll Cardiol 1998;32(5):1486–588. A summary is available from the National Guidelines Clearinghouse (www.guidelines.gov)
- Braunwald E, ed. Heart Disease: a textbook of cardiovascular medicine, 5th edn. Philadelphia, PA: WB Saunders, 1997
- Etchells E, Bell C, Robb K. Does this patient have an abnormal systolic murmur? JAMA 1997;277(7):564–71.
- Lester SJ, Heilbron B, Gin K, et al. The natural history and rate of progression of aortic stenosis. Chest 1998;113(4):1109–14.
- Oswalt JD. Acceptance and versatility of the Ross procedure. Curr Opin Cardiol 1999;14(2):90–4.

CONTRIBUTORS

Yul D Ejnes, MD, FACP
Mark B Stockman, MD
Nancy Sweitzer, MD

ATRIAL FIBRILLATION

SUMMARY INFORMATION

DESCRIPTION

- The most common type of cardiac arrhythmia, defined by irregular ventricular pulse and apical–radial mismatch
- May be paroxysmal or persistent or permanent
- Underlying pathology is generally present
- There are multiple causes – treatment of some will result in patient reverting to sinus rhythm
- An important cause of thromboembolism, particularly stroke, especially in the elderly
- Overall, 40/1000 patients with atrial fibrillation will have a stroke each year

URGENT ACTION

- If hemodynamic state has been compromised by the rhythm disturbance (hypotension, overt cardiac failure, syncope), urgently hospitalize (or refer to cardiologist) for investigation and management. May require urgent DC cardioversion
- If patient has experienced an associated condition that is potentially life-threatening (e.g. myocardial infarction, thromboembolic stroke, thyrotoxicosis, peripheral emboli), urgent referral to an intensivist or subspecialist may be appropriate

KEY! DON'T MISS!

- Need to distinguish atrial fibrillation with aberrancy from ventricular tachycardia
- Ventricular tachycardia can be a life-threatening emergency, and patients are at risk of recurrence and sudden cardiac death

BACKGROUND

ICD9 CODE
- 427.3 Atrial fibrillation and flutter
- 427.31 Atrial fibrillation
- 427.32 Atrial flutter

SYNONYMS
AF, AFib

CARDINAL FEATURES
Irregularly irregular pulse with radial–apical mismatch.

CAUSES
Common causes
3–11% of patients have idiopathic or 'lone' atrial fibrillation (diagnosis of exclusion) where there is no evidence of heart disease and all investigations are normal.

Cardiac causes (organic heart disease):
- Most common cause is hypertension – especially where left ventricular hypertrophy is present. Left atrium may dilate secondary to left ventricular dilatation and trigger atrial fibrillation; alternatively, hypertension may be associated with underlying heart disease, itself a risk factor for atrial fibrillation
- Coronary heart disease
- Rheumatic heart disease, especially mitral valve stenosis. This combination increases the risk of stroke 18-fold
- Nonrheumatic valvular heart disease; risk of stroke in these patients increased 5.6 times
- Sick sinus syndrome
- Pre-excitation syndromes with accessory conduction pathways (e.g. Wolff–Parkinson–White syndrome – recognized by short PR interval of <0.12 s on ECG – and delta waves on ECG when the patient is in sinus rhythm). Suspect in young patient with extremely fast atrial fibrillation
- Idiopathic dilated and hypertrophic cardiomyopathy

Noncardiac causes:
- Thyrotoxicosis, even where classic signs of overactive thyroid are absent (e.g. elderly may present with weight loss, apathy, and unexplained atrial fibrillation)
- Acute infections, especially pneumonia in the elderly
- Acute excess alcohol intake – the 'holiday heart syndrome' in healthy people with otherwise normal hearts. Caused by the release of catecholamines, especially norepinephrine, from the adrenals and epinephrine from cardiac stores. The main metabolite of ethanol increases systemic and myocardial catecholamines; its metabolites also prolong the PR, QRS, and QT intervals directly
- Chronic excess alcohol intake. Alcohol withdrawal also increases catecholamine release
- Lung carcinoma
- Other thoracic or pulmonary pathology (e.g. pleural effusion)
- Postoperative problems (especially after thoracotomy or coronary artery bypass grafting)

Rare causes
Cardiac causes:
- Cardiomyopathy – alcoholic and hypertrophic
- Pericardial disease, such as effusion, constrictive pericarditis
- Atrial septal defect
- Atrial myoma

Noncardiac causes:

- Pulmonary embolism
- Drugs (e.g. digoxin toxicity, sumatriptan)

EPIDEMIOLOGY

Incidence and prevalence

INCIDENCE

2% over 20 years.

PREVALENCE

- Overall, around 20 per 1000 of the population
- Increases with age
- Over 65 years, 50/1000

Demographics

AGE

- Uncommon in those under 50 years
- Roughly doubles in incidence with each decade over 40 years
- Occurs in 5 per 1000 people aged 50–59 years
- Increases to 88 per 1000 cases in people aged 80–89 years
- Rare in children

GENDER

More common in males than females.

GENETICS

Rare genetic cases exist – there is an autosomal-dominant form of familial atrial fibrillation, caused by a mutation on chromosome 10; this may be suspected in younger patients who have a strong family history. However, in an overwhelming majority of patients, no specific genetic pattern exists.

DIFFERENTIAL DIAGNOSIS

- Most important to distinguish atrial fibrillation from the other supraventricular tachycardias (atrial flutter, atrial extrasystoles, atrial tachycardia), especially where there is a rapid atrial rhythm with rapid ventricular response as treatment for atrial fibrillation can worsen some other arrhythmias significantly
- Important also to distinguish atrial fibrillation from other tachyarrhythmias such as ventricular tachycardia and Wolff–Parkinson–White syndrome
- Sinus tachycardia may mimic atrial fibrillation
- It is worth remembering that lone atrial fibrillation is a diagnosis of exclusion when there is no evidence of heart disease and all investigations are normal
- Key distinguishing feature of atrial fibrillation is variability in the R-R intervals on ECG trace
- If heart rate is very high try carotid sinus massage to slow rate (if no carotid bruits), or increase rate of recording trace on ECG machine
- If in any doubt, refer ECG to cardiologist for interpretation

Lone atrial fibrillation

FEATURES

- Most often manifest as isolated or recurrent episodes of paroxysmal atrial fibrillation; a few cases have chronic rhythm disturbance
- More common when patient is under 50 years of age
- May be precipitated by stress, alcohol ('holiday heart'), stimulants, or smoking
- Possibly gives small increase in morbidity or mortality if patient is under 65 years, even if no other cardiovascular risk factors present
- Beware of this diagnosis in the elderly – consider subclinical coronary heart disease or subtle clinical conditions such as cardiomyopathy, sick sinus syndrome, Wolff–Parkinson–White syndrome, or apathetic hyperthyroidism

Atrial flutter

FEATURES

- Atria discharge in a coordinated fashion, due to a re-entry circuit, giving an atrial rate of 250–300 beats/min
- Commonly, alternate atrial impulses are conducted to the ventricles, giving a pulse rate of 150 (called 2:1 AV conduction)
- Other conduction patterns are possible, especially after drugs such as digoxin, adenosine, or verapamil, which increase atrioventricular block, giving 3:1 or 4:1 block, or with intrinsic AV conduction disease
- Rarely 1:1 conduction (i.e. all atrial impulses conducted to ventricles)
- Where atrioventricular block is variable, rhythm may be confused with atrial fibrillation
- ECG shows characteristic F ('flutter') waves giving a saw-tooth pattern on ECG (especially leads II, III, and aVF or V1)

Atrial extrasystoles

FEATURES

- Common
- Cause irregular pulse with long pauses between beats as sinus node is 'reset' by the extrasystole
- Extrasystoles arising from several sites are common in lung disease
- ECG is diagnostic

Sinus tachycardia

FEATURES

- Sinus rhythm of more than 100 beats/min
- Slow onset and ending
- Distinguishable from atrial fibrillation by presence of P waves before each QRS complex (best seen in leads II or VI), but can be hard to see if rate is very fast

Atrial tachycardia

FEATURES

- Atrial rate is slower, usually 120–250 beats/min
- Atrioventricular block, which may be variable, may coexist and is commonly seen in digoxin toxicity
- ECG features absence of saw-tooth appearance and abnormally shaped P waves at regular rate. Best seen in V1; narrow QRS complexes unless pre-existing conduction defect present

Atrioventricular nodal re-entrant tachycardia

FEATURES

- Re-entry circuit in atrioventricular node
- Atrial and ventricular rates of 130–240 beats/min
- ECG shows regular rhythm with normal QRS complexes, P waves follow QRS complex and are inverted in II, III, and aVF, or P waves may not be seen

Wolff–Parkinson–White syndrome

Distinguishing features of Wolff–Parkinson–White syndrome are as follows.

FEATURES

- Young, otherwise healthy patients
- Suspect if patient has atrial fibrillation with a ventricular rate >200 beats/min, with no other cause for fibrillation
- Drugs such as digoxin or verapamil worsen the ventricular rate by blocking atrioventricular node impulses and increasing conduction through accessory pathway
- ECG shows short P-R interval (up to 0.10 s) and wide QRS complex with slurred take-off due to diagnostic delta wave
- Refer to cardiologist for investigation and possible ablation of abnormal pathways

Ventricular tachycardia

Distinguishing features of ventricular tachycardia are as follows.

FEATURES

- Atrial fibrillation with bundle branch block on QRS complexes may look like ventricular tachycardia
- Key distinguishing feature is irregularity of the R-R interval in atrial fibrillation
- Axis is usually Northwest (minus 90 to minus 180º) in ventricular tachycardia
- Other features for ventricular tachycardia include: AV dissociation with P waves progressing through the QRS complexes, and QRS axis width >0.14 if associated with a right bundle branch block and >0.16 if associated with a left bundle branch block
- Key feature of ventricular tachycardia is AV dissociation, but up to 20% of ventricular tachycardia may have 1:1 AV conduction
- Must distinguish from supraventricular tachycardia with aberrancy and Wolff–Parkinson–White syndrome in atrial fibrillation

SIGNS & SYMPTOMS

Signs

- Pulse is irregularly irregular in rhythm, rate, and volume as only occasional impulses penetrate atrioventricular node

- First heart sound of variable loudness
- Absent a- waves in jugular venous pulse
- Apical–radial pulse mismatch develops when rate is rapid as not all ventricular contractions transmit an arterial pulse

Symptoms

- Usually related to hemodynamic consequences of rate (too fast or, rarely, too slow)
- Asymptomatic in up to 20% of patients
- Palpitations – may be paroxysmal or chronic
- Dyspnea
- Reduced exercise tolerance – lethargy, fatigue, shortness of breath on exertion
- Heart failure
- Chest pain, including myocardial ischemia or angina
- Dizziness
- Syncope; this is rare unless patient has sick sinus syndrome or Wolff–Parkinson–White syndrome, in which hypotension may occur

ASSOCIATED DISORDERS

- Hypertension
- Rheumatic heart disease
- Coronary heart disease
- Diabetes mellitus (in children; in adults: type I or type II)
- Hyperthyroidism

KEY! DON'T MISS!

- Need to distinguish atrial fibrillation with aberrancy from ventricular tachycardia
- Ventricular tachycardia can be a life-threatening emergency, and patients are at risk of recurrence and sudden cardiac death

CONSIDER CONSULT

- Age <30 years
- Emergency DC cardioversion needed and not otherwise available
- Syncope associated with fibrillation
- Patient with moderate to severe or resistant heart failure
- Patients with atrial fibrillation due to a pre-excitation syndrome, such as Wolff–Parkinson–White syndrome
- Most patients will require echocardiography for assessment (to confirm those with valvular heart disease) and referral may be needed if not otherwise available

INVESTIGATION OF THE PATIENT

Direct questions to patient

Q **Are the symptoms there all the time or do they come and go?** It is important to distinguish between permanent and paroxysmal atrial fibrillation as the management of each is different

Q **What seems to bring them on?** May suggest cause and appropriate treatment

Q **Do you get tightness in your chest? Air hunger? Do you get palpitations at rest?** Distinguish anxiety disorders

Q **How far can you walk? Has the distance changed?** Exercise intolerance is a common presentation of atrial fibrillation but anxiety symptoms may not be affected by exercise

Q **Any shortness of breath? Cough? Swelling of your ankles?** The dysrhythmia may be affecting cardiac output and causing heart failure

Q **Has your weight changed?** If weight has increased, consider fluid retention related to heart failure; if weight has decreased, consider thyrotoxicosis

Q **Any chest pain?** Atrial fibrillation may be contributing to coronary heart disease

- **Q** **Have you felt dizzy/blacked out?** Consider sick sinus syndrome in older person
- **Q** **Are you taking any medications?** Especially consider digoxin, theophylline preparations, sympathomimetics, tricyclic antidepressants and other anticholinergics, migraine treatments (e.g. sumatriptan). Look for nonprescription agents that may contain catecholamines or theophylline compounds. Drugs that affect potassium channels, such as terfenadine, cisapride, and astemizole, can interact with prescription agents resulting in serious arrhythmias

Contributory or predisposing factors

- **Q** **Is there a history of predisposing factors?** Hyperthyroidism, hypertension, hyperlipidemia, acute myocardial infarction
- **Q** **Any history of heart problems?** Rheumatic heart disease, valve disease, ischemia, murmur
- **Q** **Do you smoke? Does anyone in your family have heart disease?** Risk factors for heart disease should be explored
- **Q** **How much alcohol do you drink?** Heavy intake can precipitate paroxysmal fibrillation

Family history

Overall, the family history is not useful since atrial fibrillation is relatively common and inherited etiology is rare. However, in a young patient with atrial fibrillation, obtain the family history.

Examination

- **Is the patient inappropriately anxious?** Excessive anxiety may cause palpitations
- **Check the blood pressure**, including postural change, and look for widened pulse pressure
- **Count apical rate** and note rhythm and compare with radial pulse – deficit in atrial fibrillation
- **Look for evidence of hyperthyroidism** – exophthalmos, goiter, tremor – although absent signs do not exclude the diagnosis
- **Check neck vessels** – carotid upstroke, jugular vein for distension and cannon waves
- **Listen for signs of lung disease**
- **Check heart for additional sounds** including clicks, murmurs (especially mitral stenosis and regurgitation), third heart sound. Lateral decubitus positioning may help
- **Inspect legs for edema and tenderness** – signs of heart failure
- **Conduct a neurologic examination** to detect any subtle signs of secondary stroke (neurologic deficits)

Summary of investigative tests

- The 12-lead ECG is diagnostic except in paroxysmal atrial fibrillation between attacks, but it can be difficult to interpret; refer for cardiologist opinion before commencing nonurgent treatment if results unclear
- Thyroid function tests may show clinically silent hyperthyroidism to be the cause of atrial fibrillation and are particularly important in the elderly
- Echocardiography is useful to diagnose and document structural heart disease as cause of atrial fibrillation; it can also predict the likelihood of successful DC cardioversion in an individual patient. Transesophageal echo can show the presence of intra-atrial thrombus, which increases the risk of a stroke complicating the procedure. Echocardiography is essential to exclude otherwise silent disorders if a diagnosis of 'lone atrial fibrillation' is contemplated
- Chest radiography may indicate cardiac structural causes of atrial fibrillation such as mitral valve disease as well as complications, particularly heart failure
- Abnormal serum potassium levels can potentiate arrhythmias, particularly if the patient is taking, or about to start, digoxin
- Renal function tests may indicate impaired renal function, which may require medication dosages to be adjusted
- A hemoglobin level may suggest anemia as differential diagnostic of palpitations
- Transesophageal echocardiography is superior to transthoracic cardiac echocardiography if intra-atrial thrombus is suspected
- CT scan of the brain is useful if neurologic examination is suggestive of a secondary stroke

DIAGNOSTIC DECISION

- ECG is the definitive test. Can be difficult to interpret and diagnostic uncertainty is a reason to refer to a cardiologist
- Diagnostic accuracy is important as some drugs used in atrial fibrillation may worsen similar arrhythmias
- Prompt diagnosis improves the chance of successful cardioversion – the ideal outcome

Guidelines

Prystowsky EN, Benson DW, Fuster V, et al. Management of patients with atrial fibrillation. A statement for healthcare professionals from the subcommittee on electrocardiography and electrophysiology, American Heart Association. Circulation 1996;93:1262–77

CLINICAL PEARL(S)

'48-h rule' – if atrial fibrillation has been present for more than 48h (or the time cannot be determined accurately), avoid stroke by not converting the rhythm until risk of clot is low (unless hemodynamic emergency).

THE TESTS

Body fluids

FULL BLOOD COUNT

Description

Venous blood sample.

Advantages/Disadvantages

Advantages:

- Excludes anemia as cause of palpitations
- Useful baseline if anticoagulation contemplated

Normal

Hemoglobin 14.4g/dL.

Abnormal

Hemoglobin below 14.4g/dL.

Cause of abnormal result

- Anemia (multiple potential causes)
- Hemorrhage – especially consider if patient taking warfarin
- Keep in mind the possibility of a false-positive result

SERUM ELECTROLYTES

Description

Venous blood sample.

Normal

- Potassium 3.8–5.0mEq/L (3.8–5.0mmol/L)
- Aim for potassium level >4mEq/L if patient is taking digoxin

Abnormal

Below 3.8mEq/L (3.8mmol/L).

Cause of abnormal result

- If low, look for diuretic therapy, and other causes of hypokalemia
- Keep in mind the possibility of a false-positive result

Drugs, disorders, and other factors that may alter results
Thiazide and loop diuretics may lower serum potassium.

Tests of function

RENAL FUNCTION TESTS

Description
Venous blood sample.

Advantages/Disadvantages
Advantages:
- Allows for rapid, relatively inexpensive means of indirectly measuring renal function – identifies renal failure when creatinine above normal range
- Provides baseline measurement of renal function
- If renal function impaired, a reduced dosage of several antiarrhythmic drugs should be prescribed, including digoxin and verapamil

Disadvantages:
- Renal function may be impaired despite normal creatinine result
- No diagnostic role in atrial fibrillation

Normal
- Urea: 15–40mg/dL (2.5–6.6mmol/L)
- Serum creatinine: 0.7–1.4mg/dL (62–124mcmol/L), although local laboratory should be consulted because normal ranges vary; also affected by sex and body mass
- Serum potassium: 3.5–5mEq/L
- Serum calcium: 8.8–10.3mg/dL
- Serum phosphate: 2.5–5mg/dL
- Creatinine clearance: 75–124mL/min

Abnormal
Values higher than normal.

Cause of abnormal result
- Renal failure
- Keep in mind the possibility of a false-positive result

Drugs, disorders, and other factors that may alter results
Chronic renal failure.

THYROID FUNCTION TESTS

Description
Measures plasma levels of thyroid hormones and pituitary thyroid-stimulating hormone.

Advantages/Disadvantages
Advantage: may confirm hyperthyroidism in otherwise asymptomatic patient.

Normal
- Plasma thyroxine (T4): 5.5–12.5mcg/dL (70–160nmol/L)
- Thyroid stimulating hormone (TSH): 1–4mU/L
- Tri-iodothyronine (T3): 70–170ng/dL (1.1–2.6nmol/L)

Abnormal

- T3 or T4 high; TSH low or undetectable
- Low values of T4/high values of TSH suggesting hypothyroidism may be found, but are not related to atrial fibrillation

Cause of abnormal result

- Hyperthyroidism
- Factitious hyperthyroidism
- Keep in mind the possibility of a false-positive result

RESTING 12-LEAD ECG

Description

12-lead resting ECG.

Advantages/Disadvantages

Advantages:

- Diagnostic of condition and some underlying causes (such as coronary heart disease)
- Noninvasive

Disadvantage: may be difficult to interpret, especially if other rate or rhythm abnormalities also present.

Abnormal

- Absent P waves
- P waves replaced by irregular 'F' (fibrillatory) waves especially seen in V1 lead
- Variability in the R-R intervals on ECG trace

Cause of abnormal result

- Loss of normal atrial contractions (no P waves) which are replaced by disordered atrial activation front (fibrillatory waves)
- Varying conduction of atrial impulse through AV node gives uneven ventricular rate

Drugs, disorders, and other factors that may alter results

- Interpretation of ECG may be confused by coexistence of other rhythm disorders, such as Wolff–Parkinson–White syndrome, heart block, presence of ventricular extrasystoles
- Digoxin treatment alters the appearance of the ECG, giving an inverted T wave with a steep take-off from a depressed ST segment; the P-R interval is prolonged and the Q-T segment shortened

Imaging

CHEST X-RAY

Advantages/Disadvantages

Advantages:

- May give information about complications of atrial fibrillation (e.g. heart failure)
- May indicate cause of atrial fibrillation (e.g. structural heart disease)

Abnormal

May show signs of:

- Heart failure (upper lobe venous diversion, Kerley B lines, pleural effusion)
- Cardiac enlargement
- Structural disease such as mitral stenosis (straight left heart border, prominent left atrial appendage, dilated left atrium, calcified valve)
- In a young patient, may show atrial septal defect (cardiomegaly, prominent hila, pulmonary plethora)

Cause of abnormal result
- Heart failure
- Cardiac enlargement
- Structural disease such as mitral stenosis
- Atrial septal defect
- Keep in mind the possibility of a false-positive result

ECHOCARDIOGRAPHY
Advantages/Disadvantages
Advantages:
- Noninvasive
- Diagnostic of structural disease including valvular heart disease, left atrial myxoma
- Documents left atrial size and left ventricular systolic function, and hence predicts likely success of cardioversion
- Can demonstrate the presence of intra-atrial thrombus – especially transesophageal echo
- Can help predict stroke: independent predictors include left ventricular dysfunction, dilated left atrium

Disadvantage: requires specialized equipment and training to interpret.

Abnormal
- Enlarged left atrium
- Thickening of the left ventricular walls
- Reduced left ventricular ejection fraction
- Valvular abnormalities
- Presence of intracardiac thrombus

Cause of abnormal result
- Intra-atrial thrombus
- Hypertensive changes to the heart
- Structural heart disease (e.g. valvular disease)
- Left atrial myxoma
- Congenital heart disease
- Keep in mind the possibility of a false-positive result

CT SCAN OF THE BRAIN
Description
Noninvasive tomography of the brain.

Advantages/Disadvantages
Advantage: useful in identifying occurrence of cerebrovascular accident.

Abnormal
Focal density or hemorrhage of the brain.

Cause of abnormal result
Cerebrovascular accident.

Drugs, disorders, and other factors that may alter results
If cerebrovascular accident is recent, CT scan may be normal.

TREATMENT

CONSIDER CONSULT

- Hemodynamic emergency or urgency (syncope or near-syncope, angina, or severe dyspnea)
- Structural heart disease requiring further assessment
- Bleeding while on anticoagulation
- Side-effects from cardiac medications (e.g. torsade de pointes)
- Thromboembolic disease

IMMEDIATE ACTION

Rapid ventricular rate causing symptoms requires intravenous drug loading.

MANAGEMENT ISSUES

Goals

- Diagnose and treat any underlying disease
- Improve quality of life – including reassurance for patients with 'lone atrial fibrillation', 'holiday heart', as appropriate
- Reduce symptoms; in acute-onset atrial fibrillation, cardioversion to sinus rhythm is ideal. With longer-standing arrhythmia, aim for ventricular rate control and anticoagulation as an alternative
- Trials to determine optimal management philosophy for chronic atrial fibrillation are awaited. At present, rhythm control (cardioversion and drugs to restore and maintain sinus rhythm) and rate control (ventricular rate control and anticoagulation) are equally valid
- Both alternatives have risks and benefits; patient preference is important
- Limit major complications, especially thromboembolism and cardiomyopathy due to chronic tachyarrhythmia
- Limit adverse effects of treatment

Management in special circumstances

- Younger patients who have structurally normal hearts ('lone atrial fibrillation') have a very low risk of stroke and should be managed accordingly with aspirin instead of warfarin
- In patients with congestive heart failure, an acute decompensation may trigger atrial fibrillation

COEXISTING DISEASE

Look for and treat coexisting disease if possible, as this may reverse atrial fibrillation.

COEXISTING MEDICATION

Check that the patient is not using a nonprescription medication that includes catecholamines or theophylline compounds, or medications that prolong the QT interval (terfenadine, cisapride, or astemizole).

SPECIAL PATIENT GROUPS

Pregnancy:

- Atrial fibrillation is uncommon during pregnancy if patient is free of structural heart disease
- Beta-blockers are preferable to calcium channel blockers
- If DC cardioversion is needed, this is usually not associated with fetal complications
- However, warfarin is associated with fetal anomalies; hence subcutaneous heparin is preferred

PATIENT SATISFACTION/LIFESTYLE PRIORITIES

- Warn patients that, even with optimal treatment, rhythm disturbance can recur. Patients may continue to experience some symptoms, and the drugs themselves can have significant side-effects
- Patients with paroxysmal atrial fibrillation should avoid precipitating dietary factors, such as alcohol and caffeine

SUMMARY OF THERAPEUTIC OPTIONS

Choices

- Therapeutic aims are to improve quality of life by controlling the dysrhythmia and to prevent complications, particularly stroke
- In most cases, medical management achieves these aims, although many of the options have serious side-effects and require careful balancing of risks and benefits as well as long-term close monitoring
- Must be aware that all antiarrhythmic drugs can also be proarrhythmic and may promote potentially serious arrhythmias, especially ventricular tachycardia
- Lifestyle changes may prevent some attacks, particularly where the arrhythmia is associated with alcohol or caffeine ingestion
- Resistant cases, particularly where there are other indications such as coronary heart disease requiring surgery, may benefit from surgery or radiofrequency ablation of AV node and pacemaker implantation

Management strategies for patients with atrial fibrillation:

- Conversion to sinus rhythm using DC cardioversion or pharmacologic agents. In cases where atrial fibrillation is due to hyperthyroidism, reversion to sinus rhythm may follow appropriate endocrine treatment. However, this is often a long delay and may not be helpful in immediate decision-making
- Treat any concomitant conditions such as hyperthyroidism or heart failure
- When sinus rhythm achieved, maintenance medical treatment is usually required
- Where this is not possible, control of the rate improves symptom control. A number of pharmacologic agents exist, but many have serious side-effects (including increased mortality with class I antiarrhythmics) and require close monitoring
- Prevention of stroke using oral anticoagulants, usually warfarin
- In resistant cases, surgery may be useful in selected cases or radioablation of aberrant conduction pathways or radioablation of the AV node and permanent pacemaker may be considered if ventricular rate cannot be controlled with drugs

Pharmacologic management:

- Cardiac glycosides (e.g. digoxin) – well-known and relatively safe option, particularly if patient has heart failure. Useful in rate control, but not FDA approved for conversion of the rhythm. However, may need to be used in combination with a beta-blocker (e.g. metoprolol) or calcium channel blocker (e.g. verapamil) in selected patients
- Antiarrhythmic agents (flecainide, propafenol, sotalol, amiodarone). These drugs are used to control ventricular rate, convert atrial fibrillation to sinus rhythm and maintain it, prevent paroxysms of atrial fibrillation and to control symptoms. Type Ic antiarrthymics (flecainide and propafenol) should not be used in patients with structural heart disease because of higher mortality
- Class Ia antiarrhythmics (fast sodium channel blocker, procainamide) can also have serious adverse effects including proarrhythmic potential and should only be started with the patient under close supervision
- Class III antiarrhythmics (which prolong repolarization) control the rate. Some (e.g. sotalol) have beta-blockade effects useful in patients with coronary heart disease and hypertension
- Amiodarone has become more popular, especially in Europe, and is better tolerated than previously thought (although can still have many side-effects)
- Class IV antiarrhythmics (calcium channel blockers, such as verapamil) offer good rate control but rarely achieve conversion to sinus rhythm and can worsen arrhythmias in some patients
- All antiarrhythmic medications should be started under supervision of a knowledgeable physician. Individual patient circumstances are extremely important in choosing drug therapy

Guidelines for the medical prevention of stroke, an important corollary of atrial fibrillation management, are available from the National Guidelines Clearinghouse, and the American College of Chest Physicians (5th ACCP consensus conference on antithrombotic therapy. Chest 1998;114(5 Suppl):439S–769S). These guidelines state:

- In patients under age 65 and without previous embolism, poor left ventricular function or other major risk factors, long-term aspirin is recommended
- For all other patients, long-term warfarin is strongly recommended (target INR (international normalized ratio) 2.5), but risks of anticoagulation must be balanced against benefits for individual patients

Guidelines

Prystowsky EN, Benson DW, Fuster V, et al. Management of patients with atrial fibrillation. A statement for healthcare professionals from the subcommittee on electrocardiography and electrophysiology, American Heart Association. Circulation 1996;93:1262–77

The American Academy of Family Physicians has published the following information:

- Dell'orfano JT, Luck JC, Wolbrette DL, Patel H. Drugs for conversion of atrial fibrillation. Am Fam Physician 1998;58(2):471–80
- Akhtar W, Reeves W, Movahed A. Indications for anticoagulation in atrial fibrillation. Am Fam Physician 1998;58(1):130–6

Clinical pearl(s)

- Digoxin should be avoided as a sole agent for rate control given its limited effectiveness and narrow therapeutic window. It is not effective when vagal tone is increased, and another AV nodal agent is often needed
- Amiodarone is preferred in post myocardial infarction patients and for those with ventricular dysfunction
- Note that quinidine and amiodarone both increase serum digoxin levels
- Anticoagulation for 4–6 weeks before converting the rhythm is warranted if the duration of atrial fibrillation is more than 48h

Never

- Do not use type Ic drugs (e.g. flecainide) in patients with a history of coronary artery disease or structural heart abnormality
- Do not use type Ia drugs (e.g. procainamide) or sotalol in patients with a history of torsade de pointes
- Do not use class Ia agents until the heart rate is controlled

FOLLOW UP

It is important to monitor patients for drug side-effects and interactions and spontaneous reversion to fibrillation.

Plan for review

Patients on long-term warfarin need monitoring of prothrombin time or INR monthly (or more often, if clinically indicated). Some drug therapy can be guided by serum drug levels. Since many patients with atrial fibrillation have associated medical conditions, continued review of interactions, electrolytes, etc, is needed.

Information for patient or caregiver

All patients on warfarin need detailed instruction on monitoring, dietary issues with vitamin K-containing foods, signs of excessive anticoagulation. All patients should be instructed on what to do if symptoms recur despite medical therapy.

DRUGS AND OTHER THERAPIES: DETAILS

Drugs

WARFARIN

Indication is for full anticoagulation to reduce risk of embolism; aspirin is a less effective alternative.

Dose

- Must be individualized, using international normalized ratio (INR)
- Aim to keep INR between 2.0–3.0 (up to 4.0 under special circumstances) using regular blood tests
- Multiple manufacturers of warfarin; sometimes bioavailability issues become important for a given patient

Efficacy

- Requires full anticoagulation for maximum efficacy
- Many studies have shown that warfarin prevents 20–30 primary strokes per 1000 patient-years of treatment at a cost of 6–8 serious bleeding episodes
- Several multicenter trials have demonstrated that after a first thromboembolic episode, warfarin prevents 80 secondary strokes per 1000 life-years of treatment

Risks/Benefits

Risks:

- Use caution alongside infection and trauma; diverticulitis, renal, and hepatic disease; hypertension, congestive heart failure, and tuberculosis; thyroid disease and diabetes mellitus; protein C deficiency, polyarteritis, and vasculitis
- Use caution in the elderly, children, and nursing mothers

Benefit: Reduced risk of embolism.

Side-effects and adverse reactions

- Gastrointestinal: cramps, diarrhea, vomiting
- CNS: fatigue, headache
- Genitourinary: gonadal dysfunction
- EENT: blurred vision
- Skin: contact dermatitis
- Metabolic: altered thyroid, pituitary, and adrenal hormones
- Musculoskeletal: weakness

Interactions (other drugs)

- Acetaminophen ▪ Allopurinol ▪ Amiodarone ▪ Aminoglutethimide ▪ Aspirin ▪ Azathioprine ▪ Barbiturates ▪ Bile acid-binding resins ▪ Carbamazepine ▪ Cephalosporins ▪ Chloramphenicol ▪ Chloral hydrate ▪ Clofibrate ▪ Co-trimoxazole ▪ Danazole ▪ Dextrothyroxine ▪ Disulfiram ▪ Ethanol ▪ Ethchlorvynol ▪ Fluconazole ▪ Fluorouracil ▪ Gemfibrozil ▪ Glutethimide ▪ Griseofulvin ▪ Glucagon ▪ Heparin ▪ Isoniazid ▪ Metronidazole ▪ Nalidixic acid ▪ Neomycin ▪ NSAIDs ▪ Oral contraceptives ▪ Phenytoin ▪ Propafenones ▪ Propoxyphene ▪ Quinidines ▪ Quinolones ▪ Rifampin ▪ Salicyclates ▪ Sertraline ▪ Sulfonamides ▪ Sulfonylureas ▪ Testosterone derivatives

Contraindications

- Active bleeding ▪ Bacterial endocarditis ▪ Cerebral hemorrhage ▪ Eclampsia ▪ Hemorrhagic blood dyscrasias ▪ Hemorrhagic tendencies ▪ Hypertension ▪ Pericarditis ▪ Recent surgery presenting heightened risk of bleeding ▪ Pregnancy and threatened abortion ▪ Hypertension ▪ Gastrointestinal ulceration ▪ Ulcerative colitis ▪ Visceral carcinoma

Evidence

Warfarin therapy is safe and effective in preventing thromboembolic complications in patients with nonrheumatic atrial fibrillation.

- A RCT (nonblinded) compared warfarin with placebo in the treatment of nonrheumatic atrial fibrillation. The incidence of stroke was decreased in patients receiving warfarin, and the frequency of serious bleeding events was similar for both groups [1] *Level P*
- Patients with nonrheumatic AF were treated with either warfarin, aspirin, or placebo. The patients who received warfarin had a significantly lower incidence of thromboembolic complications and vascular mortality. Warfarin therapy caused nonfatal bleeding complications more often than aspirin [2] *Level P*
- Another RCT compared warfain with placebo in patients with AF. Warfarin-treated patients had a relative risk reduction of 37% for primary outcome event (nonlacunar stroke, nonCNS embolism, and fatal or intracranial hemorrhage) [3] *Level P*

Acceptability to patient

- Some patients find compliance, regular blood tests, and lifestyle restrictions (e.g. diet) difficult to maintain. Drug is ineffective and may be dangerous to use unless the former are observed
- May not be suitable for elderly patients who are forgetful or at risk of falls

Follow up plan

When INR is stable, patient requires INR check every 4–6 weeks; if INR is outside required range, checks should be done more often until control is achieved.

Patient and caregiver information

- Patient must carry anticoagulation warning card at all times
- Must be aware of restrictions on other medications including nonprescription drugs as well as dietary interactions
- Must be aware of risk of hemorrhage

AMIODARONE

- Class III antiarrhythmic
- Prolongs refractoriness of all myocardial tissues
- Weak beta-blocker action
- Treatment should be initiated in a hospital

Dose

Acute treatment (intravenous):

- Intravenous 150–300mg over 1–2min in emergency
- Intravenous infusion 5mg/kg over 20min as loading dose; maintenance 15–20mg/kg over 24h. Start oral dose as soon as possible and overlap oral treatment by 2 days

Chronic treatment (oral):

- Loading dose: 200–400mg three times daily for 1 week, then 200–400mg twice daily for 1 week
- Maintenance: 200–400mg daily (but monitor levels as dose may be less; aim for 0.5–1.5mg/L)

In resistant atrial fibrillation, 4 weeks' loading dose (600mg/day) before cardioversion then 200mg/day maintenance may successful.

Long half-life means dose adjustments are not reflected in serum levels for 1–3 months.

Efficacy

- Highly effective for conversion of atrial fibrillation and maintenance in sinus rhythm
- Up to 75% success rate with intravenous infusion (equivalent to DC conversion success rate)

Risks/Benefits

Risks:

- Should be used only by physicians with access to all methods of treating and monitoring arrhythmias
- Use caution with thyroid and pulmonary disease; AV block and bradycardia; electrolyte imbalances
- Owing to the hazards associated with this drug, a decision should be made in each case as to whether an implantable defibrillator might be a preferable alternative

Benefit:

- May control rhythm in patients refractory to other treatments

Side-effects and adverse reactions

- Gastrointestinal: nausea, vomiting, abdominal pains, constipation, diarrhea, hepatotoxicity, taste abnormalities
- Cardiovascular: congestive heart failure, hypotension, SA node dysfunction, bradycardia, conduction abnormalities, dysrhythmias
- Respiratory: cough, dyspnea, pulmonary fibrosis
- CNS: headache, ataxia, dizziness, fatigue, tremors, paresthesia, peripheral neuropathy
- EENT: visual disturbances, photophobia, dry eyes
- Metabolic: altered thyroid function
- Musculoskeletal: weakness
- Skin: contact dermatitis, rashes, itching, angioedema

Interactions (other drugs)

■ **Antiretroviral protease inhibitors**
■ **Antiarrhythmics (flecainide, digoxin, dofetilide, procainamide, quinidine, beta-blockers, calcium-channel blockers)** ■ **Cevimeline** ■ **Cholestyramine** ■ **Cisapride** ■ **Cyclosporine** ■ **Dextromethorphan** ■ **Fentanyl** ■ **Fosphenytoin** ■ **Gatifloxacin, grepafloxacin, moxifloxacin, sparfloxacin** ■ **Inhalation anesthetics** ■ **Irbesartan** ■ **Phenothiazines** ■ **Phenytoin** ■ **Pimozide** ■ **Sirolimus** ■ **Tramadol** ■ **Tricyclic antidepressants** ■ **Warfarin**

Contraindications

■ **Atrioventricular block** ■ **Hypotension** ■ **Hypersensitivity** ■ **Pregnancy** ■ **Severe sinus node disease with bradycardia** ■ **Syncope**

Evidence

Amiodarone may be useful in converting patients to sinus rhythm, and in preventing recurrence of atrial fibrillation.

- A RCT compared amiodarone with verapamil in patients with paroxysmal atrial fibrillation. After intravenous administration, amiodarone was found to be more effective than verapamil in converting patients to sinus rhythm [4] *Level P*
- A RCT compared amiodarone with sotalol and propafenone in the treatment of atrial fibrillation. Amiodarone is more effective than sotalol or propafenone for the prevention of recurrences of atrial fibrillation, but side-effects necessitated more patients discontinuing amiodarone than sotalol [5] *Level P*

Acceptability to patient

Significant incidence of side-effects and requirement for continuous monitoring makes drug less acceptable.

Follow up plan
- Thyroid, liver, pulmonary function tests
- Monitor for side-effects

Patient and caregiver information
- Regular blood tests required
- Avoid sun exposure

DIGOXIN
- Cardiac glycoside
- Inotrope and AV nodal blocker

Dose
- Must check renal function and potassium levels before starting drug
- Must be tailored to patient, taking account of renal function (as drug is mainly excreted through kidneys), clinical response, and serum drug levels
- Therapeutic range: 0.8–1.2mcg/L
- Loading dose: oral or intravenous, 250–500mcg every 4–6h to maximum of 1.5mg
- Halve this dose in the elderly
- Maintenance: oral 62.5–250mcg once daily
- Onset of effects 4–6h after taking drug (orally or intravenous)

Efficacy
- Usually does not convert atrial fibrillation to sinus rhythm
- Less effective in controlling ventricular rate in exercise than other drug options – may need to add beta-blocker or calcium channel blocker to slow AV nodal conduction

Risks/Benefits
Risks:
- Avoid in Wolff–Parkinson–White syndrome
- Use caution with electrolyte imbalances; with severe pulmonary disease, hepatic disease, or hypothyroidism; with sick sinus syndrome, acute myocardial infarction, or AV block
- Use caution in the elderly

Benefits:
- Within therapeutic range, it is a safe drug with few side-effects
- Lanoxin and amiodarone are the only positive inotropes for this condition, so it is useful for patients with heart failure and atrial fibrillation
- Reduces heart-failure hospitalizations

Side-effects and adverse reactions
- Gastrointestinal: bleeding, vomiting, diarrhea, nausea, discomfort
- Hematologic: eosinophilia, thrombocytopenia
- Skin: rash
- CNS: confusion, hallucinations, depression, seizures
- Cardiovascular system: atrial and ventricular fibrillation, AV block, bradycardia
- EENT: green/yellow vision

Interactions (other drugs)
- **Antidysrhythmics (calcium channel blockers, amiodarone, quinidine, propafenone)**
- **Antihypertensives** ▪ **Antimalarials** ▪ **Azole antifungals** ▪ **Benzodiazepines** ▪ **Calcium**
- **Charcoal** ▪ **Cholestyramine** ▪ **Cyclophosphamide** ▪ **Cyclosporine, tacrolimus**
- **Diuretics** ▪ **Erythromycin and tetracyclines** ▪ **Metoclopramide, cisapride** ▪ **NSAIDs**
- **Proton pump inhibitors** ▪ **St. John's wort** ▪ **Succinylcholine**

Contraindications

- **Ventricular fibrillation** ■ **SA or AV node disease** ■ **Idiopathic hypertrophic subaortic stenosis** ■ **Hypertrophic obstructive cardiomyopathy** ■ **Hypokalemia of less than 2.0**

Evidence

Digoxin is useful when rate control during exercise is less important. In patients with recent-onset AF, digoxin is not effective in restoring sinus rhythm, but ventricular rate is decreased.

- A systematic review of RCTs of rate control medications in patients with atrial fibrillation has been conducted. Digoxin is more effective than placebo in controlling heart rate at rest, but is less effective during exercise [6] *Level M*
- A RCT of patients with acute AF found that ventricular rate was reduced at 2h after administration of digoxin, but that sinus rhythm was not restored at 16h [7] *Level P*

Acceptability to patient

High.

Follow up plan

Must monitor drug levels: take blood immediately before dose (trough level) and again after 6 h (peak).

VERAPAMIL

- Calcium channel blocker
- Direct effect on AV node, increasing refractoriness and conduction time
- Class IV antiarrhythmic drug

Dose

- Loading dose: 5mg intravenously slowly over 2–3min under continuous ECG monitoring. Repeat after 5–10min if necessary
- Maintenance: intravenous infusion 5–10mg/h to maximum of 100mg/day or oral 120–480mg/day
- Stabilize patient on standard tablets, then transfer to once/day preparation

Efficacy

Action on AV node refractory period may give improved exercise capacity.

Risks/Benefits

Risks:

- Contraindicated in Wolff–Parkinson–White syndrome because increases risk of ventricular fibrillation and severe heart failure
- The vasodilatory effects of verapamil may cause hemodynamic complications in patients with a substantial outflow gradient or markedly elevated pulmonary pressure
- Use caution with congestive heart failure and hypotension; renal and hepatic disease; Duchenne muscular dystrophy; during acute phase of myocardial infarction
- Use caution in concomitant beta-blocker therapy
- Use caution in children

Side–effects and adverse reactions

- Gastrointestinal: nausea, constipation, vomiting, abdominal pain
- CNS: dizziness, flushing, headache, fatigue
- EENT: tinnitus
- Genitourinary: impotence, nocturia, polyuria, gynecomastia
- Cardiovascular: tachycardia, bradycardia, palpitations, congestive heart failure, atrioventricular block, hypotension, peripheral edema
- Skin: rash

Interactions (other drugs)

■ Antidysrhythmics (amiodarone, digoxin, disopyramide, dofetilide, encainide, flecainide, procainamide, quinidine) ■ Antihypertensives (particularly alpha- and beta-blockers) ■ Antivirals ■ Aspirin ■ Azole antifungals ■ Barbiturates ■ Benzodiazepines ■ Buspirone ■ Calcium ■ Carbamazepine ■ Cardiac glycosides ■ Cimetidine ■ Cisapride ■ Clarithromycin, erythromycin ■ Cyclosporine, tacrolimus ■ Dantrolene ■ Diclofenac ■ Doxorubicin ■ Ethanol ■ Fentanyl ■ General and local anesthetics ■ Grapefruit juice ■ Histamine H_2 antagonists ■ Imipramine ■ Lithium ■ Neuromuscular blockers ■ Phenytoin ■ Rifampin ■ SSRIs ■ Statins ■ Theophylline

Contraindications

■ Wolff–Parkinson–White syndrome ■ Cardiogenic shock ■ Heart block ■ Sick sinus syndrome
■ Severe heart failure, history of heart failure ■ Hypotension ■ Pregnancy ■ Porphyria

Evidence

Verapamil may be useful in slowing the ventricular rate in patients with atrial fibrillation.

- A systematic review of RCTs of rate control medications in patients with atrial fibrillation has been conducted. Calcium channel blockers control the heart rate in atrial fibrillation at rest and during exercise [6] *Level M*
- A RCT compared intravenous verapamil with placebo in patients with acute atrial fibrillation. The ventricular rate was reduced within 10 min of verapamil administration [8] *Level P*
- Another trial comparing verapamil with placebo in patients with atrial fibrillation or flutter found no significant diference between the treatment and control groups [9] *Level P*

Patient and caregiver information

Warn about constipation; try high-fiber diet preventively.

SOTALOL

- Nonselective beta-blocker
- Class III antiarrhythmic (can be proarrhythmic)
- Off-label indication

Dose

- Loading: 0.5–1.5mg/kg infused intravenously over at least 10min; can be repeated at 10min intervals to maximum of 640mg
- Maintenance: 80–160mg orally twice daily

Efficacy

- Effective in controlling ventricular rate without the need for other drugs
- Beta-blockade action may make it useful in patients with hypertension and coronary heart disease
- Continuation of beta-blockers after cardiac surgery may prevent recurrent atrial fibrillation

Risks/Benefits

Risks:

- Negative inotropic effect may worsen heart failure
- Proarrhythmic, especially where QT interval prolonged and/or potassium level low; risk of torsade de pointes
- May aggravate obstructive airways disease
- Can mask hypoglycemic symptoms – important for diabetics
- Peripheral vascular disease symptoms may be aggravated
- Do not withdraw sotalol treatment abruptly
- Use caution in hyperthyroidism, electrolyte imabalance, renal impairment, vasospastic angina, and pheochromocytoma
- Use caution in surgery

Side-effects and adverse reactions

- Gastrointestinal: nausea, vomiting, diarrhea, constipation
- Cardiovascular: beta-blockers must not be withdrawn suddenly in coronary heart disease – may precipitate myocardial infarction; sinus bradycardia, angina, palpitations, QT prolongation, proarrhythmic events, torsade de pointes, peripheral vasoconstriction
- CNS: fatigue, dizziness, sleep disturbances
- Respiratory: dyspnea, bronchospasm
- Metabolic: hyperglycemia
- Skin: rashes, exacerbation of psoriasis
- Hematologic: blood cell dyscrasias

Interactions (other drugs)

■ Alpha-blockers and agonists ■ Antacids ■ Antiarrhythmics (amiodarone, adenosine, disopyramide, procainamide, quinidine, dofeltilide, lidocaine, flecainide) ■ Antidepressants (tricyclic and possibly MAOIs) ■ Astemizole ■ Calcium channel blockers ■ Cevimeline ■ Cimetidine ■ Cisapride ■ Clarithromycin, erythromycin, and fluoroquinolones ■ Clonidine ■ Cocaine ■ Digoxin ■ Diuretics ■ Hypoglycemic agents ■ Insulin ■ Liothyronine ■ Neostigmine, physostigmine ■ Neuroleptics ■ NSAIDs ■ Phenothiazines ■ Pimozide ■ Reserpine ■ Tacrine ■ Terbutaline ■ Terfenadine ■ Theophylline

Contraindications

■ Sinus bradycardia ■ Sick sinus syndrome ■ Second- or third- degree AV block ■ QT prolongation syndromes ■ Heart failure ■ Hypokalemia ■ Cardiogenic shock ■ Bronchospastic disorders and asthma ■ Raynaud's disease or peripheral vascular disease

Evidence

Selected beta-blockers control the heart rate in atrial fibrillation at rest and during exercise.

- A systematic review of RCTs of rate control medications in patients with atrial fibrillation has been conducted. Trials comparing beta-blockers with placebo showed beta-blockers controlled the heart rate. There is evidence that this effect may be drug-specific, as atenolol and nadolol were the most effective beta-blockers [6] *Level M*
- A RCT compared amiodarone with sotalol and propafenone in the treatment of atrial fibrillation. Amiodarone was more effective than sotalol for the prevention of recurrences of atrial fibrillation, but side-effects necessitated more patients discontinuing amiodarone than sotalol [7] *Level P*

Acceptability to patient

Fair.

Follow up plan

Monitor potassium levels as hypokalemia increases risk of arrhythmia.

Patient and caregiver information

Warn patient with history of coronary heart disease that stopping drug suddenly risks increasing angina or may precipitate myocardial infarction or ventricular arrhythmia.

METOPROLOL

- Cardioselective beta-blocker
- Used to control rate in atrial fibrillation
- This is an off-label indication

Dose

50mg two or three times daily.

Efficacy

Effective at decreasing heart rate; slows conduction at the atrioventricular node.

Risks/Benefits

Risks:

- Proarrhythmic agent, so may cause bradycardia or heart block
- Use with caution in diabetes mellitus, thyroid disease, renal disease, peripheral vascular disease, Raynaud's syndrome
- Use with caution in pregnancy

Benefit: often effective at slowing heart rate; may be useful in combination with digoxin.

Side-effects and adverse reactions

- Gastrointestinal: nausea, dry mouth, dyspepsia, constipation
- Respiratory: bronchospasm, wheezing, dyspnea
- CNS: lethargy, depression, vivid dreams, dizziness, confusion, fatigue
- Genitourinary: impotence, sexual dysfunction
- Cardiovascular: congestive heart failure, bradycardia heart block, peripheral vascular disease
- EENT: tinnitus, visual disturbances
- Hematologic: agranulocytosis
- Metabolism: hyperglycemia, hyperlipidemia, masked hypoglycemia
- Skin: bruising, rash, alopecia

Interactions (other drugs)

- **Alpha-adrenergic blockers, beta-agonists**
- **Antidysrhythmics (amiodarone, digoxin, calcium channel blockers)**
- **Antidiabetics** ▪ **Barbiturates** ▪ **Benzodiazepines** ▪ **Clonidine** ▪ **Dipyridamole**
- **Fluoxetine** ▪ **Hypoglycemic agents** ▪ **Local anesthetics** ▪ **NSAIDs** ▪ **Phenylephrine**
- **Quinolones** ▪ **Rifampin** ▪ **Theophylline**

Contraindications

- **In treatment of myocardial infarction, patients with hypotension**
- **Bronchospastic diseases, asthma** ▪ **Cardiogenic shock** ▪ **Congestive heart failure**
- **Advanced atrioventricular heart block** ▪ **Severe bradycardia** ▪ **Hepatic disease**

Evidence

Selected beta-blockers control the heart rate in atrial fibrillation at rest and during exercise.

- A systematic review of RCTs of rate control medications in patients with atrial fibrillation has been conducted. Trials comparing beta-blockers with placebo showed beta-blockers controlled the heart rate. There is evidence that this effect may be drug-specific, as atenolol and nadolol were the most effective beta-blockers [6] *Level M*

Acceptability to patient

Generally good.

Patient and caregiver information

Patients should be advised not to discontinue metoprolol suddenly.

FLECAINIDE

- Class Ic antiarrhythmic agent
- Indicated for paroxysmal atrial fibrillation associated with disabling symptoms

Dose

- 50mg orally every 12h, increased every 4 days by 50mg every 12h if necessary
- Maximum dose: 300mg/day
- Therapeutic trough serum level is 0.2–1.0mcg/mL

Efficacy

Effective antiarrhythmic agent; decreases intracardiac conduction in all cardiac areas.

Risks/Benefits

Risks:

- Use caution in hepatic or renal impairment; respiratory depression; myasthenia gravis
- Use caution in children under 18 years old; in pregnancy and breast-feeding

Benefits: may provide good relief to patients whose atrial fibrillation is otherwise resistant to treatment.

Side-effects and adverse reactions

- Gastrointestinal: nausea, vomiting, diarrhea, constipation, flatulence, abdominal pain, taste changes, dry mouth
- Cardiovascular: angina, palpitations, edema, ventricular tachycardia, sinus bradycardia, QT prolongation, torsade de pointes, proarrhythmic effect, congestive heart failure
- Central nervous system: headache, dizziness, fatigue, asthenia, tremor, vertigo, somnolence, anxiety, insomnia, depression
- Ears, eyes, nose, and throat: visual impairment, tinnitus
- Genitourinary: impotence, urinary difficulties, loss of libido
- Hematologic: leukopenia, thrombocytopenia
- Skin: rashes, pruritus, urticaria

Interactions (other drugs)

■ Acetazolamide ■ Amiodarone ■ Antacids ■ Antiarrhythmics ■ Antidepressants (tricyclic) ■ Beta-blockers ■ Cimetidine ■ Diuretics ■ Fluoxetine ■ Quinine ■ Ritonavir ■ Verapamil

Contraindications

■ Cardiogenic shock ■ AV block, bundle branch block ■ Frequent PVCs ■ Heart failure ■ Recent myocardial infarction (MI), history of MI, and either asymptomatic ventricular ectopics or asymptomatic nonsustained ventricular tachycardia ■ Sick sinus syndrome

Acceptability to patient

Generally reasonable, given that the drug is used in patients whose atrial fibrillation is difficult to control and is causing severe symptoms.

Follow up plan

Trough plasma levels of flecainide should be monitored, especially in patients with severe renal or hepatic impairment.

PROCAINAMIDE

- Class Ia antiarrhythmic agent
- Used to suppress recurrent paroxysmal atrial fibrillation
- This is an off-label indication

Dose

- 250–500mg orally every 3–6h
- Intravenous: 100mg/5min up to 1g, with continuous ECG and blood pressure monitoring
- Therapeutic trough plasma level is 3–10mcg/mL

Efficacy

Can be effective at suppressing paroxysmal atrial fibrillation; decreases myocardial conduction velocity and excitability, and prolongs atrial refractive period and action potential.

Risks/Benefits

Risks:

- Use caution in tartrazine or sulfide sensitivity; dental disease; and in breast-feeding
- Use caution in myasthenia gravis; renal dysfunction or hepatic impairment; history of idiopathic systemic lupus erythematosus; congestive heart failure; and following myocardial infarction

Benefit: may provide good relief to patients whose atrial fibrillation is otherwise resistant to treatment.

Side-effects and adverse reactions

- Gastrointestinal: nausea, diarrhea, vomiting, abdominal pain, bitter taste
- Cardiovascular: myocardial depression, heart failure, hypotension, ventricular arrhythmias, second-degree heart block, PR and QT prolongation, torsade de pointes, angioedema
- Hematologic: neutropenia, agranulocytosis, bone marrow depression, agranulocytosis, thrombocytopenia
- CNS: dizziness, confusion, psychosis, headache, hallucinations
- Lupus erythematosus-like syndrome in prolonged therapy

Interactions (other drugs)

- Amiodarone
- Antiarrhythmics
- Antidepressants (tricyclic)
- Antihypertensives
- Captopril
- Cimetidine
- Ethanol
- Muscle relaxants
- Neostigmine
- Ofloxacin
- Phenothiazines
- Pimozide
- Pyridostigmine
- Sotalol
- Thioridazine
- Trimethoprim

Contraindications

- Heart block
- Hypotension
- Digitalis toxicity
- Torsades de pointes
- Pre-existing cytopenia or bone marrow depression
- Intramuscular injections

Acceptability to patient

Generally reasonable in short term, but often poor long term because of the development of lupus-like syndrome. Does require several doses daily even with sustained-release preparations.

Follow up plan

- Patients should have weekly complete blood count for the first 3 months of treatment and every 2–3 months after this
- ECG should be monitored to look for widening of the QRS complex or prolongation of the QT interval, especially during intravenous administration; dosage should be reduced if the QRS complex widens by more than 50%
- Serum creatinine and blood urea nitrogen should be checked periodically
- Plasma procainamide concentration should be checked periodically (procainamide plus N-acetyl-procainamide levels are totaled)

Patient and caregiver information

Report symptoms of joint swelling, skin rash, headache, personality changes (systemic lupus erythematosus symptoms).

Surgical therapy

- Cardiac surgery is generally limited to those patients who are medically refractory and severely symptomatic
- Radiofrequency ablation procedures, the Maze procedure, or ablation of pulmonary vein foci are under investigation; however ablation of the AV node with insertion of permanent pacemaker is an alternative to chronic medication therapy

MAZE OPERATION

- Aims to prevent atrial fibrillation by directing all atrial electrical activity between a series of incisions and thus restoring coordinated atrial and ventricular activity
- Claimed to result in good cardiac output and a low risk of intracardiac thrombus development
- Consider if patient severely symptomatic, but failing to respond to other treatment, or patient having concomitant surgery
- Only available in highly specialized centers

Efficacy

Usually requires permanent postoperative pacemaker.

Risks/Benefits

Risk: stroke or embolism.

Acceptability to patient

In context of cardiac surgery for other indications, acceptable.

Follow up plan

In view of risk of arrhythmia recurrence during the first 3 months postoperatively, patients require close monitoring over this period and may require short-term medical treatment.

Other therapies

DC CARDIOVERSION

- External DC shock, synchronized to the R wave
- Permits uniform repolarization after initial atrial asystole and is followed by ordered conduction throughout the heart as sinoatrial node regains role as natural cardiac pacemaker
- Requires at least 3 weeks, therapeutic anticoagulation before treatment unless atrial fibrillation is less than 48h duration or is an emergency procedure for hemodynamic reasons
- In hospitals where transesophageal echocardiography is available to exclude the presence of intra-atrial thrombus, patients can be cardioverted without the need for pretreatment anticoagulation with warfarin
- At least 4 weeks, anticoagulation is required after the procedure in all cases as normal atrial contractions are not immediately regained (atrial stunning); atrial fibrillation may also recur

Should be considered for all patients with:

- Recent-onset atrial fibrillation of less than 24–48h duration
- Failed pharmacologic cardioversion
- Successful treatment of the underlying cause (e.g. thyrotoxicosis)
- No structural abnormality of the heart, such as mitral valve disease, poor left ventricular function, or a dilated left atrium

Efficacy

- Highly successful when good technique used
- Maintained success depends on cause of atrial fibrillation – best for atrial fibrillation related to hyperthyroidism (90% success); worst when severe valvular disease (e.g. mitral regurgitation) (20% success) or other cause of left atrial enlargement over 5cm

Predictors of poor outcome:
- Atrial fibrillation for >1 year (main predictor)
- Age >50 years (controversial as independent predictor)
- Hypertension
- No correctable precipitating factor(s)
- Structural heart disease (e.g. left atrial diameter >45mm)
- Associated heart failure of New York Heart Association class II or greater

Risks/Benefits

Benefits:
- May avoid use of antiarrhythmic drugs
- Rapid return to wellbeing and premorbid exercise capacity
- May reduce risk of thromboembolism if sinus rhythm sustained

Risks:
- Peripheral emboli complicate 1–3% cases; highest risk of embolism during first 4 weeks postcardioversion. American Association of Chest Physicians recommends anticoagulation for 3 weeks before elective cardioversion (INR 2–3 for most patients; if at particularly high risk (e.g. history of thromboembolism), INR 3.0–4.5). However, anticoagulation does not completely prevent occurrence. Use intravenous heparin followed by warfarin if urgent cardioversion required
- Skin burns may occur
- Avoid if digoxin toxicity suspected or possible
- Ventricular fibrillation can follow nonsynchronized shock

Acceptability to patient
- Requires day admission for ECG monitoring and to ensure electrolytes (especially potassium) and anticoagulation levels are optimal
- Requires short general anesthetic or conscious sedation
- Some patients fear concept of electrical cardioversion

Follow up plan

Should have close routine outpatient follow up to monitor maintenance of normal sinus rhythm; this may require a Holter monitor.

Patient and caregiver information
- Elective DC cardioversion requires brief admission to hospital and short general anesthetic or conscious sedation
- No food or drink for 6–8h before procedure to reduce risk of aspiration
- If successful, may allow patient to avoid need for antiarrhythmic drugs, with their associated disadvantages and risks

RADIOFREQUENCY ABLATION OF AV NODE AND PACEMAKER IMPLANTATION
- Patients who respond poorly to drugs should be referred to be considered for radiofrequency ablation of the AV node and bundle of His using a catheter, with implantation of a permanent pacemaker
- Mainly useful for re-entry arrhythmias (e.g. Wolff–Parkinson–White syndrome)
- Also recently successful in selected patients with fibrillation, by ablating focal sources of atrial electrical activity – refer younger patients where the arrhythmia is sufficiently troublesome to require any form of treatment

Efficacy
- Very successful for rate control
- Usually successful at first treatment in re-entry syndromes

Risks/Benefits

Risks:

- Requires pacemaker to be monitored for life
- Anticoagulation still required
- Still under assessment in atrial fibrillation
- Requires specialist referral

Benefit: relatively noninvasive.

Evidence

Radiofrequency catheter ablation may be recommended for certain patients with atrial fibrillation.

- Patients with atrial tachycardia, paroxysmal atrial fibrillation associated with atrial tachycardia, and atrial fibrillation with a localized site of origin, when the tachycardia is drug resistant, or there is drug intolerance, or desire for avoidance of long-term drug therapy [10] *Level C*

Acceptability to patient

High.

Follow up plan

Pacemaker should be tested 6-monthly for life.

Patient and caregiver information

- Warn about triggering airport security
- Avoid MRI scans, electromagnetic fields

ABLATION OF CARDIAC TISSUE AROUND PULMONARY VEINS

- Recent development for treatment of paroxysmal atrial fibrillation
- Only available in specialized centers
- Needs referral to specialist

Efficacy

Successful in majority of suitable patients.

Risks/Benefits

Risks:

- Long-term efficacy is still not clear
- Invasive procedure

Benefit: successful conversion could obviate the need for chronic cardiac medication.

Evidence

Radiofrequency ablation of pulmonary vein foci may be an effective treatment for paroxysmal atrial fibrillation.

- In a prospective trial of 45 patients with frequent attacks of paroxysmal atrial fibrillation, 94% of trigger depolarizations occurred around the pulmonary veins and radiofrequency ablation of these foci rendered 62% disease-free at 8 ± 6 months [11] *Level P*
- Most paroxysms of atrial fibrillation are initiated by series of rapid discharges from the pulmonary veins. 110 patients with paroxysmal atrial fibrillation underwent radiofrequency catheter ablation targeting these triggers; 69% were free of atrial fibrillation at a follow-up of 8 ± 4 months. Six of the targeted pulmonary veins (4%) developed pulmonary vein stenosis but did not require treatment [12] *Level P*

Acceptability to patient
Moderate, owing to limited availability.

Follow up plan
Will need periodic regular follow up to confirm maintenance of normal sinus rhythm.

Patient and caregiver information
- Procedure not widely available
- New technique, so long-term outcome information not yet available

LIFESTYLE
Reduce intake of alcohol and caffeine in paroxysmal atrial fibrillation.

RISKS/BENEFITS
Risks: none unless chronic alcohol abuse (risk of precipitating atrial fibrillation and of alcohol withdrawal syndrome)

ACCEPTABILITY TO PATIENT
If concerned about arrhythmia, lifestyle changes likely to be acceptable to patient.

PATIENT AND CAREGIVER INFORMATION
- Educate patient and family about signs of heart failure
- Reassure that long-term medication is beneficial, but should be warned to watch for specific signs of toxicity and report promptly for medical attention

OUTCOMES

EFFICACY OF THERAPIES

Depends on underlying cause of arrhythmia and delay to treatment.

Evidence

- Warfarin therapy reduces the risk of stroke in patients with nonvalvular atrial fibrillation. The increased risk of bleeding does not offset the benefit [13] *Level M*
- Patients with atrial fibrillation (nonrheumatic) and recent cerebral ischemia benefit from treatment with oral anticoagulants [14] *Level M*
- Amiodarone is more effective than sotalol for the prevention of recurrences of atrial fibrillation but side-effects necessitated more patients discontinuing amiodarone than sotalol [5] *Level P*
- Digoxin is useful when rate control during exercise is less important [6] *Level M*
- Calcium channel blockers can control the heart rate in atrial fibrillation at rest and during exercise [6] *Level M*
- Selected beta-blockers can control the heart rate in atrial fibrillation at rest and during exercise [5] *Level M*
- Radiofrequency ablation of pulmonary vein foci may be an effective treatment for paroxysmal atrial fibrillation [11] *Level P*
- PDxMD is unable to cite evidence that meets our criteria for flecainide, procainamide, Maze operation, and DC cardioversion

Review period

- Young patients with no other disease can be reassured and have limited follow up
- Older patients, particularly those on medications above, require regular lifetime follow up

PROGNOSIS

Although evidence in younger patients with no other pathology is conflicting, atrial fibrillation is associated with reduced life expectancy in older patients. In some cases, antiarrhythmic drugs appear to contribute to increased mortality.

Clinical pearl(s)

- Results of prospective trials comparing the efficacy and quality of life with heart rate control and anticoagulation vs rhythm control are pending
- Uncontrolled heart rates may lead to tachycardia-mediated cardiomyopathy

Therapeutic failure

- Where pharmacologic conversion to sinus rhythm fails, it is worth considering one attempt at DC conversion, even in chronic atrial fibrillation if adverse predictors not overwhelming (see above)
- Use of antiarrhythmic drugs is frequently a balance between unwanted side-effects and rhythm control

Recurrence

Risk of recurrence is high after successful conversion to sinus rhythm, particularly in first 3 months, if no maintenance therapy commenced.

Deterioration

Continued and uncontrolled tachyarrhythmia can lead to cardiomyopathy.

Terminal illness

Associated with underlying cause of arrhythmia.

COMPLICATIONS

- Stroke is major complication
- Heart failure

CONSIDER CONSULT

- When usual drugs for atrial fibrillation fail to control rate or symptoms
- When there are frequent episodes of paroxysmal fibrillation
- If specialist consultation is needed for interpretation of echocardiography for assessment (e.g. with valvular heart disease)
- For investigation and possible ablation of abnormal pathways, ablation of AV node and permanent pacemaker, or ablation of focal atrial fibrillation

PREVENTION

Most important in paroxysmal atrial fibrillation.

RISK FACTORS

- **Alcohol:** acute alcoholic intoxication or alcohol withdrawal may precipitate paroxysmal atrial fibrillation
- **Caffeine:** may induce paroxysmal atrial fibrillation in susceptible individuals
- **Smoking:** is a risk factor for coronary heart disease, and a cause of atrial fibrillation

MODIFY RISK FACTORS

Lifestyle and wellness

TOBACCO

General advice is to avoid smoking in all cardiovascular conditions; coronary heart disease is an important cause of atrial fibrillation.

ALCOHOL AND DRUGS

Avoid alcohol in paroxysmal atrial fibrillation.

DIET

Avoid caffeine in paroxysmal atrial fibrillation.

DRUG HISTORY

It is important that the patient consults a physician, especially before taking any nonprescription medications, as these may precipitate an attack of atrial fibrillation, or interact with prescribed drugs.

SCREENING

As the population ages, the incidence of atrial fibrillation will rise. Prevention of stroke by early diagnosis of atrial fibrillation and prophylactic anticoagulation should reduce the morbidity and mortality from stroke in this group. Primary care physicians should consider screening patients complaining of palpitations or syncope, those with stroke or transient ischemic attacks, or heart failure, and those on regular diuretic therapy or digoxin.

ELECTROCARDIOGRAPHY

Simple, noninvasive diagnostic test.

Cost/efficacy

Main expense is time taken to record the ECG.

ASSOCIATIONS

The American College of Cardiology
Heart House
9111 Old Georgetown Road
Bethesda
MD 20814-1699
Tel: (800) 253-4636 or (301) 897-5400
Fax: (301) 897-9745
http://www.acc.org

Heart Failure Society of America
Box 358
420 Delaware Street S.E.
Minneapolis
MN 55455
Tel: (612) 626-3864
Fax: (612) 624-2174
http://www.hfsa.org

Canadian Cardiovascular Society
Société Canadienne de Cardiologie
222 Queen Street, Suite 1403
Ottawa, ON, K1P 5V9
Canada
Tel: (613) 569-3407
Fax: (613) 569-6574
http://www.ccs.ca

American Heart Association
National Center
7272 Greenville Avenue
Dallas
TX 75231
http://www.americanheart.org

Heart and Stroke Foundation of Canada
222 Queen Street, Suite 1402
Ottawa, ON, K1P 5V9
Canada
Tel: (613) 569-4361
Fax: (613) 569-3278
http://www.heartandstroke.ca

KEY REFERENCES

- Albers GW. Atrial fibrillation and stroke. Three new studies, three remaining questions. Arch Intern Med 1994;154:1443–8
- Alexander C, Flaker GC. Practical management of atrial fibrillation. South Med J 1999;92:1136–43
- Australian Medicines Handbook, 1st edn. Sponsored by Australasian Society of Clinical and Experimental Pharmacologists and Toxicologists, Pharmacological Society of Australia, Royal Australian College of General Practitioners, 1998
- Connolly SJ. Anticoagulation for patients with atrial fibrillation and risk factors for stroke. BMJ 2000;320:1219–20
- English KM, Channer KS. Managing atrial fibrillation in elderly people (editorial). BMJ 1999;318:1088–9

- Furberg CD, Psaty BM. Prevalence of atrial fibrillation in elderly subjects (the Cardiovascular Health Study). Am J Cardiol 1994;74:236–41
- Kannel WB, Abbott RD, Savage DD, et al. Epidemiologic features of chronic atrial fibrillation. N Engl J Med 1982;306:1018–22
- Lancaster T, Mant J, Singer DE. Stroke prevention in atrial fibrillation. BMJ 1997;314:1563–4
- Laupacis A, Albers GW, Dalen J, et al. Antithrombotic therapy in atrial fibrillation. Chest 1995;108(4 Suppl):352S–359S
- Lip GYH, Beevers DG. ABC of atrial fibrillation: history, epidemiology and importance of atrial fibrillation. BMJ 1995;311:1361–3
- Lip GYH, Beevers DG, Singh SP, Watson RDS. ABC of atrial fibrillation: aetiology, pathophysiology and clinical features. BMJ 1995;311:1425–8
- Lip GYH, Singh SP, Watson RDS. ABC of atrial fibrillation: investigation and non-drug management of atrial fibrillation. BMJ 1995;311:1562–5
- Lip GYH, Watson RDS. ABC of atrial fibrillation: differential diagnosis of atrial fibrillation. BMJ 1995;311:1495–8
- Lip GYH, Watson RDS, Singh SP. ABC of atrial fibrillation: cardioversion of atrial fibrillation. BMJ 1995;311:112–5
- McCrory DC, Matchar DB, Samsa G, et al. Physician attitudes about anticoagulation for nonvalvular atrial fibrillation in the elderly. Arch Intern Med 1995;155:277–81
- McMurray J, Rankin A. Cardiology II: Treatment of heart failure and atrial fibrillation and arrhythmias. BMJ 1994;309:1631–5
- Morgan DR, Trimble M, McVeigh GE. Atrial fibrillation associated with sumatriptan. BMJ 2000;321:275
- Peters, NS. Catheter ablation for cardiac arrhythmias. BMJ 2000;321:716–7
- Report of the Quality Standards Subcommittee of the American Academy of Neurology. Practice Parameter: Stroke prevention in patients with non-valvular atrial fibrillation. Neurology 1998;51:671–3
- Sudlow M, Rodgers H, Kenny RA, Thomson R. Identification of patients with atrial fibrillation in general practice: a study of screening methods. BMJ 1998;317:327–8
- Therapeutic options for atrial fibrillation. Cardiovascular Reviews and Reports 2000;XXI:302

Evidence references

1 The Boston Area Anticoagulation Trial for Atrial Fibrillation Investigators. The effect of low-dose warfarin on the risk of stroke in patients with nonrheumatic atrial fibrillation. N Engl J Med 1990;323:1505–11

2 Petersen P, Boysan G, Godtfredsen J, et al. Placebo-controlled, randomized trial of warfarin and aspirin for prevention of thromboembolic complications in chronic atrial fibrillation. The Copenhagen AFASAK Study. Lancet 1989;1:175–9

3 Connolly SJ, Laupacis A, Gent M, et al. Canadian Atrial Fibrillation Anticoagulation (CAFA) study. J Am Coll Cardiol 1991;18:349–55

4 Noc M, Stajer D, Horvat M. Intravenous amiodarone versus verapamil for acute conversion of paroxysmal atrial fibrillation to sinus rhythm. Am J Cardiol 1990;65:679–80. Reviewed in Clinical Evidence 2001;5:1–7

5 Roy D, Talajic M, Dorian P, et al. Amiodarone to prevent recurrence of atrial fibrillation. Canadian Trial of Atrial Fibrillation Investigators. N Engl J Med 2000;342:913–920

6 Segal JB, McNamara RL, Miller MR, et al. The evidence regarding the drugs used for ventricular rate control. J Fam Pract 2000;49:47–59

7 DAAF trial group. Intravenous digoxin in acute atrial fibrillation. Results of a randomised, placebo-controlled multicentre trial in 239 patients. The Digitalis in Acute AF (DAAF) Trial Group. Eur Heart J 1997;18:649–54. Reviewed in Clinical Evidence 2001;5:1–7

8 Aronow WS, Ferlinz J. Verapamil versus placebo in atrial fibrillation and atrial flutter. Clin Invest Med 1980;3:35–9. Reviewed in Clinical Evidence 2001;5:1–7

9 Waxman HL, Myerburg RJ, Appel R, Sung RJ. Verapamil for control of ventricular rate in paroxysmal supraventricular tachycardia and atrial fibrillation or flutter: a double-blind randomized cross-over study. Ann Intern Med 1981;94:1–6. Reviewed in Clinical Evidence 2001;5:1–7

10 Zipes DP, DiMarco JP, Gillette PC, et al. Guidelines for clinical intracardiac electrophysiological and catheter ablation procedures. A report of the American College of Cardiology/American Heart Association Task Force on Practice Guidelines (Committee on Clinical Intracardiac Electrophysiologic and Catheter Ablation Procedures). J Am Coll Cardiol 1995;26:555–73

11 Haissaguerre M, Jais P, Shah DC, et al. Spontaneous initiation of atrial fibrillation by ectopic beats originating in the pulmonary veins. N Engl J Med 1998;339:659–66

12 Shah DC, Haissaguerre M, Jais P. Catheter ablation of pulmonary vein foci for atrial fibrillation: PV foci ablation for atrial fibrillation. Thorac Cardiovasc Surg 1999;47(Suppl 3):352–6
13 Benavente O, Hart R, Koudstaal P, et al. Oral anticoagulants for preventing stroke in patients with non-valvular atrial fibrillation and no previous history of stroke or transient ischemic attacks (Cochrane Review). In: The Cochrane Library, 3, 2001. Oxford: Update Software
14 Koudstaal PJ. Anticoagulants for preventing stroke in patients with nonrheumatic atrial fibrillation and a histroy of stroke or transient ischemic attacks (Cochrane Review). In: The Cochrane Library, 3, 2001. Oxford: Update Software

FAQS

Question 1

How long should anticoagulation be continued after successful cardioversion?

ANSWER 1
4 weeks.

Question 2

What initial blood tests should be obtained to evaluate for reversible causes of atrial fibrillation?

ANSWER 2
Thyroid function tests, electrolytes.

Question 3

Can atrial fibrillation cause cardiomyopathy?

ANSWER 3
Atrial fibrillation with inadequate rate control can lead to tachycardia-mediated cardiomyopathy.

CONTRIBUTORS

Dennis F Saver, MD
John McB Hodgson, MD
Amer Adam, MD

ATRIAL SEPTAL DEFECT

SUMMARY INFORMATION

DESCRIPTION

- Congenital abnormal communication between the right and left atria
- Three anatomic types: ostium primum (10–15% of atrial septal defects – ASDs) in the lower portion of the atrial septum near the mitral and tricuspid valves, which can be deformed and malfunction; ostium secundum (70–80% of ASDs) central in the region of the fossa ovalis; and sinus venosus defect (10–15% of ASDs) posterior near the orifice of either the superior or inferior vena cava, frequently associated with partial anomalous pulmonary venous return
- 'Probe patent' foramen ovale (PFO) occurs in 25–30% of adults, a condition in which a potential communication exits between the atria. Many authors consider it to be a normal anatomic variant

URGENT ACTION

Urgent surgical intervention may be indicated in cases where there is evidence of ongoing paradoxical systemic embolization or bacterial endocarditis.

KEY! DON'T MISS!

- Once symptoms occur, significant left-to-right shunting and increased pulmonary blood flow exist, and referral is warranted for possible surgical correction before fixed pulmonary hypertension and right-to-left shunting is established
- Asymptomatic abnormalities in the young adult should be documented and followed, with particular attention to endocarditis prophylaxis in patients with ostium primum defects associated with valvular abnormalities

ICD9 CODE
429.71 Atrial septal defect.

SYNONYMS
- ASD
- Patent foramen ovale
- PFO

CARDINAL FEATURES
- Most common form of congenital heart disease, set apart from many other forms of congenital heart disease by the prolonged period of asymptomatic or near-asymptomatic disease
- Early stages: flow between the atria almost exclusively from left to right, causing volume overload of the right heart chambers and pulmonary circulation
- Third to fourth decade of life with uncorrected atrial septal defect (ASD); fatigue, dyspnea, and arrhythmias occur as pulmonary hypertension causes an increase in right heart pressures. This shunt may reverse – blood flows from right to left
- Fourth decade of life onward: increasing right-to-left shunt leads to cyanosis, ventricular dysfunction, and worsening pulmonary hypertension
- Patent foramen ovale (PFO) is usually asymptomatic, although it may present with signs and symptoms of paradoxical embolism

CAUSES
Common causes
Unknown.

Rare causes
Rarely, ASDs occur as a result of a genetically determined disorder:
- Ellis–van Creveld syndrome – small stature, shortening of distal extremities, fusion of carpal bones, hypoplastic nails, dental dysplasia, and upper lip frenula. Congenital heart disease in 50% of patients, most have ASD or single atrium. Autosomal recessive inheritance, one-third of cases associated with parental consanguinity. Most commonly seen in the US in old-order Amish of Lancaster County, Pennsylvania
- Holt–Oram syndrome – upper limb abnormalities (absent, hypoplastic, or 'digitalized' thumbs) and secundum ASD. Autosomal dominant inheritance, 50% of primary relatives also affected
- Syndrome of ASD and prolonged AV conduction – autosomal dominant inheritance
- Lutembacher's syndrome – mitral stenosis (usually secondary to rheumatic heart disease) plus ASD. 0.6–0.7% of cases of mitral stenosis and 4% of ASDs
- Noonan's syndrome – short stature, webbed neck, pectus excavatum, cryptorchidism, and autosomal dominant inheritance. Congenital heart disease (60% have valvular pulmonic stenosis); 20% of Noonan's patients with congenital heart disease have ASD

Contributory or predisposing factors
- More common in females (2:1)
- Higher incidence in patients with Down syndrome

EPIDEMIOLOGY
Incidence and prevalence
INCIDENCE

ASD occurs in 8 of every 1000 live births.

PREVALENCE

PFO is present in up to 35% of adults, and many authors consider this anatomic finding a normal variant.

FREQUENCY

9.8% of all cases of congenital heart disease and 46% of cases of congenital heart disease in adults.

Demographics

AGE

Present at birth.

GENDER

More common in females (2:1).

GENETICS

Usually occurs as a sporadic disorder but may rarely be associated with the following genetic disorders:

- Noonan's syndrome
- Down syndrome
- Ellis–van Creveld syndrome (autosomal recessive inheritance)
- Holt–Oram syndrome (autosomal dominant inheritance)
- Lutembacher's syndrome
- Syndrome of ASD and prolonged AV conduction

GEOGRAPHY

Genetic clustering of Ellis–van Creveld syndrome among old-order Amish in Lancaster County, Pennsylvania, in the US.

DIFFERENTIAL DIAGNOSIS

Mitral stenosis

In both atrial septal defect (ASD) and mitral stenosis, there is often clinical, electrocardiogram (ECG), and X-ray evidence of right ventricular enlargement and increased pulmonary vascularity.

FEATURES

- Facial cyanosis and malar flush
- Prominent jugular venous pulsations
- Atrial fibrillation may be present
- Right ventricular tap or lift
- Diastolic apical thrill
- Accentuated S1 and P2, narrow splitting of S2
- Opening snap of mitral valve audible in expiration at the cardiac apex or along the left sternal border
- Low-pitched, diastolic rumbling murmur heard best at the apex with the patient in left lateral decubitus position
- ECG suggests left atrial enlargement, right axis deviation, and right ventricular hypertrophy
- Chest X-ray shows prominence of the main pulmonary arteries and backward displacement of the esophagus by an enlarged left atrium

Primary pulmonary hypertension

Clinical features of primary pulmonary hypertension are similar to those of both mitral stenosis and ASD, with clinical, ECG, and X-ray evidence of right ventricular enlargement and increased pulmonary vascularity.

FEATURES

- Increased jugular venous pressure
- Right ventricular lift
- Increased P2
- Tricuspid regurgitant flow murmur
- Peripheral cyanosis may be present
- ECG shows right axis deviation and right ventricular hypertrophy
- Chest X-ray demonstrates enlargement of the main pulmonary arteries

SIGNS & SYMPTOMS

Signs

- Childhood disease: widely fixed splitting of S2, diastolic rumbling murmur heard best at the left sternal border caused by increased tricuspid valvular flow
- Mid-life (before age 40): wide, fixed splitting of S2, pulmonic systolic ejection murmur at the upper left sternal border, diastolic tricuspid valve flow rumble diminishes and/or disappears
- Advanced disease (after age 40): loud P2, cyanosis and clubbing, prominent pulmonary artery pulsations, irregular or rapid pulse if atrial fibrillation or supraventricular tachycardia (SVT) occurs, decreased intensity of systolic murmur as shunt reverses, diastolic pulmonic insufficiency murmur may occur, focal neurologic deficits may suggest systemic embolic phenomena
- Patent foramen ovale (PFO): no physical findings until signs of paradoxical embolism develop, such as focal neurologic deficits suggestive of embolic stroke

Symptoms

- Most patients are asymptomatic at presentation
- Exertional dyspnea and symptoms related to atrial tachycardia (palpitations, near-syncope, rarely chest pain) are the most common presenting symptoms
- Focal neurologic deficits suggestive of embolic stroke are the usual presenting symptoms of PFO

ASSOCIATED DISORDERS

Down syndrome.

KEY! DON'T MISS!

- Once symptoms occur, significant left-to-right shunting and increased pulmonary blood flow exist, and referral is warranted for possible surgical correction before fixed pulmonary hypertension and right-to-left shunting is established
- Asymptomatic abnormalities in the young adult should be documented and followed, with particular attention to endocarditis prophylaxis in patients with ostium primum defects associated with valvular abnormalities

CONSIDER CONSULT

Patients with known ASD should be evaluated with further work-up if:

- They are symptomatic
- Pulmonary to systemic flow ratio is >1.5:1.0
- There are signs of right-to-left shunting or pulmonary hypertension
- They have suspected or symptomatic coronary artery disease
- PFO and paradoxical systemic embolism are suspected

INVESTIGATION OF THE PATIENT

Direct questions to patient

Q **Do you have a history of frequent respiratory tract infections – cough, bronchitis, pneumonia?** May be the only presenting sign of ASD

Q **(If the patient is a child) Have you kept up with your peers in both growth and activity? Have you experienced unusual fatigue? Do you have significant dyspnea on exertion? Can you climb two flights of stairs without stopping?** Decreased exercise tolerance may indicate early cardiac decompensation

Q **Do you get short of breath at night when lying flat?** May be sign of pulmonary congestion, pulmonary hypertension, and progressive cardiac decompensation

Q **Do you experience palpitations, racing pulse, or irregular heart beat?** May indicate the onset of arrhythmias associated with increasing atrial volumes and pressures

Q **Have you had fainting, or near-fainting, spells?** May be subtle signs of the presence of paroxysmal arrhythmias in moderate disease or of impaired cardiac output in advanced disease

Q **Do you turn blue when you feel short of breath?** May be a sign of paroxysmal right-to-left shunting

Q **Do you ever have chest pain?** Can occur in the absence of coronary artery disease but may indicate the presence of concomitant coronary artery disease and is an indication for referral

Q **Have you experienced any episodes of sudden shortness of breath unrelated to exertion or focal numbness or weakness suggestive of transient ischemic attack (TIA) or stroke?** May be signs of embolic complications: pulmonary embolus associated with sudden changes in respiratory status or paradoxical systemic embolization associated with ASD or PFO

Contributory or predisposing factors

Q **Do you have Down syndrome?** Down syndrome is closely associated with ASD

Family history

- **Q Is there a family history of congenital heart disease or limb malformations?** Some rare genetic disorders are associated with ASD but include other physical deformities, often involving the limbs
- **Q Has anyone in the family ever required a pacemaker?** ASD and prolonged AV conduction is one inherited form of ASD
- **Q Is the family Amish?** Ellis–van Creveld syndrome is associated with ASD and is found most often in Amish populations in Lancaster County, Pennsylvania, in the US

Examination

- **Does the patient have a widely split second heart sound?**
- **Does the patient have a crescendo–decrescendo systolic murmur?** Note that this may not be heard before the age of 3 months and may diminish or disappear in late stages of disease as shunt reverses
- **Is there a prominent right ventricular impulse?** May indicate increased volume and pressure to the right side of the heart as pulmonary artery pressure rises
- **Does the patient have clubbing or cyanosis?** A late and serious finding, indicating significant right-to-left shunting and probable severe pulmonary hypertension

Summary of investigative tests

- Echocardiogram, including Doppler flow and saline contrast 'bubble' studies: diagnostic test of choice in all cases of suspected ASD or PFO
- Chest X-ray
- ECG
- Cardiac catheterization: usually performed to evaluate patients with suspected significant pulmonary hypertension, other congenital heart disease, or concomitant coronary artery disease – performed by a specialist

DIAGNOSTIC DECISION

- Tests to evaluate shunt size: physical examination findings, chest X-ray, ECG, and echocardiogram
- Definition of small shunt: absence of diastolic flow rumble, normal chest X-ray, and echocardiographic evidence of normal right ventricular size, normal interventricular septal motion, or pulmonary to systemic flow ratio of <1.5:1.0
- Definition of large shunt: presence of diastolic flow rumble, ECG evidence of right ventricular hypertrophy, chest X-ray evidence of cardiomegaly or increased pulmonary vascular markings, or echocardiographic evidence of right ventricular enlargement or paradoxical septal motion, or a pulmonary to systemic flow ratio of >1.5:1.0

Guidelines

Guidelines for evaluation and management of common congenital cardiac problems in infants, children, and adolescents. A statement for healthcare professionals from the Committee on Congenital Cardiac Defects of the Council on Cardiovascular Disease in the Young, American Heart Association. These guidelines base treatment decisions on age at presentation and shunt size.

CLINICAL PEARL(S)

- Accounts for 30% of congenital abnormalities found in adults
- Consider ASD in adults with bizarre respiratory and cardiac unexplained by routine history and physical examination
- Most adults reach their fourth decade without symptoms
- Surgical treatment is indicated if the shunt is >1.5:1, even if asymptomatic

THE TESTS
Imaging
ECHOCARDIOGRAM WITH DOPPLER FLOW SALINE CONTRAST 'BUBBLE' STUDIES

Advantages/Disadvantages

Advantages:
- Noninvasive, high sensitivity, and specific to detect ASD
- Can also assess pulmonary hypertension, concomitant valvular heart disease, chamber size, and ventricular function

Disadvantages:
- Saline 'bubble' test requires a peripheral intravenous line, associated with mild physical discomfort
- Transesophageal echocardiography may be needed to visualize the entire atrial septum, involving the risks of intravenous sedation and probe placement

Normal
- Normal chamber size and the absence of a visible defect in the atrial septum
- No Doppler-detected flow across the atrial septum during a Valsalva maneuver
- No bubble contrast appears in the left atrium in the first two to three cardiac cycles after contrast is seen in the right atrium, when agitated saline is injected in a peripheral vein during a patient Valsalva maneuver

Abnormal
- Visible ASD (note that in the case of a PFO, no visible defect may be seen and the only echocardiographic finding may be a positive Doppler flow or saline contrast study during maneuvers)
- Enlarged atria
- Paradoxical motion of the interventricular septum
- Doppler flow study indicating blood flow between the atria
- Saline contrast 'bubble' study in which contrast appears in the left atrium within one to two cardiac cycles after agitated saline is injected in a peripheral vein during Valsalva maneuver
- Significant tricuspid or pulmonic valvular regurgitation
- Reversal of flow in the hepatic veins, suggesting significant pulmonary hypertension

Cause of abnormal result
- Defect in the atrial septum does not reflect ultrasound waves on echocardiogram when the atrial septum is imaged
- Blood flow between the atria is demonstrated by Doppler flow study
- Direct communication between the atria allows saline contrast to cross directly from the right atrium and appear in the left atrium within one to two cardiac cycles, rather than via the pulmonary vascular system, which causes a normal delay of two to three cardiac cycles
- Increased blood volume in the right atrium and ventricle lead to chamber dilation
- Tricuspid and/or pulmonic valvular regurgitation is secondary to increased volume in the right ventricle and increased pressure in the pulmonary arteries
- Reversal of flow in the hepatic veins is secondary to tricuspid valvular regurgitation that occurs as the right ventricle dilates and pulmonary artery pressures increase

CHEST X-RAY

Advantages/Disadvantages

Advantages:
- Noninvasive
- Relatively inexpensive
- Low risk with little radiation exposure

Disadvantages:
- Not sensitive or specific for ASD
- Many false-positive and false-negative results

Abnormal
- Prominent right heart silhouette
- Prominence of the main pulmonary arteries

Cause of abnormal result
Increased blood flow to the right heart (from flow across the ASD) causes ventricular dilation and increases in pulmonary artery blood flow and pressure.

Other tests
ECG
Description
The ECG may demonstrate several abnormalities indicative of right ventricular overload or conduction abnormalities associated with septal structural changes. However, ECG is not diagnostic.

Advantages/Disadvantages
Advantages:
- Noninvasive
- Relatively inexpensive

Disadvantages:
- Insensitive
- Results are nonspecific to ASD

Abnormal
- Ostium secundum defects: right axis deviation, rSr' pattern in right precordial leads, right ventricular hypertrophy in children
- Ostium primum defects: prolonged PR interval, right ventricular conduction defect characterized by left axis deviation
- Sinus venosus defects: ectopic atrial pacemaker or first-degree heart block
- Any ASD: right or left ventricular hypertrophy, depending on pulmonary artery pressures

Cause of abnormal result
- Atrioventricular conduction changes related to abnormalities of the atrial septum
- Abnormal interventricular conduction and/or QRS axis secondary to elevations in pulmonary artery pressure with right and/or left ventricular overload

Drugs, disorders, and other factors that may alter results
Beta-blockers and calcium channel blockers can cause conduction delays, such as first-degree AV block.

TREATMENT

IMMEDIATE ACTION

Immediate intervention, either medical or surgical, may be indicated for patients with known atrial septal defect (ASD) who develop:

- Signs and symptoms suggestive of bacterial endocarditis
- Symptoms of coronary artery insufficiency
- Symptoms of embolism and stroke
- Significant arrhythmia with associated hemodynamic compromise

PATIENT AND CAREGIVER ISSUES

Patient or caregiver request

Patients with uncomplicated ASD may have specific questions about the following issues:

- **Are prophylactic antibiotics indicated prior to dental procedures or other surgery?** The American Heart Association Guidelines for Antibiotic Prophylaxis for Prevention of Bacterial Endocarditis do not recommend antibiotic prophylaxis for uncomplicated secundum ASD because of low incidence of endocarditis and risk of serious reactions to antibiotic therapy
- **What is the risk of stroke associated with ASD?** Risk varies with size of the defect and presence of right-to-left shunting. Specific numbers are difficult to find, but in uncorrected, small ASDs including patent foramen ovale (PFO), the risk of stroke is low (<0.8% per year)
- **Can I expect to have normal sexual relationships? Am I at increased risk of dying during sexual intercourse?** Male adolescents and young adults with congenital heart disease often have concerns about arousal and fear of dying during intercourse. Uncomplicated ASD is not associated with increased risks of adverse events during sexual activity
- **Does having an ASD affect my ability to have children?** Many adolescents and young women with congenital heart disease mistakenly believe that they cannot get pregnant. Complicated ASD may be associated with increased risks of pregnancy; patients need to be advised of risks of pregnancy and childbirth in uncorrected ASD
- **Will my own children be at increased risk of having congenital heart disease?** Yes. When one parent has congenital heart disease, the rate of recurrence in offspring is 3–5% if the mother is affected and about 1.5% if the father is affected. Highest recurrence rates are in parents with left-sided cardiac lesions and left ventricular outflow obstruction
- **If I have one child with ASD, am I more likely to have a second child with congenital heart disease?** Yes. Recurrence risk for congenital heart disease is about 2.5% if one sibling has ASD and 8% if two prior siblings have ASD
- **Will having ASD affect my employability?** Unfortunately, congenital heart disease negatively impacts employability, with one study showing a turndown rate 50% over that of other employees. Discrimination is based on fears that physical disability may impact absenteeism and the rising cost of supplying insurance benefits to employees. When a job application asks 'Do you have any conditions or disabilities that may interfere with your ability to perform the job?,' patients are not required to disclose the fact that they have ASD if it will not interfere with the job for which they are applying. One-half of employed patients with congenital heart disease do not disclose the fact when hired
- **Will I have trouble obtaining and maintaining health insurance coverage?** Large numbers of adults with congenital heart disease are uninsured or underinsured. Private health insurance usually stops coverage to dependants at age 21 unless the dependant is a full-time student. Medicaid coverage continues only for disabled patients. Patients should be encouraged to seek employment with businesses that are likely to provide healthcare coverage as an employee benefit

MANAGEMENT ISSUES

Goals

- Assessment of whether the patient has a 'significant' ASD, i.e. whether pulmonary to systemic blood flow ratio is >1.5:1.0

- Recognition of patients who should be referred for surgical management to prevent progressive pulmonary hypertension and cardiac decompensation
- Recognition and treatment of potential acute complications of ASD, such as bacterial endocarditis or systemic embolization
- Recognition of PFO as a potential source of systemic embolization

Management in special circumstances

- Patients with known ASD undergoing noncardiac surgery: increased risks of several complications following noncardiac surgery, including paradoxical embolus, atrial arrhythmias, increased left-to-right shunting (if there is significant blood loss), changes in pulmonary compliance (in cases with significantly increased pulmonary blood flow), increases in pulmonary vascular resistance with acute right ventricular overload, and bacterial endocarditis (in particular patients with primum defects and associated mitral valve abnormalities)
- Patients with known ASD or PFO and stroke: treatment choices include long-term antithrombotic therapies or mechanical closure of the atrial defect. Closure of an ASD or PFO in patients with stroke who have otherwise low risks for operative or procedural intervention is controversial
- Patients with known ASD undergoing surgery or procedures associated with bacteremia: prophylaxis not recommended by the American Heart Association for ASD patients who have uncomplicated secundum defects; otherwise, general principles for endocarditis prophylaxis should be followed
- Patients with known ASD and signs or symptoms suggestive of bacterial endocarditis: diagnosis and management per American Heart Association consensus, antibiotic therapy per American Heart Association Statement on Antibiotic Treatment of Adults with Infective Endocarditis

COEXISTING DISEASE

- Chronic obstructive pulmonary disease: increases the risk of development of changes in pulmonary compliance, the development of pulmonary hypertension, and the risk of right-to-left shunting
- Coronary artery disease: can decrease ventricular adaptation to increases in blood flow and pressure, leading to early right and/or left ventricular failure

SPECIAL PATIENT GROUPS

- Children: high rate of spontaneous closure of ostium secundum defects (up to 39%) must be weighed against the low morbidity rate of surgical closure in patients under age 25 (long-term survival rates are the same as for normal patients)
- Older adults: survival past age 40 in patients with significant ASD is <50%, with late complications of heart failure, stroke, atrial fibrillation
- Pregnant patients: pregnancy is usually well tolerated in women under age 40 with uncomplicated ASD but may be associated with right and/or left heart failure, thromboembolism, pulmonary hypertension, or significant right-to-left shunting at the time of delivery

SUMMARY OF THERAPEUTIC OPTIONS

Choices

- Patient is under age 5 at time of presentation with symptomatic large shunt: surgical closure, or medical management in anticipation of possible spontaneous closure
- Patient is under age 5 at time of presentation with asymptomatic large shunt: re-evaluate in 1 year and proceed to surgical closure if shunt is still large and/or symptoms develop
- Patient is under age 5 at the time of presentation with small, asymptomatic shunt: repeat history and physical in 2 years. Follow small, asymptomatic shunts at 5 years and 8 years after presentation with history and physical examination, then every 5 years thereafter with

chest X-ray, ECG, and echocardiogram. If shunt becomes large or symptomatic, surgical closure is indicated
- Patient is over age 5 at the time of presentation: history, physical examination, chest X-ray, ECG, and echocardiogram. Small shunts are followed every 5 years with history, examination, chest X-ray, and ECG. If shunt becomes large, symptomatic, or pulmonary hypertension is suspected, surgical closure is indicated
- Transcatheter closure of ASD is an experimental procedure that can be used for closure of secundum ASDs <20mm in diameter with a sufficient tissue rim surrounding the defect

Guidelines

Guidelines for evaluation and management of common congenital cardiac problems in infants, children, and adolescents. A statement for healthcare professionals from the Committee on Congenital Cardiac Defects of the Council on Cardiovascular Disease in the Young, American Heart Association. These guidelines base treatment decisions on age at presentation and shunt size.

Clinical pearl(s)

- Surgical treatment is indicated if the shunt is >1.5:1 even if asymptomatic
- Endocarditis prophylaxis is not needed for untreated ASD

FOLLOW UP

Plan for review

American Heart Association Guidelines:
- Patients under age 5 at presentation with uncorrected ASD: follow up at 2, 5, and 8 years after presentation, and every 5 years thereafter, with history, examination, chest X-ray, and ECG
- Patients over age 5 at presentation with uncorrected ASD: follow up every 5 years with history, examination, chest X-ray, and ECG
- Patients who undergo closure of secundum ASD: initial postoperative follow up and echocardiogram at 3 months. If history and examination are normal, follow up at 1 year and every 5 years thereafter with history, examination, and ECG. A second postclosure echocardiogram may be obtained at the 6-year visit
- If history or examination at initial postoperative follow up indicates persistent ASD, arrhythmia, or conduction abnormality, further referral may be indicated

Information for patient or caregiver

- Early closure of ASD is associated with low morbidity and mortality rates and a normal lifespan
- Delayed closure of ASD after age 25 is associated with a rise in post-treatment morbidity and mortality rates and a significant decrease in lifespan; fewer than 50% of patients survive past age 40 with uncorrected significant ASD

DRUGS AND OTHER THERAPIES: DETAILS

Surgical therapy

SURGICAL CORRECTION OF ASD

Efficacy
- Children: 30-year survival rate in children who undergo correction of ASD is the same as that of the general population (97%)
- Multiple studies have documented excellent short- and long-term outcomes in children with ASD treated surgically
- Risks increase in older patients

Risks/Benefits

Risks:
- Mortality rate in children – early surgical mortality rate approaches 0%. 30-year survival is the same as in normal controls

- Mortality rate in adults – mortality rate of surgical correction of ASD or PFO varies with age and the presence of cardiac failure and pulmonary hypertension. Surgical mortality rate is <1% in healthy patients under 45 years old and up to 10% in older patients and those with congestive heart failure and systolic pulmonary hypertension
- Postoperative complications – 5–10% residual ASD flow in children, 5–10% complete heart block after primum ASD repairs, early tamponade in 1.5% of patients, common transient arrhythmias
- Benefits of PFO closure in symptomatic patients – still controversial, with no long-term follow up studies of sufficient size to analyze benefits
- In children under the age of 8, spontaneous closure of ostium secundum defects may approach 39%. Detection of an ostium secundum defect in a child may warrant observation only if the patient is asymptomatic and the shunt is small

Evidence

There is some evidence that surgical management for patients who have ASD diagnosed after 40 years improves functioning and long-term survival.

A retrospective study examined the clinical course of patients diagnosed with ASD after the age of 40 years. Medical management was compared with surgical repair of the defect. The mortality rate (from all causes) was lower in the patients who underwent surgical repair, according to multivariate analysis. Functional deterioration due to heart failure was prevented, and 10-year survival rate was higher in the surgical group. There was no significant difference in the incidence of atrial arrhythmias or thromboembolic complications between the groups [1] *Level S*

Acceptability to patient

Surgical therapy is associated with significant discomfort and a relatively short period of recovery.

Follow up plan

- After closure of secundum ASD: initial postoperative follow up and echocardiogram at 3 months. If history and examination are normal, follow up at 1 year and every 5 years thereafter with history, examination, and ECG. A second postclosure echocardiogram may be obtained at the 6-year visit
- If history or examination at initial postoperative follow up indicates persistent ASD, arrhythmia, or conduction abnormality, further referral may be indicated

TRANSCATHETER CLOSURE OF ASD

An occlusive device is introduced intravascularly and deployed across the ASD. Most devices for which information is available are implanted under FDA-approved IDE protocols or are awaiting FDA approval.

Efficacy

Consensus regarding the use of ASD closure devices included in the American Heart Association's AHA Scientific Statement on Pediatric Therapeutic Cardiac Catheterization:

- Used for closure of secundum ASDs <20mm in diameter with a sufficient tissue rim surrounding the defect
- Not useful for sinus venosus defects, ostium primum ASDs, or secundum ASDs with significant associated congenital heart disease

Risks/Benefits

Benefits:

- Preliminary studies only; success rate is 90–95%
- Complication rate in small series is <5% but includes embolization of the device itself
- Residual leaks are common initially after the procedure but decrease with time to 5–15% at 5 years

- Less incisional discomfort over conventional surgery or minimally invasive surgery
- Earlier recovery and return to routine activities over traditional surgery
- Potentially lower costs due to abbreviated hospital and/or intensive care unit length of stay

Evidence

To date, studies have been too small to draw conclusions about safety, benefits, and relative risks of transcatheter ASD or PFO closure when compared with surgical closure. Use of transcatheter devices is considered investigational.

Acceptability to patient

May be more acceptable to patients, with less recovery time and less discomfort over conventional surgery.

EFFICACY OF THERAPIES

- Mortality rate of surgical closure of atrial septal defect (ASD) prior to age 25 is near zero, with a subsequent normal lifespan
- Mortality rate of surgical closure of ASD after age 25 is 1–10% (depending on age), has been shown to decrease functional deterioration in older patients, and is significantly superior to medical therapy in improving long-term survival, functional exercise capacity, and mean ventilatory function
- Surgical closure of ASD was associated with greatly increased mortality rates in patients with pulmonary vascular resistance >15 Wood units

Evidence

PDxMD are unable to cite evidence that meets our criteria for evidence; however, a number of comparative and longitudinal follow up studies suggest that the surgical approach may be beneficial in selected adult patients.

PROGNOSIS

- Normal cardiac function and a normal life span if repaired before age 25
- Increasing surgical morbidity and mortality rates after age 25, but overall increase in survival and improvement in functional class for all but the most complex of cases. The key is diagnosing or having a higher index of suspicion
- In patients with significant ASD (pulmonary to systemic blood flow ratio >1.5:1.0), survival past age 40 is <50% and is complicated by significant rates of atrial fibrillation (50%), cardiac failure, and stroke
- Prognosis for recurrence of stroke in patients with PFO who undergo surgical closure is at this time unknown, with no adequate long-term follow up studies

Clinical pearl(s)

- Early repair is associated with normal lifespan and function
- The key is diagnosing or having a higher index of suspicion

COMPLICATIONS

- Pulmonary hypertension: occurs in uncorrected ASD when pulmonary blood flow exceeds systemic blood flow by >1.5:1.0. Reactive hypertrophy of pulmonary blood vessels leads to permanent increases in pulmonary vascular resistance
- Cyanotic heart disease: right heart pressures increase with the development of pulmonary hypertension, flow across the ASD reverses, and blood travels from right to left, leading to systemic cyanosis
- Cardiac decompensation: cyanosis and increasing right heart pressure lead to right, and sometimes left, cardiac failure
- Paradoxical embolization across the ASD: risk increases as blood flow across the ASD reverses and travels from right to left. Occurs late in disease or with events that increase right heart pressures relative to left, such as Valsalva maneuvers, or acute hemorrhage in the face of pulmonary hypertension
- Endocarditis: occurs rarely with secundum defects and is more likely to occur when there are associated valvular heart defects

PREVENTION

MODIFY RISK FACTORS

SCREENING

Screening for unsuspected atrial septal defect (ASD) should be carried only out in patients in whom a genetic predisposition to develop ASD occurs, e.g.:

- Patients with syndromes known to have an increased rate of congenital heart disease, such as Down syndrome or Noonan's syndrome
- Primary relatives of patients with known ASD and one of the following conditions – Ellis–van Creveld syndrome, Holt–Oram syndrome, syndrome of ASD, and prolonged AV conduction

ECHOCARDIOGRAM

- Sensitive and specific test for cardiac structural abnormalities
- Can both rule in or out the presence of ASD and detect other associated cardiac abnormalities
- Assesses cardiac function for the presence of complications such as atrial thrombosis, pulmonary hypertension, and right or left ventricular functional deterioration

Cost/efficacy

- Noninvasive and relatively inexpensive
- Sensitive and specific for detection of cardiac structural abnormalities

ASSOCIATIONS

American Heart Association
National Center
7272 Greenville Avenue
Dallas, TX 75231
Tel: (800)-242-8721
http://www.americanheart.org

Children's Health Information Network: Congenital Heart Disease
1561 Clark Drive
Yardley, PA 19067
Tel: (215)-493-3068
E-mail: mb@tchin.org
http://www.tchin.org
For information for patients and families on ASD: Surgical and Transcatheter Management: http://www.tchin.org/

KEY REFERENCES

- Chan KC, Godman MJ, Walsh K, et al. Transcatheter closure of atrial septal defect and interatrial communications with a new self-expanding nitinol double disc device (Amplatzer Septal Occluder): Multicentre UK Experience. Heart 1999;82(3):300–6
- Rao PS. Summary and comparison of atrial septal defect closure devices. Curr Interv Cardiol Rep 2000;2(4):367–76
- Agarwal SK, Ghosh PK, Mittal PK. Failure of devices used for closure of atrial septal defects: mechanisms and management. J Thorac Cardiovasc Surg 1996;112(1):21–6
- Allen HD, Beekman RH, Garson A Jr, et al. AHA Scientific Statement: Pediatric therapeutic cardiac catheterization. A statement for healthcare professionals from the Council on Cardiovascular Disease in the Young. Circulation 1998;97(6):609–25.
- Berdjis F, Brandl D, Uhlemann F, et al. Adults with congenital heart defects – clinical spectrum and management. 1996;21(5):330–6
- Bogousslavsky J, Duvuyst G, Nendaz M, et al. Prevention of stroke recurrence with presumed paradoxical embolism. J Neurol 1997;244(2):71–5
- Chavez GF, Cordero JF, Becerra JE. Leading major congenital malformations among minority groups in the United States, 1981–1986. MMWR CDC Surveill Summ 1988;37(3):17–24
- Dearani JA, Urgurlu BS, Danielson GK, et al. Surgical patent foramen ovale closure for prevention of paradoxical embolism-related cerebrovascular ischemic events. Circulation 1999;100:Suppl):II171–5
- Driscoll D, Allen HD, Atkins DL, et al. Guidelines for evaluation and management of common congenital cardiac problems in infants, children, and adolescents. Circulation 1994;90(4):2180–8
- Engle MA. Recognition and management of atrial septal defect. Heart Dis Stroke 1994;3(6):383–7
- Ferencz C, Boughman JA. Teratology, genetics and recurrence risks. Cardiol Clin 1993;II(4):557–65
- Ghisla RP, Hannon DW, Meyer RA, et al. Spontaneous closure of isolated secundum atrial septal defects in infants: an echocardiographic study. Am Heart J 1985;109(6):1327–33
- Hart EM, Garson A. Psychosocial concerns of adults with congenital heart disease: employability and insurability. Cardiol Clin 1994;II(4):711–5
- Hung J, Landzberg MJ, Jenkins KJ, et al. Closure of patent foramen ovale for paradoxical emboli: intermediate-term risk of recurrent neurological events following transcatheter device placement. J Am Coll Cardiol 2000;35(5):1311–6
- Kaplan S. Natural and postoperative history across age groups. Cardiol Clin 1993;II(4):543–56
- Konstantinides S, Geibel A, Olschewski M, et al. A comparison of surgical and medical therapy for atrial septal defect in adults. N Engl J Med 24;333(8):469–73
- Li W, Somerville J. Infective endocarditis in the grown-up congenital heart population. Eur Heart J 1998;19(1):166–73
- Mahoney LT, Truesdell SC, Krzmarzick TR, Lauer RM. Atrial septal defects that present in infancy. Am J Dis Child 1986;14(11);603–16

- Mas JL. Diagnosis and management of paradoxical embolism and patent foramen ovale. Curr Opin Cardiol 1996;11(5):519–24
- Nendaz MR, Srasin FP, Junod AF, Bogousslavsky J. Preventing stroke recurrence in patients with patent foramen ovale: antithrombotic therapy, foramen closure, or therapeutic abstention? A decision analytic perspective. Am Heart J 1998;135(3):532–41
- Romanelli AM, Pierini A, et al. Cardiovascular malformations and smoking during pregnancy: results of case-control surveillance in the Eurocat Register of Florence. Acta Paediatrica Latina 47(3):282–7
- Shibata Y, Abe T, Kuribayashi R, et al. Surgical treatment of isolated secundum atrial septal defect in patients more than 50 years old. Ann Thorac Surg 1996;62(4):1096–9
- Soliman A, Shanoudy H, et al. Increased prevalence of patent foramen ovale in patients with severe chronic obstructive pulmonary disease. J Am Soc Echocardiogr 1999;12(2):99–105
- Steele PM, Fuster V, Cohen M, et al. Isolated atrial septal defect with pulmonary vascular obstructive disease: long-term follow-up and prediction of outcome after surgical correction. Circulation 1987;76(5):1037–42
- Tikkanen J, Heninonen OP. Risk factors for atrial septal defect. Eur J Epidemiol 1992;8(4):50–5
- Braunwald E, ed. Heart disease: a textbook of cardiovascular medicine, 5th edn. Philadelphia: WB Saunders, 1997
- Otto C. The practice of clinical echocardiography. Philadelphia: WB Saunders, 1997

Websites:

- Evaluation and management of common congenital cardiac problems in infants, children, and adolescents. American Heart Association. http://www.americanheart.org/
- Pediatric therapeutic cardiac catheterization. American Heart Association. http://circ.ahajournals.org/
- ACP-ASIM online: http://www.acponline.org
- Centers for Disease Control and Prevention. Available online: http://www2.cdc.gov/

Evidence references

1 Konstantinides S, Geibel A, Olschewski M, et al. A comparison of surgical and medical therapy for atrial septal defect in adults. N Engl J Med 1995; 333:469–73. Medline

FAQS

Question 1

What is the most common finding in children with ASD?

ANSWER 1

Wide, fixed splitting of the second heart sound, sometimes associated with a diastolic tricuspid flow rumble.

Question 2

Should all ASDs be closed?

ANSWER 2

General consensus is that after age 4 any significant ASD should be closed to prevent late complications. In older populations, morbidity and mortality rates are decreased by ASD closure, except in those with significant pulmonary hypertension.

Question 3

Do patients with ASDs require endocarditis prophylaxis for dental procedures and surgery?

ANSWER 3

Uncomplicated secundum defects do not require endocarditis prophylaxis. Prophylaxis should be provided in other types of ASD, particularly primum defects with associated valvular abnormalities.

Question 4

If my patient with PFO presents with stroke or other signs of systemic embolism, should he/she undergo surgery to close the PFO?

ANSWER 4

Long-term follow up of patients with PFO and stroke who undergo surgical or transcatheter closure of the PFO is lacking in sufficient numbers to provide a clear cut answer. Alternative therapies include antithrombotic therapy (either antiplatelet or anticoagulant drugs) or no therapy.

Question 5

What is the mortality rate associated with surgical closure of an ASD before the age of 25, and what is the prognosis for patients who have undergone successful closure?

ANSWER 5

The mortality rate of surgical closure of ASD prior to age 25 is near zero. These estimates are based on published case series from experienced surgical centers, and extrapolation to all centers may not be appropriate. Mortality rate of surgical closure of ASD after age 25 is 1–10% (depending on age). Normal cardiac function and a normal lifespan are expected if the defect is repaired before age 25.

CONTRIBUTORS

Martin L Kabongo, MD, PhD
John McB Hodgson, MD, FACC, FSCAI
James Orford, MD

ATRIOVENTRICULAR BLOCK

SUMMARY INFORMATION

DESCRIPTION

- A disturbance in the conduction of impulses from the atrium to the ventricles
- Severity ranges from first-degree atrioventricular (AV) block, in which a long PR interval on the ECG indicates delayed conduction, to third-degree or complete AV block, in which there is complete failure of conduction between the atria and the ventricles. In this case the atria and ventricles beat independently and at different rates
- Minor degrees of AV block are usually asymptomatic and do not require treatment other than that for any underlying heart disease; patients with more severe AV block may experience symptoms of hypoperfusion with syncope or Stokes–Adams attacks – such patients are at risk of sudden death from asystole
- Drugs have very little part to play in the management of AV block. If treatment is required, a temporary or permanent pacemaker should be inserted

URGENT ACTION

- Refer immediately for pacemaker insertion if there are symptoms of heart failure or hypoperfusion (syncope, dizziness, shortness of breath, and hypotension)
- Transcutaneous pacing, if available, is useful during the prehospital phase for symptomatic patients or patients with AV block secondary to acute myocardial infarction
- Intravenous atropine may improve the cardiac output in patients with complete AV block and type I second-degree AV block
- If pacing is not available and the patient does not respond to atropine, isoproterenol (beta-adrenergic agonist) should be given intravenously
- Isoproterenol should be used with great caution, if at all, in patients with acute myocardial infarction

KEY! DON'T MISS!

Patients with complete AV block are at risk of asystole. They should be referred for immediate pacemaker insertion.

ICD9 CODE

- 426.11 First-degree heart block
- 426.13 Mobitz type I heart block
- 426.12 Mobitz type II heart block
- 426.0 Complete heart block

SYNONYMS

- Heart block
- Wenckebach block (Mobitz type I block)
- Mobitz type II block
- Third-degree block

CARDINAL FEATURES

- A disturbance in the conduction of impulses from the atrium to the ventricles
- First-degree atrioventricular (AV) block: delayed conduction through the AV node. Usually asymptomatic but prolonged PR interval (>0.20s) on the ECG
- Second-degree AV block: failure of some (but not all) impulses to conduct from atria to ventricles. In Mobitz type I (Wenckebach) block there is progressive prolongation of the PR interval until an impulse fails to conduct, causing a regular pattern of dropped beats; in Mobitz type II block, there is a periodic failure of conduction without progressive PR-interval prolongation
- Complete or third-degree AV block is characterized by complete failure of atrioventricular conduction. Atria and ventricles beat independently and at their own rates. The ventricular escape rhythm is characteristically slow: <40 beats/min in acquired complete AV block
- Minor degrees of AV block are usually asymptomatic and do not require treatment other than that for any underlying heart disease
- Patients with more severe AV block may experience symptoms of hypoperfusion with syncope or Stokes–Adams attacks. They are at risk for sudden death from asystole
- Drugs have very little part to play in the management of AV block. If treatment is required, a temporary or permanent pacemaker should be inserted

CAUSES

Common causes

- Physiologic: first- and second-degree atrioventricular (AV) block may be an incidental finding in healthy children. Increased vagal tone in well-trained athletes may cause type I second-degree AV block
- Drugs (e.g. digitalis, quinidine, procainamide, calcium channel blockers, beta-blockers)
- Degenerative change within the conducting system
- Myocardial ischemia or infarction
- Cardiac surgery (e.g. mitral valve surgery)
- Congenital AV block

Rare causes

- Congenital heart disease
- Acute rheumatic fever
- Sarcoidosis
- Tick-borne illness, including Lyme disease
- Aortic valve disease

EPIDEMIOLOGY

Incidence and prevalence

First-degree atrioventricular block is present in 16 per 1000 young adults and is usually of no clinical significance.

FREQUENCY

Worldwide, over 100,000 pacemakers are implanted each year in patients with atrioventricular block.

Demographics

AGE

Patients may present at any age from neonates with congenital atrioventricular block to the elderly, in whom the cause is more likely to be ischemic or degenerative.

GENDER

Both sexes are affected.

RACE

All racial groups are affected.

DIFFERENTIAL DIAGNOSIS

The differential diagnoses of syncope are as follows.

Vasovagal syncope

Inappropriate vasodilation and excess vagal tone, usually mediated by central nervous system.

FEATURES

- Preceded by inactivity, emotional strain, kneeling, cough, pain, micturition
- Warning symptoms of dizziness, sweating

Orthostatic hypotension

Associated with getting up from a lying or sitting position.

FEATURES

Associated with:

- Diabetes mellitus (autonomic insufficiency)
- Parkinson's disease

Sinus node disease

Sick sinus syndrome, also known as 'tachy-brady' syndrome.

FEATURES

- Occurs in the elderly
- Intermittent sinus bradycardia, sinus pauses
- Episodic atrial fibrillation

Ventricular tachycardia

Ventricular tachycardia occurs in the setting of known coronary artery disease.

FEATURES

- Shortness of breath
- Syncope
- May proceed to ventricular fibrillation and sudden death

Aortic stenosis

Inadequate cardiac output due to stenotic valve; exacerbated by postural changes.

FEATURES

- Shortness of breath on exertion
- Syncope

Grand mal epilepsy

Central nervous system electrical disturbance. The main features of epilepsy are as follows.

FEATURES

- Tonic-clonic movements
- Aura
- Tongue biting and urinary incontinence

Vertebrobasilar disease

Usually due to vertebral artery atherosclerosis.

FEATURES
- History of cardiovascular disease
- Syncope precipitated by neck movements

Myocardial infarction
The main features of myocardial infarction are as follows.

FEATURES
- Crushing central chest pain
- Pain radiates into jaw and arm
- Sweating and nausea
- History of ischemic heart disease

Stroke
The following main features of stroke may occur suddenly, and are indicative of stroke.

FEATURES
- Numbness or weakness of face, arm, or leg, especially on one side of the body
- Confusion and difficulty with speaking or understanding
- Loss of vision or difficulty seeing in one or both eyes
- Difficulty with walking, dizziness, loss of balance, or coordination
- Severe headache with no known cause

Atrial fibrillation
Atrial fibrillation and supraventricular tachycardia seldom cause syncope, but may cause dizziness, particularly in the elderly and in patients with impaired cardiac function. If a supraventricular tachycardia causes hypotension, syncope may occur.

FEATURES
- Palpitations (most common)
- Nonuniform, irregular rhythm on cardiac auscultation
- Fatigue, dizziness, light-headedness in some patients
- Asymptomatic (rare)

SIGNS & SYMPTOMS
Signs
First-degree atrioventricular (AV) block:
- The heart rate is normal and there are often no clinical signs
- The first heart sound may be quieter than normal (consequence of prolonged PR interval)
- A long *a–c* wave interval may be visible in the jugular venous pulse

In second-degree AV block, dropped beats are a feature:
- Some patients with type I second-degree AV block have a regular pattern of dropped beats, e.g. every third or fourth beat is dropped and 'grouped beats' are seen on the ECG
- With each successive beat in the group ('Wenckebach group'), heart rate may increase (often imperceptibly), the first heart sound may diminish, and the *a–c* interval in the jugular venous pulse widens. When a beat is dropped, the *a* wave is not followed by a *v* wave
- Type II second-degree AV block is associated with occasional dropped beats. When the beat is dropped the *a* wave in the jugular venous pulse is not followed by a *v* wave

Complete AV block is associated with bradycardia:
- Heart rate is usually less than 40 beats/min in acquired cases but may be faster with a congenital etiology. The heart rate is usually regular

- Beat-by-beat changes in the PR interval are associated with variable intensity of the first heart sound and a variable relationship between the *a* and *v* waves in the jugular venous pulse
- Very large *a* waves may be visible in the jugular venous pulse when atrial and ventricular contractions coincide

Symptoms

Many patients, particularly with first- and second-degree atrioventricular (AV) block, are asymptomatic. Symptoms are a consequence of poor cardiac output and are more common in complete AV block:

- Lethargy, postural hypotension, breathlessness
- Syncope, dizziness, and acute heart failure tend to be confined to patients with a ventricular rate <40 beats/min
- Asystole leading to Stokes–Adams attacks or sudden death

KEY! DON'T MISS!

Patients with complete atrioventricular block are at risk of asystole. They should be referred for immediate pacemaker insertion.

INVESTIGATION OF THE PATIENT

Direct questions to patient

Q **Do you suffer from palpitations or an irregular heart beat?** Patients may be aware of dropped beats

Q **Do you become short of breath easily?** An inappropriately slow heart rate may reduce exercise tolerance

Q **Do your ankles swell up?** May suggest congestive heart failure

Q **Are you taking any medication?** Ask particularly about antiarrhythmic and antianginal drugs

Q **Do you tend to feel dizzy or faint? Have you lost consciousness at any time?** Syncope or Stokes–Adams attacks indicate a need for immediate referral

Q **Do you have problems lying flat in bed?** May suggest congestive heart failure

Contributory or predisposing factors

Q **Have you suffered a previous cardiac event?** Myocardial ischemia or infarction (especially an inferior or anterior wall myocardial infarction) may interrupt the blood supply to the atrioventricular node resulting in transient or permanent AV block

Q **Are you taking any medication?** Beta-blockers, digoxin, and antiarrhythmic drugs may precipitate AV block

Examination

- Assess radial pulse for rate, rhythm, and character
- Watch jugular venous pulse and note character and timing of *a* and *v* waves
- Check lying and sitting blood pressure to identify postural hypotension
- Examine the heart: check apex beat for position and character (especially first sound) and listen for valvular murmurs
- Check for evidence of pulmonary edema or peripheral pitting edema
- Perform a neurologic examination to identify focal neurologic deficits

Summary of investigative tests

- Diagnosis rests principally on the 12-lead electrocardiogram or continuous electrocardiographic monitoring. As well as identifying the presence and severity of atrioventricular block, it may also provide useful information about any underlying cardiac disease
- In some patients when the degree of atrioventricular block is not readily apparent, 24-h Holter monitoring may be ordered by a specialist

DIAGNOSTIC DECISION

Diagnosis rests on the ECG appearance:

- First-degree atrioventricular (AV) block is characterized by a prolonged PR interval (>0.2s). Every P wave is followed by a QRS complex and the ventricular rate is regular
- Type I second-degree AV block is characterized by the PR interval becoming longer with each beat until one P wave fails to conduct and is not followed by a QRS complex. There may be a recurring ratio of conducted to nonconducted P waves (e.g. 3:1)
- Type II second-degree AV block is characterized by the PR interval being normal (<0.2s) and constant, but occasional P waves failing to conduct and not being associated with a QRS complex
- Complete AV block is characterized by both P waves and QRS complexes being present, but they are unrelated in time and have different rates. A ventricular pacemaker above the bundle of His is associated with narrow QRS complexes, whereas a pacemaker at or below the bundle of His produces a wide QRS complex

CLINICAL PEARL(S)

Type II second-degree atrioventricular block usually progresses to complete heart block.

THE TESTS

Other tests

ELECTROCARDIOGRAPHY

Description

12-lead ECG with rhythm strip on leads II and V1.

Advantages/Disadvantages

Advantages:

- Inexpensive
- Readily available
- Noninvasive
- Safe

Normal

- The normal PR interval in adult patients measures 0.14–0.2s
- Each P wave should be followed by a QRS complex

Abnormal

- A regular but prolonged PR interval (>0.2s) indicates first-degree atrioventricular (AV) block
- Second-degree AV block exists when some, but not all, of the P waves are not followed by a QRS complex
- Atrial premature beats that fail to conduct because they occur during the normal refractory period of the AV node do not indicate AV block
- Progressive lengthening of the PR interval until one QRS complex is dropped indicates type I second-degree AV block. A regular pattern of dropped beats (e.g. every third or fourth P wave fails to transmit) may be apparent on longer recordings
- A regular PR interval with irregularly dropped QRS complexes indicates type II second-degree AV block
- A slow regular ventricular rate, as measured by the RR interval, with a highly variable PR interval indicates complete AV block. The ventricular rate is usually <40 beats/min in acquired cases, although it may be higher with congenital etiology. There is no relationship between the P waves and the QRS complexes. The QRS complexes may be normal or wide, depending on the site of the dominant escape pacemaker (ventricle or AV junction)

- Differentiating between type I and type II second-degree AV block on the basis of the ECG is usually straightforward, but in some cases subtle or exceptional changes may create confusion, and referral may be necessary
- Keep in mind the possibility of a falsely abnormal result

Drugs, disorders, and other factors that may alter results

Some commonly used medications reduce conduction at the atrioventricular (AV) node and may induce type I second-degree AV block:

- Digitalis
- Quinidine
- Procainamide
- Calcium channel blockers
- Beta-blockers

A high resting vagal tone (e.g. in athletes) may also be sufficient to reduce AV node conduction.

TREATMENT

CONSIDER CONSULT

- Refer immediately for specialist evaluation and possible pacemaker insertion if there are symptoms of heart failure or hypoperfusion (syncope, dizziness, shortness of breath, and hypotension)
- Refer all patients with complete atrioventricular block. Apart from some asymptomatic patients with congenital etiology, a pacemaker will be required in all cases
- Type II second-degree AV block is never a normal variant and is associated with a number of acute and chronic cardiac conditions. Patients should be referred for urgent specialist opinion and pacemaker insertion in most cases
- Underlying heart disease, if present, may require referral
- First-degree and type I second-degree AV block in otherwise healthy young patients tend to be benign and referral is not typically necessary

IMMEDIATE ACTION

- Transcutaneous pacing, if available, is useful during the prehospital phase for symptomatic patients or patients with AV block secondary to acute myocardial infarction
- Intravenous atropine may improve the cardiac output in patients with complete AV block and type I second-degree AV block. It is not effective in type II second-degree block but is unlikely to cause further deterioration
- If pacing is not available and the patient does not respond to atropine, isoproterenol (beta-adrenergic agonist) should be given intravenously
- Asymptomatic patients with first-degree and type I second-degree AV block do not usually require treatment

PATIENT AND CAREGIVER ISSUES

Patient or caregiver request

- **Will electrical equipment interfere with a pacemaker?** Most domestic equipment will not cause any problems, but some medical equipment and industrial equipment may do so. Avoid magnetic fields, such as those from magnetic resonance imaging (MRI). Seek appropriate guidance
- **Will I be able to exercise with a pacemaker?** Your exercise tolerance will probably improve with a pacemaker, although very strenuous exercise may be limited. Contact sports are best avoided as your pacemaker could be damaged

The American Heart Association (www.americanheart.org) has published information sheets on heart block and pacemakers for patients.

MANAGEMENT ISSUES

Goals

- Maintain cardiac output and blood pressure
- Prevent profound bradycardia or asystole
- Identify and treat any underlying cardiac disease

Management in special circumstances

COEXISTING DISEASE

Acute myocardial infarction:

- Ischemic injury can produce any degree of atrioventricular (AV) block
- First-degree and type I second-degree AV block should be monitored in case of progression, but treatment is not usually needed
- Indications for pacemaker insertion in type II second-degree or complete AV block do not necessarily depend on the presence of symptoms

- After inferior infarction the requirement for pacing is almost always temporary, but permanent pacing is more likely to be required after anterior infarction
- Mortality is high and reflects the degree of myocardial damage

COEXISTING MEDICATION

Antiarrhythmic drugs (e.g. digitalis, quinidine, procainamide, calcium channel blockers, beta-blockers) may have an etiologic role in atrioventricular block, and should normally be discontinued.

SPECIAL PATIENT GROUPS

Pregnant women:
- Patients may remain asymptomatic and have an uncomplicated pregnancy and labor
- If symptoms develop during pregnancy, a temporary or permanent pacemaker can be inserted. Temporary pacer placement under ECG and echocardiographic guidance minimizes the exposure to ionizing radiation
- Submammary placement of the pacemaker may minimize discomfort as the breasts and abdomen grow during pregnancy
- There are numerous reports of successful pregnancy after pacemaker insertion

Children:
- Atrioventricular block in children is usually congenital
- Most children are asymptomatic and do not require treatment
- If the heart rate is <50 beats/min, syncope is likely and a pacemaker is recommended. Extreme bradycardia may contribute to the frequency of Stokes–Adams attacks

PATIENT SATISFACTION/LIFESTYLE PRIORITIES

The elderly:
- The majority of pacemakers are implanted into elderly patients, and in general they are very well tolerated

Younger patients:
- Strenuous exercise may be limited by congenital complete atrioventricular block. Exercise tolerance may improve after pacemaker insertion, depending on the type of pacemaker used. Contact sports risk damage to the pacemaker

Operation of permanent pacemakers may be adversely affected by electromagnetic radiation. Patients should be advised of the risks associated with:
- Power generators
- Arc welding equipment
- Powerful motors
- Magnetic resonance imaging
- Extracorporeal shock-wave lithotripsy
- Therapeutic radiation
- Short-wave or microwave diathermy

An information sheet for patients with pacemakers is available from the American Heart Association (www.americanheart.org).

SUMMARY OF THERAPEUTIC OPTIONS

Choices

Asymptomatic patients with first-degree or type I second-degree atrioventricular (AV) block do not usually require treatment other than discontinuation of drugs that have a potential etiologic role:

- Digitalis
- Antiarrhythmic drugs (quinidine, procainamide)
- Calcium channel antagonists
- Beta-blockers

- If treatment is required, the first choice is insertion of a pacemaker
- Transcutaneous pacing, if available, is an effective temporary measure while awaiting transfer to hospital
- Atropine and other anticholinergic drugs may be used as a temporary measure before pacemaker implantation, but have no place in long-term management
- Patients who do not respond to atropine may be treated with the beta-adrenergic agonist isoproterenol. However, isoproterenol should be used with extreme caution or not at all in patients with acute myocardial infarction

Guidelines

The American College of Cardiology and American Heart Association have drawn up Guidelines for Implantation of Cardiac Pacemakers and Antiarrhythmia Devices [1]. Permanent pacing is indicated for all cases of permanent or intermittent complete or type II second-degree AV block, symptomatic cases of second-degree block, asymptomatic type I second-degree AV block at or below the bundle of His, and exercise-induced complete or second-degree AV block without reversible ischemia.

Clinical pearl(s)

- Discontinue all medications that affect atrioventricular conduction
- Refer to specialist if the patient has profound bradycardia or evidence of cerebral hypoperfusion, low cardiac output, or hypotension

FOLLOW UP

After pacemaker insertion, specialist follow up usually includes assessment of battery status, pacing threshold and pulse width, sensing function, and lead integrity. The frequency of follow up is determined by a number of factors, including coexisting cardiovascular or medical problems, the age of the pacemaker, and the results of transtelephonic testing.

Patients who do not require pacemaker insertion should be reviewed periodically by the primary care physician in order to ensure that their clinical and ECG condition has not deteriorated.

Information for patient or caregiver

- An information sheet for patients with pacemakers is available from the American Heart Association.

General:

- Strenuous exercise may be limited by congenital complete atrioventricular block
- Depending on the type of pacemaker used, exercise tolerance may improve after pacemaker insertion. Contact sports should be avoided because the pacemaker may get damaged
- The pacemaker will need to be checked periodically to ensure that it is functioning properly and that the battery is not expiring
- When the battery is nearing the end of its life, the pacemaker will need to be replaced. Depending on the type of pacemaker fitted and its programming, it should last from 5 to 12 years

Electromagnetic radiation:

- Permanent pacemakers may not function properly after exposure to electromagnetic radiation. Patient should inform their physician if they are likely to come into contact with any of the following: power generators, arc welding equipment, powerful motors, magnetic resonance imaging (MRI), extracorporeal shock-wave lithotripsy (treatment for kidney stones), therapeutic radiation (e.g. radiotherapy for treating tumors), short-wave or microwave diathermy

DRUGS AND OTHER THERAPIES: DETAILS

Drugs

ATROPINE

Atropine may be given as an intravenous bolus for the emergency management of complete or type I second-degree atrioventricular (AV) block. It may be ineffective in type II block but is unlikely to cause clinical deterioration. Suitable for short-term treatment only, e.g. during transfer to hospital.

Dose

- 0.3–0.6mg intravenous bolus, repeated after 5min if necessary
- Maximum dose 2mg

Efficacy

The administration of atropine often improves AV nodal block, but it may worsen conduction if the level of the block is below the AV node. Therefore, if the level of block is in the His–Purkinje system, conduction block may worsen to 3:1 or higher after atropine administration.

Risks/Benefits

- Benefit: Atropine therapy may be instituted promptly (intravenous bolus) in emergency situations
- Risks: Use caution in pregnancy and extreme caution in gastrointestinal infection

Side-effects and adverse reactions

- Cardiovascular: angina, ectopic ventricular beats, paradoxical bradycardia, tachycardia, atrioventricular depression, hypotension
- CNS: anxiety, insomnia, headache, ataxia, hallucinations, dizziness, drowsiness, confusion, delirium, coma
- Gastrointestinal: nausea, vomiting, constipation, xerostomia
- Genitourinary: retention of urine
- EENT: blurred vision, cycloplegia, mydriasis
- Hematologic: leukocytosis

Interactions (other drugs)

■ Amantadine ■ Antihistamines ■ Antimuscarinics ■ Clozapine ■ Cyclobenzaprine ■ Digoxin ■ Disopyramide ■ Domperidone ■ Ketoconazole ■ Levodopa ■ Monoamine oxidase inhibitors ■ Metoclopramide ■ Mexiletine ■ Nitrates ■ Opiate agonists ■ Parasympathomimetics ■ Phenothiazines ■ Potassium salts ■ Procainamide ■ Tricyclic (and related) antidepressants

Contraindications

■ Prostatic hypertrophy/urinary tract obstruction ■ Angle closure glaucoma ■ Prostatic hypertrophy ■ Myasthenia gravis ■ Gastrointestinal obstruction ■ Hypersensitivity to belladonna alkaloids ■ Acute myocardial infarction and ulcerative colitis (both relatively contraindicated) ■ Tachycardia ■ Thyrotoxicosis ■ Bleeding

ISOPROTERENOL

Isoproterenol is a beta-adrenergic agonist that stimulates both $beta_1$ and $beta_2$ receptors. It is used as a temporary measure before pacemaker implantation in patients who have not responded to atropine.

Dose

- Initial intravenous bolus 0.02–0.06mg (1–3mL of 1:50,000 dilution); subsequent boluses 0.01–0.2mg (0.5–10mL of 1:50,000 dilution)
- Alternatively, give by intravenous infusion: 5mcg/min initially, titrate dose according to response. Usual range 2–20mcg/min

Efficacy

- Note that isoproterenol is currently not available in the US
- May be effective for cardiovascular support before pacemaker implantation

Risks/Benefits

Benefit: is used in patients who have not responded to atropine and who require immediate cardiovascular support.

Risks:

- Use caution in pregnancy and breast-feeding, the elderly, and children
- Use caution in hyperthyroidism, diabetes, coronary artery disease, coronary insufficiency, patients sensitive to amines, and hypovolemia
- Use extreme caution in severe/uncontrolled hypertension, and pheochromocytoma

Side-effects and adverse reactions

- CNS: anxiety, headache, tremors, nervousness, weakness, insomnia, dizziness
- Cardiovascular: angina, ventricular tachycardia, palpitations, hypertension, hypotension, tachydysrhythmias
- Respiratory: pulmonary edema
- Gastrointestinal: nausea, vomiting
- Respiratory: cough
- Skin: flushing, sweating

Interactions (other drugs)

▪ Aminoglycosides ▪ Amphotericin B ▪ Antihypertensive agents ▪ Beta-blockers ▪ Bretylium ▪ Cardiac glycosides ▪ Corticosteroids ▪ Diuretics ▪ Entacapone ▪ Ergot alkaloids ▪ Guanethidine ▪ Halogenated anesthetics ▪ Insulin ▪ Levodopa ▪ MAOIs ▪ Methylxanthine derivatives ▪ Nitrates ▪ Oxytocic agents ▪ Penicillins ▪ Sympathomimetics ▪ Thyroid hormones ▪ Tricyclic antidepressants

Contraindications

▪ Tachycardia or heart block due to digitalis intoxication ▪ Use with extreme caution, if at all, in patients with acute myocardial infarction or angina pectoris ▪ Tachydysrhythmias ▪ Ventricular dysrhythmias that need inotropic therapy ▪ Sulfite hypersensitivity

Surgical therapy

PACEMAKER IMPLANTATION

Pacemaker implantation is the first choice for patients who require treatment. Temporary pacing may suffice for patients with an acute illness, e.g. during Lyme disease or after inferior myocardial infarction.

Guidelines published by the American College of Cardiology and the American Heart Association recommend permanent pacing for:

- All cases of permanent or intermittent, complete, or type II second-degree atrioventricular (AV) block
- Symptomatic cases of second-degree block
- Asymptomatic type I second-degree AV block at or below the bundle of His
- Exercise-induced complete or second-degree AV block without reversible ischemia

Efficacy

- There are no data from randomized clinical trials regarding the efficacy of pacemaker insertion
- Data from some nonrandomized studies strongly suggest that permanent pacing improves survival in complete atrioventricular (AV) block, especially if syncope has occurred

Evidence

There is no evidence from randomized controlled clinical trials, although data from some nonrandomized studies strongly suggest that permanent pacing improves survival in complete atrioventricular (AV) block, especially if syncope has occurred [1] *Level C*

Acceptability to patient

- Patient acceptability of implanted pacemakers is generally excellent
- Some power-generating equipment and medical devices may need to be avoided
- Exercise capacity may be impaired

Follow up plan

- Follow up after pacemaker implantation is generally undertaken by the specialist
- Follow up issues include assessment of battery status, pacing threshold and pulse width, sensing function, and lead integrity
- The frequency of follow up is determined by a number of factors, including coexisting cardiovascular or medical problems, the age of the pacemaker, and the results of transtelephonic testing

Patient and caregiver information

- Exercise tolerance may improve after pacemaker insertion, depending on the type of pacemaker used, but overexertion remains inadvisable. Contact sports risk damage to the pacemaker
- Electromagnetic radiation may adversely affect operation of permanent pacemakers. This may create occupational difficulties for patients who work with power generators, arc welding equipment, or powerful motors
- Certain medical procedures may also interfere with pacemaker operation and patients should always be advised to discuss their pacemaker before undergoing magnetic resonance imaging, extracorporeal shock-wave lithotripsy, therapeutic radiation, or short-wave or microwave diathermy

An information sheet for patients with pacemakers is available from the American Heart Association.

Other therapies

TRANSCUTANEOUS PACING

Transcutaneous pacing is an emergency measure for treatment of asystole or hemodynamically significant bradycardia

- High-impedance electrodes with a large surface area are placed on the anterior and posterior chest walls. The electrical stimuli are of high current (50–100mA) and long duration (20–40ms)

- Demand pacing is possible by sensing the surface ECG
- For definitive treatment, patients will require an implanted pacemaker

Risks/Benefits

Risks:

- Failure to pace: unless there is severe metabolic disturbance, failure to pace is almost always due to incorrect electrode placement
- Unpleasant for patient

Benefits:

- Suitable for use outside the hospital setting
- Avoids the possible complications of an invasive procedure (e.g. infection, phlebitis, thrombosis)

Acceptability to patient

- Patients may experience severe pain due to skeletal muscle stimulation
- Analgesics may help, but some patients are unable to tolerate this form of pacing

OUTCOMES

EFFICACY OF THERAPIES

- An implanted pacemaker should remain highly effective throughout its life
- Precautions against pacemaker malfunction should be taken prior to exposure to sources of electromagnetic radiation

Evidence

PDxMD are unable to cite evidence that meet our criteria for evidence.

Review period

- Follow up after pacemaker implantation is generally undertaken by the specialist. The frequency will depend on multiple factors, including coexisting cardiovascular or medical problems, the age of the pacemaker, and the results of transtelephonic testing
- Implanted pacemakers need to be replaced when the battery is coming to the end of its life. Depending on the type of pacemaker and the way it has been programmed, replacement will be necessary every 5–12 years

PROGNOSIS

- Following pacemaker implantation, the prognosis is good for patients with complete or second-degree type II atrioventricular (AV) block
- Asymptomatic second-degree type I AV block and first-degree AV block are generally considered to be benign conditions with a good prognosis, even without active treatment

Clinical pearl(s)

- Asymptomatic Wenckebach block has a good prognosis
- Type II second-degree AV block often progresses to complete heart block
- Asymptomatic first-degree AV block, asymptomatic Wenckebach block, and AV block expected to resolve (e.g. drug toxicity or Lyme disease) are contraindications for permanent pacing

PREVENTION

RISK FACTORS

Antiarrhythmic drugs may depress normal conduction of impulses through the atrioventricular node and bundle of His.

MODIFY RISK FACTORS

Lifestyle and wellness

DRUG HISTORY

- Monitor patients on antiarrhythmic medication. Atrioventricular block may develop in patients taking digitalis without signs of toxicity
- Monitor patients' heart rates if they are taking beta-blockers or calcium channel blockers

PREVENT RECURRENCE

Reassess coexisting disease

INTERACTION ALERT

The following agents may precipitate or aggravate atrioventricular block:

- Antiarrhythmic drugs (e.g. digitalis, quinidine, procainamide)
- Antihypertensive/antianginal therapy (e.g. beta-blockers, calcium channel antagonists)

ASSOCIATIONS

American Heart Association
National Center
7272 Greenville Avenue
Dallas, TX 75231
Tel: (800) AHA-USA1
www.americanheart.org

The American College of Cardiology
Heart House
9111 Old Georgetown Road
Bethesda, MD 20814-1699
Tel: (800) 253-4636 or (301) 897-5400
Fax: (301) 897-9745
www.acc.org

European Society of Cardiology
The European Heart House
2035 Rte des Colles
B.P. 179, Les Templiers
FR-06903 Sophia Antipolis
France
Tel: (492) 94-7600
Fax: (492) 94-7601
www.escardio.org

KEY REFERENCES

- Beers MH, Berkow R, eds. Arrhythmias. In: The Merck Manual, section 16, chapter 25. Whitehouse Station, NJ: Merck, 2000 (www.merck.com)
- Gregoratos G, Cheitlin MD, et al. ACC/AHA Guidelines for implantation of cardiac pacemakers and antiarrhythmia devices. J Am Coll Cardiol 1998;31:1175–209
- Wagner GS. Atrioventricular block. In: Marriott's practical electrocardiography, 9th edn. Baltimore, MD: Lippincott Williams and Wilkins, 1994
- Yealy DM, Delbridge, TR. Dysrhythmias. In: Rosen: Emergency medicine: Concepts and clinical practice, 4th edn. St Louis, MO: Mosby-Year Book, 1998
- Zipes DP. Specific arrhythmias: diagnosis and treatment. In: Braunwald E, ed. Heart disease: a book of cardiovascular medicine, 5th edn. Philadelphia, PA: WB Saunders

Guidelines

1 Gregoratos G, Cheitlin MD, et al. ACC/AHA guidelines for implantation of cardiac pacemakers and antiarrhythmia devices: a report of the American College of Cardiology/American Heart Association Task Force on Practice Guidelines (Committee on Pacemaker Implantation). J Am Coll Cardiol 1998;31(5):1175–209

FAQS

Question 1

Is type I second-degree atrioventricular block associated with poor exercise tolerance, and is it an indication to place a permanent pacemaker?

ANSWER 1

No. Type I second-degree atrioventricular block is seldom associated with symptoms and as an isolated finding is not an indication for placement of a permanent pacemaker.

Question 2
Can myocardial ischemia or infarction be complicated by varying degrees of atrioventricular block?

ANSWER 2
Yes. Atrioventricular block due to inferior ischemia or infarction is commonly reversible and does not require emergency placement of a permanent pacemaker. A temporary pacemaker may be required if atrioventricular block is hemodynamically significant. The use of medications to increase heart rate and cardiac output during the acute phase of myocardial infarction should be avoided. Atrioventricular block due to anterior ischemia or infarction may be permanent and may require placement of a permanent pacemaker.

Question 3
What are the most important interventions to consider when treating a patient with hemodynamically significant bradycardia?

ANSWER 3
- Intravenous fluids
- Oxygen
- Transcutaneous pacing
- Atropine
- Isoproterenol
- Dopamine
- Temporary pacemaker

Question 4
What are the classes of drugs that may precipitate or aggravate atrioventricular block?

ANSWER 4
- Beta-blockers
- Calcium channel blockers
- Digitalis glycosides
- Antiarrhythmics

Question 5
Is an atrial premature beat that fails to conduct through the atrioventricular node an early sign of atrioventricular block and the need for a pacemaker?

ANSWER 5
No. The normal atrioventricular node has an intrinsic refractory period. An atrial premature beat that reaches the atrioventricular node during this refractory period will not be conducted. This is a normal electrophysiologic phenomenon and is not an indication for a pacemaker.

CONTRIBUTORS
Joseph E Scherger, MD, MPH
John McB Hodgson, MD, FACC, FSCAI
James Orford, MD

CARDIAC TAMPONADE

SUMMARY INFORMATION

DESCRIPTION

- Physiologic phenomenon of reduced cardiac output resulting from the compression of cardiac chambers by accumulation of fluid within the pericardial space
- Tamponade can result from the acute (rapid) or chronic (slow) accumulation of fluid
- May present as a life-threatening emergency that requires, and usually responds well to, urgent treatment with pericardiocentesis

URGENT ACTION

- Cardiac tamponade is a medical emergency
- In a situation in which the patient is in extremis (e.g. following trauma, or cardiac arrest with electromechanical dissociation), emergency pericardiocentesis may need to be performed before hospital admission
- Prehospital oxygen and cardiac monitoring should be initiated if possible
- Rapid administration of intravenous fluids should be instituted

KEY! DON'T MISS!

Tension pneumothorax in trauma patients may cause signs similar to those of tamponade and should be considered in the differential diagnosis. If available, immediate chest X-ray examination will clarify the diagnosis.

ICD9 CODE
423.9 Unspecified diseases of the pericardium.

SYNONYMS
Pericardial tamponade.

CARDINAL FEATURES
- Compression of cardiac chambers by fluid in the pericardial space leading to their impaired dilation and filling and so to reduced stroke volume and, as a consequence, a dangerous reduction in cardiac output
- It is a life-threatening emergency, a significant cause of fatalities after chest wall trauma, and one of the causes of electromechanical dissociation at cardiac arrest
- Acute tamponade results from the rapid accumulation of pericardial fluid. Patients are critically ill with distended neck veins, reduced systolic pressure, and distant or absent heart sounds (Beck's triad)
- Chronic cases are more likely to occur in patients with pre-existing pericardial disease or as a complication of a predisposing medical condition. Presentation is with dyspnea, reduced exercise tolerance, sequelae of low cardiac output, venous distention, pulsus paradoxus, distant or absent heart sounds, and clear lung fields
- Diagnosis is by clinical picture, echocardiography, and cardiac catheterization
- Rapid relief is obtained by pericardiocentesis, even of small volumes (15–20mL), which should be performed by a specialist guided by echocardiography
- Rarely, urgent pericardiocentesis may have to be performed by the primary care physician in certain life-threatening scenarios (e.g. cardiac arrest or with a patient in extremis)

CAUSES
Common causes
Acute (as little as 200mL of rapidly accumulating fluid may cause tamponade):
- Trauma – penetrating wounds or steering wheel injury cause hemopericardium
- Aortic dissection
- Myocardial rupture after myocardial infarction and/or treatment with thrombolytics or heparin
- Iatrogenic – central line insertion, pacemaker insertion
- After cardiothoracic surgery
- After cardiac resuscitation

Chronic (over 1L of effusion can accumulate slowly before causing tamponade):
- Malignancy – lung, breast, lymphoma, leukemia
- Idiopathic pericarditis
- Viral pericarditis – coxsackievirus group B, influenza, echo, herpes, HIV
- Uremia
- Bacterial and fungal infection (e.g. *Staphylococcus aureus, Mycoplasma tuberculosis)*

Rare causes
Chronic:
- Dressler's syndrome – postmyocardial infarction fever, pleuritis, and pericarditis
- Myxedema
- Collagen-vascular diseases – rheumatoid arthritis, systemic lupus erythematosus
- Radiation
- Over-anticoagulation

Serious causes

Cardiac tamponade is itself a life-threatening sequelae of many serious conditions such as:

- Myocardial rupture after infarction
- Aortic dissection
- Malignancies
- Tuberculosis

Contributory or predisposing factors

- Pre-existing pericardial disease (e.g. pericarditis)
- Pre-existing medical condition that may involve the pericardium (e.g. malignancy, end-stage renal disease)

EPIDEMIOLOGY

Incidence and prevalence

FREQUENCY

- Occurs in 2% of penetrating chest wall trauma
- Pericardial effusions, which may lead to tamponade, occur in 20% of patients with uremia

DIFFERENTIAL DIAGNOSIS

Can be confused with other disorders that exhibit venous distention pulsus paradoxus and clear lung fields.

Chronic obstructive pulmonary disease

The distinguishing features of chronic obstructive pulmonary disease are as follows:

FEATURES

- History of dyspnea and exposure to toxic agent (e.g. tobacco, dusts, coal, silica)
- May have chronic history of cough and sputum production with acute (often infective) exacerbations
- Heart sounds often clear but may be muffled by emphysematous lung

Pneumothorax

The distinguishing features of pneumothorax are as follows:

FEATURES

- Often sudden and spontaneous
- Occurs most frequently in tall, thin males of 20–40 years of age
- Sudden, sharp, pleuritic chest pain with dyspnea
- Ipsilateral chest signs – reduced expansion and breath sounds and hyper-resonant percussion note; mediastinal shift away from side of tension pneumothorax

Constrictive pericarditis

The distinguishing features of constrictive pericarditis are as follows:

FEATURES

- Clinically very similar to cardiac tamponade
- Rigid pericardium leads to same impaired cardiac filling and reduced output
- Has a more chronic course with gradual onset of symptoms and development of hepatomegaly, ascites, and pedal edema
- Kussmaul's sign (jugular venous pressure increases on inspiration)
- Pericardial knock following second heart sound may be present
- Chest X-ray examination shows rim of pericardial calcification in 50% of cases
- Echocardiogram shows thickened pericardium but normal ventricular contraction

Restrictive cardiomyopathy

The distinguishing features of restrictive cardiomyopathy are as follows:

FEATURES

- Myocardial dysfunction most frequently due to amyloid infiltration, myocardial fibrosis, or radiation
- Clinically similar to chronic tamponade or constrictive pericarditis with congestive heart failure (right heart failure can predominate)
- Tricuspid regurgitation murmur is common
- Associated with arrhythmias (including atrial fibrillation) and left axis deviation on ECG
- Echocardiogram shows increased wall thickness and Doppler flow evidence of diastolic dysfunction
- Kussmaul's sign may be present

Right ventricular infarction

The distinguishing features of right ventricular infarction are as follows:

FEATURES

- Occurs after acute inferior myocardial infarction
- Diagnosed by history, right-sided ECG findings, and cardiac enzyme studies
- Heart sounds should be clearly audible, and added sounds may be present, such as right ventricular third sound
- Pulmonary congestion may occur
- Very sensitive to nitrate administration (hypotension)

Pulmonary embolism

Massive pulmonary embolism can resemble tamponade.

FEATURES

- Acute dyspnea, pleuritic chest pain, and possibly hemoptysis
- Jugular venous pressure will be raised, and there may be prominent a-waves
- Heart sounds should be clear. A right ventricular gallop may be present. The pulmonic component of the second heart sound should be increased
- Consider in patients with appropriate risk factors
- Diagnosis is by ventilation perfusion studies or, definitively, pulmonary angiography
- Lower extremity venous Doppler studies or D-dimer measurement may provide supportive evidence

Hypovolemia/shock

FEATURES

- Distinguished by examination of jugular venous pressure – raised in cardiac tamponade and low in shock/dehydration states, although tamponade may rarely occur in low-volume states without the usual venous distention
- In shock, clinical findings in keeping with the cause are present (e.g. pulmonary edema in cardiac failure, fever in sepsis)
- Heart sounds should be clear in hypovolemic/shocked patients, although difficult to separate due to tachycardia

Cardiogenic shock

Shock caused by the failure of the heart to maintain adequate outflow.

FEATURES

- May be sudden in onset, or after a period of worsening heart failure
- Many causes, including cardiac tamponade, but also myocardial infarction, valve dysfunction, arrhythmia (e.g. rapid atrial fibrillation, ventricular tachycardia), pulmonary embolus, tension pneumothorax

SIGNS & SYMPTOMS

Signs

Consider tamponade in a cardiac arrest situation when the rhythm observed is electromechanical dissociation.

Acute:

- Patient may be stuporous
- Cold exremities
- Tachypnea and tachycardia
- Beck's triad of decreased systemic arterial pressure, raised central venous pressure, and a quiet (distant) or silent heart

Chronic:

- Acutely ill but not usually in extremis
- Cold extremities
- Tachypnea and tachycardia
- Decreased systolic blood pressure
- Narrow pulse pressure
- Pulsus paradoxus (a more than 10mmHg fall in systolic blood pressure during inspiration or, in severe cases, disappearance of palpable pulses during inspiration); absence of pulsus paradoxus does not exclude a tamponade
- Raised jugular venous pressure with a characteristic prominent *x* descent and absent *y* descent
- Kussmaul's sign (jugular venous pressure rises with inspiration), but this is a nonspecific finding
- Pericardial friction rub is more likely with small pericardial effusions but can rarely occur with a large effusion
- Soft, distant heart sounds
- Clear lung fields
- Right upper quadrant tenderness (due to hepatic engorgement) or soft, tender liver edge

Symptoms

- Dyspnea – main symptom in chronic cases
- Minimal exercise tolerance
- May progress rapidly to restlessness and agitation, coma, and cardiac arrest (electromechanical dissociation)
- Chest pain
- Abdominal pain

KEY! DON'T MISS!

Tension pneumothorax in trauma patients may cause signs similar to those of tamponade and should be considered in the differential diagnosis. If available, immediate chest X-ray examination will clarify the diagnosis.

CONSIDER CONSULT

All patients in whom cardiac tamponade is suspected should be referred urgently:

- Nontraumatic cases to internal medicine or cardiology
- Traumatic cases to trauma surgery or cardiothoracic surgery
- Investigations are best performed by the appropriate specialist

INVESTIGATION OF THE PATIENT

Direct questions to patient

In trauma cases the history may not be available from the patient but diagnosis may be suspected by the site of the penetrating injury. There may be a history of recent procedure in iatrogenic cases (central line, pacemaker insertion, postbypass surgery). Other history can be used to identify chronic etiology:

- Q **Has there been a sudden increase in breathlessness or deterioration in exercise tolerance?** If sudden, may indicate acute tamponade; if gradual, then more likely to be due to a slow accumulation of fluid
- Q **Has the patient suffered sudden chest pain?** Consider acute myocardial infarction with rupture and aortic dissection
- Q **Has the patient had sharp chest pains?** Consider pericarditis
- Q **Has the patient suffered fevers, myalgia, or other symptoms of viral or bacterial infection?** May indicate infectious pericarditis
- Q **Has the patient suffered night sweats and weight loss?** Consider tuberculosis, malignancies
- Q **Has the patient had any abdominal pain?** Hepatomegaly resulting from tamponade causes right upper quadrant pain

Contributory or predisposing factors

- **Q** **Is there a recent history of trauma?** Particularly penetrating wounds to chest wall but also blunt injuries and contusion
- **Q** **Is there a history of pre-existing pericardial disease?** Pericarditis or neoplastic involvement of the pericardium may predispose to tamponade
- **Q** **Has there been a recent myocardial infarction?** Consider Dressler's syndrome
- **Q** **Is there a pre-existing medical condition that may involve the pericardium?** Consider malignancy and end-stage renal failure

Examination

- **Examine for cardiac output.** Tamponade may present as a cardiac arrest scenario
- **Establish whether the patient is in extremis.** In this case there may be a need to perform urgent unguided pericardiocentesis
- **Check for any evidence of trauma to chest wall.** Consider penetrating wounds particularly, but also other injuries, such as steering wheel trauma
- **Check for evidence of a low cardiac output state.** Cold peripheries, tachycardia, low systolic blood pressure, low pulse pressure
- **Examine the jugular venous pressure.** In chronic cases there may be characteristic prominent *x* descent and absent *y* descent of the jugular venous pressure. Also look for Kussmaul's sign (a paradoxical rise in the jugular venous pressure during inspiration)
- **Check for evidence of distended neck veins and clear lung fields.** Distended neck veins and a raised jugular venous pressure are seen secondary to back pressure on the heart. The lungs are clear in the acute situation
- **Are the heart sounds audible and, if so, are there any added sounds?** In cardiac tamponade the heart sounds are classically, but not always, distant or silent. No extra heart sounds should be heard other than a pericardial rub, which is usually, but not always, associated with a small effusion
- **Examine for evidence of Beck's triad in acute cases (i.e. low systolic pressure, distended neck veins, and distant or absent heart sounds).** Beck's triad indicates that the patient is critically ill
- **Can pulsus paradoxus be demonstrated?** Either with blood pressure recording or palpation of peripheral pulses
- **Examine the abdomen for signs of chronic venous distention?** Engorged and tender liver may be palpated

Summary of investigative tests

In the primary care setting, there is usually no time for investigation. The following tests may be useful in determining the etiology of a pericardial effusion and tamponade:

- ECG – performed on all suspected cases of cardiac tamponade. The findings are often suggestive but not diagnostic
- Chest X-ray examination – performed on all suspected cases, although not a very specific aid to diagnosis
- Echocardiogram – performed on all suspected cases by a specialist
- Cardiac catheterization – performed by a cardiologist usually in nontraumatic cases when immediate surgery is not necessary

In cases of nontraumatic tamponade when the etiology of the pericardial fluid (effusion) is unknown, the following blood tests are useful:

- Complete blood count may point to possible causes of pericardial effusion
- Blood urea nitrogen may reveal uremia, which can cause pericardial effusion
- Erythrocyte sedimentation rate (ESR) – a raised ESR can occur in many causes of pericardial effusion
- Thyroid function tests may reveal hypothyroidism, which can cause pericardial effusion

- Antinuclear antibodies – a positive result may point to rheumatoid arthritis or lupus as the etiology of the pericardial effusion
- Purified protein derivative can be used as a screening test for tuberculosis exposure

DIAGNOSTIC DECISION

- The diagnosis of cardiac tamponade is based on history and clinical findings supported by investigations
- Echocardiography is extremely useful in identifying pericardial effusion and its hemodynamic effect, and in guiding pericardiocentesis
- Right-sided cardiac catheterization and intrapericardial pressure measurement is the investigation of choice for definitive diagnosis and guiding pericardiocentesis

Guidelines

- Mueller HS, Chatterjee K, Davis KB, et al. Present use of bedside right heart catheterization in patients with cardiac disease. J Am Coll Cardiol 1998,32(3):840–64. Available online at the American College of Cardiology website [1]
- Cheitlin MD, Alpert JS, Armstrong WF, et al. ACC/AHA guidelines for the clinical application of echocardiography. Echoardiography 1997;95(6):1686–744. Available online at the American College of Cardiology website [2]

CLINICAL PEARL(S)

- The diagnosis of pericardial tamponade is primarily a clinical diagnosis. When there is hemodynamic compromise, further investigations should not delay prompt treatment
- Nitrates should be avoided (they lower preload and worsen hypotension)
- Rapid administration of intravenous fluids should be initiated

THE TESTS

Body fluids

COMPLETE BLOOD COUNT

Description

Venous blood sample.

Advantages/Disadvantages

- Advantages: simple, inexpensive test
- Disadvantage: nonspecific

Normal

- Hemoglobin: male 13.5–18.0g/dL; female 11.5–16.0g/dL
- White cell count: 4.0–11.0x10^9/L
- Platelet count: 150–400x10^9/L

Abnormal

Results outside normal reference range.

Cause of abnormal result

- Anemia – malignancy, tuberculosis
- Leukocytosis – bacterial infection
- Lymphocytosis – viral infection, Hodgkin's disease, chronic lymphatic leukemia

BLOOD UREA NITROGEN

Description

Random venous blood.

Advantages/Disadvantages
Advantages: inexpensive and readily available.

Normal
8–18mg/dL (3–6.5mmol/L).

Abnormal
>18mg/dL (>6.5mmol/L).

Cause of abnormal result
Uremia may be the cause of pericardial effusion and therefore tamponade.

ERYTHROCYTE SEDIMENTATION RATE
Description
Rate of sedimentation of red blood cells in anticoagulated blood over a 1h period.

Advantages/Disadvantages
Advantages: inexpensive and readily available (can be measured in office).

Normal
- Males: 0–15mm/h
- Females: 0–20mm/h

Abnormal
- Males: >0–15mm/h
- Females: >0–20mm/h

Cause of abnormal result
Raised ESR can occur in many causes of pericardial effusions – infections including tuberculosis, malignancy, collagen-vascular diseases, and myocardial infarction.

THYROID FUNCTION TESTS
Description
Random venous blood sample.

Advantages/Disadvantages
- Advantages: readily available
- Disadvantage: nonspecific for cardiac tamponade

Normal
- Thyroid-stimulating hormone (TSH): 2–11mcU/mL (2–11mU/L); new 'sensitive' TSH assays have different ranges
- Thyroxine (T4): 4–11mcg/dL (51–142nmol/L)

Abnormal
Hypothyroidism – raised TSH and reduced T4.

Cause of abnormal result
Myxedema (hypothyroidism) may be the cause of pericardial effusion.

Drugs, disorders, and other factors that may alter results
Lithium and amiodarone can cause elevated levels of TSH in some patients.

RHEUMATOID FACTOR

Description

Random venous blood sample.

Advantages/Disadvantages

- Advantage: inexpensive
- Disadvantage: may not be available in all laboratories

Normal

Normally rheumatoid factor (RF) titer is negative.

Abnormal

RF titer >1:20 is positive.

Cause of abnormal result

Positive RF points to the cause of pericardial effusion as being related to rheumatoid arthritis or systemic lupus erythematosus.

Drugs, disorders, and other factors that may alter results

Rheumatoid factor may be increased in:

- Rheumatoid arthritis
- Systemic lupus erythematosus
- Multiple myeloma
- Sarcoidosis
- Sjögren's syndrome
- Pulmonary fibrosis
- Various chronic inflammatory processes
- Old age

ANTINUCLEAR ANTIBODIES

Description

Random venous blood sample.

Advantages/Disadvantages

- Advantage: inexpensive
- Disadvantage: may not be available in all laboratories

Normal

Normally antinuclear antibody (ANA) titer is <1:20.

Abnormal

ANA titer >1:20 is positive.

Cause of abnormal result

Positive ANA points to lupus, especially if titer >1:160.

Drugs, disorders, and other factors that may alter results

Phenytoin, ethosuximide, hydralazine, carbamazepine, penicillin cause positive results (drug-induced lupus).

Imaging

CHEST X-RAY

Advantages/Disadvantages

- Advantages: inexpensive and readily available
- Disadvantages: in acute cases there may be no change in heart size because more than 250mL of pericardial fluid must build up before cardiac shadow is seen to enlarge

Abnormal

- In acute cardiac tamponade the heart size can be normal
- In chronic cases (with effusions larger than 250mL) the cardiac shadow may be enlarged and may have a characteristic globular or water-bottle shape
- Pulmonary congestion is very unusual

Cause of abnormal result

The globular/water-bottle-shaped heart seen in cardiac tamponade secondary to chronic pericardial effusions is similar to the heart shadow seen in dilated cardiomyopathy.

ECHOCARDIOGRAM

Advantages/Disadvantages

Advantages:

- Noninvasive
- Can differentiate tamponade from constrictive pericarditis and right ventricular infarction, and can identify other pathology – extracardiac hematoma or tumor
- Can guide pericardiocentesis

Disadvantage: may need specialized knowledge to interpret

Abnormal

- The presence of excess pericardial fluid
- Diastolic collapse of right atrium and right ventricle suggests physiologic tamponade
- Paradoxical septal motion with respiration
- Abnormal filling pattern on Doppler flow study

Cause of abnormal result

Pericardial effusions and their hemodynamic sequelae can be seen.

Special tests

PURIFIED PROTEIN DERIVATIVE

Description

Purified protein derivative (PPD) is an intradermal injection that screens for exposure to tuberculosis.

Advantages/Disadvantages

- Advantage: screening test for tuberculosis exposure
- Disadvantage: may be negative if the patient is anergic – patient should have an anergy control placed at the same time

Normal

No local reaction at 48h.

Abnormal

Inflammatory reaction resulting in edema at injection site.

Cause of abnormal result

If the patient has been previously infected with tuberculosis, the injection site will demonstrate inflammation.

Drugs, disorders, and other factors that may alter results

May be negative if patient is anergic – patient should have an anergy control placed at the same time.

Other tests

RIGHT-SIDED CARDIAC CATHETERIZATION

Description

- Performed by a specialist
- Simultaneous intrapericardial and intracardiac chamber pressure measurements are taken to confirm diagnosis in chronic case where diagnosis is in doubt

Advantages/Disadvantages

Advantages:

- Provides definitive diagnosis
- Guides pericardiocentesis
- Allows the detection of coexisting hemodynamic problems

Disadvantages: complications include arrhythmias, systemic and cardiac thromboembolism, infection, trauma to heart and vessels (e.g. dissection).

Abnormal

- Diastolic equalization of pressures so that pulmonary artery diastolic pressure, right ventricular diastolic pressure, right atrial pressure, and intrapericardial pressure are almost identical
- Loss of the *y* descent in the atrial tracing with preserved respiratory variation of venous pressures

Cause of abnormal result

Diastolic equalization of pressure is typical of cardiac tamponade.

Drugs, disorders, and other factors that may alter results

- Chronic pericardial effusion and myocardial restrictive processes can have similar results
- Fluid loading or assessing ventricular pressure interdependence may be required for differential diagnosis

ECG

Advantages/Disadvantages

Advantages:

- Simple, noninvasive
- Results are immediate

Disadvantage: findings may not be diagnostic because abnormal findings can mimic other cardiac abnormalities.

Abnormal

- May show low-voltage QRS complexes, ST-segment elevation, and PR-segment depression of pericarditis
- Electrical alternans is pathognomonic of cardiac tamponade and is characterized by alternating levels of ECG voltage of the P wave, QRS complex, and T waves
- Possible bradycardia or pulseless electrical activity

Cause of abnormal result

Pressure on the myocardium from a large effusion.

TREATMENT

PATIENT AND CAREGIVER ISSUES

Health-seeking behavior

Has there been a delay in seeking treatment? Patients at risk from predisposing conditions should be educated to report early warning symptoms and signs.

MANAGEMENT ISSUES

Goals

- To restore some function to the cardiovascular system of a patient in extremis using pericardiocentesis and hemodynamic support until admitted to hospital. Even removing 20mL of fluid may improve cardiac output
- In all patients – to ensure urgent referral and transfer to a specialist for full assessment and treatment
- To follow up treated patients to detect early signs of recurrence

Management in special circumstances

COEXISTING DISEASE

The underlying cause for the cardiac tamponade will need to be appropriately managed. If the tamponade is secondary to trauma, assessment for other injuries and treatment is necessary.

SUMMARY OF THERAPEUTIC OPTIONS

Choices

- Percutaneous needle pericardiocentesis – ideally performed by a specialist with echocardiographic guidance or during cardiac catheterization. Rarely, it has to be performed by a primary care practitioner in the emergency scenario of a cardiac arrest or a patient in extremis
- Immediate cardiothoracic surgery may be necessary in traumatic cases, postmyocardial infarction rupture, and in a patient with dissecting aorta as the only life-saving treatment. Intravenous saline/colloids and pericardiocentesis are important for establishing hemodynamic stability
- Pericardiotomy and pericardiectomy are surgical procedures used in large or recurrent effusions; virtually always needed if effusion is due to malignancy (performed by a thoracic surgeon)
- Note that advanced life support (cardiopulmonary resuscitation, vasopressor agents, pericardiocentesis) is needed for a cardiac arrest, and hemodynamic support with intravenous saline and colloids, and possibly urgent pericardiocentesis for unstable or moribund patients

Never

- Agents that lower preload such as nitrates and diuretics are contraindicated
- Beta-blockers should be avoided
- Positive-pressure ventilation should be avoided if possible (depresses cardiac output even further)

FOLLOW UP

Plan for review

- Aim of follow up is to monitor for early evidence of recurrence of problem that led to cardiac tamponade
- Acutely, by clinical assessment, chest X-ray examination, and echocardiography
- Any pericardial drainage catheter should be left in place for 18–24h with frequent assessment for reaccumulation of fluid
- Long-term review is recommended at monthly intervals initially
- Follow up will depend on the cause and the treatment

Information for patient or caregiver

Patient should be advised to report any symptoms that may represent recurrence as soon as they occur.

DRUGS AND OTHER THERAPIES: DETAILS

Surgical therapy

PERCUTANEOUS NEEDLE PERICARDIOCENTESIS

- Indicated when there is rapid deterioration of hemodynamic state or for diagnostic collection of fluid
- Ideally, should be performed by a cardiologist using echocardiography or cardiac catheterization, with fluoroscopy for guidance, and with hemodynamic and electrocardiographic monitoring
- May have to be performed unguided by primary care practitioner as necessary in life-threatening emergencies (cardiac arrest and moribund patients)
- Unguided pericardiocentesis – best with patient's head and thorax tilted up; if possible perform under ECG monitoring; if time allows use aseptic technique and 1% lidocaine to infiltrate skin and deep tissues; intravenous access and resuscitation equipment at ready; use pericardiocentesis kit if available; otherwise introduce an 18-gauge catheter needle (or an 18-gauge spinal needle) at 45° angle just below and left of xiphisternum and aim for tip of left scapula; aspirate continuously; evacuate pericardial contents through three-way tap; withdraw needle when clinical improvement is noted or ECG shows ST-segment depression, which would indicate penetration had reached the myocardium; catheter can be sutured and left for continuous drainage

Efficacy

- Sometimes the withdrawal of only small volumes of fluid, as little as 20mL, will produce marked clinical improvement
- Pericardiocentesis during catheterization relieves tamponade in approximately 60% of patients; surgical procedures may be needed in other patients
- Pericardiocentesis with echocardiography has been shown to provide pericardial fluid in 91% of patients with effusions and relieves tamponade in 61% of patients if performed during cardiac catheterization
- Echo-guided aspiration at a community hospital was 100% successful, with no patients needing emergency surgical attention
- At a university hospital, emergency echo-guided aspiration for tamponade complicating catheter-based procedures was 99% successful with a 3% complication rate (no deaths). Further surgical therapy was needed in 18%

Risks/Benefits

Risks:

- Complications (risk <5%) include hemopericardium; laceration of ventricle or coronary artery; arrhythmias (ventricular fibrillation in particular); pneumothorax; puncture of aorta, esophagus, and/or peritoneum
- In unguided pericardiocentesis these risks are much higher
- Risk of complications is high and poor success rate with hemopericardium when blood enters the pericardial space as quickly as it is aspirated. Surgical correction, if possible, is necessary in such patients

Benefits:

- Benefits are a rapid relief of tamponade; allows the taking of fluid for cytologic and other analysis to determine cause of effusion if unknown; long-term catheter can be placed in situ if large, reaccumulating effusions (tuberculosis, malignancy)

Acceptability to patient

Pericardiocentesis is usually an urgent, life-saving single procedure.

Follow up plan

Immediate follow up with repeat echocardiography and X-ray examinations and then follow up to detect recurrence of effusion.

Patient and caregiver information

Patients should be advised to report symptoms that may reflect reaccumulation of pericardial fluid early, before the development of tamponade.

PERICARDIOTOMY AND PERICARDIECTOMY

- Performed by cardiothoracic specialist
- Used in large and recurrent pericardial effusions or tamponade, usually due to malignancy
- Procedures are surgical/subxiphoid pericardiotomy (pericardial window) and limited/complete/partial pericardiectomy
- May have similar results with a percutaneous balloon pericardiotomy performed in the catheterization laboratory

Efficacy

- Subxiphoid pericardiotomy – permits therapeutic drainage of fluid, collection of fluid for laboratory analysis, and pericardial biopsy if necessary; can be performed under local anesthesia
- 30-day mortality rate has been found to be up to 15.5%; it is higher in patients with malignant effusions than in those with benign effusions

Risks/Benefits

Risks: 30-day mortality rate has been found to be up to 15.5%; it is higher in patients with malignant effusions than in those with benign effusions.

Benefits: Subxiphoid pericardiotomy permits therapeutic drainage of fluid, collection of fluid for laboratory analysis, and pericardial biopsy if necessary; can be performed under local anesthesia

Acceptability to patient

Subxiphoid pericardiotomy is possible using local anesthetic and therefore may be more acceptable to patients requiring the procedure.

Follow up plan

Postprocedure echocardiography and chest X-ray examinations will be necessary immediately after the surgery and then usually during the monthly follow up.

Patient and caregiver information

To report symptoms suggestive of reaccumulation of fluid as early as possible to ensure appropriate management before tamponade recurs.

OUTCOMES

EFFICACY OF THERAPIES

- After emergency pericardiocentesis for catheter-based procedural tamponade, there may be a need for surgical intervention. Initial catheter-based injuries may lead to a significant mortality rate
- Percutaneous balloon pericardiotomy for tamponade or large effusion is durable. Most patients do not suffer from recurrent tamponade

Evidence

PDxMD are unable to cite evidence that meets our criteria for evidence.

PROGNOSIS

- Depends on underlying cause
- Good prognosis expected with appropriate treatment of penetrating injuries
- Prognosis depends markedly on rapid identification of tamponade
- Other factors that favor a good prognosis are a minor perforation, isolated right ventricular wounds, and systolic pressure >50mmHg

Therapeutic failure

- Drainage of pericardial fluid will almost always improve the hemodynamic situation
- However, in cases due to penetrating wounds, ventricular rupture, or dissecting aorta, only cardiothoracic repair will be effective

Recurrence

- If recurrence occurs after the initial pericardiocentesis, then the patient should be urgently referred for repeat pericardiocentesis and/or consideration for pericardiotomy or pericardiectomy
- Recurrence of pericardial effusion after the surgical treatment of traumatic tamponade is sometimes associated with a fever. This is termed the postcardiotomy syndrome and usually responds to aspirin or other nonsteroidal anti-inflammatory drugs, but steroid therapy is sometimes required

Terminal illness

Terminally ill patients who develop cardiac tamponade (malignancies) may benefit greatly from palliative pericardiocentesis. Sclerosis may prevent recurrence.

COMPLICATIONS

- Untreated will result in cardiac arrest (usually electromechanical dissociation)
- Constrictive pericarditis can occur in 10–15% of patients with prior pericarditis
- Constrictive pericarditis is sometimes a complication of traumatic tamponade
- Recurrent pericardial effusions with fever are a complication of traumatic tamponade and termed the postpericardiotomy syndrome
- Complications of pericardiocentesis (bleeding, pneumothorax)

CONSIDER CONSULT

- All treated cases of cardiac tamponade in whom there is evidence of recurrence should be referred urgently back to the specialist for repeat pericardiocentesis and/or consideration of pericardiotomy/pericardiectomy
- Patients with terminal illnesses who develop tamponade may benefit from repeated palliative pericardiocentesis or pericardiotomy/pericardiectomy

PREVENTION

PREVENT RECURRENCE

- Ensure that underlying condition is treated adequately
- Close monitoring of patient for early clinical and radiologic evidence of recurrence of pericardial effusion

RESOURCES

ASSOCIATIONS

American College of Cardiology
Heart House
9111 Old Georgetown Road
Bethesda, MD 20814-1699
Phone: (800) 253-4636 or (301) 897-5400
Fax: (301) 897-9745
http://www.acc.org/

American Heart Association
National Center
7272 Greenville Avenue
Dallas, TX 75231
Phone: (800)-AHA-USA1
http://www.americanheart.org/

KEY REFERENCES

- Lorell BH. Chapter 43 – Pericardial diseases. Cohn PF. Chapter 44 – Traumatic heart disease. In: Braunwald E, ed. Heart disease: textbook of cardiovascular medicine, 5th edn. St Louis, MO: WB Saunders, 1997, p1486–95 and 1535–36
- Gibson DG, Bradley RD. Chapter 15.20 – Pericardial tamponade. Treacher DF. Chapter 16 – Intensive care. In: Weatherall DJ, Ledingham JGG, Warrel DA, eds. Oxford textbook of medicine, 3rd edn. Oxford, UK: Oxford University Press, 1996, p2476–8 and 2570–1
- Kern ML. The handbook of cardiac catheterization, 3rd edn. St Louis, MO: Mosby, 1999, p446–54
- Yang et al. In: Davis FA. From catheterization data to hemodynamic parameters, 3rd edn. 1988, p302–13

Guidelines

1 Mueller HS, Chatterjee K, Davis KB, et al. Present use of bedside right heart catheterization in patients with cardiac disease. J Am Coll Cardiol 1998;32(3):840–64. Available online at the American College of Cardiology website

2 Cheitlin MD, Alpert JS, Armstrong WF, et al. ACC/AHA guidelines for the clinical application of echocardiography. Echocardiography 1997;95(6):1686–744. Available online at the American College of Cardiology website

FAQS

Question 1

Will less than 200mL of fluid in the pericardial space usually not result in hemodynamically significant cardiac tamponade?

ANSWER 1

False. The rapid accumulation of even small amounts of fluid within the pericardial space may compromise right ventricular filling and cardiac output, and result in hemodynamically significant cardiac tamponade.

Question 2

What is the characteristic hemodynamic feature of cardiac tamponade noted at the time of right heart catheterization?

ANSWER 2
Equalization of the diastolic pressures – right atrial pressure, right ventricular diastolic pressure, pulmonary artery diastolic pressure, and intrapericardial pressure are almost identical.

Question 3
Is it true that pericardiocentesis should be performed only in the cardiac catheterization laboratory or operating room and after confirmation by echocardiography or right heart cardiac catheterization?

ANSWER 3
No. Unguided pericardiocentesis at the bedside is indicated in cases of severe hemodynamic compromise of cardiac arrest.

Question 4
Will a chest X-ray examination reveal enlargement of the cardiac silhouette in all cases of hemodynamically significant cardiac tamponade?

ANSWER 4
No. The chest X-ray examination is not a sensitive test for the presence of cardiac tamponade. Effusions of less than 200mL may not result in radiographic cardiomegaly yet may be hemodynamically significant if they accumulated rapidly.

Question 5
What is the physiologic basis of pulsus paradoxus?

ANSWER 5
Pulsus paradoxus is an exaggeration of normal cardiac physiology. During inspiration the intrathoracic pressure drops, facilitating venous return to the thorax and filling of the right ventricle. This transient increase in filling of the right ventricle results in bulging of the interventricular septum and reduced left ventricular filling, with reduced left ventricular stroke volume, cardiac output, and systemic blood pressure.

CONTRIBUTORS
Dennis F Saver, MD
John McB Hodgson, MD, FACC, FSCAI
James Orford, MD

CARDIOMYOPATHY

SUMMARY INFORMATION

DESCRIPTION

- Disease of the heart muscle that results in abnormal cardiac function. Arrhythmias and sudden death are common in hypertrophic cardiomyopathy and right ventricular dysplasia
- Distinct from heart muscle impairment caused by hypertension, coronary atherosclerosis, valvular dysfunction, or abnormalities of the pericardium
- Dilated cardiomyopathy: heart's cavity is enlarged and the systolic function of one or both ventricles is impaired
- Hypertrophic cardiomyopathy: characterized by left ventricular hypertrophy that is disproportionate to the hemodynamic load
- Restrictive cardiomyopathy: marked by restricted filling and reduced diastolic volume of either or both ventricles, with normal or near-normal wall thickness
- Relatively uncommon, can occur in the young, and tends to be progressive
- A leading cause of heart transplantation

URGENT ACTION

- Presentation with congestive heart failure or cardiac arrest is a medical emergency
- Prompt evaluation is needed for patients with a history of syncope

KEY! DON'T MISS!

- Signs and symptoms of pulmonary emboli or stroke suggest thrombi formation in the cardiac chambers. Thrombus is frequently found in the apices of either ventricle in dilated cardiomyopathy
- In all patients with unexplained syncope with exercise and in a young people with cardiac arrest, hypertrophic cardiomyopathy and right ventricular dysplasia should be considered in the differential diagnosis

ICD9 CODE
425.1 Hypertrophic obstructive cardiomyopathy; 425.4 Other primary cardiomyopathies; 425.5 Alcoholic cardiomyopathy; 746.84 Hypertrophic congenital cardiomyopathy

SYNONYMS
- Congestive cardiomyopathy (dilated cardiomyopathy)
- Idiopathic hypertrophic subaortic stenosis (hypertrophic cardiomyopathy)
- Hypertrophic obstructive cardiomyopathy (hypertrophic cardiomyopathy)
- Muscular subaortic stenosis (hypertrophic cardiomyopathy)
- Arrhythmogenic right ventricular dysplasia (hypertrophic cardiomyopathy)

CARDINAL FEATURES
- Dilated cardiomyopathy: dilated cardiac chambers and systolic dysfunction in the absence of congenital, coronary, valvular, or pericardial heart disease
- Hypertrophic cardiomyopathy: abnormal left ventricular wall stiffness that causes impaired diastolic filling
- Restrictive cardiomyopathy: restricted filling and diminished diastolic volume of either or both ventricles, with normal or near-normal wall thickness and systolic function

CAUSES
Common causes
Dilated cardiomyopathy
- Alcoholism
- Tachycardia-induced dilated cardiomyopathy. Seen in patients with prolonged sinus tachycardia (either sinus rhythm or a supraventricular tachycardia) or atrial fibrillation or flutter with rapid ventricular response
- Drug abuse, including cocaine, methamphetamine, and heroin
- Medically prescribed drugs, including certain chemotherapeutic drugs (anthracyclines) and phenothiazines
- Infection with human immunodeficiency virus (HIV), and exposure to antiretroviral agents used to treat AIDS
- Pregnancy, particularly during the peripartum period in women with pre-eclampsia or multiple births
- Genetic: Pattern of familial inheritance is evident in up to 20% of instances of otherwise idiopathic dilated cardiomyopathy
- Hemochromatosis
- Infectious disease (coxsackievirus, adenovirus, cytomegalovirus, Rocky Mountain spotted fever, Q fever, toxoplasmosis, trichinosis, leptospirosis, Lyme disease, Chagas' disease)

Hypertrophic cardiomyopathy
- Most cases have a genetic origin, caused by a number of possible genotypic abnormalities.
- A variant form of the gene encoding the beta heavy chain of cardiac myosin is the most commonly identified cause
- Certain mutations causing hypertrophic cardiomyopathy may be associated with an increased risk of sudden death

Restrictive cardiomyopathy
- Infiltrative and storage disorders, most typically amyloidosis, but also glycogen storage disease, sarcoidosis, and hemochromatosis, eosinophilic endomyocardial disease
- Idiopathic

Rare causes

Dilated cardiomyopathy

- Exposure to toxins, including heavy metals, cobalt, organic solvents, and mercury
- Nutritional deficiency involving thiamine, selenium, carnitine, or taurine
- Endocrine disorders, including hypothyroidism, hyperthyroidism, adrenal cortical insufficiency, acromegaly
- Electrolyte disturbances including potassium deficiency and magnesium deficiency
- Connective tissue disease: systemic lupus erythematosus, polyarteritis nodosa, rheumatoid arthritis, scleroderma, and dermatomyositis
- Hematologic disorders, including sickle-cell anemia and thalassemia
- Muscular dystrophies; Duchenne, Becker-type and myotonic
- Sarcoidosis
- Idiopathic disease is diagnosed in a significant minority of cases

Hypertrophic cardiomyopathy

- Idiopathic

Restrictive cardiomyopathy

- Myocarditis
- Cardiac transplantation
- Pseudoxanthoma elasticum
- Loeffler's eosinophilic endomyocardial fibrosis
- Gaucher's disease (in children only)
- Myocardial fibrosis following cardiac surgery
- Radiation
- Scleroderma
- Endomyocardial fibrosis
- Toxic effects of anthracyclines
- Carcinoid heart disease and metastatic cancer

Contributory or predisposing factors

- Alcoholism
- Drug addiction
- AIDS
- Myocarditis
- Sarcoidosis
- Cancer affecting the heart or being treated with radiation or chemotherapeutic drugs (increased risk of cardiomyopathy occurs in patients with pre-existing decrease in systolic function who receive chemotherapy with anthracyclines)

EPIDEMIOLOGY

Incidence and prevalence

INCIDENCE

Dilated cardiomyopathy: 1.48 per 1000.

PREVALENCE

- Dilated cardiomyopathy: estimated 9.2 per 1000
- Hypertrophic cardiomyopathy: estimated 0.5–2.0 per 1000
- Restrictive cardiomyopathy is the most rarely encountered form of heart muscle disease in Western countries

Demographics

AGE

- Ischemic cardiomyopathy has a higher incidence in the elderly (since it is due to coronary artery disease)
- The nonischemic cardiomyopathies can occur at younger ages. A young person presenting with a cardiomyopathy of unknown etiology has a low likelihood of coronary artery disease, so nonischemic cardiomyopathy should be suspected. It can occur at all ages, including childhood
- Hypertrophic cardiomyopathy most commonly presents in the third decade of life, although it may occur throughout the lifespan. Among children, the condition is most likely to present in the second decade
- Risk of sudden death due to hypertrophic cardiomyopathy is greatest in those younger than age 30

GENDER

- Dilated cardiomyopathy occurs more frequently in males than in females (about 3:1)
- Hypertrophic cardiomyopathy is slightly more prevalent among males, although its inheritance is not sex-linked. Females with the disease tend to present at an earlier age than males

RACE

Dilated cardiomyopathy occurs more frequently in African-Americans than in caucasians (about 2.5:1).

GENETICS

- Hypertrophic cardiomyopathy is generally inherited as an autosomal dominant trait with variable penetrance and expressivity. Echocardiography shows disease in about one-fourth of first-degree relatives of patients with this condition
- Different genetic mutations have a different prognosis. Troponin T mutations have an increased risk of sudden death, which can occur without evidence of significant left ventricular hypertrophy
- A minority of cases reflect a sporadic, nonfamilial form of the disease
- Up to 30% of instances of otherwise idiopathic dilated cardiomyopathy suggest familial inheritance
- Familial inheritance is not characteristic of restrictive cardiomyopathy

GEOGRAPHY

Restrictive cardiomyopathy is more prevalent in tropical Africa than in the Western world.

DIAGNOSIS

DIFFERENTIAL DIAGNOSIS

Magnetic resonance imaging may be required to distinguish between the following disorders.

Coronary artery disease

FEATURES

- Ischemia
- More commonly presents at older ages than does nonischemic cardiomyopathy

Primary mitral valve disease

FEATURES

- History of mitral valve prolapse or rheumatic fever
- Significant mitral valve calcification is common
- Frequent atrial fibrillation in comparison to dilated cardiomyopathy
- Ventricular function is less severely depressed than would be expected in dilated cardiomyopathy

End-stage aortic valve disease

FEATURES

- Murmur of severe aortic stenosis is usually detectable
- Diastolic murmur may disappear when left ventricular end-diastolic pressure is severely elevated
- Note: Invasive cardiac examination is sometimes necessary for this differential diagnosis

Hypertensive heart disease

FEATURES

- Usually reflects severe, chronic systolic and diastolic hypertension
- Diastolic heart failure, rather than systolic dysfunction, is typical of this disorder
- Left ventricular hypertrophy is linked to severe, chronic hypertension
- Asymmetric septal hypertrophy or hypertensive hypertrophy cardiomyopathy
- Senile septal hypertrophy is seen in elderly hypertensive patients and can cause some degree of outflow obstruction. It is more common in women
- Previous blood pressure readings show chronic hypertension

'Athlete's heart'

FEATURES

- Lengthy athletic training may produce heart changes resembling some features of hypertrophic cardiomyopathy. However, the hypertrophy is concentric and decreases with deconditioning
- In contrast to patients with hypertrophic cardiomyopathy, athletes with this condition are unlikely to have family members with the disorder
- In 'athlete's heart,' left ventricular filling is not impaired

Amyloidosis

FEATURES

- Multiorgan involvement is common, including peripheral neuropathy, renal disease, hematologic abnormalities, and intestinal malabsorption
- Causes a restrictive-type cardiomyopathic picture

Valvular and subvalvular aortic stenosis

FEATURES

- A characteristic harsh systolic murmur is present, occasionally with thrill along left sternal border, often radiating to the neck

- The characteristic features of significant aortic stenosis are exertional dyspnea, angina pectoris, syncope, and heart failure, but patients may be asymptomatic until the fifth to seventh decade
- Left ventricular hypertrophy is usually present, owing to the increasingly higher left ventricular pressure that is required to drive blood across the obstructed valve

Chronic mitral regurgitation
FEATURES
- Hyperdynamic apical beat
- Holosystolic apical murmur that radiates to the base of the heart or to the left axilla
- Lacks the brisk carotid upstroke of hypertrophic cardiomyopathy

Infundibular pulmonic stenosis
FEATURES
- Dyspnea and syncope
- Prominent jugular *a* wave
- Midsystolic murmur with pulmonary ejection sound
- Lacks the brisk carotid upstroke of hypertrophic cardiomyopathy
- Signs of right ventricular failure

Ventricular septal defect
FEATURES
- Often congenital
- Dyspnea and fatigue
- Hyperdynamic apical beat with thrill along the left lower border of the midsternal border
- Holosystolic murmur with S3 and loud P2

Constrictive pericarditis
FEATURES
- Fibrous scarring of the pericardium
- Unlike restrictive cardiomyopathy, which tends to affect left ventricular filling disproportionately, constrictive pericarditis involves both ventricles equall.
- Pericardial ‘knock’ is often heard at the apex during diastole

SIGNS & SYMPTOMS
Signs
Dilated cardiomyopathy
Findings are similar to those of congestive heart failure:
- Increased jugular venous pressure
- Small pulse pressure
- Pulmonary rales
- Peripheral edema
- Presence of S3 and/or S4
- Hepatojugular reflux
- Resting tachycardia
- Pale or cyanotic extremities
- Cardiomegaly, typically with an increase in left ventricular mass without an increase in left ventricular wall thickness

Hypertrophic cardiomyopathy
- Large, dominant *a* waves in the jugular venous pulse
- Brisk, forceful carotid upstroke
- Bifid apical systolic impulse (spike and dome)

- Point of maximal impulse is prominent and prolonged, possibly with a triple impulse
- Harsh systolic ejection murmur heard across the precordium that varies with maneuvers: Valsalva maneuver (strain phase) or abrupt standing accentuates the outflow murmur, while squatting or isometric hand grip reduces the murmur
- Left ventricular lift and a loud S4 (in asymptomatic patients, these may be the primary signs of the disorder). An S3 may also be heard

Restrictive cardiomyopathy
- Elevated jugular venous pressure with prominent *x* and *y* descents
- Kussmaul's sign may be evident
- Presence of a loud S3
- Regurgitant murmurs
- Pulmonary congestion
- Edema
- Ascites
- Heart size is normal or slightly enlarged

Symptoms
Dilated cardiomyopathy
- Dyspnea
- Orthopnea
- Weakness
- Leg edema
- Syncope

Hypertrophic cardiomyopathy
- Dyspnea on exertion
- Angina
- Syncope or presyncope after exercise
- Palpitations
- Patients are frequently asymptomatic

Restrictive cardiomyopathy
- Dyspnea
- Fatigue
- Leg edema

KEY! DON'T MISS!
- Signs and symptoms of pulmonary emboli or stroke suggest thrombus formation in the cardiac chambers. Thrombus is frequently found in the apices of either ventricle in dilated cardiomyopathy
- In all patients with unexplained syncope with exercise and in a young people with cardiac arrest, hypertrophic cardiomyopathy and right ventricular dysplasia should be considered in the differential diagnosis

CONSIDER CONSULT
- Unexplained syncope or cardiac arrest, particularly in the young
- Unexplained congestive heart failure in the absence of coronary heart disease

INVESTIGATION OF THE PATIENT
Direct questions to patient
Q **Do you experience extreme fatigue, difficulty in breathing when lying down, or shortness of breath?** Evidence of heart failure with pulmonary congestion requires immediate treatment, even before the cause is definitively ascertained

- **Q Do you have heart palpitations?** Ventricular arrhythmias may be present in any of the cardiomyopathies. They are a frequent cause of sudden death from this disorder
- **Q Do your symptoms tend to worsen after exercise?** This is a characteristic of hypertrophic cardiomyopathy but also can be seen with all forms of cardiomyopathy
- **Q Have you fainted or felt in danger of fainting?** This may also signal hypertrophic cardiomyopathy or right heart dysplasia
- **Q Have you experienced dizziness?** Possibly associated with hypertrophic cardiomyopathy or right heart dysplasia
- **Q Did your symptoms emerge gradually or suddenly?** Symptoms of dilated cardiomyopathy often develop gradually, although this is not always the case. In patients with a sudden onset of symptoms, dilated cardiomyopathy may have been exacerbated by a clinical event that placed increased demands on the heart, such surgery or infection

Contributory or predisposing factors

- **Q What is your intake of alcohol and exposure to drugs such as cocaine and heroin?** Dilated cardiomyopathy due to drugs or toxins may be reversed if patient becomes totally abstinent from the causative agent
- **Q Are you pregnant, or have you recently had a child?** Dilated cardiomyopathy may occur during the last 6 weeks of pregnancy or during the first 3 months after delivery. Peripartum cardiomyopathy tends to be associated with pre-eclampsia or multiple births
- **Q Have you had, or do you have, cancer?** If so, what treatments have you received? Cancer affecting the heart may be a cause of cardiomyopathy. Radiation, as well as certain chemotherapeutic drugs, may also cause the disorder
- **Q Do you have AIDS?** If so, what drugs are you taking for the condition? Cardiomyopathy is common among AIDS patients, both because of HIV-induced myocarditis and because of drugs such as zidovudine (also known as azidothymidine) and interferon alfa, which are used to treat the disorder
- **Q Have you had inflammatory heart disease?** Viral myocarditis is often a cause of acute dilated cardiomyopathy. This etiology is often found in children and adolescents
- **Q Have you had recent flu-like symptoms?** Viral cardiomyopathy can have a flu-like illness prior to the onset of heart failure symptoms
- **Q Have you undergone heart surgery?** In distinguishing between restrictive cardiomyopathy and constrictive pericarditis, patients who have undergone a heart operation are more likely to have constrictive pericarditis. However, those who have received a heart transplant are more likely to have restrictive cardiomyopathy

Family history

- **Q Do you have a family member with a heart disorder, or who has experienced similar symptoms?** Hypertrophic cardiomyopathy typically displays familial inheritance. Although most instances of dilated cardiomyopathy are not hereditary, a substantial minority of cases do suggest familial inheritance
- **Q Have any members of your family died abruptly, possibly before reaching old age?** Sudden death may be a result of cardiomyopathy; screening of relatives is particularly important families with hypertrophic cardiomyopathy

Examination

All patients reporting paroxysmal nocturnal dyspnea, orthopnea, or new-onset dyspnea on exertion should be evaluated for signs of congestive heart failure.

Dilated cardiomyopathy may present with the following signs:

- Tachypnea
- Tachycardia
- Hypertension
- Hypoxia

- Pulmonary rales
- Presence of an S3 or S4
- Jugular venous distension
- If congestive heart failure is evident, begin treatment immediately

If examination reveals elevated jugular venous pressure with prominent *x* and *y* descents, check for Kussmaul's sign as a further possible sign of restrictive cardiomyopathy.

For patients presenting with exertional dyspnea and chest pain, possibly accompanied by syncope, near-syncope, dizziness, palpitations, or orthopnea, listen to heart sounds for indications of hypertrophic cardiomyopathy:

- Large, dominant *a* waves in the jugular venous pulse
- Brisk, forceful carotid upstroke
- Bifid apical systolic impulse
- Harsh systolic ejection murmur
- Left ventricular lift and a loud S4

If systolic murmur is present, perform maneuvers to check for variability in accordance with hypertrophic cardiomyopathy. Valsalva maneuver or abrupt standing accentuates the outflow murmur; squatting or isometric hand grip reduces the murmur.

Summary of investigative tests

- Complete blood count
- Serum chemistry
- Measurement of thyroid stimulating hormone levels is indicated in patients with atrial fibrillation and unexplained heart failure
- Chest X-ray
- Electrocardiogram can signal dilated and hypertrophic cardiomyopathies and rule out ischemia
- Transthoracic Doppler echocardiography can confirm the diagnosis of hypertrophic cardiomyopathy, help distinguish between restrictive cardiomyopathy and constrictive pericarditis, and exclude valvular heart disease
- Magnetic resonance imaging may distinguish between constrictive disease and restrictive cardiomyopathy
- Computed tomography also may distinguish between constrictive disease and restrictive cardiomyopathy
- Noninvasive stress testing is recommended only for patients who have a high probability of underlying ischemic heart disease, prior myocardial infarction, or extensive hibernating myocardium, or evaluation for possible heart transplantation
- Cardiac catheterization (typically performed by a specialist) can assist in diagnosing hypertrophic cardiomyopathy and in distinguishing restrictive cardiomyopathy from constrictive pericarditis
- Right ventricular endomyocardial biopsy (performed by a specialist) is occasionally used to distinguish between myocarditis and idiopathic dilated cardiomyopathy; a normal result does not rule out cardiomyopathy

CLINICAL PEARL(S)

Kussmaul's sign cannot distinguish between restrictive cardiomyopathy and constrictive pericarditis, since it can be present in both conditions.

THE TESTS

Body fluids

COMPLETE BLOOD COUNT

Description

Venous blood.

Advantages/Disadvantages

- Ease of collection of sample
- Routine laboratory test

Normal

- Red blood cells: 4.33–5.67x10^{12}/L
- White blood cells: 3.83–11.0x10^{9}/L
- Neutrophils: 1.94–7.78x10^{9}/L
- Lymphocytes: 1.08–3.10x10^{9}/L
- Monocytes: 0.240–0.870x10^{9}/L
- Eosinophils: 0.028–0.531x10^{9}/L
- Basophils: 0.011–0.106x10^{9}/L
- Platelets: 156–352x10^{9}/L

Abnormal

- Elevated white cell counts
- Elevated eosinophil count
- Keep in mind the possibility of a false-positive result

Cause of abnormal result

- Systemic infection
- An elevated eosinophil count may indicate eosinophilic endomyocardial disease

SERUM CHEMISTRY

Description

Venous blood for measurement of electrolytes, blood urea nitrogen (BUN), creatine, phosphate, magnesium, calcium, and albumin levels.

Advantages/Disadvantages

- Ease of collection of sample
- Routine laboratory test

Normal

- Serum sodium: 3–5mEq/L (3–5mmol/L)
- Serum potassium: 135–147mEq/L (135–147mmol/L)
- Serum chloride: 95–105mEq/L (95–105mmol/L)
- Serum carbon dioxide: 24–30mEq/L (24–30mmol/L)
- Blood urea nitrogen (BUN): 8–18mg/dL (3–6.5mcmol/L)
- Serum creatinine: 0.6–1.2mg/dL (120–420mcmol/L)
- Serum phosphate: 2.5–5mg/dL (0.8–1.6mmol/L)
- Serum magnesium: 1.8–3.0mg/dL (0.80–1.20mmol/L)
- Serum calcium: 8.8–10.3mg/dL (2.2–2.58mmol/L)
- Serum albumin: 4–6g/dL (40–60g/L)

Abnormal

- Values outside the normal range
- Keep in mind the possibility of a false-positive result

THYROID-STIMULATING HORMONE LEVELS

Description

Venous blood.

Advantages/Disadvantages
- Ease of collection of sample
- Routine laboratory test

Normal
2–11mcU/mL (2–11mU/L)

Abnormal
- Values outside the normal range
- Keep in mind the possibility of a false-positive result

Cause of abnormal result
- Thyroid disease
- Some drugs (e.g. amiodarone)

Imaging

CHEST X-RAY
Advantages/Disadvantages
- Cardiomegaly may signal dilated cardiomyopathy
- X-ray may also indicate pulmonary congestion
- Not necessarily helpful in diagnosing hypertrophic or restrictive cardiomyopathy

Abnormal
- Cardiomegaly, atrial enlargement, pulmonary congestion
- Keep in mind the possibility of imaging artifacts

Cause of abnormal result
- Cardiomegaly is a sign of dilated cardiomyopathy
- Atrial enlargement frequently occurs in hypertrophic cardiomyopathy and restrictive disease; heart size may range from normal to enlarged
- Pulmonary congestion is commonly seen in restrictive cardiomyopathy; cardiomegaly may be mild or absent

TRANSTHORACIC DOPPLER ECHOCARDIOGRAPHY
Advantages/Disadvantages
- Can confirm the diagnosis of cardiomyopathy
- Can define area and degree of obstruction in hypertrophy cardiomyopathy
- May help distinguish between restrictive cardiomyopathy and constrictive pericarditis
- Enables exclusion of valvular heart disease and cardiomyopathy due to coronary artery disease

Abnormal
- Asymmetric hypertrophy of the left ventricle usually in the septum and left ventricular outflow obstruction, possibly with systolic anterior motion of the mitral valve leaflet is indicative of hypertrophic cardiomyopathy
- Keep in mind the possibility of false-positive results

Other tests

ELECTROCARDIOGRAM
Advantages/Disadvantages
Can signal dilated and hypertrophic cardiomyopathies and rule out ischemia.

Abnormal

- In dilated cardiomyopathy, results are often nonspecific
- In hypertrophic cardiomyopathy, unexplained left ventricular hypertrophy is generally evident; left atrial enlargement and nonspecific repolarization abnormalities or a strain pattern may also be present. Lateral T-wave inversion may indicate apical HCM
- In restrictive cardiomyopathy, procedure shows nonspecific repolarization changes
- Keep in mind the possibility of false-positive results

NONINVASIVE STRESS TESTING

Advantages/Disadvantages

Assists diagnosis of ischemia.

Abnormal

- Arrhythmias, ST-segment changes, blood pressure symptoms, angina symptoms, dyspnea
- Keep in mind the possibility of false-positive results

Cause of abnormal result

Ischemia.

TREATMENT

CONSIDER CONSULT

For dilated cardiomyopathy, refer when:
- Conventional therapy fails to halt progression of symptoms
- Invasive procedure required
- Acute myocarditis
- Symptomatic ventricular tachyarrhythmias

For hypertrophic cardiomyopathy, refer for:
- Genetic counseling and assessment of risk of sudden death
- Children or young adults with asymptomatic disease and family history of sudden death
- Patients reporting syncopal spells
- Patients with nonsustained ventricular tachycardia on ambulatory monitoring
- Competitive athletes with a heart murmur or ECG signs of significant hypertrophy
- Patients being considered for myectomy or dual-chamber pacing, due to refractory heart failure or anginal symptoms
- Patients with angina or heart failure

For restrictive cardiomyopathy most patients should be referred to a cardiologist.

IMMEDIATE ACTION

Congestive heart failure, regardless of etiology, requires immediate treatment.

MANAGEMENT ISSUES

Goals

- Remove complicating factors
- Halt disease progression
- Avert sudden cardiac death

Management in special circumstances

COEXISTING MEDICATION

Phenothiazines and anthracyclines may cause cardiac dilation.

SPECIAL PATIENT GROUPS

Athletes: Those with significant hypertrophy, hypertrophy combined with family history of sudden death, or evidence of marked outflow tract gradient at rest should not participate in competitive sports.

Pregnant women: Subsequent pregnancies are considered high risk in women who experienced peripartum cardiomyopathy and failed to regain normal heart size and function. Cardiology referral is recommended for all women with cardiomyopathy who are considering pregnancy.

Elderly patients: Increased likelihood of having other diseases that add to complications of cardiomyopathy and its treatment, depending on the comorbidity.

Children: Those with hypertrophic cardiomyopathy that becomes symptomatic in childhood are at heightened risk of sudden death. Family counseling, education, and screening are advisable.

SUMMARY OF THERAPEUTIC OPTIONS

Choices

Guidelines: The American College of Cardiology/American Heart Association Task Force have produced Practice Guidelines for the Evaluation and Management of Heart Failure. These are available at the website of the American College of Cardiology, and have been published (ACC/AHA practice guidelines for evaluation and management of heart failure. J Am Coll Cardiol 1995;26:1376–98).

There are lifestyle measures that are helpful in patients with cardiomyopathy.

Dilated cardiomyopathy:

- Angiotensin-converting enzyme (ACE) inhibitors for all patients with significantly reduced left ventricular ejection fraction. Note: If the patient cannot take these drugs, hydralazine and isosorbide dinitrate are advised
- Digoxin should be given to patients who do not adequately respond to ACE inhibitors and diuretic drugs, as well as those with atrial fibrillation and rapid ventricular rates
- Diuretics for fluid overload
- Anticoagulants for patients with atrial fibrillation or history of systemic or pulmonary embolism
- Beta-blockers for high-risk patients following acute myocardial infarction
- Amiodarone can reduce ventricular arrhythmias and may be of value in high-risk patients
- An implantable cardioverter–defibrillator may prevent sudden death in high-risk patients who have failed pharmacologic therapy
- Cardiac transplantation can improve quality of life and survival rates in patients under age 60 years with intractable congestive heart failure

Hypertrophic cardiomyopathy:

- Beta-blockers: typically the initial treatment
- Verapamil: sometimes prescribed to patients who do not respond to beta-blockers alone or who do not tolerate them; can be used with beta-blockers, although the advantage of combination therapy over single-drug therapy is unproven. Close observation for hypotension (particularly in patients with outflow tract obstruction) and for heart block is essential, especially if verapamil is added to beta-blockers
- Diuretics: may be added to beta-blockers or verapamil if congestive heart failure persists. However, they should be used cautiously because many patients with hypertrophic cardiomyopathy require high filling pressures for sufficient ventricular filling
- Anticoagulants: indicated in patients who have persistent atrial fibrillation or evidence of cardiac thrombi
- Amiodarone can prevent recurrences of atrial fibrillation and may be of benefit in patients at high risk of life-threatening tachyarrhythmias
- Surgical myotomy/myectomy, or removal of part of the myocardium in the outflow tract, is an option for patients with a large gradient (greater than 50mmHg) and severe congestive heart failure that is unresponsive to medical therapy
- Pacemaker therapy, using dual-chamber pacing, may be beneficial, but the evidence is not strong
- An implantable cardioverter–defibrillator may prevent sudden death in high-risk patients (patients with a history of sustained ventricular tachycardia or a ventricular fibrillation cardiac arrest, a significant family history of sudden death, frequent episodes of nonsustained ventricular tachycardia, or genetic testing indicating the presence of a high-risk mutation)

Restrictive cardiomyopathy:

Treatment for restrictive cardiomyopathy should be administered by a specialist.

- Diuretics
- Anticoagulants
- Amiodarone can reduce ventricular arrhythmias and may be of value in high-risk patients
- Pacemaker therapy may be necessary due to the increased prevalence of advanced conduction system disease and the poor tolerance of bradyarrhythmias in patients with restrictive cardiomyopathy
- An implantable cardioverter–defibrillator may prevent sudden death in high-risk patients who have failed pharmacologic therapy
- Cardiac transplantation is an option for patients with refractory symptoms

Clinical pearl(s)

Early diagnosis and treatment of hemochromatosis may improve hemodynamic function in patients with heart failure secondary to the disease.

FOLLOW UP

Plan for review

- Dilated cardiomyopathy: regular follow up is needed to monitor electrolytes and assess effectiveness of therapy
- Hypertrophic cardiomyopathy: regular monitoring of medication and side-effects
- Restrictive cardiomyopathy: patients should be followed by a specialist

Information for patient or caregiver

Dilated cardiomyopathy

- In disease caused by alcoholism or substance abuse, patients should be informed of the risks of these behaviors and the potential to reverse early stages of disease
- Obtain regular medical care
- Adequate rest
- Moderate exercise
- Low sodium diet
- Daily monitoring of weight

Hypertrophic cardiomyopathy

- Obtain regular medical care
- Avoid alcohol
- Avoid dehydration
- Educate about the risk of sudden death, particularly if symptoms begin in childhood
- Family members of high-risk patients might consider learning cardiopulmonary resuscitation
- Family members should be screened and genetic counseling provided
- Support should be given on the problems of living with a chronic disease

Restrictive cardiomyopathy

- Obtain regular medical care
- Restrict salt intake

DRUGS AND OTHER THERAPIES: DETAILS

Drugs

RAMIPRIL

Dose

1.25–5mg twice daily gradually increased to 5mg

Risks/Benefits

Use with caution in patients with hypertrophic cardiomyopathy or aortic stenosis; unsafe during pregnancy.

Side-effects and adverse reactions

- CNS: anxiety, dizziness, headache, paresthesia
- Cardiovascular: angina, hypotension, postural hypotension, palpitations
- Gastrointestinal: constipation, nausea, dry mouth, pancreatitis
- Respiratory: cough, asthma, dyspnea
- Genitourinary: sexual dysfunction
- Hematologic: agranulocytosis, neutropenia, thrombocytopenia
- Metabolic: hyperkalemia, hyponatremia, hypoglycemia
- Musculoskeletal: arthralgia, arthritis, myalgia
- Skin: alopecia, pruritus, rash

Interactions (other drugs)

■ Allopurinol ■ Alpha-adrenergic blockers ■ Aspirin ■ Cyclosporin ■ Insulin ■ Iron ■ Lithium ■ Loop diuretics ■ NSAIDs ■ Potassium/potassium-sparing diuretics

Contraindications

■ Bilateral renal artery stenosis ■ Pregnancy

Evidence

The American College of Cardiology/American Heart Association Task Force has produced Practice Guidelines for the Evaluation and Management of Heart Failure. These are available at the website of the American College of Cardiology, and have been published (ACC/AHA practice guidelines for evaluation and management of heart failure. J Am Coll Cardiol 1995; 26:1376–98). In its guidelines for patients with left ventricular systolic dysfunction, this task force recommends ACE inhibitors 'for all patients with significantly reduced left ventricular ejection fraction unless contraindicated.'

Patient and caregiver information

Do not use salt substitutes containing potassium.

DIGOXIN

Dose

Adult oral dose: 0.125–0.5mg daily.

Efficacy

Recommended for two groups of patients: those who do not respond adequately to ACE inhibitors and diuretics, and those with atrial fibrillation and rapid ventricular rates.

Risks/Benefits

- Reduces hospitalizations due to heart failure.
- Use caution with hypokalemia, hypomagnesia, hypercalcemia
- Use caution with hypothyroidism and hepatic disease
- Use caution with severe pulmonary disease
- Use caution with sick sinus syndrome, acute myocardial infarction, AV block and Wolff–Parkinson–White syndrome
- Use caution in the elderly

Side-effects and adverse reactions

- CNS: confusion, hallucinations, depression, seizures
- Cardiovascular: atrial fibrillation, AV block, bradycardia, ventricular fibrillation
- EENT: green/yellow vision
- Gastrointestinal: hemorrhagic necrosis of the intestine, vomiting
- Hematologic: eosinophilia, thrombocytopenia
- Skin: rash

Interactions (other drugs)

■ Alprazolam ■ Amiodarone ■ Amphotericin B diuretics ■ Azole antifungals ■ Bepridil ■ Beta-blockers ■ Calcium ■ Carvedilol ■ Charcoal ■ Cholestyramine ■ Cyclosporin/cyclophosphamide ■ Hydroxychloroquine ■ Macrolides ■ Metoclopramide ■ Propafenone ■ Proton pump inhibitor ■ Quinine ■ Spironolactone ■ Succinylcholine ■ Tacrolimus ■ Tetracyclines

Contraindications

■ Ventricular fibrillation ■ SA or AV node disease ■ Idiopathic hypertrophic subaortic stenosis ■ Hypokalemia of less than 2.0 ■ Hypersensitivity reaction

Evidence

The American College of Cardiology/American Heart Association Task Force has produced Practice Guidelines for the Evaluation and Management of Heart Failure. These are available at the website of the American College of Cardiology, and have been published (ACC/AHA practice guidelines for evaluation and management of heart failure. J Am Coll Cardiol 1995; 26:1376–98). In recommendations for patients with left ventricular systolic dysfunction, this task force cites two groups of patients who should receive digoxin:

- Those who are not adequately responsive to ACE inhibitors and diuretics
- Those with atrial fibrillation and rapid ventricular rates

Acceptability to patient

Good.

Follow up plan

Clinical assessment to monitor response every 3 months or as indicated.

FUROSEMIDE

Loop diuretic.

Dose

- Adult oral dose: 20–400mg daily
- Child oral dose: 1–6mg/kg per dose up to four times daily

Efficacy

Proven to be efficacious.

Risks/Benefits

- Reduces fluid congestion
- Use caution with diabetes mellitus and gout
- Use caution with renal and liver disease
- Use caution with systemic lupus erythematosus
- Use caution with pregnancy and nursing mothers

Side-effects and adverse reactions

- CNS: dizziness, headache, paresthesia
- Cardiovascular: chest pain, circulatory collapse
- EENT: blurred vision
- Gastrointestinal: ischemic hepatitis, vomiting, pancreatitis
- Genitourinary: glycosuria, hyperuremia, bladder spasm
- Hematologic: agranulocytosis, leukopenia, thrombocytopenia
- Metabolic: hyperglycemia
- Skin: e.rythema multiforme, exfoliative dermatitis, urticaria

Contraindications

Anuria

Evidence

The American College of Cardiology/American Heart Association Task Force has produced Practice Guidelines for the Evaluation and Management of Heart Failure. These are available at the website of the American College of Cardiology, and have been published (ACC/AHA practice guidelines for evaluation and management of heart failure. J Am Coll Cardiol 1995; 26:1376–98). This task force recommends diuretics for patients with left ventricular systolic dysfunction who display fluid overload.

Acceptability to patient
Good.

Follow up plan
Clinical assessment every 3 months or as indicated.

Patient and caregiver information
- Take with milk or food
- Take early in the day

WARFARIN
Oral anticoagulant.

Dose
Adult oral dose: 2–10mg daily dependent on international normalized ratio (INR) determinations.

Efficacy
Recommended for patients with atrial fibrillation or history of systemic or pulmonary embolism

Risks/Benefits
- Use caution with infection and trauma
- Use caution with diverticulitis, renal and hepatic disease
- Use caution with hypertension, congestive heart failure, and tuberculosis
- Use caution with thyroid disease and diabetes mellitus
- Use caution with elderly, children, and nursing mothers
- Use caution with protein C deficiency, polyarteritis, and vasculitis

Side-effects and adverse reactions
- CNS: fatigue, headache
- EENT: blurred vision
- Gastrointestinal: cramps, diarrhea, vomiting
- Genitourinary: gonadal dysfunction
- Metabolic: altered thyroid, pituitary, and adrenal hormones
- Musculoskeletal: weakness
- Skin: contact dermatitis

Interactions (other drugs)
■ Acetaminophen ■ Allopurinol ■ Amiodarone ■ Aminoglutethimide ■ Aspirin ■ Azathioprine ■ Barbiturates ■ Bile acid-binding resins ■ Carbamazepine ■ Cephalosporins ■ Chloramphenicol ■ Chloral hydrate ■ Clofibrate ■ Co-trimoxazole ■ Danazol ■ Dextrothyroxine ■ Disulfiram ■ Ethanol ■ Ethchlorvynol ■ Fluconazole ■ Fluorouracil ■ Gemfibrozil ■ Glutethimide ■ Griseofulvin ■ Glucagon ■ Oral contraceptives ■ Phenytoin ■ Propafenones ■ Propoxyphene ■ Quinidines ■ Quinolones ■ Rifampin ■ Salicylates ■ Sertraline ■ Sulfonamides ■ Sulfonylureas ■ Testosterone derivatives

Contraindications
■ Active bleeding ■ Bacterial endocarditis ■ Cerebral hemorrhage ■ Eclampsia ■ Hemorrhagic blood dyscrasias ■ Hemorrhagic tendencies ■ Hypertension ■ Pericarditis ■ Recent surgery presenting heightened risk of bleeding ■ Pregnancy and threatened abortion ■ Hypertension ■ Gastrointestinal ulceration ■ Ulcerative colitis ■ Visceral carcinoma

Evidence
The American College of Cardiology/American Heart Association Task Force has produced Practice Guidelines for the Evaluation and Management of Heart Failure. These are available at the website of the American College of Cardiology, and have been published (ACC/AHA practice guidelines for evaluation and management of heart failure. J Am Coll Cardiol 1995; 26:1376–98). In its guidelines for patients with left ventricular systolic dysfunction, this task force recommends anticoagulants for patients with atrial fibrillation, as well as those with history of systemic or pulmonary embolism.

Acceptability to patient
Good, but care is required in following the dosage schedule.

Follow up plan
Monitor INR (international normalized ratio).

Patient and caregiver information
- Strict adherence to dosage schedule is necessary
- Avoid alcohol and aspirin

ATENOLOL
Dose
50mg daily increasing to 100mg daily.

Efficacy
Reduces heart rate and cardiac output; frequently used to treat hypertrophic cardiomyopathy.

Risks/Benefits
- Risk of depressing myocardial contractility
- Benefits: beta-blockers, when given in adequate dosages, help to prevent anginal attacks by reducing myocardial oxygen demand and the severity of ischemia
- Use with caution in diabetes mellitus, thyroid disease, renal disease
- Use with caution in chronic obstructive pulmonary disease
- Use with caution in peripheral vascular disease

Side-effects and adverse reactions
- CNS: lethargy, depression, and vivid dreams
- Cardiovascular: bradycardia, congestive heart failure, heart block, peripheral vascular disease
- EENT: dry eyes, sore throat
- Respiratory: bronchospasm, dyspnea, wheezing
- Gastrointestinal: ischemic colitis, nausea, dry mouth
- Hematologic: agranulocytosis, thrombocytopenia
- Metabolism: hyperglycemia, hyperlipidemia, masked hypoglycemia
- Skin: alopecia, bruising, rash

Interactions (other drugs)
- Adenosine
- Amoxicillin, ampicillin
- Antacids
- Calcium channel blockers
- Clonidine
- Dipyridamole
- Lidocaine
- Neostigmine
- NSAIDs
- Physostigmine
- Prazosin
- Tacrine
- Theophylline
- Verapamil

Contraindications
- Asthma
- Cardiogenic shock
- Congestive heart failure
- Heart block
- Sinus bradycardia

Evidence
A meta-analysis concluded that low-dose beta-blockers are beneficial in the treatment of patients with ischemic or idiopathic cardiomyopathy. They appear to improve New York Heart Association functional class and left ventricular ejection fraction. (Zarembski DG, Nolan PE, Slack MK, Lui CY. Meta-analysis of the use of low-dose beta-adrenergic blocking therapy in idiopathic or ischemic dilated cardiomyopathy. Am J Cardiol 1996;77:1247–50.)

Acceptability to patient
Good.

Follow up plan
Clinical assessment every 3 months or as indicated.

METOPROLOL
Dose
50–100mg daily

Risks/Benefits
- Benefits: beta-blockers, when given in adequate dosages, help to prevent anginal attacks by reducing myocardial oxygen demand and the severity of ischemia
- Use with caution in diabetes mellitus, thyroid disease, renal disease
- Use with caution in chronic obstructive pulmonary disease
- Use with caution in peripheral vascular disease
- Use with caution in pregnancy

Side-effects and adverse reactions
- CNS: lethargy, depression, and vivid dreams
- Cardiovascular: bradycardia, congestive heart failure, heart block, peripheral vascular disease
- EENT: Tinnitus
- Respiratory: bronchospasm, dyspnea, wheezing
- Gastrointestinal: constipation, nausea, dry mouth, dyspepsia
- Genitourinary: impotence, sexual dysfunction
- Hematologic: agranulocytosis
- Metabolism: hyperglycemia, hyperlipidemia, masked hypoglycemia
- Skin: alopecia, bruising, rash

Interactions (other drugs)
- Amiodarone ■ Antidiabetics ■ Antipyrine ■ Barbiturates ■ Benzodiazepines ■ Calcium channel blockers ■ Cimetidine ■ Clonidine ■ Dipyridamole ■ Lidocaine ■ NSAIDs ■ Phenylephrine ■ Physostigmine ■ Prazosin ■ Quinolones ■ Rifampin ■ Theophylline ■ Verapamil

Contraindications
- Asthma ■ Cardiogenic shock ■ Congestive heart failure ■ Heart block ■ Sinus bradycardia

VERAPAMIL
Dose
Adult oral dose: 80–420mg daily.

Efficacy
Shown to improve symptoms in some patients with hypertrophic cardiomyopathy who were unresponsive to beta-blockers.

Risks/Benefits

- The vasodilatory effects of verapamil may cause hemodynamic complications in patients with a substantial outflow gradient or markedly elevated pulmonary pressure
- Use caution with congestive heart failure and hypotension
- Use caution with renal and hepatic disease
- Use caution with Duchenne's muscular dystrophy
- Use caution in children

Side-effects and adverse reactions

- CNS: dizziness, headache
- Cardiovascular: AV block, bradycardia, congestive heart failure, hypotension
- Gastrointestinal: constipation, vomiting
- Genitourinary: nocturia, polyuria
- Skin: rash

Interactions (other drugs)

■ Alpha-blockers ■ Amiodarone ■ Barbiturates ■ Benzodiazepines ■ Beta-blockers ■ Calcium ■ Carbamazepine ■ Cimetidine ■ Cyclosporine/tacrolimus ■ Diclofenac ■ Digitalis ■ Doxorubicin ■ Encainide ■ Ethanol ■ Imipramine ■ Lithium ■ Neuromuscular ■ Quinidine ■ Rifampin ■ Theophylline

Contraindications

■ Cardiogenic shock ■ Heart block ■ Severe heart failure ■ Hypotension ■ Pregnancy ■ Sick sinus syndrome

Acceptability to patient

Good.

Follow up plan

Clinical assessment every 3 months or as indicated.

AMIODARONE

Antidysrhythmic.

Dose

Adult oral dose: 600–1600mg daily in gradually decreasing doses.

Efficacy

Suppresses arrhythmias.

Risks/Benefits

- Should be used only by physicians with access to all methods of treating and monitoring arrhythmias. Treatment should be initiated in a hospital
- Use caution with thyroid and pulmonary disease
- Use caution with AV block and bradycardia
- Use caution in electrolyte imbalances
- Owing to the hazards associated with this drug, a decision should be made in each case in regard to whether an implantable defibrillator might be a preferable alternative

Side-effects and adverse reactions

- CNS: Ataxia, dizziness, fatigue, headache, paresthesia, peripheral neuropathy, tremors
- Cardiovascular: bradycardia, congestive heart failure, hypotension, sinoatrial node dysfunction
- Respiratory: cough, dyspnea, pulmonary fibrosis

- EENT: blurred vision, corneal microdeposits, optic neuritis, photophobia
- Gastrointestinal: abdominal pains, constipation, diarrhea, hepatotoxicity, taste abnormalities, vomiting
- Metabolic: altered thyroid function
- Musculoskeletal: weakness
- Skin: contact dermatitis

Interactions (other drugs)

- Aprindine ■ Beta-adrenergic blockers ■ Calcium channel blockers ■ Cholestyramine ■ Cimetidine ■ Cyclosporin ■ Digitalis ■ Flecainide ■ Oral anticoagulants ■ Phenytoin ■ Procainamide ■ Quinidine ■ Theophylline

Contraindications

- AV block ■ Hypotension ■ Hypersensitivity ■ Pregnancy ■ Syncope ■ Severe sinus node disease with bradycardia

Follow up plan

Measurement of digoxin levels as clinically appropriate to assess likelihood of digoxin intoxication.

Surgical therapy

HEART TRANSPLANTATION

Surgical therapy, including heart transplantation, may be recommended for patients with cardiomyopathy whose treatment is not alleviated by medication.

Efficacy

Dilated cardiomyopathy is the most common reason for heart transplantation. A significant drawback is the scarcity of hearts available for transplantation.

Risks/Benefits

Lifelong immunosuppression and the potential for rejection are risks of transplantation. Quality of life and survival rates may improve.

Evidence

Selection and Treatment of Candidates for Heart Transplantation, American Heart Association (www.americanheart.org/)

Patient and caregiver information

Website: www.nhlbi.nih.gov/health/public/heart/other/hrt_lung.htm Facts About Heart and Heart-Lung Transplants.

IMPLANTABLE CARDIOVERTER–DEFIBRILLATOR

Risks/Benefits

Provides an alternative to chronic antiarrhythmic therapy with potentially hazardous drugs.

ATRIOVENTRICULAR SEQUENTIAL PACING (PACEMAKER THERAPY)

Efficacy

In hypertrophic cardiomyopathy, this therapy has proven useful for some patients with outflow tract obstruction whose symptoms were not controlled by drugs. However, it is not effective for the nonobstructive form of hypertrophic cardiomyopathy.

Risks/Benefits

Poses less risk than surgical myotomy/myectomy. However, its impact on long-term survival is not yet known.

LIFESTYLE

Dilated cardiomyopathy:
- Avoid alcohol
- Avoid substance abuse (cocaine, methamphetamine, heroin)
- Take moderate exercise
- Restrict salt intake

Hypertrophic cardiomyopathy:
- Avoid alcohol
- Avoid strenuous exercise

Restrictive cardiomyopathy:
- Restrict salt intake

RISKS/BENEFITS

No risks.

ACCEPTABILITY TO PATIENT

Moderate; support may be required for patients with alcohol or substance abuse problems.

OUTCOMES

PROGNOSIS

Prognosis for all three forms of cardiomyopathy is variable.

- **Dilated cardiomyopathy:** Prognosis tends to be related to severity of disease at initial diagnosis. Five-year mortality rate has been estimated at between 40 and 80%
- **Hypertrophic cardiomyopathy**: Prognosis is particularly variable. Genetic analysis may soon assist prognosis, because certain mutations that cause this disorder correlate with specific disease outcomes
- **Restrictive cardiomyopathy:** Fewer than 10% of patients live more than 10 years after initial diagnosis

Deterioration

Refer to a specialist. Consider for heart transplantation, particularly if patient is less than 60 years old and in otherwise good health.

Terminal illness

Refer to a specialist. Consider for heart transplant, particularly if patient is less than 60 years old and in otherwise good health.

COMPLICATIONS

- Congestive heart failure
- Sudden death
- Embolic stroke or pulmonary emboli

CONSIDER CONSULT

When symptoms persist in spite of standard therapy; for management of arrhythmias; for invasive testing; for consideration of cardiac transplantation.

PREVENTION

RISK FACTORS

- **Alcohol:** Excessive alcohol can induce dilated cardiomyopathy. It should be avoided or used in moderation
- **Cocaine**: May be a cause of dilated cardiomyopathy; should be avoided

MODIFY RISK FACTORS

Lifestyle and wellness

ALCOHOL AND DRUGS

Avoidance of excessive alcohol consumption and abstinence from cocaine can avert dilated cardiomyopathy due to these substances.

FAMILY HISTORY

Those with a family history of hypertrophic cardiomyopathy should be screened for cardiomyopathy.

SCREENING

Screening for hypertrophic cardiomyopathy is important for all family members of a person who has been diagnosed with cardiomyopathy.

ASSOCIATIONS

American Heart Association
National Center
7272 Greenville Avenue
Dallas, TX 75231
http://www.americanheart.org

National Heart, Lung, and Blood Institute
P.O. Box 30105
Bethesda, MD 20824-0105
Telephone: (301) 592-8573
Fax: (301) 592-8563
http://www.nhlbi.nih.gov/

American College of Cardiology
Heart House
9111 Old Georgetown
Bethesda, MD 20814-1699
Telephone: (800) 253-4636
Fax: (301) 897-9745
http://www.acc.org

KEY REFERENCES

- Goldman L, Braunwald E. Primary cardiology. Philadelphia: WB Saunders,1998
- Guidelines for the Evaluation and Management of Heart Failure. Report of the American College of Cardiology/American Heart Association Task Force on Practice Guidelines (Committee on Evaluation and Management of Heart Failure) (http://www.acc.org/)
- Kushwaha SS, Fallon JT, Fuster V. Restrictive cardiomyopathy. New Engl J Med 1997;336:267–76
- Spirito P, Seidman CE, McKenna WJ, Maron BJ. The management of hypertrophic cardiomyopathy. New Engl J Med 1997;336:775–85
- Dec GW, Fuster V. Idiopathic dilated cardiomyopathy. New Engl J Med 1994;331:1564–75

CONTRIBUTORS

Yul D Ejnes, MD, FACP
Mark B Stockmann, MD
Elizabeth Jackson, MD

DEEP VEIN THROMBOSIS

SUMMARY INFORMATION

DESCRIPTION

- Occurrence of thrombi in the deep veins of the extremities or pelvis
- Physical findings alone are not reliable for diagnosis
- Pain, edema, erythema in affected extremity may be present
- Treatment consists of acute and chronic anticoagulation

URGENT ACTION

- As thromboembolism is an important complication of deep vein thrombosis (DVT), achieving therapeutic anticoagulation with heparin within 24h of presentation significantly reduces the occurrence of this complication
- Less commonly, referral for immediate surgery for phlegmasia cerulea dolens may be necessary if extremity is cyanotic

KEY! DON'T MISS!

Physical examination is generally aimed at the vascular system. However, the physical examination is often inaccurate: 50% of patients with symptoms attributable to DVT have been found to have a diagnosis other than DVT.

ICD9 CODE

451.1 Thrombosis of deep vessels of lower limb
451.11 Thrombosis of femoral vein
451.19 Thrombosis of other (femoropopliteal, tibial, popliteal)
451.8 Thrombosis of other sites
451.81 Thrombosis of iliac vein
451.83 Thrombosis of deep veins of upper extremities

SYNONYMS

DVT, venous thrombosis, deep venous thrombophlebitis, phlegmasia cerulea dolens, phlegmasia alba dolens, iliofemoral thrombophlebitis, Paget–Schroetter syndrome (spontaneous upper extremity deep vein thrombosis), axillosubclavian vein thrombosis (ASVT).

CARDINAL FEATURES

- Clinical findings are not reliable for diagnosis and a lack of physical findings is common
- Pain and swelling in affected extremity may be present
- If lower extremity, particularly the calf, is affected, pain with dorsiflexion of ipsilateral foot may be elicited (Homan's sign)
- Discoloration of lower extremity with pain, edema, and petechiae (phlegmasia cerulea dolens) – rare

CAUSES

Common causes

- Endothelial injury exposes collagen, precipitating platelet aggregation and tissue thromboplastin release (e.g. surgery)
- Endothelial injury in the setting of stasis (i.e. immobility) or hypercoagulability (inherited or acquired) initiates the coagulation mechanism

Rare causes

- Behçet's syndrome, a multisystem autoimmune disease characterized by recurrent oral and genital ulceration
- Paroxysmal nocturnal hemoglobinuria

Serious causes

- Trauma to extremities (e.g. surgery)
- Cancers of lung, pancreas, gastrointestinal tract, genitourinary tract, and breast

Contributory or predisposing factors

Virchow's triad: venous stasis, vascular damage, hypercoagulability.

Venous stasis:

- Bed rest for longer than 3 days
- Recent surgery that required more than 30min anesthesia, especially surgery involving lower leg or pelvis or gynecologic surgery
- Trauma, especially to pelvis and/or extremities
- Pregnancy and early postpartum period
- Obesity
- Age greater than 60 years
- Prolonged sitting with the legs dependant while traveling (especially on flights longer than 4h)

Vascular damage:
- Indwelling catheters
- Injection of irritating substances
- Thromboangitis obliterans
- Septic phlebitis

Hypercoagulability:
- Exogenous estrogen including oral contraceptives and estrogen replacement therapy
- Cancer, especially lung, pancreatic, gastrointestinal, genitourinary, breast, and myeloproliferative disease
- History of thromboembolic disease
- Congestive heart failure
- Nephrotic syndrome

EPIDEMIOLOGY
Incidence and prevalence
INCIDENCE
1.6 cases per 1000 per year.

PREVALENCE
Exact number of cases unknown because of frequency of inaccurate clinical diagnosis and because DVT may be silent and may resolve spontaneously.

FREQUENCY
- Occurs in more than 50% of patients undergoing orthopedic surgery, especially if it involves the hip or knee
- Occurs in 10–40 % of patients undergoing surgery to chest or abdomen

Demographics
AGE
Usually occurs in people over 60 years of age.

GENDER
Male to female ration is 1.2:1.

GENETICS
- Family history of hypercoagulability including: antithrombin III deficiency, protein C deficiency, protein S deficiency, lupus anticoagulant, dysfibrinogenemias, anticardiolipin antibody, hyperhomocysteinemia, homocystinuria, factor V Leiden mutation, prothrombin gene mutation (G20210A), high levels of factor XI
- Family history of deep vein thrombosis, varicose veins

DIFFERENTIAL DIAGNOSIS

Postphlebitic syndrome

FEATURES

In affected extremity:

- Pain
- Presence/absence of warmth/erythema
- Presence of varicose veins
- Negative non-invasive studies
- Stasis pigmentation
- Subcutaneous tissue induration

Superficial thrombophlebitis

FEATURES

- Palpable subcutaneous vein
- Tender cord with erythema, edema
- Linear induration, redness, tenderness that follows vein
- No edema
- Low-grade fever

Ruptured Baker's cyst

FEATURES

- Aseptic inflammation of gastrocnemius–semimembranosus bursa
- Tenderness at site
- Pain with joint movement
- Palpable fibrocartilaginous bodies

Cellulitis

FEATURES

- Superficial inflammation of skin
- Erythema, warmth, tenderness in affected area
- Common causative organisms: staphylococci, *Haemophilus influenzae*, *Vibrio vulnificus*

Lymphangitis

FEATURES

- Inflammation of lymphatic vessels
- Associated with bacterial cellulitis
- May or may not be related to skin trauma
- Linear erythematous streaks extend proximately to regional lymph nodes
- Lymphadenitis and fever
- Usually caused by group A streptococcal infection of skin in people with lymphedema and superficial fungal infections

Achilles tendinitis

FEATURES

- Pain upon wakening that improves with increased activity
- Pain at onset of exercise that improves with further exercise
- Tenderness at site when tendon squeezed

Varicose veins

FEATURES

- Tortuous superficial veins with incompetent valves
- May be painful, warm to touch

Lymphedema

FEATURES

- Painless edema initially relieved with elevation of extremity
- Usually unilateral
- In lower extremity may cause loss of ankle contour
- Associated with hard, thick, leathery skin
- Prone to cellulitis, lymphangitis

Arterial insufficiency

FEATURES

- Claudication in calves, feet, and/or hands
- Trophic nail changes if upper extremity involved
- Absent or intermittent pulses
- Ulcers common at extremities

SIGNS & SYMPTOMS

Signs

- Unilateral edema and/or warmth – if calf vein or partial occlusion, edema is local; if entire iliofemoral vein involved, edema or warmth may be more generalized
- A difference in calf circumference of at least 1.5cm is present in up to 80% of patients with deep vein thrombisis (DVT), but is not specific.

In affected extremity:

- Tenderness
- Warmth
- Palpable cord
- If the lower extremity is involved, a positive Homan's Sign not specific: found in <1/3 patients with DVT and in 50% of patients without DVT
- Prominent superficial veins

Symptoms

- Swelling in affected extremity
- Pain in affected extremity on standing
- Pain on dorsiflexion of ipsilateral foot if lower extremity involved
- May be asymptomatic

ASSOCIATED DISORDERS

- Pulmonary thrombembolism
- Chronic venous insufficiency
- Clotting disorders: antithrombin III deficiency, protein C deficiency, protein S deficiency, lupus anticoagulant, dysfibrinogenemias, anticardiolipin antibody, hyperhomocysteinemia, homocystinuria, factor V Leiden mutation, prothrombin gene mutation (G20210A), high levels of factor XI

KEY! DON'T MISS!

Physical examination is generally aimed at the vascular system. However, the physical examination is often inaccurate: 50% of patients with symptoms attributable to DVT have been found to have a diagnosis other than DVT.

INVESTIGATION OF THE PATIENT

Direct questions to patient

Q **Have you had this before?** Edema and prominent superficial veins in a patient with prior DVT may be a sign of chronic venous insufficiency

- **Q Have you had any recent injury to the affected area?** Effects of trauma, particularly pain and swelling, may mimic DVT
- **Q How long have the symptoms been present?** Symptoms of DVT usually arise over hours to a few days
- **Q Are you currently taking aspirin, high doses of vitamin A, heparin, or coumadin?** These drugs will affect clotting studies

Contributory or predisposing factors

- **Q Is there a history or recent prolonged bed rest or a long flight?**
- **Q Has there been recent trauma to the extremity?**
- **Q Has there been recent surgery or manipulation (catheter placement) involving the extremity, or gynecologic or pelvic surgery?**
- **Q Is the patient obese?**
- **Q Does the patient take any exogenous estrogen (include oral contraceptives, infertility drugs, estrogen replacement)?** These are known to increase the risk of thrombosis
- **Q If female, is the patient pregnant or had a history of recurrent fetal loss?**
- **Q Is the patient taking tamoxifen?** This is known to increase the risk of thrombosis
- **Q Is there a personal history of cancer?**

Family history

- **Q Is there a family history of clotting disorders?**
- **Q Is there a family history of deep vein thrombosis or venous thromboembolism?**
- **Q Is there a family history of varicose veins?**

Examination

- **Is there pain, warmth, tenderness, palpable cord in affected extremity?**
- **Check respiration: if dyspnea or chest pain is present, may have pulmonary embolism.** 10% of DVTs present as pulmonary embolism
- **Check temperature: low-grade fever is common with DVT; high-grade fever is more indicative of infections (cellulitis, lymphangitis)**
- **Check color of affected extremity: if cyanotic this is indicative of substantial iliofemoral venous obstruction**
- **Are superficial collateral veins visible on the affected extremity?**
- **Signs of ascites or hepatomegaly may be present if associated hepatic vein thrombosis is present**
- **Less commonly, deep venous thrombosis may be the first manifestation of malignancy.** Rectal and stool examination for occult blood as well as pelvic examination in women is prudent

Summary of investigative tests

- Coagulation studies (prothrombin time and activated partial thromboplastin time). Disturbances in blood counts or coagulation times may signify underlying hematologic problem as well as affecting treatment (heparin-induced thrombocytopenia). Baseline coagulation studies must be obtained before anticoagulation is started
- Platelet count. Low platelet counts may predispose to thrombus formation. Baseline platelet count must be obtained before anticoagulation is started
- D-dimer test. Can be rapidly measured by enzyme-linked immunosorbent assays. Useful, if negative, in excluding DVT if used in combination with a normal compression ultrasound or impedance plethysmography (IPG). Its main limitation is that patients with comorbid disease may have falsely abnormal D-dimer assays
- Venous compression ultrasound plus Doppler is a useful non-invasive test that should be repeated (when clinically indicated) to monitor the progress of a suspected acute DVT. Repeat ultrasound after 3–7 days is useful to diagnose patients with calf vein thrombi who subsequently develop proximal thrombosis

- Impedance plethysmography is a sensitive and non-invasive means of diagnosing DVT. A normal result does not exclude DVT. It should be repeated after 2–7 days to diagnose patients with calf vein thrombi who subsequently develop proximal thrombosis
- Contrast venography has traditionally been considered the most accurate means of diagnosing and evaluating a DVT, but it is an invasive and painful procedure
- Plasma protein C, protein S, antithrombin III, lupus anticoagulant, fibrinogen, anticardiolipin antibody, plasma homocysteine and factor V Leiden levels are useful in young patients with DVT, patients who have recurrent DVT without obvious cause, and patients with DVT who have a family history of the disorder

DIAGNOSTIC DECISION

- The known utility of conventional noninvasive studies (e.g. compression ultrasonography and impedance plethysmography) as well as experience with magnetic resonance imaging (MRI) has decreased the need for contrast venography
- Ultrasound and IPG are reliable diagnostic tests for symptomatic proximal lower-extremity venous thrombosis, but are limited in patients with asymptomatic lower-extremity thrombosis
- The clinical examination by itself cannot confirm or exclude the diagnosis of deep venous thrombosis

The American Heart Association guidelines divide deep vein thromboses as follows:

- High probability: classic clinical feature plus one risk factor – 80% of these patients had DVT
- Low probability: no classic clinical features and no risk factors – only 5% had DVT
- Intermediate: presentation does not fit either high or low probability. DVT is confirmed by one of three tests: venography, impedance plethysmography, venous ultrasound

Guidelines

- American Heart Association. Management of deep vein thrombosis and pulmonary embolism. Council on Thrombosis (in consultation with the Council on Cardiovascular Radiology). Circulation 1996;93:2212–45 [1]
- American Thoracic Society. The diagnostic approach to acute venous thromboembolism. Clinical practice guideline. Am J Respir Crit Care Med 1999;160:1043–66 [2]
- Institute for Clinical Systems Improvement. Venous thromboembolism. Cardiovascular Steering Committee. Bloomington (MN): ICSI, 2001. Available at the National Guidelines Clearinghouse [3]

CLINICAL PEARL(S)

Repeat noninvasive testing (IPG, compression ultrasound), when clinically indicated, is recommended for patients with an initial normal result in order to diagnose those with calf vein thrombi who subsequently develop proximal thrombosis.

THE TESTS

Body fluids

D-DIMER

Description

Blood by finger-stick.

Advantages/Disadvantages

- Easy to obtain sample
- Sensitivity >80%
- Negative predictive value >90%
- Specificity only about 30%
- Latex assay not as accurate as enzyme-linked immunosorbent assay (ELISA)
- False-positive after surgery, trauma

Normal

- Varies with assay kit – normal is below cutoff point established by assay
- Normal reading useful in excluding deep vein thrombosis and pulmonary embolism only in low-probability patients

Abnormal

- Varies with assay kit – abnormal is above cutoff point established by assay
- Keep in mind the possibility of a false-positive result

Cause of abnormal result

- Excessive or inadequate anticoagulation
- Malignancy or recent surgery may cause elevated levels

Drugs, disorders, and other factors that may alter results

- Recent surgery
- Recent trauma
- Estrogen (oral contraceptive, infertility drugs, hormone replacement therapy)
- Anticoagulants

Tests of function

PROTHROMBIN TIME (PT) (INTERNATIONAL NORMALIZED RATIO – INR)

Description

Blood.

Advantages/Disadvantages

- Wide availability
- Monitors anticoagulation therapy
- International normalized ratio (INR) can be used to monitor patients on anticoagulant therapy for >2 weeks – it takes into account laboratory differences so is a more standard measure
- Normal value for PT is based on control that varies between laboratories
- Normal value for INR is dependent upon instrumentation
- Influenced by aspirin

Normal

Prothrombin time (PT):

- ±2s of control
- Control should be 11–16s
- International normalized ratio (INR) 2.0–3.0 (for patients on standard-dose anticoagulant therapy)

Abnormal

Prothrombin time (PT):

- >2s above or below control
- International normalized ratio (INR) <2.0 or >3.0 (for patients on standard-dose anticoagulant therapy)
- Keep in mind the possibility of a false-positive result

Cause of abnormal result
Excessive or inadequate anticoagulation.

Drugs, disorders, and other factors that may alter results
- Salicylates
- Anticoagulants (overdose or omission)
- Decreased dietary vitamin K, rarely
- Prematurity in infants
- Disorders of fat absorption: obstructive jaundice, fistulas, sprue, steatorrhea, celiac disease, colitis, chronic diarrhea
- Idiopathic familial hypoprothrombinemia
- Hypofibrinogenemia
- Lupus anticoagulant

ACTIVATED PARTIAL THROMBOPLASTIN TIME (APTT)
Description
Blood.

Advantages/Disadvantages
- Best single screening test for coagulopathies
- Monitors anti-coagulant therapy
- May not detect mild clotting defects

Normal
25–28s.

Abnormal
- Less than 25s or more than 28s
- Keep in mind the possibility of a false-positive result

Cause of abnormal result
Prolonged by excessive or inadequate anticoagulation.

Drugs, disorders, and other factors that may alter results
- Clotting factor defect in I, II, V, VIII, IX, X, XI, or XII (mixing equal parts patient plasma with normal plasma corrects result if factor deficiency is present)
- Presence of clotting factor inhibitors – usually antibody against factor VIII – prolongs result
- Lupus anticoagulant prolongs result
- Extremely low or high hematocrit
- Collection aberrations: contamination of specimen with ethylenediamine tetra-acetic acid (EDTA), clots in specimen, partially filled collection tube
- Drugs that decrease heparin action: antihistamines, digitalis, nicotine, penicillin, protamine, tetracycline, phenothiazine
- Warfarin

PLATELET COUNT
Description
Blood.

Advantages/Disadvantages
- Determines presence of adequate numbers of platelets to assist in clotting
- Does not give any qualitative information about platelet function

Normal
- 140,000–340,000/mm^3 (Rees–Ecker)
- 150,000–350,000/mm^3 (Coulter counter)

Abnormal
- Below 140,000/mm^3 cu/mm or above 450,000/mm^3
- Keep in mind the possibility of a false-positive result

Cause of abnormal result
Pseudothrombocytopenia.

Drugs, disorders, and other factors that may alter results
An increased platelet count may be caused by:
- Recent surgery (especially splenectomy), severe trauma, substantial acute hemorrhage, thrombotic episode
- Myeloproliferative disease such as polycythemia vera, chronic myelogenous leukemia (CML), agnogenic myeloid metaplasia, essential thrombocythemia
- Metastatic cancer

A decreased platelet count may be caused by:
- Exposure to ionizing radiation
- Infection
- Hypersplenism
- Disorders that cause decreased platelet production (e.g. aplastic anemia, myelophthisis)
- Nutritional deficiencies (e.g. of folate, vitamin B12)
- Infections (e.g. AIDS, subacute bacterial endocarditis, septicemia, typhus, rubella, infectious mononucleosis)
- Disorders causing increased platelet consumption (thrombotic thrombocytopenic purpura, disseminated intravascular coagulation, septicemia, toxemia of pregnancy, massive blood loss)
- Hypersplenism
- Inherited syndromes (e.g. Allport's, Bernard–Soulier, Chediak–Higashi, Ehlers–Danlos, May–Hegglin, Wiskott–Aldrich, Glanzmann's thrombasthenia, Hermansky–Pudlak, thrombocytopenia, absent radius bones)

VENOUS COMPRESSION ULTRASOUND / DUPLEX ULTRASOUND (ULTRASOUND PLUS DOPPLER)

Advantages/Disadvantages
- Noninvasive
- Not painful
- Duplex ultrasound can identify Baker's cyst, hematoma, abscess and other causes of pain and edema
- Reliable in detecting lower-extremity venous thrombosis proximally in symptomatic individuals
- Resolution may be poor
- Poor sensitivity in isolated or nonocclusive calf vein thrombi
- Unable to differentiate between old and new thrombus
- Requires skilled operator
- Difficult to detect nonoccluding thrombus
- Less reliable in asymptomatic individuals
- Normal test should be repeated after 3–7 days (when clinically indicated) to diagnose patients with calf vein thrombi who subsequently develop proximal thrombosis

Normal
Vascular lumen can be compressed.

Abnormal

- Vascular lumen cannot be compressed
- Absence of Doppler signals
- Keep in mind the possibility of imaging artifacts
- Presence of an echogenic band in vascular lumen

Cause of abnormal result

Lack of compressability of vascular lumen and absence of Doppler signal secondary to occlusion of lumen.

Drugs, disorders, and other factors that may alter results

- Baker's cyst
- Hematoma
- Patients with pelvic malignancy or abscess may have noncompressible femoral veins when venous thrombosis is absent

CONTRAST VENOGRAPHY

Advantages/Disadvantages

- Reference standard
- Detects about 50% of symptomatic calf vein thrombosis
- Painful
- Invasive
- Increased possibility of phlebitis, new thrombosis, renal failure, and allergic reaction to contrast
- Imaging of deep femoral vein in thigh and internal iliac vein is dependent upon technique and skill
- Allergy to contrast material may occur

Normal

No thrombosis detected.

Abnormal

- Visualization of intraluminal filling defect
- Keep in mind the possibility of imaging artifacts

Cause of abnormal result

Abnormal luminal flow or turbulence.

Drugs, disorders, and other factors that may alter results

- Prior contrast study within 24h
- Inadequate study or poor visualization of the vein

IMPEDANCE PLETHYSMOGRAPHY

Advantages/Disadvantages

- Noninvasive
- Not painful
- Good sensitivity and specificity for proximal DVT in symptomatic patients
- Not sensitive for calf vein thrombosis, non-occlusive proximal vein thrombosis or thrombosis above the inguinal ligament in the iliofemoral vein
- Serial IPG (repeat test after 2–7 days when clinically indicated) is useful to diagnose patients with calf vein thrombi who subsequently develop proximal thrombosis

Normal

Changes in blood flow are within normal limits as measured by standard graphs.

Abnormal

- Lower-extremity venous outflow slowed
- Venous capacitance increased
- Keep in mind the possibility of imaging artifacts

Cause of abnormal result

- Venous obstruction from prior venous disease
- Poor filling from severe arterial disease
- Raised venous pressure from congestive heart failure

Drugs, disorders, and other factors that may alter results

- Congestive heart failure
- Increased central venous pressure
- Acute arterial insufficiency
- Inadequate study

TREATMENT

CONSIDER CONSULT

Consider referral when:

- Anticoagulant therapy is thought to be unsafe or has been ineffective in the past refer for inferior vena caval interruption
- Recurrent deep vein thrombosis (DVT) or contraindications to anticoagulation is present (placement of a Greenfield filter in the inferior vena cava may be indicated)
- Anticoagulation therapy fails or initial laboratory results indicate hypercoagulable state (refer to hematology for investigation of possible underlying coagulopathy)

IMMEDIATE ACTION

Achieving therapeutic anticoagulation within 24h of presentation reduces risk of thromboembolic complications.

MANAGEMENT ISSUES

Goals

- Prevent pulmonary embolus
- Prevent chronic venous insufficiency
- Increase fibrinolysis in certain clinical cases
- Reduce pain and swelling (postphlebitic syndrome)

Management in special circumstances

- Sudden deterioration of patient undergoing diagnostic testing or therapy may indicate pulmonary embolism, and appropriate confirmation studies and support measures should be instituted immediately
- Unexpected bleeding should be investigated as anticoagulant therapy may reveal occult disease (gastrointestinal, genitourinary, lung cancer, pancreatic cancer, breast cancer, peptic ulcer disease)

COEXISTING DISEASE

- Patients with significant thrombocytopenia on heparin may need further investigation for heparin-associated thrombocytopenia
- Patients with symptomatic pulmonary embolism and right ventricular dysfunction by echocardiography may be candidates for thrombolytic therapy

COEXISTING MEDICATION

- Use of salicylates for pain may effect laboratory test results and increase risk of bleeding
- Anticoagulants for prior DVT
- Estrogen (oral contraceptives, infertility, replacement)

SPECIAL PATIENT GROUPS

Pregnant women:

- Warfarin, nonsteroidal anti-inflammatory drugs, thrombolytics are contraindicated
- Heparin is safe to give in pregnancy (low molecular weight heparin safety not fully established). Heparin does not cross placenta. If documented DVT in previous pregnancy, consider heparin therapy starting 4–6 weeks before the time that DVT occurred in previous pregnancy

Children:

- Heparin is same dose per kg as in adults. Safety of low molecular weight heparin not fully established
- Warfarin dose is based on weight but infants may require high end of range
- Thrombolytics – same dose as adults

Elderly:

- Check all concomitant medications for salicylates. Will need more supervision with warfarin if confused

Disabled:

- If extremity paralysis involved in disability, chronic anticoagulation may be needed

Metastatic cancer:

- Indefinite anticoagulation necessary

PATIENT SATISFACTION/LIFESTYLE PRIORITIES

- Change in method of birth control for women taking oral contraceptives may be needed
- Change in estrogen replacement for menopausal women who are symptomatic may be needed
- Patients with sedentary occupations may have difficulty incorporating more movement into their day
- Patients who travel on long (more than 4h) airplane, train, or car, trips will need to incorporate exercises while they are traveling

SUMMARY OF THERAPEUTIC OPTIONS

Choices

- Heparin: initiated with intravenous bolus followed by continuous infusion for 5 days or until prothrombin time (PT) is therapeutic for 2 days; activated partial thromboplastin time (aPTT) is measured 6h after start of infusion then daily – goal is to keep it 1.8–3.0 times the normal range. Subcutaneous administration is equivalent and safe but more difficult to monitor
- Low molecular weight heparin: fixed dose given subcutaneously for 5 days or until INR is therapeutic on warfarin (2.0–3.0)
- Warfarin: initiated within 72h of heparin or low molecular weight heparin; 3-month course with dose adjusted to keep INR 2.0–3.0. Therapy may continue for 3–6 months if DVT is idiopathic, or indefinitely if there is a thrombophilic disorder; more than two documented episodes of recurrent DVT or one DVT in a patient with cancer
- Thrombolytics (streptokinase and urokinase) are contraindicated postoperatively and if patient is at high risk for bleeding. They are indicated in selected patients who have extensive proximal vein thrombosis, regardless of age
- Referral for placement of Greenfield filter or caval balloon may be needed when anticoagulant is ineffective or unsafe (e.g. anticoagulant-induced bleeding, anticipated hemorrhagic complication such as peptic ulcer disease, gastrointestinal cancer, intracranial hemorrhage, liver failure, or thrombocytopenia), failure of anticoagulant, new pulmonary embolus, extension of thrombus
- Surgical removal of thrombus can be performed for phlegmasia cerulea dolens with impending gangrene
- Removal of a subclavian catheter may be necessary to treat a deep venous thrombosis of the upper extremity

Guidelines

- American Heart Association. Management of deep vein thrombosis and pulmonary embolism. Council on Thrombosis (in consultation with the Council on Cardiovascular Radiology). Circulation 1996;93:2212–45 [1]
- American Thoracic Society. The diagnostic approach to acute venous thromboembolism. Clinical practice guideline. Am J Respir Crit Care Med 1999;160:1043–66 [2]
- Institute for Clinical Systems Improvement. Venous thromboembolism. Cardiovascular Steering Committee. Bloomington (MN): ICSI; 2001. Available at the National Guidelines Clearinghouse [3]

FOLLOW UP

Plan for review

- Activated partial thromboplastin time (aPTT) 6h after bolus heparin then daily to maintain in therapeutic range
- When warfarin in place for 2 weeks, check international normalized ratio (INR) weekly to maintain in therapeutic range

Information for patient or caregiver

Information about controllable risk factors (obesity, sedentary lifestyle) should be given.

DRUGS AND OTHER THERAPIES: DETAILS

Drugs

HEPARIN

Anticoagulant.

Dose

- Adult intravenous dose: 50–100U/kg initial infusion then 15–25U/kg, adjust to activated partial prothrombin time (aPTT)
- Child intravenous dose: 50U/kg initially then 15–25U/kg, adjust to aPTT

Efficacy

- Immediate onset if given intravenously
- Onset for subcutaneous injection: 20–60min

Risks/Benefits

- Rapid onset, consistent bioavailability in intravenous form
- Use caution with elderly and children
- Use caution with renal disease and subacute bacterial endocarditis
- Use caution with diabetes mellitus and severe hypertension
- Use caution with history of gastrointestinal cancer and peptic ulcer disease

Side-effects and adverse reactions

- CNS: fever, headache
- Cardiovascular: allergic vasospastic reactions, shock
- EENT: lacrimation, rhinitis
- Gastrointestinal: vomiting
- Genitourinary: hematuria, priapism
- Hematologic: hemorrhage, thrombocytopenia, new thrombus formation
- Metabolism: hyperlipidemia
- Musculoskeletal: osteoporosis
- Respiratory: anaphylactoid reactions, asthma
- Skin: cutaneous necrosis, alopecia, erythema, urticaria

Interactions (other drugs)

- Salicylates
- Warfarin

Contraindications

- Severe thrombocytopenia
- Uncontrolled bleeding (except disseminated intravascular coagulation (DIC))
- Suspected intracranial hemorrhage
- Shock
- Severe hypotension

Evidence

A RCT compared combination warfarin and unfractionated heparin with warfarin alone in the management of patients with proximal DVT. Patients receiving both medications had a significantly reduced recurrence rate at 6 months [4] *Level P*

Acceptability to patient

- Intravenous therapy: medium acceptability; requires hospitalization
- Subcutaneous therapy: medium acceptability; requires self-injection and follow up blood tests

Follow up plan

- Monitor activated partial thromboplastin time (aPTT) daily in hospitalized patients and aim to maintain in a therapeutic range (1.5–2.5 times normal)
- Monitor platelet count, hemoglobin/hematocrit if signs of bleeding

Patient and caregiver information

- Use soft-bristle toothbrush to avoid bleeding gums
- Use electric razor
- Avoid intramuscular injections
- Avoid contact sports
- Report signs of bleeding: urine, stool, gums, bruising

ENOXAPARIN

Low molecular weight heparin (LMWH).

Dose

Adult subcutaneous dose: 1mg/kg twice daily (treatment) and 30mg twice daily subcutaneously every 12h (prevention)

Efficacy

Onset of action 3–5h.

Risks/Benefits

- Subcutaneous injection may be given at home
- Use precaution with bleeding disorders and thrombocytopenia
- Use precaution with angiodysplastic gastrointestinal disease and active peptic ulceration
- Use precaution with bacterial endocarditis and hemorrhagic stroke
- Use precaution with recent surgery
- Use precaution with elderly and children

Side-effects and adverse reactions

- CNS: confusion, fever
- Cardiovascular: edema
- Gastrointestinal: altered liver function test results, nausea
- Hematologic: thrombocytopenia, hemorrhage, anemia
- Skin: ecchymosis, erythema/irritation at injection site, hematoma, pain

Interactions (other drugs)

No interactions recorded.

Contraindications

- Active bleeding
- Drug-related thrombocytopenia

Evidence

Low molecular weight heparins are effective in the management of deep vein thrombosis.

- Low molecular weight heparin is the preferred treatment option for initial anticoagulation in patients with DVT. It is as safe and effective as unfractionated heparin [3] *Level C*
- A systematic review found low molecular weight heparin was at least as effective as unfractionated heparin in preventing recurrence of venous thromboembolism. Hemorrhage during treatment is reduced with LMWH, and overall mortality is reduced [5] *Level M*
- LMWH was found to reduce thrombus extension in patients with proximal DVTs compared to unfractionated heparin in a systematic review [6] *Level M*
- A systematic review found symptomatic thromboembolic complications and mortality related to proximal DVTs were reduced in patients treated with LMWH compared with unfractionated heparin [7] *Level M*
- Another systematic review found that LMWH is possibly as effective as vitamin K antagonists for the prevention of symptomatic thromboembolism after an episode of DVT. LMWH is significantly safer than vitamin K antagonists, and may be a possible alternative treatment for selected patients; however, vitamin K antagonists are the treatment of choice for most patients [8] *Level M*

Acceptability to patient

Medium to high: needs to learn subcutaneous injections but they can be given at home.

Follow up plan

Laboratory monitoring is not necessary with LMWH.

Patient and caregiver information

- Learn subcutaneous injection technique into abdominal wall and alternate injection sites
- Report bleeding (skin, gums, under skin, gastrointestinal or genitourinary) to provider

WARFARIN

Dose

- 5mg by mouth for 2–4 days, then adjust according to international normalized ratio (INR) in 5–20% increments
- Usual daily dose 2–10mg
- Therapeutic INR 2.0–3.0

Efficacy

- Rapidly absorbed
- Peak activity 1.5–3 days

Risks/Benefits

- Use caution with infection and trauma
- Use caution with diverticulitis, renal and hepatic disease
- Use caution with hypertension, congestive heart failure, and tuberculosis
- Use caution with thyroid disease and diabetes mellitus
- Use caution with elderly, children, and nursing mothers
- Use caution with protein C deficiency, polyarteritis, and vasculitis

Side-effects and adverse reactions

- CNS: fatigue, headache
- EENT: blurred vision
- Gastrointestinal: cramps, diarrhea, vomiting
- Genitourinary: gonadal dysfunction

- Metabolic: altered thyroid, pituitary, and adrenal hormones
- Muscloskeletal: weakness
- Skin: contact dermatitis

Interactions (other drugs)

- Acetaminophen - Allopurinol - Amiodarone - Aminoglutethimide - Aspirin - Azathioprine - Barbiturates - Bile acid-binding resins - Carbamazepine - Cephalosporins - Chloramphenicol - Chloral hydrate - Clofibrate - Co-trimoxazole - Danazol - Dextrothyroxine - Disulfiram - Ethanol - Ethchlorvynol - Fluconazole - Fluorouracil - Gemfibrozil - Glutethimide - Griseofulvin - Glucagon - Heparin - Isoniazid - Metronidazole - Nalidixic acid - Neomycin - NSAIDs - Oral contraceptives - Phenytoin - Propafenones - Propoxyphene - Quinidines - Quinolones - Rifampin - Salicyclates - Sertraline - Sulfonamides - Sulfonylureas - Testosterone derivatives

Contraindications

- Active bleeding - Bacterial endocarditis - Cerebral hemorrhage - Eclampsia - Hemorrhagic blood dyscrasias - Hemorrhagic tendencies - Hypertension - Pericarditis - Recent surgery presenting heightened risk of bleeding - Pregnancy and threatened abortion - Hypertension - Gastrointestinal ulceration - Ulcerative colitis - Visceral carcinoma

Evidence

There is evidence for the use of warfarin in the management of deep vein thrombosis.

- Warfarin therapy should be commenced with heparin unless the patient is pregnant or thrombophilia is suspected [3] *Level C*
- A RCT compared intravenous heparin therapy for at least 5 days, with or without 3 months of warfarin therapy, in patients with isolated calf vein thrombosis. The combination therapy was more effective in reducing the extension of thrombus at 1 year [9] *Level P*
- A systematic review found that LMWH is possibly as effective as vitamin K antagonists for the prevention of symptomatic thromboembolism after an episode of DVT. LMWH is significantly safer than vitamin K antagonists, and may be a possible alternative treatment for selected patients; however, vitamin K antagonists are the treatment of choice for most patients [8] *Level M*

Acceptability to patient

High: oral medication; does require follow up laboratory work.

Follow up plan

- Monitor international normalized ratio (INR) every 4–6 weeks once in stable therapeutic range
- Increase frequency of monitoring if INR out of range
- Monitor for bleeding

Patient and caregiver information

- Need to adhere to prescribed dose and regimen
- Avoid alcohol, salicylates, and any major dietary changes
- Do not change from one brand to another without speaking to clinician

STREPTOKINASE

Thrombolytic.

Dose

Adult intravenous dose: 250,000 IU over 30min, then 100,000 IU/h for 72h.

Risks/Benefits

- Use caution with recent surgery, obstetric delivery, infection and trauma
- Use caution with subacute bacterial endocarditis and streptococcal infection
- Use caution with diabetic hemorrhagic retinopathy and bleeding disorders
- Use caution with the elderly

Side-effects and adverse reactions

- CNS: fever, headache
- Cardiovascular: hypotension, reperfusion dysrhythmias
- EENT: periorbital edema
- Gastrointestinal: nausea
- Hematologic: hemorrhage, anemia
- Respiratory: bronchospasm, dyspnea, pulmonary edema
- Skin: flushing, irritation, phlebitis at injection site, urticaria

Interactions (other drugs)

- Fibrinogen
- Lactate dehydrogenase isoenzymes

Contraindications

- Active internal bleeding
- Intracranial neoplasm
- Recent cerebrovascular accident
- Recent surgery
- Severe uncontrolled hypertension

Evidence

Thrombolytic therapy may be used in patients with extensive iliofemoral thrombotic disease who demonstrate evidence of vascular compromise [3] *Level C*

UROKINASE
Thrombolytic

Dose

Adult intravenous dose: 4400 IU/kg over 10min, then 4400 IU/kg for 12h.

Efficacy

Evidence that thrombolytic therapy is associated with reduced incidence of post-thrombotic syndrome remains controversial.

Risks/Benefits

- Fast acting
- Use caution with recent surgery, obstetric delivery, and trauma
- Use caution with subacute bacterial endocarditis and streptococcal infection
- Use caution with diabetic hemorrhagic retinopathy and bleeding disorders
- Use caution with the elderly

Side-effects and adverse reactions

- Cardiovascular: hypotension, hypertension, myocardial infarction, reperfusion dysrhythmias
- Gastrointestinal: nausea
- Hematologic: hemorrhage, surface bleeding
- Metabolism: acidosis
- Respiratory: bronchospasm, dyspnea
- Skin: rash

Interactions (other drugs)

- Anticoagulants
- Antiplatelet agents

Contraindications

- Active bleeding ▪ Intraspinal surgery ▪ Intracranial tumor ▪ Ulcerative colitis ▪ Enteritis ▪ Coagulation defects ▪ Rheumatic valvular heart disease ▪ Cerebral embolism ▪ Thrombosis or hemorrhage within 2 months ▪ Intra-arterial diagnostic procedure ▪ Surgery or trauma within 10 days ▪ Severe hypertension

Evidence

Thrombolytic therapy may be used in patients with extensive iliofemoral thrombotic disease who demonstrate evidence of vascular compromise [3] *Level C*

Acceptability to patient

Medium: requires hospitalization for intravenous therapy.

Follow up plan

- Monitor coagulation tests during therapy
- Treat bleeding with cryoprecipitate or fresh frozen plasma

Patient and caregiver information

Tell patient to report bleeding: gums, gastrointestinal tract, genitourinary tract skin.

Surgical therapy

THROMBECTOMY

Efficacy

- Rapid removal of clot in phlegmasia cerulea dolens
- Leaves endothelial surface rough – clot may reform

Risks/Benefits

- Bleeding
- Anesthesia risks
- Clot reformation
- Prevention of gangrenous complications of phlegmasia cerulea dolens

Acceptability to patient

Low because it involves surgery and hospitalization.

Follow up plan

- Monitor for clot formation
- Monitor anticoagulant therapy

Patient and caregiver information

- Signs and symptoms of recurrent clot
- Need for support stockings/anticoagulant therapy

INSERTION OF GREENFIELD FILTER

An umbrella filter inserted into the vena cava.

Efficacy

- Traps emboli from thrombus
- Patency 95%

Risks/Benefits
- Bleeding associated with placement
- Prevention of pulmonary embolus
- Can be used in situations in which bleeding prevents use of heparin therapy or if there is a contraindication to warfarin therapy

Evidence
Inferior vena cava filters may be indicated in patients with proximal DVT who have contraindications to anticoagulation, progressive thromboembolism despite adequate anticoagulation, or underlying pulmonary hypertension [3] *Level C*

Acceptability to patient
Low: requires hospitalization for placement.

Follow up plan
- Monitor anticoagulant therapy
- Assess for recurrent DVT

Patient and caregiver information
- Report bleeding from gums, gastrointestinal tract, genitourinary tract, skin
- Instruction in anticoagulant therapy may be needed

Other therapies

SUPPORT STOCKINGS

Efficacy
Along with elevation of extremity, decreases edema of affected extremity.

Risks/Benefits
- If not properly fitted may increase edema
- Support of extremity and decreased edema

Acceptability to patient
Medium: may be difficult to apply for elderly or in hot weather; not cosmetically esthetic.

Follow up plan
Check fit of stocking and peripheral pulses on follow up examination.

Patient and caregiver information
- Report increased swelling, numbness, or tingling in extremity
- Stockings must be worn daily

LIFESTYLE

- Rest with limb elevated for 4 days then gradually return to normal activity
- Wear support stockings daily
- Dietary changes to lose weight if obese

RISKS/BENEFITS
- Duration of rest period is controversial and prolonged rest may increase the risk of thrombosis
- Edema and pain are decreased

ACCEPTABILITY TO PATIENT
Low: bed rest and dietary changes are required.

FOLLOW UP PLAN
Review dietary changes and activity level at follow up appointment.

PATIENT AND CAREGIVER INFORMATION
Change in lifestyle: dietary changes to decrease obesity.

OUTCOMES

EFFICACY OF THERAPIES

- Anticoagulation for 3 months is usually effective for patients with reversible risk factors
- Therapy may be required to continue for 3–6 months if deep vein thrombosis (DVT) is idiopathic, or indefinitely if there is a thrombophilic disorder, more than two documented episodes of recurrent DVT, or one DVT in a patient with cancer
- An inferior vena cava filter is a useful treatment alternative when anticoagulation is ineffective or contraindicated
- Extensive thrombosis may be managed effectively with thrombolysis in selected patients with vascular compromise

Evidence

- Warfarin plus unfractionated heparin for patients with proximal DVT results in a significantly reduced recurrence rate at 6 months [4] *Level P*
- Low molecular weight heparin (LMWH) is at least as effective as unfractionated heparin in preventing recurrence of venous thromboembolism [10] *Level M*
- Low molecular weight heparin is at least as safe as unfractionated heparin for the management of DVT [10] *Level M*
- LMWH is possibly as effective as vitamin K antagonists for the prevention of symptomatic thromboembolism after an episode of DVT. LMWH is significantly safer than vitamin K antagonists, and may be a possible alternative treatment for selected patients; however, vitamin K antagonists are the treatment of choice for most patients [8] *Level M*
- Intravenous heparin therapy for at least 5 days with 3 months of warfarin therapy in patients with isolated calf vein thrombosis is more effective for reducing the extension of thrombus at 1 year than heparin alone [9] *Level P*

Review period

Patients should be actively monitored for bleeding and thrombocytopenia.

PROGNOSIS

Short-term prognosis of patients with proximal DVT and treated with adequate doses of anticoagulant for 3 months is good. Recurrent DVT in 5–10% of patients in 1 year after therapy; 30% at 8 years.

Therapeutic failure

- Placement of Greenfield filter (a permanent filter placed in the inferior vena cava to trap emboli)
- A caval balloon can be placed percutaneously and removed after threat of embolus decreases
- Thrombectomy: recurrent DVT is common after surgery despite anticoagulation. Thrombectomy is also used in phlegmasia cerulea dolens

Recurrence

- Greenfield filter
- Caval balloon

Terminal illness

Advanced metastatic cancer: indefinite anticoagulant therapy unless contraindicated, i.e. peptic ulcer disease, brain metastasis, gastrointestinal cancer, genitourinary cancer, liver failure, thrombocytopenia.

COMPLICATIONS

- Pulmonary embolus
- Propagation of thrombus causing obstruction leading to phlegmasia cerulea dolens and gangrene
- Hemorrhage

PREVENTION

RISK FACTORS

- **Prolonged bed rest** – promotes stasis
- **Post operative** – disrupts venous endothelium and leads to stasis
- **Trauma or surgery pelvis/extremities** – disruption of venous endothelium
- **Exogenous estrogen** – hypercoagulability
- **Cancer** – causes hypercoagulability
- **Age >60 years** – stasis
- **Pregnancy/postpartum** – disrupts venous endothelium

MODIFY RISK FACTORS

- Prolonged bed rest: if elderly or disabled, institute passive exercise that flexes muscles in extremities and support hose
- Obesity: weight-reducing diet
- Prolonged travel: support hose; exercise

Lifestyle and wellness

TOBACCO

Pregnant women who smoke may be at particular risk or women on estrogen therapy. Tobacco smoking should be discouraged.

DIET

If patient is obese, institute weight reduction diet.

PHYSICAL ACTIVITY

- If sedentary, patient should increase physical activity
- If disabled, exercises to flex muscles of extremities – either active or passive

SEXUAL BEHAVIOR

Consider barrier methods of birth control rather than oral contraceptives.

CHEMOPROPHYLAXIS

Low molecular weight heparin after major trauma, hip or pelvic surgery.

SCREENING

Screening is not necessary.

PREVENT RECURRENCE

Recurrence rate of DVT after heparin/warfarin/compression stockings is 20.3% at 8 years.

ASSOCIATIONS

The Center for Outcomes Research and the Venous Educational Institute of North American (VEIN) provide an Internet resource on venous thromboembolism at www.dvt.org.

The American Heart Association
7272 Greenville Ave
Dallas, TX 75231-4596
http://www.americanheart.org

KEY REFERENCES

- ACCP Consensus Committee on Pulmonary Embolism. Opinions regarding the diagnosis and management of venous thromboembolic disease. Chest 1998;113(2): 499–504
- Baker WF. Diagnosis of deep vein thrombosis and pulmonary embolism. Med Clin North Am 1998;82(3):459–76

Evidence references and guidelines

1 American Heart Association. Management of deep vein thrombosis and pulmonary embolism. Council on Thrombosis (in consultation with the Council on Cardiovascular Radiology). Circulation 1996;93:2212–45
2 American Thoracic Society. The diagnostic approach to acute venous thromboembolism. Clinical practice guideline. Am J Respir Crit Care Med 1999;160:1043–66
3 Institute for Clinical Systems Improvement. Venous thromboembolism. Cardiovascular Steering Committee. Bloomington (MN): ICSI, 2001. Available at the National Guidelines Clearinghouse
4 Brandjes DPM, Heijboer H, Buller HR, et al. Acenocoumarol and heparin compared with acenocoumarol alone in the initial treatment of proximal-vein thrombosis. N Engl J Med 1992;327:1485–89. Reviewed in: Clinical Evidence 2001;6:178–88
5 van den Belt AGM, Prins MH, Lensing AWA, et al. Fixed dose subcutaneous low molecular weight heparins versus adjusted dose unfractionated heparin for venous thromboembolism (Cochrane Review). In: The Cochrane Library, 1, 2002. Oxford: Update Software
6 Leisosorovicz A, Simonneau G, Decousous H, Boissel JP. Comparison of efficacy and safety of low molecular weight heparins and unfractionated heparin in initial treatment of deep venous thrombosis: a meta-analysis. BMJ 1994;309:299–304. Reviewed in: Clinical Evidence 2001;6:178–88
7 Lensing AWA, Prins MH, Davidson BL, Hirsh J. Treatment of deep venous thrombosis with low molecular weight heparins. Arch Intern Med 1995;155:601–7. Reviewed in: Clinical Evidence 2001;6:178–88
8 van der Heijden, Hutten BA, Buller HR, Prins MH. Vitamin K antagonists of low-molecular-weight heparin for the long term treatment of symptomatic venous thromboembolism (Cochrane Review). In: The Cochrane Library, 1, 2002. Oxford: Update Software
9 Lagerstedt C, Olsson C, Fagher B, et al. Need for long term anticoagulant treatment in symptomatic calf vein thrombosis. Lancet 1985;334:515–8. Reviewed in: Clinical Evidence 2001;6:178–88
10 Fitzmaurice D, Hobbs FDR, McManus R. Thromboembolism: cardiovascular disorders. In: Clinical Evidence 2001;6:178–188. London: BMJ Publishing Group

CONTRIBUTORS

Fred F Ferri MD, FACP
Mark B Stockman, MD
Elizabeth Jackson, MD

INFECTIVE ENDOCARDITIS

SUMMARY INFORMATION

DESCRIPTION

- Syndrome resulting from microbial infection of the endothelial surface of the heart (typically the cardiac valves), usually by bacteria, although fungi, rickettsiae, mycoplasmas, and chlamydiae may be the cause
- Symptoms are generally nonspecific, including fever, chills, and sweats. Signs include altered or new heart murmur, systemic emboli, and splenomegaly
- Injection drug users and patients with underlying cardiac conditions, especially prosthetic valves, are particularly susceptible
- Commonly classified as acute or subacute, although intermediate presentation is possible
- Usually fatal without effective antibiotic therapy. Treatment is generally for 2–6 weeks but can vary with pathogen, duration of fever, and whether an infected valve is native or prosthetic

URGENT ACTION

- Monitor for signs of congestive heart failure
- Initiate the first of three sequential blood cultures
- With acute disease, it is acceptable to draw multiple cultures within 1h, rather than 24h, as normally recommended
- Also with acute disease, antibiotic treatment aimed at the most likely pathogen may begin before the etiologic agent is identified (antibiotic regimen should be reassessed after the agent is known)

KEY! DON'T MISS!

- A high index of suspicion is needed in any patient with a predisposing factor and vague chronic symptoms
- Multiple blood cultures must be drawn prior to initiation of antibiotic therapy, since correct identification of the infective organism is critical to treatment success and establishing the diagnosis

ICD9 CODE

421.0 Acute and subacute endocarditis

SYNONYMS

Bacterial endocarditis.

CARDINAL FEATURES

- Syndrome resulting from microbial infection of the endothelial surface of the heart (mainly the cardiac valves). Infection typically begins when micro-organisms in the bloodstream attach to a fibrin-platelet matrix (vegetation) that has developed on a damaged cardiac valve or the mural endocardium or on synthetic materials within the heart
- Infectious organisms are usually bacteria but may be fungi, rickettsiae, mycoplasmas, or chlamydiae. Most commonly affected area is the mitral valve, followed by the aortic valve, combined mitral and aortic valve, tricuspid valve, and (rarely) the pulmonic valve. The mural endocardium may also be infected
- Symptoms are generally nonspecific: fever, chills, sweats, and anorexia. Signs include fever; heart murmur, including altered or new murmur; systemic emboli; and splenomegaly. Disease usually affects the left side of the heart, although in injection drug users, the right side is more often involved
- Acute disease has a fulminant course that progresses to valvular destruction and metastatic infection. Subacute disease develops over weeks to months, only rarely with metastatic infection
- Usually fatal unless treated with an antibiotic that is effective against the etiologic agent. Duration of therapy (generally 2–6 weeks) is influenced by the pathogen, persistence of fever, and whether the infected valve is native or prosthetic. Outpatient parenteral therapy is acceptable for selected patients with uncomplicated disease caused by penicillin-susceptible streptococci

CAUSES

Common causes

Streptococci:

- Viridans streptococci cause about 50–60% of cases in patients with native valves who are not injection drug users. Also seen in patients with prosthetic valves that have been in place for more than 60 days. Associated with subacute disease
- *Streptococcus bovis* is most likely to infect patients with native valves who have gastrointestinal malignancy or colonic polyps. Most often seen in elderly patients. Associated with subacute disease
- *S. intermedius* group can cause acute and subacute disease
- *S. pneumoniae* may cause acute infection of a normal aortic valve. Alcoholism is a risk factor. Patients may have concurrent pneumonia or meningitis
- *Streptococcus* groups A, B, C, G cause acute disease
- Enterococci are associated with genitourinary tract manipulations and are most often seen in elderly patients

Staphylococci:

- *Staphylococcus aureus* is the most frequent cause of acute disease. Seen in acutely ill patients with native valves, injection drug users, and patients with prosthetic valves implanted within the past 60 days. Among nonaddicts, it usually infects the left side of the heart. In addicts, it often infects the tricuspid valve
- Coagulase-negative staphylococci commonly infect prosthetic valves during the first year after implantation. *S. epidermidis* is the species most often involved. *S. lugdunensis*, usually community acquired, can infect native and prosthetic valves

HACEK group of Gram-negative bacilli:

- *Haemophilus parainfluenzae*, *H. aphrophilus*, *Actinobacillus actinomycetemcomitans*, *Cardiobacterium hominis, Eikenella* species, and *Kingella* species may infect prosthetic valves, particularly during initial year after implantation. Possible nonacute disease in patients with native valves

Rare causes

- Fungi (including *Candida albicans*, nonalbicans *Candida* species, *Torulopsis* (*Candida*) *glabrata*, and *Aspergillus* species): seen with open heart surgery and indwelling central venous catheters. Detected in 5–15% of instances of prosthetic valve endocarditis. Also seen in injection drug users and immunosuppressed patients
- *Pseudomonas aeruginosa*: seen in injection drug users. Can occur on prosthetic valves
- *Burkholderia cepacia*: seen in injection drug users
- *Listeria monocytogenes*: implicated in a small number of patients with abnormal left heart valves or prosthetic devices
- Gram-negative coccobacilli: including *Bartonella* and *Legionella* species, as well as *Neisseria gonorrheae* (rare in the antibiotic era). *Bartonella quintana* seen in homeless men; *Bartonella henselae* seen in cat owners. Other species associated with prosthetic valve replacement
- Atypical mycobacteria: may cause nosocomial prosthetic valve endocarditis
- Diphtheroids (usually *Corynebacterium jeikeium*): may infect prosthetic valves during first year after implantation; may also infect abnormal native valves
- Polymicrobial: *Pseudomonas* and enterococci most likely combination. Seen in injection drug users. Results in heightened risk of mortality from cardiac surgery
- *Coxiella burnetii* (Q fever): transmitted by sheep, cattle, or wild rabbits. Patients with abnormal mitral or aortic valves who experience acute, prolonged infection with this pathogen may develop subacute infective endocarditis. Culture negative
- *Chlamydia* species: culture negative

Serious causes

- *Staphylococcus aureus*: causes acute, destructive illness, often with metastatic infection and central nervous system complications. Surgery improves likelihood of survival and is often warranted with left-sided disease
- Enterococci: increasing resistance to multiple antibiotics
- *Streptococcus pneumoniae*: high mortality rate; surgery is frequently required
- *Streptococcus intermedius* group: can invade tissue and cause abscess formation
- Group B streptococci: mortality rate 40%; valve replacement often necessary
- Groups A, C, and G streptococci: acute disease with suppurative complications
- *Pseudomonas aeruginosa*: patients often require surgery
- HACEK organisms: surgery often needed for cure
- Fungi: surgery often needed for cure
- Polymicrobial: patients undergoing cardiac surgery are at high risk of mortality

Contributory or predisposing factors

Cardiac conditions:

- Prosthetic heart valve
- Previous infective endocarditis
- Rheumatic heart disease
- Valve abnormalities, including hypertrophic subaortic stenosis; mitral valve prolapse with regurgitation and/or thickened leaflets; and bicuspid, calcific, or sclerotic aortic valve changes
- Endocardial abnormalities caused by blood flow in congenital lesions (ventricular septal defect, tetralogy of Fallot, coarctation of the aorta, and patent ductus arteriosus)
- Surgically repaired intracardiac lesions
- Intracardiac pacemaker
- Hypertrophic cardiomyopathy

- Degenerative valvular disease in elderly patients
- Valvular regurgitation following exposure to appetite-suppressant drugs (fenfluramine and dexfenfluramine)
- Diabetes mellitus
- Chronic renal disease

Recent transient or prolonged bacteremia:
- Dental, pulmonary, gastrointestinal, and genitourinary procedures

Immunosuppression:
- Malignancy, AIDS, or organ transplantation
- Increased risk of fungal endocarditis

Behaviors:
- Intravenous drug abuse
- Alcoholism is a risk factor for infective endocarditis caused by *Streptococcus pneumoniae*

EPIDEMIOLOGY

Incidence and prevalence

- 1.7–3.8 cases/10,000 in US
- Nosocomial endocarditis 14–28% of cases

INCIDENCE
0.017–0.038/1000.

PREVALENCE
0.3–3 cases/1000 hospital admissions in US.

Demographics

AGE
- Most commonly found in those aged 45–65 years
- Among females, age usually below 35 years
- Among injection drug users, average age is between 27 and 37 years
- Increasing incidence among the elderly, with more than 25% of cases seen in those older than 60 years
- Rare in infancy; usually follows open heart surgery, or infected intravenous or right-heart catheters in this age group

GENDER
- Males affected about twice as often as females
- Among males, peak incidence during ages 45–65 years; among females, often occurs before age 35 years

GENETICS
- Marfan syndrome causes heightened susceptibility
- Mitral valve prolapse with myxomatous changes of the mitral valve is a genetic disorder
- There is probably a genetic predisposition for rheumatic fever

SOCIOECONOMIC STATUS
- Injection drug users are at high risk for both initial and recurrent infective endocarditis (IE). *Staphylococcus aureus* causes more than half of cases. Between 60 and 70% of cases involve the tricuspid valve, resulting in clinical presentation with pleuritic chest pain, dyspnea, cough, and hemoptysis
- Homelessness heightens risk of IE caused by *Bartonella* species

DIAGNOSIS

DIFFERENTIAL DIAGNOSIS

Acute rheumatic fever

Acute rheumatic fever is a delayed sequela of upper respiratory infection with group A streptococcus, occurring 2–3 weeks after infection.

FEATURES

- Patients with rheumatic fever may present with fever and new cardiac murmur
- Ages 5–15 years most often affected; adults more likely to have recurrent than primary disease
- Acute episodes occur 2–3 weeks after pharyngitis
- Migratory polyarthritis occurs in most cases

Atrial myxoma

Atrial myxoma is a benign gelatinous growth usually arising from the interatrial septum of the heart in the region of the fossa ovalis.

FEATURES

- Common manifestations are chest pain, dyspnea, edema, and syncope
- Patients may develop fever, cough, clubbing
- Auscultation may reveal 'tumor plop' or a mitral insufficiency murmur

Systemic lupus erythematosus

Systemic lupus erythematosus (SLE) is a chronic multisystemic disease of autoimmune origin which characteristically affects skin and joints, although any system can be involved.

FEATURES

- Cardiac involvement may emerge as endocarditis, pericarditis, or myocarditis (this is likely to emerge as opportunistic infection by bacteria or viruses as a result of immunosuppression caused by use of corticosteroids and other drugs). Cardiac manifestations in the absence of immunosuppression may be the mode of presentation
- Fever, fatigue, arthralgia, myalgia, malaise are common symptoms
- Malar 'butterfly' rash that is sensitive to sunlight is common

Acute glomerulonephritis

Acute glomerulonephritis may occur as an immunologic response to an infection, most commonly streptococcal.

FEATURES

- May emerge as a complication of infective endocarditis
- Acute syndrome usually follows 10–14 days after streptococcal infection
- Symptoms include malaise, headache, facial edema, flank pain, and cloudy urine
- Signs are hypertension, hematuria, and oliguria

Marantic endocarditis

Also called nonbacterial thrombotic endocarditis.

FEATURES

- Involves sterile vegetations on heart valves
- Usually seen in patients with a hypercoagulable state, often in association with malignancy, and in severely ill patients, including those with AIDS
- Embolic events can occur with these sterile vegetations

Pericarditis

Pericarditis is an inflammatory or infective disease of the pericardial sac, which may be acute or chronic.

FEATURES

- Chest pain usually a prominent symptom, often localized to the retrosternal region
- Dyspnea and pericardial friction rub are common manifestations

Renal cell carcinoma

Renal cell carcinoma is a tumor that spreads via the vascular system and by direct invasion into other organ structures and lymph nodes.

FEATURES

- Classic triad of symptoms consists of hematuria, abdominal mass, and flank pain
- Fever, anemia, and weight loss may be present

SIGNS & SYMPTOMS

Signs

- Fever in 85% of patients
- Cardiac murmur, including changed or new murmur: detected in about 85% of patients other than injection drug users at presentation. Most common murmurs reflect aortic, mitral, or tricuspid regurgitation. In injection drug users, disease is likely to be right-sided, and murmur is harder to detect
- Vasculitic skin lesions (more than 50% of patients): petechiae on mucosal surface or skin; hemorrhages under nails; Osler's nodes – painful, erythematous nodules on palmar surface of fingertip; Janeway lesions – nontender, erythematous, macular lesions on palms and soles. Osler's nodes and Janeway lesions predominantly occur in subacute endocarditis
- Possible ocular findings: conjunctival or retinal hemorrhages. Retinal hemorrhages may have a pale center with red halo (Roth's spots)
- Clubbing
- Splenomegaly (about 35%): more likely with subacute disease

Symptoms

- Fever
- Chills
- Fatigue
- Weakness
- Night sweats
- Weight loss
- Red spots on palms and soles
- Red, pea-sized nodules in the pads of fingers and toes
- Headaches
- Backaches
- Joint pains
- Confusion
- Shortness of breath with exertion
- Changed color of urine
- Cough
- Stroke

ASSOCIATED DISORDERS

HIV infection is detected in 27–73% of injection drug users with infective endocarditis (IE). Heightened risk of death from IE among HIV-infected injection drug users with a CD4 count below $200/mm^3$.

KEY! DON'T MISS!

- A high index of suspicion is needed in any patient with a predisposing factor and vague chronic symptoms
- Multiple blood cultures must be drawn prior to initiation of antibiotic therapy, since correct identification of the infective organism is critical to treatment success and establishing the diagnosis

CONSIDER CONSULT

- Some physicians believe that all patients with infective endocarditis should be followed by or referred to either an expert in infectious diseases or a cardiologist, and often to both, since this is a disease with a significant risk of death and the patient's condition can change abruptly
- Refer if diagnosis is uncertain
- Consider referral of pediatric patients, those with prosthetic valves, and injection drug users

INVESTIGATION OF THE PATIENT

Direct questions to patient

- **Q Did your symptoms emerge gradually or suddenly?** Acute disease usually begins in less than a week; patients are severely ill and report chills, moderately elevated temperature, myalgias, and arthralgias. Subacute disease emerges over weeks to months, and patients often have vague complaints
- **Q Do you experience fevers and/or chills?** Fever occurs in most instances of IE, although it may be absent among the elderly, severely debilitated patients, and those with congestive heart failure or chronic renal failure
- **Q Do you have night sweats?** Common occurrence in IE
- **Q Do you become short of breath with activity, or do you have difficulty breathing when you are lying down?** Possible indications of congestive heart failure
- **Q Are you generally tired or weak?** May be a primary complaint of patients with subacute IE
- **Q Do you have a cough?** Possible symptom of right-sided IE, possibly with hemoptysis or pleuritic chest pain
- **Q Do you have chest pain?** Pleuritic chest pain may reflect right-sided IE
- **Q Do you have aches and pains?** Low back pain, myalgias, and arthralgias commonly seen with IE. Severe pain of lower back may reflect enterococcal endocarditis
- **Q Have you lost weight?** Common in subacute IE
- **Q Have you noticed a change in the color of your urine?** Hematuria, which may be microscopic, occurs in >50% of patients with IE. It results from embolic lesions of the kidney

Contributory or predisposing factors

- **Q Do you use injection drugs?** Leading risk factor for IE and recurrent IE
- **Q Do you have a heart condition, including a prosthetic valve?** Important risk factor
- **Q Have you ever had infective endocarditis?** Recurrence occurs in IE; history of this condition is a major risk factor
- **Q Have you ever had rheumatic fever?** Significant risk factor
- **Q Do you have diabetes mellitus?** Recent studies suggest heightened risk
- **Q Have you had serious kidney disease?** Recent studies suggest heightened risk
- **Q Have you undergone any recent procedures in a dentist's office, doctor's office, or hospital?** Dental, pulmonary, gastrointestinal, and genitourinary procedures are possible causes of transient bacteremia that may result in IE

Examination

- **Has patient lost weight?** Weigh patient. Weight loss may indicate subacute disease
- **Does patient have fever?** Check temperature. Fever is the most common symptom of IE, but it may be absent in elderly patients and patients with congestive heart failure, severe debility, or chronic renal failure

- **Does patient have a new or altered heart murmur?** Perform auscultation. Murmurs most likely to occur with IE are those of aortic, mitral, or tricuspid regurgitation. In injection drug users, disease is likely to be right-sided, and murmurs are harder to detect
- **Does patient have signs of congestive heart failure?** Check with auscultation. Possible signs are rales, S3 gallop, jugular venous distention, edema
- **Does patient have skin manifestations?** Check skin for Osler's nodes (painful lesions of the fingers and toes), Janeway lesions (painless hemorrhagic macules on palms and soles), splinter hemorrhages on nails, and petechiae. Any of these may be associated with IE
- **Does patient have Roth's spots?** Examine eyes for pale retinal lesions surrounded by hemorrhage. Seen in a small percentage of patients with IE
- **Does patient have clubbing?** Check fingers and toes. Most often seen in patients with prolonged, untreated IE
- **Is patient's spleen enlarged?** Palpate spleen. Enlarged spleen is a possible sign of IE, seen more commonly in subacute than acute disease

Summary of investigative tests

- Blood cultures: critical for diagnosis and for identifying infectious organism
- Rheumatoid factor: positive result provides a minor diagnostic sign
- Urinalysis: may reveal hematuria
- Two-dimensional (transthoracic) echocardiogram: initial echocardiographic test for patients with native valves and in whom perivalvular disease is not suspected
- Transesophageal echocardiogram: performed when results of two-dimensional echocardiogram are negative or inconclusive, in patients with prosthetic valves, and when perivalvular disease is suspected

DIAGNOSTIC DECISION

- Criteria for the diagnosis of endocarditis are often termed the 'Duke criteria'. They incorporate pathologic, clinical, microbiologic, and echocardiographic features
- Diagnosis is considered certain if the following pathologic criteria are met: micro-organisms demonstrated in a vegetation (valvular or embolic) or cardiac abscess or pathologic lesions confirmed by histology showing active endocarditis in a vegetation or cardiac abscess
- Diagnosis is considered certain if patient fulfils two major clinical criteria, one major and three minor clinical criteria, or five minor clinical criteria

Major criteria:

- Positive blood culture: defined as either (a) two separate cultures yielding micro-organisms that typically cause IE (viridans streptococci, *Streptococcus bovis*, HACEK organisms, community-acquired *Staphylococcus aureus*, or enterococci, in the absence of a primary focus of infection), or (b) micro-organisms consistent with IE from persistently positive cultures, i.e. at least two positive cultures of blood drawn more than 12h apart, or all three of three cultures, or a majority of four or more separate cultures, with the first and last drawn at least 1h apart
- Evidence of endocardial involvement: defined as either positive echocardiogram for IE or new valvular regurgitation (worsening or changing of a pre-existing murmur does not fulfil criterion). Positive echocardiogram for IE is defined as either (a) oscillating intracardiac mass on a valve or supporting structures, in the path of regurgitant jets, or on implanted material in the absence of alternative anatomic explanation, (b) abscess, (c) new partial dehiscence of a prosthetic valve

Minor criteria:

- Predisposing heart condition or intravenous drug use
- Temperature of 38°C or above
- Vascular phenomena: major arterial emboli, septic pulmonary infarcts, mycotic aneurysm, intracranial hemorrhage, conjunctival hemorrhages, and Janeway lesions

- Immunologic phenomena: glomerulonephritis, Osler's nodes, Roth's spots, and rheumatoid factor
- Microbiologic evidence: positive blood culture but less than major criteria as designated above or serologic evidence of active infection with an organism consistent with IE
- Echocardiographic findings that are consistent with IE but do not meet the major criteria designated above

CLINICAL PEARL(S)

- The Duke criteria are constantly being re-evaluated. Less specific features of inflammation or other organ involvement may be added to these criteria in the future
- Transesophageal echo is preferred to transthoracic due to higher sensitivity and specificity
- Positive blood cultures are key to the diagnosis; multiple blood cultures must be obtained over a 12–24h period prior to beginning antibiotic therapy (particularly in subacute cases)

THE TESTS

Body fluids

BLOOD CULTURES

Description

- Obtain 3–5 sets of venous blood cultures over 24h. Each set should include one aerobic and one nonaerobic culture flask
- If patient is acutely ill, four or more cultures may be taken over a 1h period, each with a separate venipuncture
- Inform laboratory that IE is a possible diagnosis and request incubation for 3 weeks; also notify laboratory if unusual bacteria or other pathogens are suspected
- Minimum inhibitory concentration (MIC) values should be determined once a pathogen has been identified

Advantages/Disadvantages

Advantages:

- Routine laboratory procedure
- Critical to diagnosis of IE
- With the exception of highly fastidious micro-organisms, reveals the etiologic agent in more than 95% of cases

Disadvantages:

- In a small number of instances, etiologic agent is culture negative
- If antibiotic treatment was started before blood was drawn, cultures are likely to yield negative results

Normal

No micro-organisms in blood.

Abnormal

Presence of infectious agent(s).

Cause of abnormal result

- Patient fulfils a major diagnostic criterion for IE when culture results are consistent with either of the two following categories: (a) two separate cultures yield micro-organisms that typically cause IE (viridans streptococci, *Streptococcus bovis*, HACEK organisms, community-acquired *Staphylococcus aureus*, or enterococci), in the absence of a primary focus of infection, or (b) micro-organisms consistent with IE are identified from persistently positive cultures: at least two positive cultures of blood drawn more than 12h apart, or all three of three cultures, or a majority of four or more separate cultures, with the first and last drawn at least 1h apart
- Patient fulfils a minor diagnostic criteria if the above criteria are not met but patient has one or more positive blood cultures

Drugs, disorders, and other factors that may alter results

- Recent antibiotic treatment is the most common reason for culture-negative IE. In hemodynamically stable patients with subacute presentation who have received antibiotics during the past 2 weeks, treatment should be delayed for several days so that the etiologic agent can be cultured and identified
- Length of culture may be a factor in the growth of fastidious organisms, such as the HACEK group. Laboratory should incubate cultures for 3 or more weeks before cultures are confirmed negative
- Pathogen may not grow in culture media: fungi, *Brucella* species, *Legionella* species, *Coxiella burnetii*, *Chlamydia*, and *Bartonella* species

RHEUMATOID FACTOR

Description

Venous blood.

Advantages/Disadvantages

- Advantage: routine, inexpensive test
- Disadvantage: results not definitive for IE

Normal

Dilution titer below 1:80.

Abnormal

Dilution titer above 1:80.

Cause of abnormal result

Patient considered positive for rheumatoid factor, a minor diagnostic criterion for infective endocarditis.

Drugs, disorders, and other factors that may alter results

A variety of other disorders may present with positive rheumatoid factor.

URINALYSIS

Description

Urine sample.

Advantages/Disadvantages

- Advantage: inexpensive, noninvasive, and routinely available
- Disadvantage: results not necessarily helpful in confirming diagnosis

Cause of abnormal result

Microscopic hematuria may occur in glomerulonephritis, a minor criterion for endocarditis. The presence of hematuria alone is being considered for addition to the Duke criteria.

Drugs, disorders, and other factors that may alter results

A variety of disorders may cause hematuria.

Imaging

TRANSTHORACIC ECHOCARDIOGRAPHY

Advantages/Disadvantages

Advantages:

- Not invasive
- Less expensive than transesophageal echocardiography

Disadvantages:
- Less sensitive than transesophageal echocardiography
- Possible false-positive results due to sterile vegetations or thickened valves, nodules, or calcifications

Abnormal

Diagnostic findings:
- Vegetations
- Abscesses of periannular tissue
- Dehiscence of a prosthetic valve

Abnormal findings that may be seen in infective endocarditis but not diagnostic of infective endocarditis if the above findings are absent:
- Valvular regurgitation that is more than trivial or mild
- Pericardial effusion
- Alterations in a valve, valve leaflet, or chordae tendineae

Cause of abnormal result

Abnormal results with any of the following characteristics provide a major diagnostic criterion for IE: (a) oscillating intracardiac mass on a valve or supporting structures, in the path of regurgitant jets, or on implanted material in the absence of alternative anatomic explanation, (b) perivalvular abscess, or (c) new partial dehiscence of a prosthetic valve.

Drugs, disorders, and other factors that may alter results
- Patient may have vegetations that are not associated with IE, as occurs in marantic endocarditis
- Rarely, small cardiac tumors such as a fibroelastoma can mimic a vegetation

TRANSESOPHAGEAL ECHOCARDIOGRAPHY (TEE)

Advantages/Disadvantages

Advantage:
- High sensitivity

Disadvantages:
- Invasive procedure
- More expensive than two-dimensional echocardiography
- Possible false-positive results due to sterile vegetations or thickened valves, nodules, or calcifications
- The risk of a serious adverse event is about 1/1000 studies and this includes performing TEE in critically ill patients. The risks are those of upper endoscopy and include injury (perforation) of the esophagus, inadvertent passage into the trachea with vocal cord injury, and respiratory distress in patients with marginal ventilatory status or excessive sedation

Normal

No abnormalities observed.

Abnormal

Diagnostic findings:
- Vegetations
- Abscesses of periannular tissue
- Dehiscence of a prosthetic valve

Abnormal findings that may be seen in infective endocarditis but not diagnostic of infective endocarditis if the above findings are absent:

- Valvular regurgitation that is more than trivial or mild
- Pericardial effusion
- Alterations in a valve, valve leaflet, or chordae tendineae

Cause of abnormal result

Abnormal results with any of the following characteristics provide a major diagnostic criterion for IE: (a) oscillating intracardiac mass on a valve or supporting structures, in the path of regurgitant jets, or on implanted material in the absence of alternative anatomic explanation, (b) perivalvular abscess, or (c) new partial dehiscence of a prosthetic valve.

Drugs, disorders, and other factors that may alter results

Marantic endocarditis may involve sterile vegetations evident at echocardiography.

TREATMENT

CONSIDER CONSULT

- Consider referral for cardiac surgical intervention for valvular incompetence
- Consider referral if there is persistent fever or congestive heart failure

IMMEDIATE ACTION

- Central nervous system involvement requires immediate imaging and referral
- Abrupt onset of heart failure requires transfer to an intensive care unit and immediate evaluation for urgent valve surgery

PATIENT AND CAREGIVER ISSUES

Forensic and legal issues

- Failure to provide timely diagnosis and treatment may provoke a malpractice suit
- Legal issues may also be raised by failure to inform patient of necessary prophylaxis for dental and medical procedures that may cause transient bacteremia

Impact on career, dependants, family, friends

Patients may be severely ill, with the possibility of death, and require prolonged care.

Patient or caregiver request

Is outpatient care a safe alternative to prolonged hospitalization? Patients deemed appropriate for partial outpatient care (those with uncomplicated endocarditis caused by penicillin-susceptible streptococci, as well as adequate compliance and at-home care) should understand the risks and benefits of this form of treatment.

Health-seeking behavior

Has patient taken antibiotics? This may cause negative blood culture results.

MANAGEMENT ISSUES

Goals

- Eradicate infectious agent
- Address complications
- Provide prolonged monitoring
- Educate about prophylaxis

Management in special circumstances

COEXISTING DISEASE

The severity of coexisting disease and the long-term outlook may influence the decision regarding cardiac surgery.

COEXISTING MEDICATION

Use of anticoagulant therapy in patients with infective endocarditis (IE) is controversial. Some physicians advise that for IE caused by *Staphylococcus aureus* anticoagulant therapy should be discontinued until the septic phase of disease has resolved. Others suggest replacing warfarin with heparin in patients with prosthetic valves, and discontinuing aspirin.

SPECIAL PATIENT GROUPS

- Mortality increased among the elderly. Patients may require intensive care
- Injection drug users have a high rate of recurrence; accordingly, heart valve replacement should be avoided if possible
- Children, the elderly, pregnant women, terminally ill and/or debilitated patients should be overseen by a specialist

PATIENT SATISFACTION/LIFESTYLE PRIORITIES

- Patients may be fearful for their survival. Provide assurance that IE is curable in most instances
- Some patients with native valves infected by highly penicillin-susceptible streptococci may prefer a 2-week course of treatment
- Patients may request outpatient therapy following initial hospitalization. Outpatient parenteral antimicrobial therapy is considered appropriate for selected patients with uncomplicated endocarditis caused by penicillin-susceptible streptococci. Such patients must display hemodynamic stability and have a safe home environment with caregivers who can monitor temperature, pulse rate, and blood pressure each day

SUMMARY OF THERAPEUTIC OPTIONS

Choices

Antibiotic therapy:

- Aqueous crystalline penicillin G sodium: first choice for patients with native valves and highly penicillin-susceptible viridans streptococci or *Streptococcus bovis*
- Aqueous crystalline penicillin G sodium with gentamicin sulfate: first choice for patients with native valves and relatively penicillin-resistant strains of viridans streptococci or *S. bovis*; first choice for infection by enterococci; third choice for patients with native valves and highly penicillin-susceptible viridans streptococci or *S. bovis*
- Ceftriaxone sodium: first choice for patients with infection by HACEK micro-organisms; second choice for patients with native valves infected by highly penicillin-susceptible viridans streptococci or *S. bovis*
- Vancomycin hydrochloride: first choice for patients with native valve infected by methicillin-resistant staphylococci; second choice for patients with native valves and relatively penicillin-resistant viridans streptococci or *S. bovis*; second choice for beta-lactam-allergic patients with native valves infected by methicillin-susceptible staphylococci; fourth choice for patients with native valves and highly penicillin-susceptible viridans streptococci or *S. bovis*
- Ampicillin sodium with gentamicin sulfate: second choice for patients infected by either enterococci or HACEK micro-organisms
- Vancomycin hydrochloride with gentamicin sulfate: third choice for patients infected by enterococci
- Nafcillin sodium or oxacillin sodium, with optional gentamicin: first choice for methicillin-susceptible staphylococci in patients not allergic to beta-lactams and with native valves (benefit of gentamicin in this combination is not established)
- Cefazolin or other first-generation cephalosporin with optional gentamicin: first choice for methicillin-susceptible staphylococci in beta-lactam-allergic patients with native valves (benefit of gentamicin in this combination is not established)
- Vancomycin hydrochloride with rifampin and gentamicin sulfate: first choice for patients with methicillin-resistant *Staphylococcus* infecting a prosthetic valve
- Nafcillin sodium or oxacillin sodium with rifampin and gentamicin sulfate: first choice for patients with methicillin-susceptible *Staphylococcus* infecting a prosthetic valve

Surgical therapy:

- Cardiac surgery: for valve dysfunction causing moderate to severe congestive heart failure, partially dehisced unstable prosthetic valve, persistent bacteremia despite appropriate antimicrobial therapy, pathogen for which no bactericidal therapy exists, fungal infection, relapse of prosthetic valve endocarditis after appropriate antimicrobial therapy, persistent unexplained fever in culture-negative prosthetic valve infection, prosthetic valve infection by *Staphylococcus aureus*
- Extracardiac surgery: for splenic abscess and mycotic aneurysms that hemorrhage or enlarge during antibiotic treatment
- Neurosurgical intervention may be needed with increased intracranial pressure from a large embolic stroke, an intracerebral abscess, or metastatic infection of a vertebral body causing spinal cord compression

Clinical pearl(s)

- Always obtain multiple blood cultures prior to treatment
- Confirm antibiotic susceptibility and MIC once organism identified
- Diagnosis may be confirmed by examination of an embolus

Never

Never initiate antimicrobial therapy before obtaining a series of blood cultures. For acutely ill patients, these may be taken over a 1h period.

FOLLOW UP

Patient should be monitored during therapy and for the following several months. Check for complications of microbial therapy, myocardial or metastatic abscess, emboli, worsening valvular incompetence, congestive heart failure, and relapse.

Plan for review

- Patient should be monitored intensively during therapy and followed for the next several months
- During therapy, patient should be checked for adverse drug reactions. Assess gentamicin blood levels, if appropriate. Renal function should be repeatedly evaluated if an aminoglycoside is used. Perform complete blood count at least weekly for patients receiving high-dose beta-lactam antibiotics or vancomycin
- Check patients daily during the first week of antibiotic treatment for myocardial or metastatic abscess, emboli, and relapse
- Check daily for signs of worsening valvular incompetence and/or heart failure
- If patient receives outpatient parenteral therapy after an initial hospitalization, caregiver should monitor temperature, pulse rate, and blood pressure each day. Most such patients should be seen by a physician at least once weekly

Information for patient or caregiver

Infective endocarditis is an infection of tissue within the heart, usually involving one of the heart's valves. Many people who develop this condition have a prosthetic heart valve or other heart abnormality, or are injection drug users. People with infective endocarditis are usually treated with intravenous antibiotics in a hospital. Some infections may damage a heart valve so severely that it must be surgically replaced. Infective endocarditis is a very serious condition with several potential complications including death. It is curable in most instances with appropriate therapy.

DRUGS AND OTHER THERAPIES: DETAILS

Drugs

PENICILLIN G

Aqueous crystalline penicillin G sodium.

Dose

- For adults with native valves and highly penicillin-susceptible viridans streptococci or *Streptococcus bovis* (MIC below or equal to 0.1mcg/mL): 15–20 millionU/day for 4 weeks
- Prevention of infective endocarditis in patients with congenital heart disease or rheumatic or other acquired valvular heart disease when undergoing dental procedures or surgical procedures of the upper respiratory tract (for patients unable to take oral antibiotics): administer 2 millionU (50,000U/kg for children) aqueous penicillin G, except penicillin G procaine suspension, intravenously or intramuscularly 30–60min before the procedure and one millionU (25,000U/kg for children) 6h later. Doses for children should not exceed recommendations for adults for a single dose or for a 24h period

Efficacy

Bactericidal.

Risks/Benefits

Risks:

- Serious and occasional fatal hypersensitivity (anaphylactoid) reactions have been reported in patients on penicillin therapy
- Use with caution in patients with a history of significant allergies and/or asthma
- In prolonged therapy with penicillin and particularly with high dosage schedules, periodic evaluation of the renal and hematopoietic systems is recommended
- In high doses (above 10 millionU), intravenous aqueous penicillin G sodium should be administered slowly because of the adverse effects of electrolyte imbalance from the sodium content of the penicillin
- Prolonged use of antibiotics may promote overgrowth of nonsusceptible organisms, including fungi
- Risk of severe and occasionally fatal anaphylaxis

Benefit:

- Preferred over ceftriaxone for most patients above age 65 years, and for those with impairment of the eighth nerve or renal function

Side-effects and adverse reactions

- Skin: rashes ranging from maculopapular eruptions to exfoliative dermatitis, urticaria
- CNS: serum sickness-like reactions including chills, fever, edema, neuropathy, and nephropathy are rarely observed adverse reactions and are usually associated with high intravenous dosage
- Musculoskeletal: arthralgia, prostration
- Hematologic: hemolytic anemia, leukopenia, thrombocytopenia

Interactions (other drugs)

Anticoagulants.

Contraindications

History of hypersensitivity to any penicillin.

Acceptability to patient

Good.

Follow up plan

Patient should be monitored intensively during therapy and followed for the next several months.

Patient and caregiver information

If outpatient parenteral treatment is given, patient should be informed of signs of hypersensitivity.

PENICILLIN G PLUS GENTAMICIN

Combination of aqueous crystalline penicillin G sodium with gentamicin sulfate.

Dose

For adults with native valves and highly penicillin-susceptible (MIC below or equal to 0.1mcg/mL) strains of viridans streptococci and *Streptococcus bovis* (this 2-week regimen is not recommended for patients with complications, such as extracardiac foci of infection or intracardiac abscesses. It is also not recommended for patients at high risk for adverse responses to gentamicin):

- Penicillin G: 12–18 millionU/day intravenously either continuously or in six equally divided doses for 2 weeks
- Gentamicin: 1mg/kg intramuscularly or intravenously every 8h for 2 weeks

For adults with native valve and relatively penicillin-resistant (MIC between 0.1 and 0.5mcg/mL) strains of viridans streptococci and *Streptococcus bovis*:

- Penicillin G: 18 millionU/day intravenously either continuously or in six equally divided doses for 4 weeks
- Gentamicin: 1mg/kg intramuscularly or intravenously every 8h for 2 weeks

Efficacy

Bactericidal.

Risks/Benefits

Risks

Penicillin G aqueous:

- Serious and occasional fatal hypersensitivity (anaphylactoid) reactions have been reported in patients on penicillin therapy
- Use with caution in patients with a history of significant allergies and/or asthma
- In prolonged therapy with penicillin and particularly with high dosage schedules, periodic evaluation of the renal and hematopoietic systems is recommended
- In high doses (above 10 millionU), intravenous aqueous penicillin G sodium should be administered slowly because of the adverse effects of electrolyte imbalance from the sodium content of the penicillin
- Prolonged use of antibiotics may promote overgrowth of nonsusceptible organisms, including fungi
- Risk of severe and occasionally fatal anaphylaxis

Gentamicin:

- Use caution in prolonged use (may lead to overgrowth of resistant organisms)
- Use caution in pregnancy and lactation, neonates, and the elderly
- Use caution in Parkinson's disease, renal disease, hypokalemia, and hearing deficit
- Potentially toxic
- Blood levels need monitoring for safety

Side-effects and adverse reactions

Penicillin G:

- Skin: rashes ranging from maculopapular eruptions to exfoliative dermatitis, urticaria
- CNS: serum sickness-like reactions including chills, fever, edema, neuropathy, and nephropathy are rarely observed adverse reactions and are usually associated with high intravenous dosage
- Musculoskeletal: arthralgia, prostration
- Hematologic: hemolytic anemia, leukopenia, thrombocytopenia

Gentamicin:

- Cardiovascular: changes in blood pressure, palpitations
- CNS: neurotoxicity, dizziness, confusion, convulsions
- EENT: irritation, tinnitus, deafness, ototoxicity, visual disturbances
- Gastrointestinal: altered liver function tests, anorexia, nausea, vomiting
- Genitourinary: nephrotoxicity
- Hematologic: blood cell disorders
- Respiratory: respiratory depression
- Skin: rash

Interactions (other drugs)

Penicillin:

- Anticoagulants

Gentamicin:
- Amphotericin B ▪ Antibiotics (penicillins, cephalosporins, polymyxins, vancomycin) ▪ Anticholinesterases (neostigmine, pyridostigmine) ▪ Cyclosporine ▪ Loop diuretics ▪ Neuromuscular blocking agents (atracurium, vecuronium) ▪ NSAIDs ▪ Platinum compounds (carboplatin, cisplatin) ▪ Succinylcholine

Contraindications

Penicillin:
- History of hypersensitivity to any penicillin

Gentamicin:
- Hypersensitivity to gentamicin or other aminoglycosides ▪ Myasthenia gravis ▪ Pre-existing deafness ▪ Renal impairment

Follow up plan

Patient should be monitored intensively during therapy and followed for the next several months. Monitor gentamicin levels in blood.

Patient and caregiver information

Patient should be alert to possible adverse drug reactions, particularly rash and ototoxicity.

CEFTRIAXONE

Ceftriaxone sodium.

Dose
- Adult patients with native valves infected by highly penicillin-susceptible (MIC below or equal to 0.1mcg/mL) viridans streptococci or *Streptococcus bovis*: 2g once daily intravenously or intramuscularly for 4 weeks
- Adult patients with infection by HACEK micro-organisms: 2g once daily intravenously or intramuscularly for 4 weeks

Efficacy

Bactericidal.

Risks/Benefits

Risks:
- Use caution in penicillin hypersensitivity and renal disease
- Risk of pseudomembranous colitis

Side-effects and adverse reactions
- CNS: headache, sleep disturbance, confusion, dizziness
- Gastrointestinal: anorexia, nausea, diarrhea, abdominal pain, bleeding, raised liver enzymes
- Genitourinary: nephrotoxicity
- Hematologic: bone marrow suppression
- Skin: rash

Interactions (other drugs)
- Aminoglycosides ▪ Chloramphenicol ▪ Oral anticoagulants ▪ Probenecid ▪ Vancomycin ▪ Polymyxin B

Contraindications

Infants aged less than 1 month.

Acceptability to patient
Good.

Follow up plan
Patients should be monitored during and for several months after therapy.

Patient and caregiver information
Patients should be warned that injections are painful.

VANCOMYCIN
Vancomycin hydrochloride.

Dose
- For adults with native valves and highly penicillin-susceptible viridans streptococci or *Streptococcus bovis* (MIC below or equal to 0.1mcg/mL): 30mg/kg/day intravenously in two equally divided doses, not to exceed 2g/day unless serum levels are monitored. Duration of treatment is 4 weeks
- For adults with native valves and relatively penicillin-resistant viridans streptococci or *Streptococcus bovis* (MIC between 0.1 and 0.5mcg/mL): 30mg/kg/day intravenously in two equally divided doses, not to exceed 2g/day unless serum levels are monitored. Duration of treatment is 4 weeks
- For beta-lactam-allergic adults with native valves infected by methicillin-susceptible staphylococci: 30mg/kg/day intravenously in two equally divided doses, not to exceed 2g/day unless serum levels are monitored. Duration of treatment is 4–6 weeks
- For adults with native valves, with or without allergy to beta-lactams, infected by methicillin-resistant staphylococci: 30mg/kg/day intravenously in two equally divided doses, not to exceed 2g/day unless serum levels are monitored. Duration of treatment is 4–6 weeks

Efficacy
Bactericidal.

Risks/Benefits
Risks:
- Use caution in renal disease and inflammatory bowel disease
- Use caution in neonates and the elderly

Benefits:
- Can be administered to patients allergic to beta-lactams
- The only treatment recommended for methicillin-resistant staphylococci

Side-effects and adverse reactions
- Gastrointestinal: nausea
- Hematologic: neutropenia, eosinophilia, leukopenia
- Cardiovascular: cardiac arrest, cardiovascular collapse, phlebitis
- Genitourinary: renal damage
- EENT: hearing disturbances, ototoxicity
- Skin: rashes, chills, fever, 'red man's syndrome'

Interactions (other drugs)
■ Aminoglycosides ■ Amphotericin B ■ Capreomycin ■ Cidofovir ■ Cisplatin ■ Cyclosporine ■ Ethacrynic acid ■ Indomethacin ■ Methotrexate ■ Neuromuscular blockers ■ Paromomycin ■ Pentamidine ■ Polymyxin B ■ Salicylates ■ Streptozocin ■ Surfactants

Contraindications

■ Hearing deficit ■ Cidofovir (vancomycin should be discontinued 7 days before cidofovir treatment) ■ Intramuscular administration

Follow up plan

Intensive monitoring is needed for possible adverse reactions: prolonged intravenous administration may cause thrombophlebitis, rash, fever, anemia, thrombocytopenia, and in rare instances ototoxic reactions. Should be infused over at least 1h due to risk of histamine-release (red neck syndrome).

Patient and caregiver information

Patients should understand potential risks and benefits of treatment.

AMPICILLIN PLUS GENTAMICIN

Ampicillin sodium with gentamicin sulfate.

Dose

For adults infected by enterococci:

- Ampicillin sodium: 12g/day intravenously either continuously or in six divided doses for 4–6 weeks
- Gentamicin sulfate: 1mg/kg intramuscularly or intravenously every 8h for 4–6 weeks

For adults infected by HACEK micro-organisms:

- Ampicillin sodium: 12g/day intravenously either continuously or in six divided doses for 4 weeks
- Gentamicin sulfate: 1mg/kg intramuscularly or intravenously every 8h for 4 weeks

Efficacy

Bactericidal.

Risks/Benefits

Risks

Gentamicin:

- Use caution in prolonged use (may lead to overgrowth of resistant organisms)
- Use caution in pregnancy and lactation, neonates, and the elderly
- Use caution in Parkinson's disease, renal disease, hypokalemia, and hearing deficit
- Potentially toxic
- Blood levels need monitoring for safety

Ampicillin:

- Use caution in renal disease and mononucleosis
- Use caution in neonates or the elderly
- Do not administer for prolonged or repeated treatment

Benefit: combination provides a synergistic effect.

Side-effects and adverse reactions

Ampicillin:

- CNS: seizures, hallucinations, coma, anxiety
- Gastrointestinal: nausea, diarrhea, vomiting, altered liver function tests, pseudomembranous colitis
- Genitourinary: urinary problems, renal damage, candidiasis, vaginitis
- Hematologic: bleeding disorders, bone marrow depression
- Hypersensitivity reactions

Gentamicin:

- Cardiovascular system: changes in blood pressure, palpitations
- CNS: neurotoxicity, dizziness, confusion, convulsions
- EENT: irritation, tinnitus, deafness, ototoxicity, visual disturbances
- Gastrointestinal: altered liver function tests, anorexia, nausea, vomiting
- Genitourinary: nephrotoxicity
- Hematologic: blood cell disorders
- Respiratory: respiratory depression
- Skin: rash

Interactions (other drugs)

Gentamicin:

▪ Amphotericin B ▪ Antibiotics (penicillins, cephalosporins, polymyxins, vancomycin) ▪ Anticholinesterases (neostigmine, pyridostigmine) ▪ Cyclosporine ▪ Loop diuretics ▪ Neuromuscular blocking agents (atracurium, vecuronium) ▪ NSAIDs ▪ Platinum compounds (carboplatin, cisplatin) ▪ Succinylcholine

Ampicillin:

▪ Allopurinol (may increase incidence of rash) ▪ Atenolol ▪ Chloramphenicol (inhibits effect of ampicillin) ▪ Macrolide and tetracycline antibiotics (inhibit effect of ampicillin) ▪ Methotrexate ▪ Oral contraceptives ▪ Phenindione ▪ Probenecid (decreases renal tubular secretion of ampicillin) ▪ Warfarin

Contraindications

Gentamicin:

▪ Hypersensitivity to gentamicin or other aminoglycosides ▪ Myasthenia gravis ▪ Pre-existing deafness ▪ Renal impairment

Ampicillin:

▪ Hypersensitivity to penicillins

Follow up plan

Monitoring required throughout therapy, particularly for nephrotoxicity or ototoxicity associated with gentamicin, and to verify effectiveness of therapy.

Patient and caregiver information

Patients should be informed of the risks and benefits of treatment.

VANCOMYCIN PLUS GENTAMICIN

Vancomycin hydrochloride with gentamicin sulfate.

Dose

For adult patients with IE caused by enterococci:

- Vancomycin hydrochloride: 3mg/kg/day intravenously in two equally divided doses, not to exceed 2g every 2h unless serum levels are monitored, for 4–6 weeks
- Gentamicin sulfate: 1mg/kg intramuscularly or intravenously every 8h for 4–6 weeks

Efficacy

Bactericidal synergy.

Risks/Benefits

Risks:

Gentamicin:

- Use caution in prolonged use (may lead to overgrowth of resistant organisms)
- Use caution in pregnancy and lactation, neonates, and the elderly
- Use caution in Parkinson's disease, renal disease, hypokalemia, and hearing deficit
- Potentially toxic
- Blood levels need monitoring for safety

Vancomycin:

- Use caution in renal disease and inflammatory bowel disease
- Use caution in neonates and the elderly

Benefit: vancomycin is recommended for patients allergic to beta-lactams.

Side-effects and adverse reactions

Vancomycin:

- Cardiovascular system: cardiac arrest, cardiovascular collapse, phlebitis
- EENT: hearing disturbances, ototoxicity
- Gastrointestinal: nausea
- Genitourinary: renal damage
- Hematologic: neutropenia, eosinophilia, leukopenia
- Skin: rashes, chills, fever, 'red man's syndrome'

Gentamicin:

- Cardiovascular system: changes in blood pressure, palpitations
- CNS: neurotoxicity, dizziness, confusion, convulsions
- EENT: irritation, tinnitus, deafness, ototoxicity, visual disturbances
- Gastrointestinal: altered liver function tests, anorexia, nausea, vomiting
- Genitourinary: nephrotoxicity
- Hematologic: blood cell disorders
- Respiratory: respiratory depression
- Skin: rash

Interactions (other drugs)

Vancomycin:

■ Aminoglycosides ■ Amphotericin B ■ Capreomycin ■ Cidofovir ■ Cisplatin ■ Cyclosporine ■ Ethacrynic acid ■ Indomethacin ■ Methotrexate ■ Neuromuscular blockers ■ Paromomycin ■ Pentamidine ■ Polymyxin B ■ Salicylates ■ Streptozocin ■ Surfactants

Gentamicin:

■ Amphotericin B ■ Antibiotics (penicillins, cephalosporins, polymyxins, vancomycin) ■ Anticholinesterases (neostigmine, pyridostigmine) ■ Cyclosporine ■ Loop diuretics ■ Neuromuscular blocking agents (atracurium, vecuronium) ■ NSAIDs ■ Platinum compounds (carboplatin, cisplatin) ■ Succinylcholine

Contraindications

Vancomycin:

■ Hearing deficit ■ Cidofovir (vancomycin should be discontinued 7 days before cidofovir treatment) ■ Intramuscular administration

Gentamicin:
- **Hypersensitivity to gentamicin or other aminoglycosides** - **Myasthenia gravis**
- **Pre-existing deafness** - **Renal impairment**

Patient and caregiver information
Patient should understand risks and benefits of treatment.

NAFCILLIN OR OXACILLIN WITH OPTIONAL GENTAMICIN
Dose
For adults not allergic to beta-lactams, with native valves infected by methicillin-susceptible staphylococci:
- Nafcillin sodium: 500mg every 4h intravenously (or 1g every 4h for severe infection), or oxacillin sodium: 2g intravenously every 4h for 4–6 weeks

Optional addition:
- Gentamicin sulfate: 1mg/kg intramuscularly every 8h for 3–5 days

Efficacy
Bactericidal.

Risks/Benefits
Risks
Gentamicin:
- Use caution in prolonged use (may lead to overgrowth of resistant organisms)
- Use caution in pregnancy and lactation, neonates, and the elderly
- Use caution in Parkinson's disease, renal disease, hypokalemia, and hearing deficit
- Potentially toxic
- Blood levels need monitoring for safety

Nafcillin:
- Use caution in imipenem and cephalosporin hypersensitivity, hepatic disease, and history of gastrointestinal disease
- Use caution in breast-feeding

Oxacillin:
- Use caution with renal impairment, known history of hypersensitivity to any penicillin, and significant allergies and/or asthma
- Avoid prolonged or repeated treatment
- Safety and efficacy in neonates not established
- Risk of fatal anaphylactic reaction
- With intravenous administration, particularly in elderly patients, care should be taken because of the possibility of thrombophlebitis

Benefit: Addition of gentamicin is not proven to improve cure rates but thought to hasten clearing of bacteremia.

Side-effects and adverse reactions
Gentamicin:
- Cardiovascular: changes in blood pressure, palpitations
- CNS: neurotoxicity, dizziness, confusion, convulsions
- EENT: irritation, tinnitus, deafness, ototoxicity, visual disturbances
- Gastrointestinal: altered liver function tests, anorexia, nausea, vomiting
- Genitourinary: nephrotoxicity

- Hematologic: blood cell disorders
- Respiratory: respiratory depression
- Skin: rash

Nafcillin:
- CNS: seizures
- Gastrointestinal: nausea, vomiting, diarrhea, elevated hepatic enzymes, pseudomembranous colitis
- Genitourinary: interstitial nephritis, renal tubular necrosis, nephrotic syndrome
- Hematologic: neutropenia, thrombocytopenia, leukopenia
- Skin: rash, maculopapular rash, urticaria, Stevens–Johnson syndrome, purpura, vasculitis, toxic epidermal necrosis, exfoliative dermatitis, injection site reaction, phlebitis

Oxacillin:
- Cardiovascular system: phlebitis, thrombophlebitis
- CNS: fever, headache, chills
- Gastrointestinal: increased serum aspartate aminotransferase, increased serum alanine aminotransferase
- Genitourinary: hemorrhagic cystitis, interstitial nephritis, nephropathy
- Hematologic: thrombocytopenia, bone marrow suppression, eosinophilia
- Musculoskeletal: myalgia
- Skin: pruritus, rash, pain at injection site
- Other: serum sickness-like reactions

Interactions (other drugs)
Gentamicin:
▪ Amphotericin B ▪ Antibiotics (penicillins, cephalosporins, polymyxins, vancomycin) ▪ Anticholinesterases (neostigmine, pyridostigmine) ▪ Cyclosporine ▪ Loop diuretics ▪ Neuromuscular blocking agents (atracurium, vecuronium) ▪ NSAIDs ▪ Platinum compounds (carboplatin, cisplatin) ▪ Succinylcholine

Nafcillin:
▪ Aminoglycosides ▪ Probenecid ▪ Rifampin ▪ Warfarin

Oxacillin:
▪ Tetracycline (may antagonize the effect of oxacillin)

Contraindications
Gentamicin:
▪ Hypersensitivity to gentamicin or other aminoglycosides ▪ Myasthenia gravis ▪ Pre-existing deafness ▪ Renal impairment

Nafcillin:
▪ Hypersensitivity to nafcillin

Oxacillin:
▪ Hypersensitivity to any penicillin ▪ Pregnancy and breast-feeding

Follow up plan
Intensive monitoring is necessary throughout treatment.

Patient and caregiver information
Patients should understand risks and benefits of therapy.

CEFAZOLIN OR OTHER FIRST-GENERATION CEPHALOSPORIN WITH OPTIONAL GENTAMICIN

Dose

For adults allergic to beta-lactams, with native valves infected by staphylococci:

- Cefazolin: 1.0–1.5g every 6h intravenously for infective endocarditis
- Gentamicin (optional): the recommended dosage of gentamicin sulfate injectable for patients with serious infections and normal renal function is 3mg/kg/day, administered in three equal doses every 8h

Efficacy

Bactericidal.

Risks/Benefits

Risks:

(Cefazolin)

- Use caution in renal disease and penicillin hypersensitivity

(Gentamicin)

- Use caution in prolonged use (may lead to overgrowth of resistant organisms)
- Use caution in pregnancy and lactation, neonates, and the elderly
- Use caution in Parkinson's disease, renal disease, hypokalemia, and hearing deficit
- Potentially toxic
- Blood levels need monitoring for safety

Benefits:

- First-generation cephalosporins can be used by patients with a penicillin allergy that does not induce urticaria or anaphylaxis
- Short initial treatment with gentamicin may speed eradication of pathogen from vegetations and blood

Side-effects and adverse reactions

Cefazolin:

- CNS: headache, fever, dizziness
- Gastrointestinal: nausea, vomiting, diarrhea, abdominal pain, pseudomembranous colitis, anorexia
- Genitourinary: renal toxicity, proteinuria
- Hematologic: blood cell disorders, bone marrow suppression
- Respiratory: dyspnea
- Skin: rashes, pruritus, urticaria, Stevens–Johnson syndrome

Gentamicin:

- Cardiovascular system: changes in blood pressure, palpitations
- CNS: neurotoxicity, dizziness, confusion, convulsions
- EENT: irritation, tinnitus, deafness, ototoxicity, visual disturbances
- Gastrointestinal: altered liver function tests, anorexia, nausea, vomiting
- Genitourinary: nephrotoxicity
- Hematologic: blood cell disorders
- Respiratory: respiratory depression
- Skin: rash

Interactions (other drugs)

Cefazolin:

- Aminoglycosides - Aztreonam - Carbapenems - Chloramphenicol - Loop diuretics - Macrolides - Penicillins - Polymyxin B - Probenecid - Tetracyclines - Vancomycin

Gentamicin:

- Amphotericin B ■ Antibiotics (penicillins, cephalosporins, polymyxins, vancomycin) ■ Anticholinesterases (neostigmine, pyridostigmine) ■ Cyclosporine ■ Loop diuretics ■ Neuromuscular blocking agents (atracurium, vecuronium) ■ NSAIDs ■ Platinum compounds (carboplatin, cisplatin) ■ Succinylcholine

Contraindications

Cefazolin:

- Infants less than 1 month old ■ Breast-feeding ■ Colitis ■ Gastrointestinal disease ■ Intramuscular injections

Gentamicin:

- Hypersensitivity to gentamicin or other aminoglycosides ■ Myasthenia gravis ■ Pre-existing deafness ■ Renal impairment

Follow up plan

Intensive monitoring is required throughout treatment.

Patient and caregiver information

Patients should understand risks and benefits of treatment.

VANCOMYCIN WITH RIFAMPIN AND GENTAMICIN

Dose

For adults with prosthetic valve infected by methicillin-resistant staphylococci:

- Vancomycin hydrochloride 30mg/kg/day intravenously or in two or four equal doses, not to exceed 2g/day unless serum levels are monitored, for at least 6 weeks
- Rifampin 300mg orally every 8h for at least 6 weeks
- Gentamicin sulfate 1.0mg/kg intramuscularly or intravenously every 8h for 2 weeks

Efficacy

Bactericidal: cure is more likely if surgical intervention is combined with therapy.

Risks/Benefits

Risks

Gentamicin:

- Use caution in prolonged use (may lead to overgrowth of resistant organisms)
- Use caution in pregnancy and lactation, neonates, and the elderly
- Use caution in Parkinson's disease, renal disease, hypokalemia, and hearing deficit
- Potentially toxic
- Blood levels need monitoring for safety

Vancomycin:

- Use caution in renal disease and inflammatory bowel disease
- Use caution in neonates and the elderly

Rifampin:

- Rifampin resistance coupled with resistance to isoniazid and other antituberculosis agents is common in many multidrug resistant isolates in the US
- Use caution in pregnancy, hepatic impairment, renal impairment

Benefits

Rifampin:

- Rifampin has antistaphylococcal activity for infections involving foreign bodies; its use in combination with two antimicrobials deters emergence of rifampin-resistant staphylococci
- Suitable for use in children

Side-effects and adverse reactions

Vancomycin:

- Cardiovascular: cardiac arrest, cardiovascular collapse, phlebitis
- EENT: hearing disturbances, ototoxicity
- Gastrointestinal: nausea
- Genitourinary: renal damage
- Hematologic: neutropenia, eosinophilia, leukopenia
- Skin: rashes, chills, fever, 'red man's syndrome'

Gentamicin:

- Cardiovascular: changes in blood pressure, palpitations
- CNS: neurotoxicity, dizziness, confusion, convulsions
- EENT: irritation, tinnitus, deafness, ototoxicity, visual disturbances
- Gastrointestinal: altered liver function tests, anorexia, nausea, vomiting
- Genitourinary: nephrotoxicity
- Hematologic: blood cell disorders
- Respiratory: respiratory depression
- Skin: rash

Rifampin:

- CNT: fever, headache, dizziness, behavioral changes, confusion
- Gastrointestinal: nausea, vomiting, diarrhea
- Genitourinary: acute renal failure, nephritis, hematuria, orange discoloration of urine and secretions
- Hematologic: blood cell disorders
- Respiratory: shortness of breath, collapse, and shock
- Skin: rashes, urticaria, pemphigoid reaction

Interactions (other drugs)

Vancomycin:

■ Aminoglycosides ■ Amphotericin B ■ Capreomycin ■ Cidofovir ■ Cisplatin ■ Cyclosporine ■ Ethacrynic acid ■ Indomethacin ■ Methotrexate ■ Neuromuscular blockers ■ Paromomycin ■ Pentamidine ■ Polymyxin B ■ Salicylates ■ Streptozocin ■ Surfactants

Gentamicin:

■ Amphotericin B ■ Anticholinesterases (neostigmine, pyridostigmine) ■ Antibiotics (penicillins, cephalosporins, polymyxins, vancomycin) ■ Anticholinesterases (neostigmine, pyridostigmine) ■ Cyclosporine ■ Loop diuretics ■ Neuromuscular blocking agents (atracurium, vecuronium) ■ NSAIDs ■ Platinum compounds (carboplatin, cisplatin) ■ Succinylcholine

Rifampin:

■ Acetaminophen ■ Aminosalicylic acid ■ Anticoagulants ■ Antimalarials ■ Azole antifungals ■ Beta-blockers ■ Calcium channel blockers ■ Chloramphenicol ■ Clofibrate ■ Central nervous system depressants ■ Corticosteroids ■ Dapsone ■ Disopyramide ■ Hypoglycemic agents ■ Isoniazid ■ Oral contraceptives ■ Phenytoin ■ Protease inhibitors ■ Theophyllines ■ Thyroid hormone ■ Tricyclic antidepressants ■ Zidovudine

Contraindications

Vancomycin:

- Hearing deficit
- Cidofovir (vancomycin should be discontinued 7 days before cidofovir treatment)
- Intramuscular administration

Gentamicin:

- Hypersensitivity to gentamicin or other aminoglycosides
- Myasthenia gravis
- Pre-existing deafness
- Renal impairment

Rifampin:

- Hypersensitivity to rifamycins
- Rifampin should not be used if drug susceptibility tests show a high degree of resistance

Follow up plan

Intensive monitoring throughout therapy is necessary.

Patient and caregiver information

Patients should understand the risks and benefits of treatment and the reasons for extremely prolonged therapy.

NAFCILLIN OR OXACILLIN WITH RIFAMPIN AND GENTAMICIN

Dose

For adults with a prosthetic valve infected by methicillin-susceptible staphylococci:

- Nafcillin sodium 2g intravenously every 4h, for at least 6 weeks, or oxacillin sodium 2g intravenously every 4h, for at least 6 weeks
- Rifampin 300mg orally every 8h, for at least 6 weeks
- Gentamicin sulfate 1.0mg/kg intramuscularly or intravenously every 8h, for 2 weeks

Efficacy

Bactericidal: cure is more likely if surgical intervention is combined with therapy.

Risks/Benefits

Risks

Gentamicin:

- Use caution in prolonged use (may lead to overgrowth of resistant organisms)
- Use caution in pregnancy and lactation, neonates, and the elderly
- Use caution in Parkinson's disease, renal disease, hypokalemia, and hearing deficit
- Potentially toxic
- Blood levels need monitoring for safety

Nafcillin:

- Use caution in imipenem and cephalosporin hypersensitivity, hepatic disease, and history of gastrointestinal disease
- Use caution in breast-feeding

Oxacillin:

- Use caution with renal impairment, known history of hypersensitivity to any penicillin, and significant allergies and/or asthma
- Avoid prolonged or repeated treatment
- Safety and efficacy in neonates not established
- Risk of fatal anaphylactic reaction
- With intravenous administration, particularly in elderly patients, care should be taken because of the possibility of thrombophlebitis

Rifampin:

- Rifampin resistance coupled with resistance to isoniazid and other antituberculosis agents is common in many multidrug-resistant isolates in the US
- Use caution in pregnancy, hepatic and renal impairment

Side-effects and adverse reactions

Gentamicin:

- Cardiovascular: changes in blood pressure, palpitations
- CNS: neurotoxicity, dizziness, confusion, convulsions
- EENT: irritation, tinnitus, deafness, ototoxicity, visual disturbances
- Gastrointestinal: altered liver function tests, anorexia, nausea, vomiting
- Genitourinary: nephrotoxicity
- Hematologic: blood cell disorders
- Respiratory: respiratory depression
- Skin: rash

Nafcillin:

- CNS: seizures
- Gastrointestinal: nausea, vomiting, diarrhea, elevated hepatic enzymes, pseudomembranous colitis
- Genitourinary: interstitial nephritis, renal tubular necrosis, nephrotic syndrome
- Hematologic: neutropenia, thrombocytopenia, leukopenia
- Skin: rash, maculopapular rash, urticaria, Stevens–Johnson syndrome, purpura, vasculitis, toxic epidermal necrosis, exfoliative dermatitis, injection site reaction, phlebitis

Oxacillin:

- Cardiovascular: phlebitis, thrombophlebitis
- CNS: fever, headache, chills
- Gastrointestinal: increased serum aspartate aminotransferase, increased serum alanine aminotransferase
- Genitourinary: hemorrhagic cystitis, interstitial nephritis, nephropathy
- Hematologic: thrombocytopenia, bone marrow suppression, eosinophilia
- Musculoskeletal: myalgia
- Skin: pruritus, rash, pain at injection site
- Other: serum sickness-like reactions

Rifampin:

- CNS: fever, headache, dizziness, behavioral changes, confusion
- Gastrointestinal: nausea, vomiting, diarrhea
- Genitourinary: acute renal failure, nephritis, hematuria, orange discoloration of urine and secretions
- Hematologic: blood cell disorders
- Respiratory: shortness of breath, collapse, and shock
- Skin: rashes, urticaria, pemphigoid reaction

Interactions (other drugs)

Gentamicin:

- Amphotericin B ■ Anticholinesterases (neostigmine, pyridostigmine)
- Antibiotics (penicillins, cephalosporins, polymyxins, vancomycin)
- Anticholinesterases (neostigmine, pyridostigmine) ■ Cyclosporine ■ Loop diuretics
- Neuromuscular blocking agents (atracurium, vecuronium) ■ NSAIDs
- Platinum compounds (carboplatin, cisplatin) ■ Succinylcholine

Nafcillin:
- Aminoglycosides ▪ Probenecid ▪ Rifampin ▪ Warfarin

Oxacillin:
- Tetracycline (may antagonize the effect of oxacillin)

Rifampin:
- Acetaminophen ▪ Aminosalicylic acid ▪ Anticoagulants ▪ Antimalarials ▪ Azole antifungals ▪ Beta-blockers ▪ Calcium channel blockers ▪ Chloramphenicol ▪ Clofibrate ▪ Central nervous system depressants ▪ Corticosteroids ▪ Dapsone ▪ Disopyramide ▪ Hypoglycemic agents ▪ Isoniazid ▪ Oral contraceptives ▪ Phenytoin ▪ Protease inhibitors ▪ Theophyllines ▪ Thyroid hormone ▪ Tricyclic antidepressants ▪ Zidovudine

Contraindications

Gentamicin:
- Hypersensitivity to gentamicin or other aminoglycosides ▪ Myasthenia gravis ▪ Pre-existing deafness ▪ Renal impairment

Nafcillin:
- Hypersensitivity to nafcillin

Oxacillin:
- Hypersensitivity to any penicillin ▪ Pregnancy and breast-feeding

Rifampin:
- Hypersensitivity to rifamycins ▪ Rifampin should not be used if drug susceptibility tests show a high degree of resistance

Acceptability to patient

Patient may need support adjusting to the need for extremely prolonged therapy.

Patient and caregiver information

Patients should understand the need for prolonged therapy.

Surgical therapy

CARDIAC SURGERY

Performed to correct the following: valve dysfunction causing moderate-to-severe congestive heart failure, partially dehisced unstable prosthetic valve, persistent bacteremia despite appropriate antimicrobial therapy, pathogen for which no bactericidal therapy exists, fungal infection, relapse of prosthetic valve endocarditis after appropriate antimicrobial therapy, persistent unexplained fever in culture-negative prosthetic valve infection, prosthetic valve infection by *Staphylococcus aureus*.

Efficacy
- May sustain heart function
- The valvular incompetence can be corrected in the majority of cases. Large perivalvular abscesses may preclude an adequate repair

Risks/Benefits

Risk: mortality from surgery; however, surgery may be life-saving.

Acceptability to patient
Patients who are generally severely ill may be fearful of death from surgery.

Follow up plan
Monitoring in an intensive care unit is needed.

Patient and caregiver information
Patients should understand the risks and benefits of surgery.

EXTRACARDIAC SURGERY
May be necessary for splenic abscess and mycotic aneurysms, including cranial aneurysms, that rupture or enlarge during or after antimicrobial therapy.

Efficacy
May prevent death from complications of IE.

Risks/Benefits
Risk: death from surgery, although surgery may be necessary to prolong life.

Acceptability to patient
Patient may be extremely ill.

Follow up plan
Intensive monitoring needed, possibly in an intensive care unit.

Patient and caregiver information
Patients should understand risks and benefits of procedure.

LIFESTYLE

For appropriate patients, discontinuation of injection drug use.

RISKS/BENEFITS
Injection drug use presents a significant threat for initial and recurrent IE.

ACCEPTABILITY TO PATIENT
Compliance is often extremely difficult.

PATIENT AND CAREGIVER INFORMATION
Patient should understand the dangers of injection drug use and the availability of resources for ending this behavior.

OUTCOMES

EFFICACY OF THERAPIES

- About half of patients become afebrile within 3 days of initiation of antibiotic therapy, and nearly 90% are expected to defervesce after 2 weeks of therapy
- Fever is likely to be prolonged in patients with infective endocarditis (IE) due to *Staphylococcus aureus*, Gram-negative bacilli, and culture-negative pathogens

Review period

Frequent monitoring is needed throughout antibiotic therapy, which may exceed 6 weeks, and for the following months.

PROGNOSIS

- For native valve IE, mortality rates range from 16 to 27%. Increased risk of death is associated with advanced age, underlying diseases, infection of aortic valve, development of congestive heart failure or renal failure, and CNS complications
- For prosthetic valve IE, the overall mortality rates are 33–45% with a higher mortality in patients with mechanical valves and somewhat lower mortality in patients with tissue valves; these are decreasing over time as treatment improves

Clinical pearl(s)

- Systemic emboli occur in 22–55% of cases with up to 65% of these involving the CNS. Most occur within the first 2–4 weeks of therapy, with a marked decline once successful antibiotic therapy is initiated
- Large vegetations (>1cm) seen on left-sided valves are the most likely to embolize, but *Staphylococcus aureus* or fungal infection is associated with a high rate of embolism regardless of vegetation size. When large vegetations are seen on the anterior mitral valve leaflet, prophylactic surgery should be considered
- Any conduction abnormality on ECG should be considered possible evidence of a perivalvular abscess and should be evaluated promptly

Therapeutic failure

Only failure to sterilize the area(s) of infection should be considered a therapeutic failure.

Recurrence

Patients who have recovered from IE are at an increased risk for this disorder in the future. Referral to a specialist is appropriate.

Deterioration

Rapid referral to a specialist; possible surgery or intensive care.

Terminal illness

- Patient should receive intensive care with appropriate referrals and possible surgery
- Surgery may be delayed (and sometimes withheld) if patient has developed a serious complication, such as severe embolic cerebral damage, which makes recovery unlikely

COMPLICATIONS

- Congestive heart failure secondary to valvular incompetence
- Arterial embolization: most commonly affecting coronary arteries, kidneys, brain, and spleen
- Mycotic aneurysms in abdominal aorta and splenic, coronary, and pulmonary arteries
- Perivalvular abscess

CONSIDER CONSULT

- Refer for the following: neurologic complications, arterial embolic event, cerebral or peripheral mycotic aneurysm, apparent culture-negative IE, IE caused by an unusual organism or an unusually resistant organism (such as *Enterococcus*), left-sided IE caused by *Staphylococcus aureus*

PREVENTION

RISK FACTORS
Injection drug use greatly increases risk of infective endocarditis (IE).

MODIFY RISK FACTORS
Lifestyle and wellness
ALCOHOL AND DRUGS

Injection drug use greatly increases risk of IE.

SCREENING
Screening is inappropriate. Both acute and subacute disease manifest rapidly, even though the symptoms of subacute disease may be comparatively subtle.

PREVENT RECURRENCE
History of IE is itself a risk factor for development of this disorder. Patients should use antimicrobial prophylaxis prior to dental and medical procedures with the potential to cause temporary bacteremia. Some evidence suggests that improved gum care to prevent gingivitis may have a slight deterrent effect.

RESOURCES

ASSOCIATIONS

American College of Cardiology
Heart House
9111 Old Georgetown Rd
Bethesda, MD 20814-1699
Tel: (800) 253-4636
Fax: (301) 897-9745
www.acc.org

KEY REFERENCES

- Karchmer AW. Infective endocarditis. In: Braunwald E, Zipes DP, Libby P, eds. Heart disease: a textbook of cardiovascular medicine, 6th edn. Philadelphia: WB Saunders, 2001
- Bayer AS, et al. AHA Scientific Statement. Diagnosis and management of infective endocarditis and its complications. Circulation 1998;98:2936–48
- Ad Hoc Writing Group of the Committee on Rheumatic Fever, Endocarditis, and Kawasaki Disease, American Heart Association. Diagnosis and management of infective endocarditis and its complications. Available at: http://www.americanheart.org
- Wilson WR, Karchmer AW, Dajani AS, et al. Antibiotic treatment of adults with infective endocarditis due to streptococci, enterococci, staphylococci, and HACEK micro-organisms 1995. Available at: http://www.americanheart.org/
- Karchmer AW. Approach to the patient with infective endocarditis. In: Goldman L, Braunwald E, eds. Primary cardiology. Philadelphia: WB Saunders, 1998
- Cunha BA, Johnson DH, Klein NC. Infective endocarditis. In: Noble J, Greene HL II, Levinson W, et al, eds. Textbook of primary care medicine, 3rd edn. St. Louis: Mosby, 2001
- Dunmire SM. Infective endocarditis and acquired valvular heart disease. In: Rosen P, Barkin R, Danzl DF, et al, eds. Emergency medicine: concepts and clinical practice, 4th edn. St. Louis: Mosby, 1998
- Giessel BE, Koenig CJ, Blake RL Jr. Management of bacterial endocarditis. Am Fam Physician 2000;61:1725–32, 1739
- Rehm SJ. Outpatient intravenous antibiotic therapy for endocarditis. Infect Dis Clin North Am 1998;12:880–901
- Harris GD, Steimle J. Compiling the identifying features of bacterial endocarditis. Postgrad Med 2000;107. Available at http://www.postgradmed.com
- Salem DN, Hartnett Daudelin D, Levine HJ, et al. Antithrombotic therapy in valvular heart disease. Chest 2001;119 (1 Suppl):207S–219S
- Strom BL, Abrutyn E, Berlin JA, et al. Risk factors for infective endocarditis: oral hygiene and nondental exposures. Circulation 2000;102:2842–8
- Lederman MM, Sprague L, Wallis RS, Ellner JJ. Duration of fever during treatment of infective endocarditis. Medicine 1992;71:52–7

FAQS

Question 1

If I suspect that my patient has endocarditis and they are on warfarin for a prosthetic valve, what should I do with the warfarin?

ANSWER 1

Unless cerebral emboli have occurred, they should be maintained on anticoagulation with heparin and the warfarin should be discontinued.

Question 2

What is the chance my patient will have a mycotic aneurysm?

ANSWER 2

Infections of the vascular wall are uncommon, but when they occur they most often affect the cerebral circulation. The incidence of intracerebral mycotic aneurysms is around 5%. Unfortunately the mortality rate in such cases is 60%, rising to 80% if rupture occurs.

Question 3

My patient is a drug addict and presented with pulmonary infiltrates. How are they best managed?

ANSWER 3

These patients often have *Pseudomonas* infection of the tricuspid valve, with emboli to the lungs. Careful evaluation of all valves is needed. If the left-sided valves are involved, surgery will be required for a cure.

Question 4

I am confident that my patient has endocarditis, but the cultures have been negative. What should I do?

ANSWER 4

If the patient is not toxic, antibiotics should be withheld for up to 4 days, and repeat cultures obtained. Antibiotic binding resins may be used in these samples. HACEK organisms may be difficult to isolate and your laboratory should take special steps to look for these organisms. *Bartonella* species and *Abiotrophia* species also require special culture techniques. Serology for *Brucella*, *Bartonella*, *Chlamydia*, or *Coxiella burnetii*, polymerase chain reactions, and special staining techniques may also be useful in obtaining a diagnosis. Be sure that your laboratory continues to incubate the cultures for 3–4 weeks.

Question 5

My patient is recovering from endocarditis. Do they need antibiotics for future procedures?

ANSWER 5

Patients once treated for endocarditis are at risk for recurrent infections. They should all receive appropriate antibiotic prophylaxis.

CONTRIBUTORS

Joseph E Scherger, MD, MPH
John McB Hodgson, MD, FACC, FSCAI
Robert C Bahler, MD

CONGESTIVE HEART FAILURE

SUMMARY INFORMATION

DESCRIPTION

- Syndrome in which the heart cannot pump enough oxygenated blood to meet the metabolic needs of the tissues or can do so only from an elevated filling pressure
- Congestive heart failure may be left-sided, in which pulmonary edema is a predominant symptom, or right-sided, often with hepatomegaly and systemic edema. In many instances, both sides of the heart are involved
- Congestive heart failure may also be characterized as systolic and/or diastolic. In systolic heart failure, the left ventricular ejection fraction is reduced. In diastolic heart failure, the left ventricle systolic function is preserved but the altered ventricle compliance results in a high filling pressure. This distinction should be made during the diagnostic evaluation because the two conditions are treated with different agents

URGENT ACTION

Severe heart failure or heart failure that has suddenly developed or suddenly worsened is a potential emergency that requires hospital admission.

KEY! DON'T MISS!

- The two most helpful signs noted during the examination are orthopnea and either an elevated jugular venous pulse or a positive hepatojugular reflux. These signs have a high diagnostic accuracy
- When the symptom of heart failure is predominantly fatigue, the condition may be overlooked

BACKGROUND

ICD9 CODE
428.0 Congestive heart failure

SYNONYMS
- Heart failure
- Cardiac failure
- CHF

CARDINAL FEATURES
- Left ventricular failure is characterized by fatigue, dyspnea, weakness, cough, cardiac enlargement, pulmonary rales, a positive hepatojugular reflux, and an S3 or S4 gallop rhythm
- Right-sided heart failure is associated with edema, elevated jugular venous pressure, an S3 gallop over the right ventricle, and hepatomegaly
- Congestive heart failure involving failure of both sides of the heart is marked by a combination of the above symptoms

CAUSES
Common causes
Left-sided heart failure:
- Ischemic heart disease (myocardial infarction is the most common cause of heart failure in the US)
- Hypertension (untreated or inadequately treated hypertension is the second most common cause of heart failure in the US)
- Valvular disease (aortic stenosis, aortic insufficiency, mitral insufficiency)
- Cardiomyopathy
- High-output states (anemia, hyperthyroidism)
- Congenital heart disease
- Arrhythmias (especially atrial fibrillation)
- Volume overload

Right-sided heart failure (note: the most common cause of right-sided heart failure is left-sided heart failure):
- Chronic pulmonary disease
- Pulmonary embolism
- Pulmonary hypertension
- Valvular disease (mitral stenosis)

Rare causes
- Uncommon high-output states (Paget's disease of bone, beriberi)
- Valvular disease (tricuspid incompetence, pulmonary stenosis)
- Isolated right ventricular cardiomyopathy
- Hyperthyroidism
- Vitamin deficiency
- Myocarditis
- Toxic substances
- Illicit drugs, including cocaine and amphetamines

Serious causes
- Acute myocardial infarction
- Rupture of the intraventricular septum

- Acute valvular incompetence
- Pulmonary embolism
- Cardiac tamponade
- Acute fulminant myocarditis

Contributory or predisposing factors

- Acute myocardial infarction
- Arrhythmias, especially atrial fibrillation
- Infective endocarditis
- Anemia
- Hypertension
- Obesity
- Cigarette smoking
- Alcoholism
- Hyperthyroidism
- Pregnancy
- Infection, especially pulmonary infection
- Pulmonary embolism
- Diabetes
- Physical inactivity
- Depression

EPIDEMIOLOGY

Incidence and prevalence

- Between 1 and 4 new cases per 1000 of the population per year
- 10 or more new cases per 1000 of the population per year over 65 years of age

INCIDENCE

- Approximately 10–20 per 1000 of the population
- 50 or more per 1000 of the population over 65 years of age

PREVALENCE

- Heart failure occurs at some stage in most cases of severe heart disease, whatever the underlying cause
- It is the most common inpatient diagnosis in the US for patients over 65 years of age
- Heart failure patients visit their family practitioner on average two or three times per year

FREQUENCY

- Heart failure occurs at some stage in most cases of severe heart disease, whatever the underlying cause
- It is the most common inpatient diagnosis in the US for patients over 65 years of age
- Heart failure patients visit their family practitioner on average two or three times per year

Demographics

AGE

Increases with age.

GENDER

- More common in men than women in those between 40 and 75 years of age
- The sexes are equally commonly affected in those over 75 years of age

GENETICS

- Dilated and hypertrophic forms of cardiomyopathy may run in families
- Susceptibility to myocardial infarction, which is a frequent cause of congestive heart failure, may have a genetic component
- Hypertension is frequently familial
- Hemochromatosis can lead to both a cardiomyopathy and accelerated coronary artery disease

DIAGNOSIS

DIFFERENTIAL DIAGNOSIS

Chronic obstructive pulmonary disease

Irreversible lung disease caused predominantly by smoking. The main features of chronic obstructive pulmonary disease are as follows:

FEATURES

- Smoking is by far the most common etiology
- Diagnosis in a nonsmoker is extremely unlikely unless there is a family history of $alpha_1$-antitrypsin deficiency
- Dyspnea that varies widely in severity from day to day is unlikely to be of cardiac origin; it may be due to exacerbations of chronic bronchitis
- Chronic obstructive pulmonary disease often coexists with congestive heart failure

Asthma

Reversible airway obstruction. The main features of asthma are as follows:

FEATURES

- May be associated with atopy
- May be seasonal
- Dyspnea may vary widely in severity from day to day (in which case it is unlikely to be cardiac in origin)
- Patient may be able to identify triggers
- Moist rales are not a feature

Cirrhosis

Irreversible liver disease usually caused by alcohol or the hepatitis virus. The main features of cirrhosis are as follows:

FEATURES

- Cirrhosis occurs in long-standing liver disease
- Usually accompanied by the stigmata of liver disease
- Liver function tests may be abnormal
- Excess alcohol intake and infection with hepatitis B virus are the most common etiologies

Nephrotic syndrome

Renal disease affecting the basement membrane of the kidney. The main features of nephrotic syndrome are as follows:

FEATURES

- Heavy proteinuria
- Hypoalbuminemia
- Hypercholesterolemia is almost always present
- Peripheral edema, eyelid swelling, and ascites can occur

SIGNS & SYMPTOMS

Signs

Mild heart failure:

- Mild tachypnea
- Faint gallop rhythm (third heart sound)
- Rales at lung bases (often absent)
- Positive hepatojugular reflux

Moderate heart failure:

- Tachypnea and dyspnea at rest
- Cool extremities
- Diastolic hypertension
- Raised jugular venous pressure
- Cardiomegaly
- Pleural effusion
- Prominent rales at lung bases that may extend to the mid-lung fields
- Peripheral edema, initially in dependant areas (feet and ankles in ambulant patients, the sacrum in bed-bound patients) and then in other areas as the heart failure worsens

Severe heart failure:

- Diaphoresis
- Confusion
- Cyanosis
- Cough productive of frothy or pink sputum
- Alternating pulse (pulsus alternans)
- Hypotension
- Narrow pulse pressure from a reduced stroke volume
- Marked hypertension during pulmonary edema
- Narrow pulse pressure from a reduced stroke volume
- Marked hypertension during pulmonary edema
- Loud pulmonary component of the second heart sound
- Prominent gallop
- Ascites
- Severe peripheral edema
- Cheyne–Stokes respiration (hyperventilation alternating with apnea) in very severe heart failure

Symptoms

Mild heart failure:

- Fatigue
- Dyspnea with ordinary exertion
- Nocturia
- Decreasing exercise capacity

Moderate heart failure:

- Dyspnea at rest
- Orthopnea
- Nonproductive cough, especially at night
- Wheezing, especially at night, in a person with no history of asthma and in the absence of pulmonary infection
- Paroxysmal nocturnal dyspnea

Severe heart failure:

- Patient is likely to be too distressed or mentally obtunded to give a full history
- Severe orthopnea

ASSOCIATED DISORDERS

- Ischemic heart disease
- Hypertension
- Valvular heart disease (aortic stenosis, aortic incompetence, mitral stenosis, mitral incompetence)
- Cardiomyopathy
- Anemia

- Hyperthyroidism
- Atrial fibrillation
- Chronic obstructive pulmonary disease (chronic bronchitis or emphysema)
- Pulmonary thromboembolism
- Pulmonary hypertension

KEY! DON'T MISS!

- The two most helpful signs noted during the examination are orthopnea and either an elevated jugular venous pulse or a positive hepatojugular reflux. These signs have a high diagnostic accuracy
- When the symptom of heart failure is predominantly fatigue, the condition may be overlooked

CONSIDER CONSULT

- All patients with new-onset congestive heart failure
- The high risks of congestive heart failure in pregnancy mandate a referral
- Pediatric and geriatric patients
- Patients with renal or pulmonary disease, diabetes mellitus, or coexisting cardiac valve or arrhythmia disorders
- Patients with simultaneous congestion and ischemia should be evaluated in a hospital
- Progression of symptoms and/or signs of congestive heart failure

INVESTIGATION OF THE PATIENT

Direct questions to patient

Q **Do you experience fatigue or shortness of breath?** Exertional dyspnea and fatigue are usually the first symptoms of congestive heart failure (both left- and right-sided) that has progressed gradually to the symptomatic stage. Progression to orthopnea or paroxysmal nocturnal dyspnea is highly suggestive of heart failure. Patient should be queried about the ability to walk, climb stairs, and carry packages. Inability to dress or bathe without stopping to rest usually signals severe heart failure

Q **Is your sleep disturbed by problems with breathing?** Orthopnea – the symptom most sensitive to baseline elevation of left ventricular filling pressure – usually manifests as dyspnea in the supine position. A patient's spouse may describe Cheyne–Stokes respirations, which are cycles of hyperventilation and hypoventilation or apnea during sleep

Q **Do you have a cough?** A dry cough may occur with moderate impairment; cough productive of frothy and/or pink sputum suggests severe impairment

Q **Is your sleep disturbed by a frequent need to urinate?** Nocturia is a common sign of heart failure, due to increased renal perfusion and mobilization of peripheral edema when the patient is supine

Q **Do you have chest pain when lying down?** Nocturnal angina may result from increased cardiac work associated with increased venous return. Subendocardial perfusion can become impaired due to the high left ventricular filling pressures in the supine position

Q **Have you experienced sustained heart palpitations, dizziness, fainting, or near-fainting?** Arrhythmias may be the initial manifestation of congestive heart failure. Most patients with both congestive heart failure and cardiac dysrhythmias should be rapidly referred to a specialist

Q **Have you noted any swelling of your lower limbs?** Peripheral edema is a nonspecific but possible sign of congestive heart failure. Many patients describe an inability to wear usual shoes

Q **Have you experienced abdominal swelling or discomfort, lack of appetite, or a sensation of fullness after eating only small amounts of food?** These symptoms may indicate systemic venous congestion. They are often accompanied by hepatomegaly. Weight loss can be marked

Contributory or predisposing factors

Q **Do you have angina, or have you ever had a heart attack?** Coronary artery disease is responsible for 75% of cases of congestive heart failure with decreased left ventricular function

- **Have you ever been diagnosed with high blood pressure?** Hypertension may be an important contributor to heart failure
- **Have you ever been told that you have a heart problem?** Most forms of heart disease can eventually lead to heart failure; congenital heart disease and valvular heart disease are causes for particular suspicion
- **Do you have diabetes?** Diabetes mellitus is a risk factor for congestive heart failure
- **Are you pregnant?** Pregnancy may cause peripartum cardiomyopathy or aggravate pre-existing valvular disease
- **Do you smoke?** Smoking is a major risk factor for many of the etiologies of heart failure
- **Are you anemic?** Severe anemia can cause congestive heart failure, and even mild anemia aggravates congestive heart failure
- **How much alcohol do you consume?** Heavy alcohol consumption may cause dilated cardiomyopathy; consumption of even two drinks daily may worsen pre-existing heart failure
- **What drugs are you taking?** Pre-existing heart failure may be exacerbated by first-generation calcium antagonists and antiarrhythmic agents, which severely depress myocardial contractility. Nonsteroidal anti-inflammatory drugs (NSAIDs) can heighten the symptoms of heart failure by causing fluid retention and impairment of renal function
- **Have you recently discontinued any medications or made dietary changes?** Increased sodium intake can precipitate heart failure in patients with asymptomatic left ventricular dysfunction. Discontinuing cardiac medications that are known to alleviate signs and symptoms of congestive heart failure can result in acute worsening of symptoms
- **Have you used cocaine or amphetamines?** Illicit drug use may precipitate acute heart failure
- **Do you have a history of thyroid disease?** Both hyperthyroidism and hypothyroidism may impair cardiac function

Family history

- **Do you have a family history of heart attacks?** Provides cause for heightened suspicion of coronary artery disease, the leading cause of congestive heart failure with decreased left ventricular function
- **Does a close relative have any type of congenital heart disease?** Affirmative answer could suggest congenital heart disease, which may be hereditary
- **Have any family members been diagnosed with cardiomyopathy?** Hypertrophic cardiomyopathy is usually inherited, and dilated cardiomyopathy sometimes runs in families

Examination

- **Does patient's general appearance suggest possible severe disease that may necessitate rapid hospitalization?** Assess patient's general appearance for resting dyspnea, cyanosis, cachexia, and severe mental distress/confusion
- **Does patient have abnormal blood pressure or heart rate?** Record blood pressure and heart rate. Blood pressure may range from high to low in patients with congestive heart failure. A slight elevation in diastolic arterial pressure may reflect increased adrenergic activity. Systolic arterial pressure and pulse pressure may be reduced in severe heart failure, particularly when the stroke volume is abnormally low. Tachycardia may signal heart failure, particularly in the decompensated state. A weak, thready pulse (narrow pulse pressure) and pulsus alternans (alternating weak and strong pulse) signal decreased left ventricular function. Raised systolic arterial blood pressure occur in patients with prior hypertension, and this reflects the marked increase in sympathetic activity in severe congestive heart failure
- **Does patient have edema?** Check patient's weight for possible unexplained rapid increase, and examine for edema. Among ambulatory patients, this is usually first seen in the feet or ankles. In bedridden patients, edema may occur in the sacral area. Patients with advanced heart failure may have anasarca-massive and generalized edema
- **Does patient have jugular venous distention?** Check for jugular venous distention while patient lies with the upper body elevated at a 45° angle. A positive finding is consistent with congestive heart failure

- **Does patient have probable cardiomegaly?** Identify the point of maximal impulse of the left ventricle. This point is usually in the midclavicular line at the fifth intercostal space. It should be identified with the patient in a semi-recumbent position. Cardiomegaly typically displaces this maximal impulse downward and laterally
- **Does patient have heart sounds suggestive of congestive heart failure?** Perform auscultation to check for an S3 gallop, which is highly suggestive of congestive heart failure. A fourth heart sound (S4) may be evident in patients with heart failure and left ventricular hypertrophy; however, elderly patients may have a soft S4 gallop without clinically significant heart disease. Auscultation should also seek to detect murmurs, which may shed light on the cause of heart disease
- **Does patient have pulmonary congestion?** Perform auscultation. Inspiratory rales suggest congestive heart failure of at least moderate severity. These start at the lung bases and are heard progressively higher as disease progresses. Bubbling rales accompanied by wheezes occur with acute pulmonary edema
- **Does patient have hepatojugular reflux?** This is associated with both left- and right-sided congestive heart failure. To check for this sign, gradually compress the right upper quadrant or any region of the abdomen. The compression should be firm yet gentle and continued for up to 1min while observing the patient's neck veins. Advise the patient to breathe normally. Expansion (further elevation) of the jugular veins during the period of compression indicates that the systemic veins are unable to dilate (hyperadrenergic state) and accept the blood that has been redistributed from the visceral veins. Also, the right ventricle may not be able to accept the increased venous return
- **Does patient have congestive hepatomegaly?** Palpate the patient's liver. The liver may enlarge before edema occurs elsewhere. If enlargement is recent, the liver is usually tender
- **Does patient have ascites?** Detection of shifting dullness is helpful but not very sensitive for small amounts of ascites. In most instances, ascites reflects long-standing systemic venous hypertension

Summary of investigative tests

- Complete blood count: all patients with suspected congestive heart failure
- Serum chemistry: all patients with suspected congestive heart failure
- Thyroid-stimulating hormone levels: all patients above 65 years of age with heart failure without an obvious cause; all patients who have atrial fibrillation or other indications of thyroid disease
- Liver enzymes test
- Chest X-ray: all patients with suspected congestive heart failure
- Transthoracic two-dimensional echocardiography: the key diagnostic test for all patients with suspected congestive heart failure
- Electrocardiography: all patients with suspected congestive heart failure. It is particularly helpful when one suspects cardiac ischemia, past myocardial infarction, or cardiac dysrhythmias. A normal electrocardiogram is very rare in congestive heart failure, and, if present, the diagnosis should be questioned

The assay for brain natriuretic peptide (BNP), which is released from the left ventricle in the presence of either systolic or diastolic dysfunction, is rapidly becoming available. Elevations of this hormone can be diagnostic for congestive heart failure and may soon become the best screening laboratory test for congestive heart failure.

DIAGNOSTIC DECISION

The wide variation in signs and symptoms of congestive heart failure and the broad spectrum in the severity of cardiac dysfunction have made it difficult to provide precise diagnostic criteria. Useful criteria have emerged from the Framingham Study and are as follows:

Major criteria:

- Paroxysmal nocturnal dyspnea
- Distention of the jugular veins (elevated central venous pressure)
- Hepatojugular reflux
- Rales
- Radiographic cardiomegaly
- Acute pulmonary edema
- S3 gallop
- Weight loss >4.5kg in 5 days in response to treatment

Minor criteria:

- Bilateral ankle edema
- Nocturnal cough
- Dyspnea on ordinary exertion
- Pleural effusion
- Tachycardia

The diagnosis of congestive heart failure requires two major and one minor criteria or one major and two minor criteria. The minor criteria can be used only when there is not another condition present that would explain their presence.

In the present era it would be appropriate to add to the above criteria that there should be objective evidence of cardiac dysfunction by either echocardiography or cardiac catheterization.

Guidelines

- Guidelines for the evaluation and management of heart failure: report of the American College of Cardiology/American Heart Association Task Force on Practice Guidelines (Committee on Evaluation and Management of Heart Failure). Circulation 1995;92:2764–84. J Am Coll Cardiol 1995;26:1376–98. Available at the National Guideline Clearinghouse [1]
- Information on the Framingham Study (http://rover.nhlbi.nih.gov/about/framingham/) is available at the National Heart, Lung and Blood Institute

The American Academy of Family Physicians has produced the following information:

- Shamsham F, Mitchell J. Essentials for the diagnosis of heart failure. Am Fam Physician 2000;61:1319–28 [2]
- Chavey WE, Blaum CS, Bleske BE, et al. Guideline for the management of heart failure caused by systolic dysfunction: Part I. Guideline development, etiology and diagnosis. Am Fam Physician 2001;64:769–74 [3]

CLINICAL PEARL(S)

- The diagnosis of congestive heart failure may become evident by observing the patient during the history. You may note that the patient speaks only in short phrases due to dyspnea. Mild diaphoresis and peripheral cyanosis are easily seen and an elevated jugular venous pulse can be detected with the patient seated in front of you
- Be aware that some patients tolerate poor left ventricular systolic function very well (especially if their blood pressure is low) and often complain more of fatigue than congestive symptoms

THE TESTS

Body fluids

COMPLETE BLOOD COUNT

Description

Venous blood.

Advantages/Disadvantages

Advantages:

- Ease of collection of sample
- Routine laboratory test
- Inexpensive

Normal

- Red blood cells (RBCs): 4.33–5.67x10^{12}/L
- White blood cells (WBCs): 3.83–11.0x10^9/L
- Neutrophils: 1.94–7.78x10^9/L
- Lymphocytes: 1.08–3.10x10^9/L
- Monocytes: 0.230–0.870x10^9/L
- Eosinophils: 0.028–0.531x10^9/L
- Basophils: 0.011–0.106x10^9//L
- Platelets: 156–352x10^9/L

Abnormal

- Elevated WBC counts
- Elevated eosinophil counts
- Reduced RBC counts
- Keep in mind the possibility of a false-positive result

Cause of abnormal result

- Systemic infection
- An elevated eosinophil count may indicate eosinophilic endomyocardial disease
- Anemia may cause heart failure to worsen; severe anemia may cause heart failure

SERUM CHEMISTRY

Description

Venous blood for measurement of electrolytes, blood urea nitrogen, creatinine, glucose, phosphate, magnesium, calcium, and albumin levels.

Advantages/Disadvantages

Advantages:

- Ease of collection of sample
- Routine laboratory test
- Inexpensive

Normal

- Serum sodium: 135–147mEq/L (135–147mmol/L)
- Serum potassium: 3–5mEq/L (3–5mmol/L)
- Serum chloride: 95–105mEq/L (95–105mmol/L)
- Serum carbon dioxide: 24–30mEq/L (24–30mmol/L)
- Blood urea nitrogen: 8–18mg/dL (3–6.5mcmol/L)
- Serum creatinine: 0.6–1.2mg/dL (120–420mcmol/L)
- Serum phosphate: 2.5–5mg/dL (0.8–1.6mmol/L)
- Serum magnesium: 1.8–3.0mg/dL (0.80–1.20mmol/L)
- Serum calcium: 8.8–10.3mg/dL (2.2–2.58mmol/L)
- Serum albumin: 4–6g/dL (40–60g/L)
- Serum glucose: fasting <120mg/dL

Abnormal

- Values outside the normal range
- Keep in mind the possibility of a false-positive result

Cause of abnormal result

- Blood urea nitrogen and creatinine levels may be elevated in patients with congestive heart failure, reflecting either prerenal azotemia or pre-existing renal dysfunction
- Magnesium depletion can occur in diabetics, with excessive alcohol intake and with chronic diuretic administration

Drugs, disorders, and other factors that may alter results

Prolonged use of kaliuretic diuretics may cause hypokalemia, and potassium-sparing diuretics and angiotensin-converting enzyme (ACE) inhibitors may lead to hyperkalemia. Hypomagnesemia is associated with diuretic use and diabetes.

THYROID-STIMULATING HORMONE (TSH)

Description

Venous blood.

Advantages/Disadvantages

Advantages:

- Ease of collection of sample
- High-sensitivity TSH is now a routine laboratory test

Normal

0.4–5U/mL.

Abnormal

- Values outside the normal range
- Keep in mind the possibility of a false-positive result

Cause of abnormal result

- Thyroid disease
- Some drugs, including amiodarone
- Incorrect dosage of thyroid replacement therapy

Drugs, disorders, and other factors that may alter results

- Thyroid disease
- Some drugs, including amiodarone

LIVER ENZYMES

Description

Venous blood: aspartate aminotransferase (AST), alanine aminotransferase (ALT), bilirubin, alkaline phosphatase, prothrombin time (PT).

Advantages/Disadvantages

Advantages:

- Ease of collection of sample
- Routine laboratory test
- Inexpensive

Cause of abnormal result

With liver congestion, serum transaminase and bilirubin levels may become elevated. Increased PT may occur with chronic congestive hepatomegaly.

Drugs, disorders, and other factors that may alter results

The distinction between primary liver disease and hepatic dysfunction secondary to congestive heart failure can be confusing.

Imaging

CHEST X-RAY

Description

Chest X-ray useful to obtain images of the lung fields and heart.

Advantages/Disadvantages

Advantages:

- Provides rapid information
- Inexpensive, routine procedure

Normal

Normal lung fields and heart size.

Abnormal

- Cardiomegaly, usually signaled by a cardiothoracic ratio above 0.50 on a posteroanterior view
- Absence of free space between the cardiac silhouette and the sternum on a lateral view (absence of this space is suggestive of right ventricular enlargement)
- Signs of increased pulmonary venous pressure, including linear densities reflecting interstitial edema and a redistribution of flow to the upper lung zones (antler sign)
- Pleural effusion
- Enlarged pulmonary arteries

Cause of abnormal result

Congestive heart failure may cause any of the above abnormalities. However, predominantly diastolic dysfunction does not necessarily result in altered heart size.

TRANSTHORACIC TWO-DIMENSIONAL ECHOCARDIOGRAPHY

Description

Useful to image the functioning and size of the heart.

Advantages/Disadvantages

Advantages:

- Assesses left ventricular size, mass, and function
- Differentiates between systolic and diastolic dysfunction
- Indicates structural heart disease, such as valvular and congenital abnormalities
- Reveals regional wall motion abnormalities, which when present suggest damage from coronary artery disease
- Estimates the systolic pulmonary arterial pressure
- Provides an overall assessment of the severity of cardiac dysfunction, which provides prognostic information

Normal

Normal size and function of heart.

Abnormal

Signs of systolic dysfunction:

- Low ejection fraction (<0.40 is definitely abnormal, 0.4–0.45 is generally considered abnormal, and 0.45–0.50 is borderline)
- Segmental wall motion abnormalities
- Dilated ventricle

Signs of diastolic dysfunction:

- Left ventricular hypertrophy
- Dilated left atrium

- Normal or near-normal ejection fraction
- Reversal of the normal pattern of flow velocity across the mitral valve

Signs of damage from coronary artery disease:
- Regional wall motion abnormalities with or without a dilated left ventricle

Congenital abnormalities.
Valvular disease.

Cause of abnormal result
- Left ventricular hypertrophy and/or dilation may lead to increased voltages
- Low voltage may occur with chronic constrictive pericarditis, cardiac tamponade, cardiac amyloidosis, or severe chronic obstructive pulmonary disease
- Myocardial infarction pattern indicates that ischemic heart disease may be responsible for heart failure
- Left bundle branch block or other intraventricular conduction delays are seen with ischemic heart disease and nonischemic cardiomyopathy
- Left atrial enlargement is common with many types of left heart disease

Special tests

ELECTROCARDIOGRAM

Description
Useful to image the size and function of the heart.

Advantages/Disadvantages
Advantages:
- Routine procedure
- Noninvasive
- May suggest reasons for the cause of heart failure

Disadvantage: Findings are not specific for congestive heart failure.

Normal
Normal size and function of heart.

Abnormal
- Voltage criteria for left ventricular hypertrophy (SV1 + RV5 or RV6 35 V)
- Left atrial enlargement
- T-wave abnormalities
- Low voltage
- Myocardial infarction pattern
- Left bundle branch block or other intraventricular conduction delays

Cause of abnormal result
- Left ventricular hypertrophy and/or dilation may lead to increased voltages
- Low voltage may occur with chronic constrictive pericarditis, cardiac tamponade, cardiac amyloidosis, or severe chronic obstructive pulmonary disease
- Myocardial infarction pattern indicates that ischemic heart disease may be responsible for heart failure
- Left bundle branch block or other intraventricular conduction delays are seen with ischemic heart disease and nonischemic cardiomyopathy
- Left atrial enlargement is common with many types of left heart disease

TREATMENT

CONSIDER CONSULT

- Most patients benefit from combined care with a cardiologist and a generalist
- Patients with combined congestion and hypoperfusion are managed best in a hospital
- Patients with rapid decline in serum sodium to below 130mEq/L
- Patients whose serum creatinine rises at least 2-fold to above 2.5mg/dL

IMMEDIATE ACTION

Immediate hospitalization needed for:

- Patients with pulmonary edema or respiratory distress while seated
- Patients without known hypoxemia who develop arterial desaturation to below 90%
- Patients with systolic blood pressure below 75mmHg
- Patients who display mental confusion due to hypoperfusion

Urgent hospitalization needed for:

- Patients with new indications of simultaneous congestion and hypoperfusion
- Patients with increasing dyspnea not responding to diuretic therapy
- Patients with anasarca, severe hepatic distention, or tense ascites
- Patients with severe, worsening noncardiac conditions, such as renal dysfunction or pulmonary disease, who become decompensated
- New onset of atrial fibrillation

PATIENT AND CAREGIVER ISSUES

Forensic and legal issues

- Failure to provide timely diagnosis and treatment may be grounds for a lawsuit
- Patients who are near death should have an opportunity to discuss advance directives, such as a living will

Impact on career, dependants, family, friends

- Many patients with congestive heart failure can continue to work if large physical demands are not part of the job
- Counseling is required since the patient and family need to be aware of the shortened life expectancy associated with congestive heart failure
- Family members and caregivers should understand the importance of the patient's complex drug regimen, the risks of sudden cessation of these therapies, the extreme importance of diet, and the requirement for moderate physical activity

Patient or caregiver request

Are any alternative therapies appropriate for congestive heart failure? Clinical trials of ubiquinone (Q10) for congestive heart failure have shown conflicting results; efficacy is considered modest at best, and no side-effects have been reported. Extracts of the hawthorn plant have been approved in Germany for mild cardiac insufficiency, but no randomized, placebo-controlled trials have assessed this agent in the US. L-carnitine has been reported in one controlled trial to lessen symptoms in idiopathic dilated cardiomyopathy. The importance of a number of factors that affect endothelial function is being explored, including arginine supplements, higher intakes of vitamin C, and sources of omega-3 fatty acids.

MANAGEMENT ISSUES

Goals

- Improve cardiac function when possible
- Reduce mortality rate
- Improve patient's quality of life

Management in special circumstances

COEXISTING DISEASE

- Patients with coexisting renal or pulmonary disease may require a specialist to develop a treatment regimen that relieves cardiac symptoms while preserving renal and pulmonary function
- Patients with coexisting diabetes should attempt strict glucose control since progression of the diabetic cardiomyopathy is more rapid in poorly controlled diabetics; referral may be appropriate
- Depression is associated with worsened prognosis for congestive heart failure; it should be identified and treated
- Persistent anemia worsens congestive heart failure and must be treated

COEXISTING MEDICATION

- All NSAIDs may lead to fluid retention and worsening congestive heart failure. These drugs reduce renal glomerular filtration rate (GFR)
- Patients with concomitant treatment for hypothyroidism may have an exacerbation of congestive heart failure if the thyroid replacement therapy is excessive

SPECIAL PATIENT GROUPS

Elderly patients:

- Commonly present with anorexia, generalized weakness, and fatigue
- Due to aging circulation, elderly patients usually should not have a target systolic blood pressure below 90mmHg
- Therapy may be complicated by coexisting disorders, such as renal or pulmonary impairment or orthostatic hypotension. Referral may be necessary to optimize treatment
- An appropriate goal is to achieve normal to slightly elevated but stable jugular venous pressure, creatinine, and blood urea nitrogen
- Quality of life is improved and hospitalizations are reduced when elderly patients are treated with a team of specialists in heart failure and geriatrics

Pregnant patients should be referred to a specialist.

Pediatric patients should be referred to a specialist.

PATIENT SATISFACTION/LIFESTYLE PRIORITIES

Treatment should improve patients' abilities to pursue lifestyle priorities.

SUMMARY OF THERAPEUTIC OPTIONS

Choices

- Angiotensin-converting enzyme (ACE) inhibitor: a priority for all patients with systolic heart failure unless absolutely contraindicated. May also be used for patients with diastolic heart failure. Lisinopril and ramipril are used commonly for heart failure. ACE inhibitors are likely to be useful in diastolic heart failure, particularly when hypertension is a contributing factor
- Angiotensin II inhibitor: may be indicated when an ACE inhibitor is not tolerated due to angioedema or a refractory cough. Candesartan is an example of an angiotensin II inhibitor
- Beta-adrenergic blocker (beta-blocker): indicated for all patients with systolic heart failure except for those who have dyspnea at rest, are hemodynamically unstable, or cannot tolerate beta-blockers. Also appropriate for diastolic heart failure
- Spironolactone: indicated for all patients with systolic dysfunction and dyspnea at rest or with a recent history of dyspnea at rest. Its use in diastolic heart failure has not been specifically studied, but patients with near-normal left ventricular ejection fraction appeared to benefit similarly to those with depressed ejection fractions in the RALES trial
- Diuretics: all symptomatic patients with congestive signs

- Digoxin: patients with systolic heart failure accompanied by atrial fibrillation. Also for those with systolic heart failure with persistent symptoms or recurrent hospitalizations who are concurrently using ACE inhibitors, beta-blockers, diuretics, and spironolactone. Should be avoided in patients with diastolic dysfunction
- Nitrates: patients with diastolic dysfunction and pulmonary congestion
- Valve replacement or repair: patients with heart failure caused by a dysfunctional valve
- Cardiac transplantation or left ventricular assist devices: patients with complex heart failure not responding to treatment
- Lifestyle changes: reduced salt intake, daily weighing, and moderate exercise

Guidelines

- Guidelines for the evaluation and management of heart failure: report of the American College of Cardiology/American Heart Association Task Force on Practice Guidelines (Committee on Evaluation and Management of Heart Failure). Circulation 1995;92:2764–84. J Am Coll Cardiol 1995;26:1376–98. Available at the National Guideline Clearinghouse [1]

The American Academy of Family Physicians has produced the following information:

- Chavey WE, Blaum CS, Bleske BE, et al. Guideline for the management of heart failure caused by systolic dysfunction: part II. Treatment. Am Fam Physician 2001;64:1045–54 [4]
- Hoyt RE, Bowling LS. Reducing readmissions for congestive heart failure. Am Fam Physician 2001;63:1593–8 [5]

Clinical pearl(s)

All the clinical trials of the standard medications for congestive heart failure have used the drugs at their optimal daily dosages. It is essential to strive to achieve optimal dosages of each drug.

Never

- Fail to monitor renal function while up-titrating each of the heart failure drugs
- Stop trying to optimize treatment in patients with difficult-to-manage congestive heart failure

FOLLOW UP

- Follow up is needed to assess effectiveness of treatment and to monitor the response
- During the titration of the ACE inhibitor and beta-blocker, the interval between visits should not exceed 2–3 weeks
- Renal function should be measured at each visit

Information for patient or caregiver

- Daily weighing is essential for all patients as an indication of possibly worsened condition. Patients should have a defined target weight and should contact their physician if weight increases by >3lb in 1 week
- Patients should learn when to contact their physician or seek emergency care: new swelling of feet or abdomen, worsening shortness of breath, worsening cough, persistent nausea/vomiting, sudden dizziness not related to changes in body position, and prolonged palpitations
- Low-salt diet: sodium intake should be 2–3g/day
- Moderate exercise for ambulatory patients; patients should understand the difference between moderate and strenuous exercise, and should know that moderate exercise helps rather than harms the heart
- Patients should consult physician about any over-the-counter (OTC) drugs and should avoid NSAIDs
- Patients should be informed of possible adverse effects of any medications and should contact their physician if such effects occur
- Patients should understand that the benefits of some medications, such ACE inhibitors, beta-blockers, and spironolactone, may not be immediately apparent

- Support stockings may be helpful with edema, particularly if there is a component of venous insufficiency
- Patients may need intermittent rest each day to prevent excessive fatigue

DRUGS AND OTHER THERAPIES: DETAILS

Drugs

LISINOPRIL

Lisinopril is used extensively in patients with congestive heart failure.

Dose

Lisinopril: starting dose 5mg daily; target dose 5–20mg daily.

Efficacy

- Improvement of symptoms and decreased mortality rate for patients with systolic dysfunction
- Efficacy not proven for diastolic dysfunction, but these drugs may improve passive left ventricular diastolic properties, possibly by causing regression of left ventricular hypertrophy and interstitial collagen

Risks/Benefits

Risk: Use caution in renal impairment, hypotension, aortic stenosis, hyperkalemia, and neutropenia.

Benefits:

- Reduces morbidity and mortality rates in symptomatic and asymptomatic patients
- Improves exercise tolerance in symptomatic patients

Side-effects and adverse reactions

- Cardiovascular: orthostatic hypotension and syncope, angina, palpitations, sinus tachycardia
- CNS: headache, dizziness, fatigue
- EENT: cough
- Gastrointestinal: nausea, vomiting, diarrhea, constipation, abdominal pain
- Genitourinary: renal damage, impotence
- Hematologic: neutropenia, agranulocytosis, aplastic and hemolytic anemia, pancytopenia, thrombocytopenia
- Metabolic: hyperkalemia, hyponatremia
- Skin: angioedema, maculopapular rash

Interactions (other drugs)

- Allopurinol
- Azathioprine
- Heparin
- Insulin
- Iron
- Lithium
- NSAIDs
- Antihypertensives (loop and potassium-sparing diuretics, prazosin, terazosin, doxazosin)
- Potassium
- Sodium
- Trimethoprim

Contraindications

- Pregnancy
- Angioedema
- Hypotension
- Children

Evidence

- A systematic review found that ACE inhibitors reduced mortality rates compared with placebo for patients with NYHA class II heart failure or worse. Similar benefit was found with different ACE inhibitors [6] *Level M*
- Another systematic review of patients with heart failure or left ventricular dysfunction found that ACE inhibitors significantly reduced mortality rates, readmission for heart failure, and reinfarction compared with placebo. The benefits began soon after the start of therapy and persisted long-term [7] *Level M*

Acceptability to patient

Patients should understand that the benefits of ACE inhibitors may not be evident for several weeks. Moreover, this drug should not necessarily be discontinued because of cough – cough may diminish as treatment progresses. When cough is refractory or angioedema develops, the benefits of the ACE inhibitor can usually be achieved with an angiotensin II blocker.

Follow up plan

Blood pressure and renal function need to be measured prior to each escalation of dosage.

Patient and caregiver information

- Patients should understand that the benefits of ACE inhibitors may not be immediately evident
- This drug should not necessarily be discontinued because of cough – cough may diminish as treatment progresses

RAMIPRIL

Ramipril is a useful ACE inhibitor in congestive heart failure.

Dose

Ramipril: starting dose 1.25–2.5mg twice daily; target dose 5mg twice daily.

Efficacy

- Improvement of symptoms and decreased mortality rate for patients with systolic dysfunction
- Efficacy not proven for diastolic dysfunction, but these drugs may improve passive left ventricular diastolic properties, possibly by causing regression of left ventricular hypertrophy and interstitial collagen

Risks/Benefits

Risk: Use caution in renal impairment, hypotension, aortic stenosis, hyperkalemia, and neutropenia.

Benefits:

- Reduces morbidity and mortality rates in symptomatic and asymptomatic patients
- Improves exercise tolerance in symptomatic patients

Side-effects and adverse reactions

- Cardiovascular: orthostatic hypotension and syncope, angina, palpitations, sinus tachycardia
- CNS: headache, dizziness, fatigue
- EENT: cough
- Gastrointestinal: nausea, vomiting, diarrhea, constipation, abdominal pain
- Genitourinary: renal damage, impotence
- Hematologic: neutropenia, agranulocytosis, aplastic and hemolytic anemia, pancytopenia, thrombocytopenia
- Metabolic: hyperkalemia, hyponatremia
- Skin: angioedema, maculopapular rash

Interactions (other drugs)

- Antihypertensives (loop and potassium-sparing diuretics, prazosin, terazosin, doxazosin)
- Allopurinol
- Azathioprine
- Heparin
- Insulin
- Iron
- Lithium
- NSAIDs
- Potassium
- Sodium
- Trimethoprim

Contraindications

- Pregnancy
- Angioedema
- Hypotension
- Children

Evidence

- A systematic review found that ACE inhibitors reduced mortality rates compared with placebo for patients with New York Heart Association (NYHA) class II heart failure or worse. Similar benefit was found with different ACE inhibitors [6] *Level M*
- Another systematic review of patients with heart failure or left ventricular dysfunction found that ACE inhibitors significantly reduced mortality rates, readmission for heart failure, and reinfarction compared with placebo. The benefits began soon after the start of therapy and persisted long-term [7] *Level M*
- A large randomized controlled trial showed that ramipril significantly reduced the risk of heart failure in high risk people (people with vascular disease or diabetes plus one other cardiovascular risk factor) [8] *Level P*
- Ramipril has been shown to reduce the combined risk of myocardial infarction, reduced all-cause mortality, and improved the left ventricular function [8] *Level P*

Acceptability to patient

Patients should understand that the benefits of ACE inhibitors may not be evident for several weeks. Moreover, this drug should not necessarily be discontinued because of cough – cough may diminish as treatment progresses. When cough is refractory or angioedema develops, the benefits of the ACE inhibitor can usually be achieved with an angiotensin II blocker.

Follow up plan

Blood pressure and renal function need to be measured prior to each escalation of dosage.

Patient and caregiver information

- Patients should understand that the benefits of ACE inhibitors may not be immediately evident
- This drug should not necessarily be discontinued because of cough – cough may diminish as treatment progresses

CANDESARTAN AND LOSARTAN

- Angiotensin II inhibitor
- Useful if a patient cannot tolerate an angiotensin I agent, usually due to the refractory cough or angioedema
- Not licensed for heart failure

Dose

Adult oral starting dose is 8–32mg daily.

Efficacy

- Limited evidence for losartan use in patients with heart failure
- Used only if angiotensin I agent not tolerated by the patient

Risks/Benefits

- Limited evidence for losartan to be used in patients with heart failure
- Used if angiotensin I agent not tolerated by the patient
- Monitoring of renal function necessary
- Less effective in African-Americans

Side-effects and adverse reactions

- Cardiovascular: flushing, palpitations, and tachycardia
- CNS: anxiety, depresion, drowsiness, dizziness, fatigue, headache, light-headedness, parethesia, and vertigo
- EENT: epistaxis
- Hematologic: decreased hematocrit and purpura
- Musculoskeletal: back pain and myalgia
- Skin: facial edema, angioedema, and diaphoresis
- Respiratory: cough and upper respiratory infection

Interactions (other drugs)

- Fluconazole
- Lithium
- Rifampin
- Cimetidine
- Phenobarbital

Contraindications

- Pregnancy
- Hypotension

Evidence

Systematic reviews have shown angiotensin II receptor antagonists are as effective as ACE inhibitors in reducing all-cause mortality [9] *Level M*

Acceptability to patient

- Patients should understand that the benefits of angiotensin II inhibitors may not be evident for several weeks
- Candesartan is not licensed for use in heart failure and patients should be informed

Follow up plan

Blood pressure and renal function need to be measured prior to each escalation of dosage.

Patient and caregiver information

- Patients should be informed that the benefits of angiotensin II inhibitors may not be evident for several weeks
- Candesartan is not licensed for use in heart failure and patients should be informed
- Patients should be informed to stop the medication immediately if wheezing, facial swelling, or rashes develop

BETA-BLOCKERS

- Bisoprolol, carvedilol and metoprolol succinate are used in controlled heart failure
- These drugs are used under the specialist as careful monitoring of the patient is required
- Their use is relatively novel in the treatment of heart failure and evidence is limited in their effectiveness

Dose

- Bisoprolol: starting dose 2.5–5mg once daily; target dose 10mg once daily
- Carvedilol: starting dose 3.125mg twice daily; target dose 25mg twice daily
- Metoprolol succinate: starting dose 12.5–25mg once daily; target dose 200mg once daily

Efficacy

- Beta-blockers decrease mortality rates and improve symptoms of systolic dysfunction
- Large trials of beta-blockers in diastolic congestive heart failure have not been performed, but some benefit is likely since beta-blockers may slow heart rate, control blood pressure, prevent myocardial ischemia, and induce regression of left ventricular hypertrophy

Risks/Benefits

Risks:

- Use caution in pregnancy and breast-feeding
- Use caution in diabetes mellitus, liver and renal impairment, AV block, myasthenia gravis
- Do not withdraw abruptly in angina

Side-effects and adverse reactions

- Cardiovascular: hypotension, bradycardia, conduction abnormalities, heart failure, peripheral vasoconstriction
- CNS: fatigue, sleep disturbances
- EENT: dry eyes

- Gastrointestinal: nausea, vomiting
- Respiratory: bronchospasm
- Skin: rashes, exacerbation of psoriasis

Interactions (other drugs)

■ Adenosine (may cause bradycardia) ■ Amoxicillin (reduced atenolol availability) ■ Antacids (reduced atenolol availability) ■ Calcium channel blockers (see dihydropyridine and verapamil) ■ Clonidine (exacerbation of rebound hypertension upon discontinuation of clonidine) ■ Digoxin (concomitant slowing of AV node conduction) ■ Dihydropyridines (additive hemodynamic effects; increased serum concentration of atenolol) ■ Lidocaine (increased serum lidocaine possible) ■ Neostigmine (may cause bradycardia) ■ NSAIDs (reduced antihypertensive effects of atenolol) ■ Physostigmine (bradycardia aggravated ■ Prazosin (first-dose response to prazosin may be enhanced by beta-blockade) ■ Tacrine (may cause bradycardia) ■ Theophylline (antagonistic pharmacodynamic effects) ■ Verapamil (enhanced effects of both drugs)

Contraindications

■ Pheochromocytoma ■ Metabolic acidosis ■ Asthma ■ Second- or third-degree AV block, sick sinus syndrome, marked bradycardia, hypotension, cardiogenic shock, peripheral arterial disease, uncontrolled heart failure, Prinzmetal's angina

Evidence

- Beta-blockers are effective in reducing death and hospitalization when added to ACE-inhibitors
- A systematic review found that beta-blockers were more effective than placebo in reducing the combined outcome of death or hospitalization in patients' heart failure secondary to idiopathic dilated cardiomyopathy or ischemic heart disease. Trials of patients following acute myocardial infarction were excluded [10] *Level M*
- A randomized controlled trial (RCT) compared additional bisoprolol vs placebo in people with NYHA class III–IV heart failure. A significant reduction in mortality rate (including sudden death) at 1.3 years led to early termination of the trial [11] *Level P*
- Another RCT found that additional metoprolol (controlled release) was significantly more effective than placebo in reducing mortality rate at 1 year in patients with NYHA class II–IV. This trial was also stopped early [12] *Level P*
- An RCT compared carvedilol with placebo (in addition to background therapy with digoxin, diuretics, and ACE inhibitors) in the treatment of patients with mild, moderate, and severe heart failure. A significant reduction in mortality rate was noted in the treatment group, and the trial was terminated early. The risk of hospitalization due to cardiovascular causes was also significantly reduced. Worsening heart failure secondary to treatment was more common in the placebo group than the carvedilol group [13] *Level P*

Acceptability to patient

Generally good.

Follow up plan

Periodic monitoring of renal function is necessary since there may be transient worsening of congestive heart failure and renal function.

Patient and caregiver information

- Patients should be cautioned not to discontinue any beta-blocker abruptly
- Patients should be warned to take the immediate-release preparation of metoprolol medication with food to slow absorption and minimize the risk of orthostatic hypotension

SPIRONOLACTONE

Spironolactone is a loop diuretic.

Dose

100mg daily (range 25–100mg daily); this dose may need to be reduce in patients with renal or hepatic disease.

Efficacy

Decreases mortality rate and improves symptoms.

Risks/Benefits

Risks:

- Spironolactone is a potassium-sparing diuretic; therefore use caution with potassium supplements and hyponatremia
- Use caution in renal and hepatic impairment, diabetes, acidosis, dehydration, menstrual problems, and gynecomastia
- Use caution in pregnancy and in the elderly

Side-effects and adverse reactions

- Cardiovascular: hypotension, bradycardia
- CNS: headache, drowsiness
- Gastrointestinal: nausea, vomiting, diarrhea, bleeding, abdominal pain
- Genitourinary: menstrual irregularities, gynecomastia, hirsutism, impotence
- Metabolic: hyperkalemia, hyponatremia, acidosis
- Skin: rashes, pruritus

Interactions (other drugs)

- ACE inhibitors
- Ammonium chloride
- Anticoagulants
- Lithium
- Mitotane
- Angiotensin II receptor antagonists
- Cardiac glycosides
- Carbenoxolone
- Salicylates
- Cyclosporine, tacrolimus
- Disopyramide
- Potassium

Contraindications

- Severe renal disease
- Anuria
- Hyperkalemia
- ACE inhibitors and angiotensin receptor antagonists in antikaliuretic therapy

Evidence

An RCT compared spironolactone with placebo in patients with heart failure (NYHA class III–IV). Patients were also taking ACE inhibitors and loop diuretics, and most were also taking digoxin. Mortality rate was significantly reduced in patients receiving spironolactone at 2 years, and the trial was ceased prematurely. The frequency of hospitalization due to heart failure was also reduced, and a significant symptomatic improvement was noted in the spironolactone group [10]
Level P

Acceptability to patient

The drug is usually very well tolerated, and the cost is very low.

Follow up plan

- Measure blood pressure before initiating spironolactone and at regular intervals throughout therapy
- Monitor serum electrolytes
- Weigh patient regularly throughout therapy
- Check for mental changes and lethargy
- Monitor for gynecomastia
- Monitoring should be carried out at onset of treatment and 1–2 weeks after starting treatment
- If there are no problems in the first 2 weeks, the patient should be re-evaluated in 2–3 months

Patient and caregiver information
Patient should limit high-potassium foods and eliminate salt substitutes containing potassium chloride. Drug should be taken with food.

DIURETICS
- Thiazide diuretics: hydrochlorothiazide and metolazone
- Loop diuretics: bumetanide, ethacrynic acid, furosemide, and torsemide

Dose
- Hydrochlorothiazide: starting dose 25mg daily; target dose 25–100mg daily
- Metolazone: starting dose 5mg/day; target dose 5–20mg daily
- Bumetanide: starting dose 0.5–1mg/day; maximum dose 10mg daily
- Ethacrynic acid: starting dose 50mg/day; target dose 25–200mg once or twice daily
- Furosemide: starting dose 20–80mg/day; maximum dose 600mg daily
- Torsemide: starting dose 10–20mg/day; maximum dose 200mg daily

These dosages are appropriate for both systolic and diastolic heart failure. The challenge is to find the optimal maintenance dosage in that there is tremendous variation between patients. The severity of congestive heart failure, the patient's salt intake, and the absorption of the drug are variables that affect the appropriate dosage.

Efficacy
Diuretics are always efficacious when the proper dosages are given.

Risks/Benefits
Risks:
- Use caution in diabetes mellitus, renal and liver disease, systemic lupus erythematosus, hypertension, gout, porphyria
- Use caution in pregnancy and nursing mothers

Benefit: reduces fluid congestion.

Side-effects and adverse reactions
- Cardiovascular: chest pain, circulatory collapse, orthostatic hypotension
- CNS: dizziness, headache, paresthesia, fever
- EENT: visual disturbances, ototoxicity, tinnitus, hearing impairment, thirst
- Gastrointestinal: ischemic hepatitis, vomiting, pancreatitis, nausea, diarrhea, anorexia
- Genitourinary: glycosuria, hyperuricemia, bladder spasm, polyuria
- Hematologic: blood disorders
- Metabolic: hyperglycemia, hyponatremia, hypokalemia, hypomagnesemia, hypovolemia, hypochloremia, hypercholesterolemia, hypertriglyceridemia
- Skin: erythema multiforme, exfoliative dermatitis, urticaria

Interactions (other drugs)
▪ **ACE inhibitors** ▪ **Alpha-adrenergic antagonists** ▪ **Amphotericin** ▪ **Tubocurarine** ▪ **Antibiotics (aminoglycosides, polymyxins, vancomycin, cephalosporins)** ▪ **Antidiabetics** ▪ **Antidysrhythmics (amiodarone, cardiac glycosides, disopyramide, flecainide, mexiletine, quinidine, sotalol)** ▪ **Beta$_2$-adrenergic agonists** ▪ **Carbenoxolone** ▪ **Phenobarbital** ▪ **Cholestyramine, colestipol** ▪ **Cisplatin** ▪ **Clofibrate** ▪ **Corticosteroids** ▪ **Phenytoin** ▪ **Diuretics (thiazides, metolazone, acetazolamide)** ▪ **Lignocaine** ▪ **Lithium** ▪ **NSAIDs** ▪ **Pimozide** ▪ **Reboxetine** ▪ **Selective serotonin reuptake inhibitors (SSRIs)** ▪ **Terbutaline**

Contraindications

- Renal failure with anuria
- Hepatic coma

Acceptability to patient

- Good because of possible rapid alleviation of congestion
- Patient may wish to time medication so diuresis does not disrupt sleep

Follow up plan

- When drug is administered parenterally, careful monitoring of blood pressure and vital signs is necessary
- Elderly patients require close observation during brisk diuresis
- Monitor blood count, serum electrolytes, CO_2, blood urea nitrogen, blood sugar, and uric acid
- Check for hypomagnesemia
- Monitoring should be daily during active diuresis
- When a stable treatment regimen has been established, these parameters should be routinely checked three to four times per year

Patient and caregiver information

- Patients should be informed of appropriate salt and fluid intake
- Daily ingestion of potassium-rich foods may be appropriate
- If the patient is already receiving an ACE inhibitor and/or spironolactone, caution must be exercised in the daily potassium intake since both these drugs lead to potassium reabsorption by the kidney
- Patients should report muscle cramps or weakness

DIGOXIN

Dose

Starting dose: 250mcg/day; target dose 62.5–350mcg daily.

Efficacy

Improves symptoms and decreases hospitalization rates in patients with symptomatic heart failure associated with systolic dysfunction.

Risks/Benefits

Risks:

- Use caution with electrolyte imbalances
- Use caution with severe pulmonary disease, hepatic disease, hypothyroidism, sick sinus syndrome, acute myocardial infarction, AV block
- Avoid in Wolff–Parkinson–White syndrome
- Use caution in the elderly

Benefit: reduces heart-failure hospitalizations

Side-effects and adverse reactions

- Cardiovascular: atrial and ventricular fibrillation, AV block, bradycardia
- CNS: confusion, hallucinations, depression, seizures
- EENT: green/yellow vision
- Gastrointestinal: bleeding, vomiting, diarrhea, nausea, discomfort
- Hematologic: eosinophilia, thrombocytopenia
- Skin: rash

Interactions (other drugs)

- Antidysrhythmics (calcium channel blockers, amiodarone, quinidine, propafenone)
- Antihypertensives ■ Antimalarials ■ Azole antifungals ■ Benzodiazepines ■ Calcium

Contraindications

- Ventricular fibrillation ■ SA or AV node disease ■ Idiopathic hypertrophic subaortic stenosis
- Hypertrophic obstructive cardiomyopathy ■ Hypokalemia of <2.0

Evidence

- A systematic review compared digitalis glycosides with placebo in patients with heart failure and sinus rhythm. Patients were also receiving diuretics, ACE inhibitors, and beta-blockers. There was no difference in mortality rate associated with digitalis, but lower rates of hospitalization and deterioration were noted [15] *Level M*
- A RCT compared digoxin with placebo in patients with NYHA class I–III heart failure. Patients were already taking ACE inhibitors (94%) or diuretics (82%). Digoxin reduced the number of patients hospitalized for worsening heart failure over 37 months but did not reduce all-cause mortality rate compared with placebo [16] *Level P*

Acceptability to patient

Well tolerated by most patients with congestive heart failure.

Follow up plan

- In the absence of renal dysfunction, the usual maintenance dose is 0.25mg daily. A steady state is achieved after 5–10 days of treatment. Measurement of blood level at that time will indicate whether the dose needs to be adjusted
- Monitor serum potassium and magnesium

Patient and caregiver information

- Patients should understand the need for monitoring and follow up, and should report pulse below value indicated by physician
- Drug must be taken precisely as directed. Patients should be aware of signs of toxicity

NITRATES

- Include isosorbide mononitrate, isosorbide dinitrate, and nitroglycerin sublingual or transcutaneous
- The combination of hydralazine and isosorbide dinitrate has been shown to improve symptoms and cause a slight reduction in mortality rate
- It is unclear as to which of the two drugs was most important or whether the combination was essential for the mortality benefit
- Extensive clinical experience affirms the utility of nitrates to relieve symptoms

Dose

- Isosorbide dinitrate: usually introduced at 5–20mg, three times daily; may be gradually increased to 40mg three times daily
- Isosorbide mononitrate: dosage range from 30 to 120mg/day in single or divided doses depending on the preparation used; 20mg twice daily for immediate-release tablets
- Nitroglycerin, sublingual: 0.3–0.6mg. Patient may self-administer when rapid, temporary relief of pulmonary congestion is required. In an emergency can be taken every few minutes until other therapy is available
- Nitroglycerin, transdermal: dosage range is 0.2–0.8mg/h. The Nitropatch should be used for approximately 12h daily, either in the daytime or throughout the night for relief of nocturnal symptoms

Efficacy

Alleviate symptoms of pulmonary congestion.

Risks/Benefits

Risks:
- Risk of severe hypotension
- Risk of aggravation of angina caused by hypertrophic cardiomyopathy

Benefit: helps alleviate symptoms of pulmonary congestion, although these agents do not prolong survival.

Side-effects and adverse reactions
- Cardiovascular: postural hypotension, tachycardia, atrial fibrillation, crescendo angina, dysrhythmias, palpitations, postural hypotension, rebound hypertension
- CNS: headache, confusion, anxiety, agitation, dizziness, flushing

Interactions (other drugs)

■ Sildenafil: enhances hypotensive effect; combination should be avoided
■ Ergot alkaloids: opposition to coronary vasodilatory effects of nitrates ■ Ethanol: additive vasodilation could cause hypotension ■ Metronidazole: ethanol contained in intravenous nitroglycerin preparations could cause disulfiram-like reaction in some patients

Contraindications

■ Hypotension ■ Hypertrophic obstructive cardiomyopathy ■ Aortic stenosis
■ Cardiac tamponade ■ Constrictive pericarditis ■ Mitral stenosis

Acceptability to patient
- The relief of symptoms is paramount for many patients
- Excessive dosage of nitrates can cause headache and/or postural hypotension and even syncope

Follow up plan
- Monitor drug's effectiveness, and ensure that patient is receiving a dose that is effective yet is not causing side-effects
- The proper dosage is impossible to forecast for any individual patient

Patient and caregiver information
- Patient should be aware of possible light-headedness and/or headache, and instructed to reduce the dosage if either of these symptoms should occur
- Avoid drinking alcohol
- Sildenafil should never be taken in conjunction with nitrates – the interaction can be fatal

Surgical therapy

VALVE REPLACEMENT OR REPAIR

Efficacy
- Usually reverses heart failure in patients who develop heart failure because of impaired valvular function
- Comparisons of survival with and without mitral valve surgery were carried out in the 1970s, and surgical treatment was clearly superior to continued medical management
- Aortic stenosis as the cause of congestive heart failure is always fatal, usually within 1 year. Thus valve replacement is the only therapy that can prolong the duration and quality of life in this situation
- Valve surgery undertaken for either severe aortic insufficiency or severe mitral insufficiency results in clinical improvement

Risks/Benefits
Risk: Depends on the specific type of valve surgery and comorbid conditions.

Benefits:
- Reversal of heart failure
- Prolongation of life

Evidence
Evidence for mitral valve replacement and repair is available.

Acceptability to patient
Patients may be fearful of surgery but aware of the need for treatment.

Follow up plan
Supervised by surgeon.

Patient and caregiver information
Patient should understand the life-saving potential of surgery.

CARDIAC TRANSPLANTATION
Efficacy
Provides good quality of life for appropriate patients.

Risks/Benefits
Benefit: potentially life-saving; however, this option is limited by the donor heart supply.

Acceptability to patient
Some patients may reject this option.

Follow up plan
Monitoring should be supervised by a cardiac surgeon and cardiologist.

Patient and caregiver information
Patient should receive extensive counseling about the decision to undergo this procedure and about survival after the procedure.

LIFESTYLE
- Moderate exercise for ambulatory patients
- Reduced salt intake (2–3g sodium/day)
- Avoid NSAIDs
- Wear support stockings to reduce edema when venous insufficiency is also present
- Check weight daily: patient should have a target weight and should contact physician if weight gain exceeds 3lb/week
- Alcohol consumption should be markedly limited

RISKS/BENEFITS
- Risk: NSAIDs cause fluid retention and may interact with ACE inhibitors to impair renal function

Benefits:
- Moderate exercise: prevents physical deconditioning and improves endothelial function, resulting in less vasoconstriction
- Salt restriction: reduces fluid retention

- Support stockings help enhance venous return and reduce edema due to venous stasis
- Daily weighing provides an excellent signal of excess fluid retention; fluid retention may be a sign of dietary indiscretion, improper use of diuretics, or possible worsening cardiac function

ACCEPTABILITY TO PATIENT

Patients need the above information to be reinforced at each visit and with written materials.

FOLLOW UP PLAN

- Patient should be monitored to assess compliance
- Weigh patient at each visit

PATIENT AND CAREGIVER INFORMATION

- Patients should understand the reason for salt restriction
- They should know that moderate exercise helps rather than harms the heart, although strenuous exercise such as lifting excessive weight may be harmful
- Patients should be advised to contact their physician if weight gain exceeds 3lb/week

EFFICACY OF THERAPIES

Evidence

- Angiotensin-converting enzyme (ACE) inhibitors reduce mortality rates compared with placebo for patients with New York Heart Association (NYHA) class II heart failure or worse. Similar benefits are seen with different ACE inhibitors [6] *Level M*
- Patients with heart failure or left ventricular dysfunction have significantly reduced mortality rates, readmission for heart failure, and ischemic events when treated with ACE inhibitors. The benefits begin soon after the start of therapy and persist long-term [7] *Level M*
- Systematic reviews have shown angiotensin II receptor antagonists are as effective as ACE inhibitors in reducing all-cause mortality [9] *Level M*
- Beta-blockers are effective in reducing death or hospitalization in patients with heart failure secondary to idiopathic dilated cardiomyopathy or ischemic heart disease. Trials of patients following acute myocardial infarction were excluded from this systematic review [10] *Level M*
- RCTs have found that the addition of beta-blockers to ACE inhibitors in people with heart failure reduces mortality rates [11–13] *Level P*
- Spironolactone has been shown to be effective when added to an ACE inhibitor in patients with severe heart failure. Reduction of mortality rates and frequency of hospitalization due to heart failure, and a significant symptomatic improvement, has been found with spironolactone [14] *Level P*
- A systematic review found that digitalis reduced hospitalization for worsening heart failure, although a reduction in mortality rate was not achieved [15] *Level P*
- There is no evidence to support the use of calcium channel blockers for the treatment of heart failure [17]
- Prescribed exercise training improves functional capacity and quality of life in people with heart failure. The rate of adverse cardiac events may also be reduced [17] *Level P*

Review period

6 months.

PROGNOSIS

- Prognosis depends on severity of illness and underlying cause of congestive heart failure. The overall 5-year mortality rate is approximately 50%
- For patients with diastolic heart failure and preserved left ventricular systolic function, the annual mortality rate is 3–11%. Mortality rate is highest among the elderly and among patients with coexisting coronary artery disease
- For patients with systolic heart failure, left ventricular ejection fraction is a prognostic indicator. Patients with an ejection fraction below 20% have a predicted 3-year mortality rate of nearly 50%, and those with an ejection fraction of 30–35% have a predicted 3-year mortality rate of about 25%
- Cardiac transplantation has a 5-year survival rate in excess of 70% at many centers

Clinical pearl(s)

- Always search for underlying causes of congestive heart failure that are remedial. Examples are thyrotoxicosis, myocardial ischemia, and undetected valvular disease or valvular disease that is more severe than evidenced by the clinical examination
- Exacerbations of congestive heart failure are not always due to worsening of the underlying heart disease. Other factors that are often relevant are major psychosocial stresses, depression, and anemia

Therapeutic failure

Refer to specialist if patient fails to show improvement.

Deterioration

Refer to specialist or hospitalize if necessary.

Terminal illness

Refer to specialist. Help patient optimize daily quality of life.

COMPLICATIONS

- Death
- Anorexia, weight loss, and malnutrition
- A cycle of inactivity leading to deconditioning, which further reduces activities

CONSIDER CONSULT

- Clinical deterioration or failure to improve with treatment
- Patient is a candidate for cardiac surgery or transplantation
- Patients with progression of symptoms despite standard therapies

PREVENTION

RISK FACTORS

- Coronary artery disease and myocardial infarction
- Hypertension
- Excessive alcohol consumption
- Obesity and diabetes mellitus type II

MODIFY RISK FACTORS

- For prevention of coronary artery disease: low-fat diet, regular exercise, and smoking cessation
- Identify and treat hypertension
- Avoid smoking cigarettes
- Weight reduction and exercise both decrease the incidence of diabetes
- Weight reduction, salt restriction, and exercise all reduce blood pressure and the incidence of hypertension

Lifestyle and wellness

TOBACCO

Cigarette smoking is a risk factor for coronary artery disease, which in turn can result in congestive heart failure.

ALCOHOL AND DRUGS

Alcohol and cocaine are associated with increased risk of congestive heart failure.

DIET

A low-fat diet is important to prevention of coronary artery disease.

PHYSICAL ACTIVITY

Regular exercise is a deterrent of hypertension, diabetes, and coronary artery disease.

FAMILY HISTORY

Family history of heart attack or dilated cardiomyopathy may increase a person's risk of developing congestive heart failure.

SCREENING

- Screening is not appropriate in asymptomatic patients
- Patients at high risk of congestive heart failure include the elderly, those with prior myocardial infarction, and those with poorly controlled hypertension
- It is probable that in the near future we will be able to screen such individuals with an inexpensive blood assay for brain natriuretic peptide

BRAIN NATRIURETIC PEPTIDE (BNP)

Cost/efficacy

- Current data indicate a high diagnostic accuracy for congestive heart failure
- When this test is applied to high-risk populations, such as patients presenting with dyspnea to an emergency department, the cost/efficacy ratio is favorable

PREVENT RECURRENCE

Always be sure there is not an underlying cardiac condition that can be fully corrected.

Reassess coexisting disease

- For coexisting renal or pulmonary disease, referral to a specialist is appropriate
- In patients with diabetes mellitus, increased control of glucose may be advisable
- Even mild anemia worsens congestive heart failure. From 30% to 40% of functional class III and IV patients have concomitant anemia. Referral to a hematologist may be needed, particularly if the cause of the anemia is an erythropoietin deficiency

ASSOCIATIONS

American Heart Association
7272 Greenville Avenue
Dallas, TX 75231
Tel: (800) 242-8721
www.americanheart.org

American College of Cardiology
Heart House
9111 Old Georgetown Road
Bethesda, MD 20814-1699
Tel: (800) 253-4636
Fax: (301) 897-9745
www.acc.org

KEY REFERENCES

- Chavey WE II, Blaum CS, Bleske BE, et al. Guideline for the management of heart failure caused by systolic dysfunction: Part I. Guideline development, etiology and diagnosis. Am Fam Physician 2001;64:769–74
- Chavey WE II , Blaum CS, Bleske BE, et al. Guideline for the management of heart failure caused by systolic dysfunction: Part II. Treatment. Am Fam Physician 2001;64:1045–54
- Spencer KT, Lang RM. Diastolic heart failure: what primary care physicians need to know. Postgrad Med 1997;101:63–73
- Shamsham F, Mitchell J. Essentials of the diagnosis of heart failure. Am Fam Physician 2000;61:1319–28
- Chavey WE II. The importance of beta blockers in the treatment of congestive heart failure. Am Fam Physician 2000;62:2453–62
- Morelli V, Zoorob R. Alternative therapies: Part II. Congestive heart failure and hypercholesterolemia. Am Fam Physician 2000;62:1325–30
- Baker DW, Hayes RP, Massie BM, Craig CA. Variations in family physicians' and cardiologists' care for patients with heart failure. Am Heart J 1999;138:826–34
- Stevenson LW, Braunwald E. Recognition and management of patients with heart failure. In: Goldman L, Braunwald E, eds. Primary cardiology. Philadelphia: WB Saunders, 1998
- Packer M, O'Connor CM, Ghali JK, et al. Effect of amlodipine on morbidity and mortality on severe chronic heart failure. Prospcctive Randomized Amlodipine Survival Evaluation Study Group. N Engl J Med 1996;335:1107–14. Reviewed in: Clinical Evidence 2001;6:50–69
- Gheorghiade M, Benatar D, Konstam MA, et al. Pharmacotherapy for systolic dysfunction: a review of randomized clinical trials. Am J Cardiol 1997;80(Suppl 8B):14–27H

Evidence references and guidelines

1 Guidelines for the evaluation and management of heart failure: report of the American College of Cardiology/American Heart Association Task Force on Practice Guidelines (Committee on Evaluation and Management of Heart Failure). Circulation 1995;92:2764–84. J Am Coll Cardiol 1995;26:1376–98. Available at the National Guidelines Clearinghouse

2 Shamsham F, Mitchell J. Essentials for the diagnosis of heart failure. Am Fam Physician 2000;61:1319–28

3 Chavey WE, Blaum CS, Bleske BE, et al. Guideline for the management of heart failure caused by systolic dysfunction: Part I. Guideline development, etiology and diagnosis. Am Fam Physician 2001;64:769–74

4 Chavey WE, Blaum CS, Bleske BE, et al. Guideline for the management of heart failure caused by systolic dysfunction: Part II. Treatment. Am Fam Physician 2001;64:1045–54

5 Hoyt RE, Bowling LS. Reducing readmissions for congestive heart failure. Am Fam Physician 2001;63:1593–8

6 Garg R, Yusuf S. Overview of randomized trials of angiotensin-converting enzyme inhibitors on mortality and morbidity in patients with heart failure. Collaborative Group on ACE Inhibitor Trials. JAMA 1995;273:1450–6. Reviewed in: Clinical Evidence 2001;6:50–69

7 Flather M, Yusuf S, Kober L, et al. Long-term ACE-inhibitor therapy in patients with heart failure or left-ventricular dysfunction: a systematic overview of data from individual patients. The ACE-inhibitor Myocardial Infarction Collaborative Group. Lancet 2000;355:1575–81. Reviewed in: Clinical Evidence 2001;6:50–69

8 Heart Outcome Prevention Evaluation Study Investigators. Effects of angiotensin-converting enzyme inhibitor, ramipril, on cardiovascular events in high risk patients. N Engl J Med 2000;342:145–53. Reviewed in: Clinical Evidence 2001;6:50–69
9 McKelvie R, Yusuf S, Pericak D, et al. Comparison of candesartan, enalapril, and their combination in congestive heart failure: randomized evaluation of strategies for left ventricular dysfunction (RESOLVD pilot study). Circulation 1999;100:1056–64. Reviewed in: Clinical Evidence 2001;6:50–69
10 Lechat P, Packer M, Chalon S, et al. Clinical effects of beta-adrenergic blockade in chronic heart failure: a meta-analysis of double-blind, placebo-controlled, randomized trials. Circulation 1998;98:1184–91. Reviewed in: Clinical Evidence 2001;6:50–69
11 CIBIS-II Investigators and Committees. The cardiac insufficiency bisoprolol study II (CIBIS II): a randomized trial. Lancet 1999;353:9–13. Reviewed in: Clinical Evidence 2001;6:50–69
12 Effect of metoprolol CR/XL in chronic heart failure: Metoprolol CR/XL Randomized Intervention Trial in Congestive Heart Failure (MERIT-HF). Lancet 1999;353:2001–7. Reviewed in: Clinical Evidence 2001;6:50–69
13 Packer M, Bristow MR, Cohn JN, et al. The effect of carvedilol on morbidity and mortality in patients with chronic heart failure. US Carvedilol Heart Failure Study Group. N Engl J Med 1996;334:349–55. Medline
14 Pitt B, Zannad F, Remme WJ, et al. The effects of spironolactone on morbidity and mortality in patients with severe heart failure. Randomized Aldactone Evaluation Study Investigators. N Engl J Med 1999;341:709–17. Reviewed in: Clinical Evidence 2001;6:50–69
15 Hood WB Jr, Dans AL, Guyatt GH, et al. Digitalis for treatment of congestive heart failure in patients in sinus rhythm (Cochrane Review). In: The Cochrane Library, 1, 2002. Oxford: Update Software
16 Digitalis Investigation Group. The effect of digoxin on mortality and morbidity in patients with heart failure. N Engl J Med 1997;336:525–33. Reviewed in: Clinical Evidence 2001;6:50–69
17 McKelvie R. Heart failure: Cardiovascular disorders. Reviewed in: Clinical Evidence 2001;6:50–69. London: BMJ Publishing Group

FAQS

Question 1

What should be the first therapeutic steps for a patient in severe respiratory distress?

ANSWER 1

A full set of vital signs should be followed by a quick lung examination. If rales and wheezes are heard, sublingual nitroglycerin may be very effective in temporizing while transport to a hospital can be arranged. Intravenous dobutamine can also be administered in a dose of 2.5–5.0mcg/kg/min.

Question 2

Should patients with congestive heart failure be allowed to travel?

ANSWER 2

These patients are at higher risk of deep vein thrombosis. If they need to travel, frequent stops and short walks should be taken to avoid acute thrombosis.

Question 3

Should all patients with new-onset congestive heart failure undergo cardiac catheterization?

ANSWER 3

This is controversial. If the systolic function is segmentally depressed or moderately depressed globally, many cardiologists recommend angiography to screen for correctable coronary artery disease. If the systolic function is severely depressed, this recommendation is less well supported because few therapeutic options exist.

Question 4
When should a patient be admitted to the hospital?

ANSWER 4
Usually, hospital admissions occur at times of clinical symptom decompensation; however, it is often better to admit the patient before he/she acutely decompensates. Good clues are rapid weight gain (>4lb in 2–3 days), rising creatinine or blood urea nitrogen levels, worsening edema not responsive to increased oral furosemide, concomitant illness (e.g. influenza, bleeding). Several days in the hospital for a tune-up at this stage may prevent an emergent admission (and the patient anxiety associated with an acute decompensation).

Question 5
How often should I check the echocardiogram?

ANSWER 5
If the patient's symptoms are stable, once every 1–2 years is appropriate. If clinical changes occur, the echo should be repeated. In valvular disease, more frequent echocardiograms may be indicated (in conjunction with cardiology consultation).

CONTRIBUTORS
Randolph L Pearson, MD
John McB Hodgson, MD, FACC, FSCAI
Robert C Bahler, MD

HYPERLIPIDEMIA

SUMMARY INFORMATION

DESCRIPTION

- A group of disorders characterized by an excess of serum cholesterol, triglycerides, and lipoproteins
- Familial hyperlipidemias determined genetically
- Diseases, inappropriate diet, and hyperlipidemic drugs can be associated with hyperlipidemia
- Hyperlipidemia is an important risk factor for atherosclerosis and coronary heart disease
- Total serum cholesterol: <200mg/dL is 'desirable,' 201–239mg/dL is 'borderline high,' >240mg/dL is 'high'
- Evidence states that a reduction of total cholesterol by 25% reduces the progression of coronary atherosclerosis

KEY! DON'T MISS!

Patients with relatives diagnosed with hypercholesterolemia, with familial hyperlipidemia, or with atherosclerosis should be screened for hyperlipidemia.

BACKGROUND

ICD9 CODE
272.4 Hyperlipidemia.

SYNONYMS
- High blood cholesterol
- High blood triglycerides
- Hypercholesterolemia
- Hypertriglyceridemia

CARDINAL FEATURES
- A group of disorders characterized by an excess of serum cholesterol, triglycerides, and lipoproteins
- Familial hyperlipidemia is determined genetically
- Hyperlipidemia can be associated with disease, inappropriate diet, hyperlipidemic drugs, including corticosteroids and beta-blockers
- Associated diseases include insulin-dependent diabetes mellitus, non-insulin dependent diabetes mellitus, hypothyroidism, Cushing's syndrome
- Hyperlipidemia is an important risk factor for atherosclerosis and coronary heart disease
- Total serum cholesterol: <200mg/dL is 'desirable,' 201–239mg/dL is 'borderline high,' >240mg/dL is 'high'
- Evidence states that a reduction of total cholesterol by 25% reduces the progression of coronary atherosclerosis

CAUSES
Common causes
- Abnormal regulation of low-density lipoprotein (LDL) receptors, which is aggravated by: excess of saturated fats in the diet, obesity, sedentary lifestyle
- May be genetically inherited with polygenetic factors

Rare causes
- Familial combined hypercholesterolemia with raised lipids and cholesterol
- Familial hypercholesterolemia with raised cholesterol
- Familial hypertriglyceridemia where triglycerides are markedly raised and cholesterol is mild to moderately raised
- Remnant hyperlipoproteinemia with marked combined hyperlipidemia
- Lipoprotein lipase deficiency with extremely raised triglycerides and moderately raised cholesterol

Serious causes
Homozygous familial hypercholesterolemia.

Contributory or predisposing factors
- Insulin-dependent diabetes mellitus
- Noninsulin-dependent diabetes mellitus
- Hypothyroidism
- Cushing's syndrome
- Certain types of renal failure
- Drugs, including oral contraceptives, hormones, corticosteroids, certain diuretics, and beta-blockers

Dietary causes include:
- Fat intake per total calories greater than 40%
- Saturated fat intake per total calories greater than 10%
- Cholesterol intake greater than 300mg per day
- Habitual excessive alcohol use, obesity

EPIDEMIOLOGY
Demographics
AGE
- Total and LDL cholesterol rise about 20% in males between 20 and 50 years of age
- Total and LDL cholesterol rise steadily about 30% in females between 20 and 60 years of age
- Younger females have lower levels than males
- Homozygous familial hypercholesterolemia manifests itself from birth

GENDER
Incidence is higher among men than women.

RACE
- Total cholesterol and LDL levels are similar in caucasians and African-Americans
- Triglycerides are lower, and high-density lipoprotein (HDL) levels are higher in the African-American population
- Ethnicity determines absolute risk of coronary disease for given levels of cholesterol
- Asian-Indians have the highest risk
- Chinese have the lowest risk
- Europeans have an intermediate risk

GENETICS
- Familial combined hyperlipidemia: 3/1000; inheritance is likely to involve multiple genetic etiologies
- Familial hypercholesterolemia: heterozygotes (2/1000 people) and homozygotes (1/1,000,000) with gene inherited as an autosomal dominant defect
- Familial hypertriglyceridemia: 1/1000, most likely inherited as an autosomal dominant defect
- Lipoprotein lipase deficiency: a very rare autosomal recessive condition

GEOGRAPHY
- Differences in mean levels of plasma lipids for different populations around the world and within different ethnic groups in North America
- Differences in plasma lipid levels can be partly explained by dietary and lifestyle differences

SOCIOECONOMIC STATUS
- Awareness of dietary factors that affect plasma lipid levels increases with higher educational levels
- Low-cost food items are often higher in saturated fats and lower in nutritional value

DIFFERENTIAL DIAGNOSIS

- Lipid metabolism is altered in a number of physiologic and pathologic conditions
- Secondary hyperlipidemia causes include glycogen storage disease types I and II

Diabetes mellitus

- Hyperglycemia resulting from imbalance between glucose levels and insulin activity
- The types are known as insulin-dependent diabetes mellitus (type I) and noninsulin-dependent diabetes mellitus (type II)
- Due to multiple causes

FEATURES

- A significant number of diabetics have raised plasma triglycerides
- Type I diabetics typically have normal lipid values if controlled
- Type I diabetics may have an underlying lipid abnormality
- Type II diabetics frequently have elevated cholesterol and triglyceride levels
- Abnormal lipoprotein composition is seen even in patients with normal cholesterol and triglyceride levels
- Oral glucose tolerance test under standard conditions differentiates diabetes mellitus from impaired glucose tolerance

Obesity

- Body mass index is >25
- Prevalence rising rapidly throughout the world

FEATURES

- In obese patients with mild glucose intolerance, hyperlipidemia may be due to triglyceride and very-low-density lipoprotein (VLDL) over-production
- HDL levels are generally low in obese patients
- Weight reduction improves glucose tolerance and reduces insulin resistance and triglyceride levels
- Glucose intolerance, hypertension, gout, high triglyceride levels, and low HDL levels are diagnostic of metabolic 'syndrome X,' leading to a high risk of atherosclerotic disease

Hypothyroidism

Hypothyroidism is caused by inadequate secretion of thyroid hormone.

FEATURES

- Results in a rise in circulating low-density lipoprotein (LDL) and total cholesterol levels secondary to LDL-receptor downregulation
- May also cause high triglyceride levels
- May also result in marked hyperlipidemia if it occurs in genetically disposed people
- There is usually a rapid fall in lipid levels in response to treatment with thyroxine

Chronic renal failure

- Progressive decrease in renal function >3 months
- Leads to subsequent accumulation of waste products

FEATURES

- Raised levels of plasma triglycerides, LDL, and intermediate-density lipoprotein (IDL) cholesterol occur in chronic renal failure due to decreased triglyceride lipolysis and remnant clearance
- VLDL production may be increased, but HDL levels tend to be low

- Cardiovascular disease is a frequent complication in patients receiving hemodialysis partly due to hyperlipidemia
- The lipoprotein abnormalities often disappear after successful renal transplantation
- Hyperlipidemia may persist if the patient has to remain on high doses of corticosteroids
- Drug treatment must be adjusted for renal function impairment

Liver disease

Liver disease can be due to various causes and leads to metabolic abnormalities.

FEATURES

- Severe liver disease is accompanied by various disorders of lipid metabolism
- The lipoproteins may be of abnormal composition, such as lipoprotein X
- Plasma triglycerides may be raised
- HDL levels are often low
- Underlying alcohol abuse must be considered because it is under-reported
- All of these changes may be fully reversible if the inflammatory liver disease has not progressed to cirrhosis

Nephrotic syndrome

Characterized by high protein excretion, peripheral edema, and metabolic abnormalities.

FEATURES

- The causes of this hyperlipidemia are unclear
- Overproduction of VLDLs and LDLs seems to occur, and their plasma levels are usually raised
- HDL level may be very low if urinary losses are high
- The subfraction of HDLs, which is inversely related to coronary heart disease risk, is particularly reduced
- Low cholesterol levels may be a marker of poor prognosis
- The diet advised for a patient with nephrotic syndrome and severe hyperlipidemia will need to be specially designed for the individual patient
- Drug treatment must be adjusted for renal function

SIGNS & SYMPTOMS

Signs

- Familial hypercholesterolemia is characterized by xanthomas on the extensor tendons of the hands, the Achilles tendons, and at the insertion of the patella tendon
- Corneal arcus commonly occurs in familial and other types of hypercholesterolemia
- Half arcus in a young person is very suggestive of familial hypercholesterolemia
- Xanthelasma may be found in patients with normal cholesterol as well as with familial or common hypercholesterolemias

Symptoms

There are no symptoms of hyperlipidemia.

ASSOCIATED DISORDERS

- Atherosclerosis
- Coronary artery disease

KEY! DON'T MISS!

Patients with relatives diagnosed with hypercholesterolemia, with familial hyperlipidemia, or with atherosclerosis should be screened for hyperlipidemia.

CONSIDER CONSULT

- Patients diagnosed with familial hypercholesterolemia
- Patients with comorbidities that would complicate treatment
- Patients known or suspected to suffer from significant clinical atherosclerosis should be referred to a vascular specialist for determination of disease progression and possible surgical intervention. However, dietary therapy (and in some cases drug treatment) should begin immediately

INVESTIGATION OF THE PATIENT

Direct questions to patient

- Q **Have you ever had your blood cholesterol level checked?** Patients may have already been tested for their cholesterol level. If the level was high, ask whether they have started treatment of any kind
- Q **Do you smoke?** This is an important risk factor for coronary artery disease
- Q **Do you have high blood pressure?** Hypertension is another important risk factor for coronary artery disease

Contributory or predisposing factors

- Q **Have you been diagnosed with pancreatitis, diabetes, hypothyroidism, Cushing's disease, or renal disease?** These medical conditions may predispose to high cholesterol levels
- Q **Are you pregnant?** Pregnancy can be associated with hyperlipidemia
- Q **Do you drink alcohol at all, and, if so, how much?** Alcohol use can contribute to hyperlipidemia. It is important to establish the quantity and type of alcohol consumed as well as how often
- Q **What are the compositions of your typical meals?** Diets that are high in fat can lead to hyperlipidemia. It is important to establish dietary habits so that modification can be used if required
- Q **Do you exercise, and what is your occupation?** A sedentary lifestyle can contribute to obesity, which may be associated with hyperlipidemia
- Q **Are you taking any medication?** Several common medications can contribute to hyperlipidemia. These include the oral contraceptive pill, hormones, steroids, as well as some diuretics and beta-blockers

Family history

- Q **Does anyone in your family (including parents, uncles, aunts, brothers, or sisters) have high cholesterol or fat levels in their blood?** It is important to establish whether there is any familial tendency toward hyperlipidemia
- Q **Does anyone in your family suffer from heart disease, hypertension, or diabetes?** It is important to establish absolute risk for coronary artery disease by assessing all known risk factors

Examination

- **Is the patient obese?** Obesity, high-fat diet, and a sedentary lifestyle can contribute to hyperlipidemia
- **Does the patient present with xanthomas, corneal arcus, xanthelasmas?** Check the patient for signs of familial hyperlipidemia
- **Check the blood pressure, palpate for heart enlargement, and listen for murmurs or bruits.** Examine for signs of cardiovascular disease. It is of paramount importance to assess the other cardiovascular risk factors as well as hyperlipidemia
- **Check the patient's blood sugar level?** Diabetics may have raised lipids if their diabetes is poorly controlled, and diabetes is also a major risk factor for coronary heart disease (CHD)

Summary of investigative tests

- Fasting or nonfasting cholesterol and triglyceride levels. Both these tests are essential for differential diagnosis of hyperlipidemia
- Screening can be done in the nonfasting state and should include measurements of total cholesterol and HDL concentrations

DIAGNOSTIC DECISION

- Diagnosis is made by finding elevated lipid levels in the blood
- There are four major classes of lipoproteins, and each must be quantified in order to distinguish between type of lipid disorder
- Triglyceride
- Chylomicrons (principally triglyceride)
- VLDL (principally triglyceride)
- HDL (principally phospholipid – inversely associated with CHD)
- LDLs are principally made up of cholesterol and are most strongly associated with CHD
- Secondary hyperlipidemia needs to be excluded
- Characterization of the primary hyperlipidemia is needed
- A precise diagnosis is essential for correct prognosis, genetic counseling, life-long diet, and drug treatments

CLINICAL PEARL(S)

- Children of patients with cardiovascular atherosclerosis need lipid levels tested
- Aim to distinguish primary from secondary hyperlipidemias because the former has a greatly increased risk of cardiovascular disease

THE TESTS

Body fluids

FASTING TRIGLYCERIDE LEVEL

Description

- The patient should have fasted for 12h
- Two or three lipid analyses are needed because of the biologic variation observed within individuals
- Blood sampling techniques and the use of plasma samples (plasma levels are 3–4% lower than serum samples) should be standardized to aid consistency of results
- Venous blood sample

Advantages/Disadvantages

- Advantage: quick, easy, and cheap
- Disadvantage: can have false-negative or false-positive result

Normal

- 100–190mg/dL (0.11–2.2mmol/L)
- Normal values are dependent on age

Abnormal

- >190mg/dL (>2.2mmol/L)
- Keep in mind the possibility of a falsely abnormal result

Cause of abnormal result

Greater than normal levels may indicate:

- Cirrhosis
- Familial hyperlipoproteinemia (rare)
- Hypothyroidism

- Low protein in diet and high carbohydrates
- Poorly controlled diabetes mellitus
- Nephrotic syndrome
- Pancreatitis

Lower than normal levels may indicate:
- Malabsorption syndrome
- Malnutrition
- Hyperthyroidism
- Low-fat diet

Drugs, disorders, and other factors that may alter results
- Pregnancy is usually associated with elevated cholesterol level
- Drugs that can increase triglyceride levels include cholestyramine, estrogen, oral contraceptives, beta-blockers, thiazide diuretics
- Drugs that can decrease triglyceride levels include ascorbic acid (vitamin C), asparaginase, lipid-lowering medication

CHOLESTEROL LEVEL

Description
- Individuals with clinical CHD should proceed to a full lipid profile
- The patient should have fasted and should not have exercised for 12h, and should sit for 5min before the blood sample is drawn
- Levels should be obtained 1 month apart and the average calculated
- Lipid profile is recommended for initial assessment of diabetics and hypertensives
- Venous blood sample

Advantages/Disadvantages
- Advantages: quick, easy, and cheap
- Disadvantage: can have false-negative or false-positive result

Normal
- Normal values tend to increase with age
- Premenopausal women have lower levels than men of the same age
- Total cholesterol of less than 200mg/dL (5.2mmol/L) is desirable
- For cholesterol in HDL, the recommended value is greater than 45mg/dL
- Cholesterol in LDL should be less than 130mg/dL

Abnormal
- Total cholesterol of 200–239mg/dL is borderline high and >240mg/dL is high
- Cholesterol in HDL <40mg/dL is low and >60mg/dL is high
- Cholesterol in LDL 130–159mg/dL is borderline high and >160mg/dL is high
- Keep in mind the possibility of a falsely abnormal result

Cause of abnormal result

Increased levels may indicate:
- Biliary cirrhosis
- Familial hyperlipidemias
- High-cholesterol diet
- Hypothyroidism
- Nephrotic syndrome
- Uncontrolled diabetes

Decreased levels may indicate:
- Hyperthyroidism
- Liver disease
- Malabsorption
- Pernicious anemia
- Sepsis

Drugs, disorders, and other factors that may alter results
- Pregnancy is usually associated with elevated cholesterol levels
- Oophorectomy may increase cholesterol levels
- Drugs that may increase cholesterol levels include adrenocorticotrophic hormone (ACTH), anabolic steroids, beta-blockers, corticosteroids, epinephrine, oral contraceptives, phenytoin, sulfonamides, thiazide diuretics, vitamin D
- Drugs that may decrease cholesterol levels include allopurinol, androgens, captopril, chlorpropamide, erythromycin, isoniazid, monoamine oxidase inhibitors (MAOIs), neomycin, niacin, dietary nitrates

IMMEDIATE ACTION

- Patients who are obese or have any of the clear risk factors for hyperlipidemia should be placed on dietary therapy immediately
- Patients with known coronary artery disease and high low-density lipoprotein level (>130mg/dL) should be considered for early drug therapy

PATIENT AND CAREGIVER ISSUES

Impact on career, dependants, family, friends

- If one parent has familial hypercholesterolemia, there is a 50% chance that any children will inherit the gene and have the condition. The risk is probably the same in familial combined hyperlipidemia
- In families with familial combined hyperlipidemia, testing should not be performed until the offspring are in their late teens or early twenties
- Although heterozygous familial hypercholesterolemia can often be diagnosed at birth, testing between 4 and 6 years of age is more sensible. The results should be interpreted by someone with experience in diagnosis of this condition in children

Patient or caregiver request

- **What is cholesterol?** It is a fat that is carried in the bloodstream
- **What is coronary heart disease?** Narrowing of the blood vessels that supply the heart muscle
- **What is the difference between the types of hypercholesterolemia?** The common form is much more prevalent than the familial form. The mode of inheritance of familial hypercholesterolemia is known, whereas the common form has polygenetic inheritance. Most importantly, familial hypercholesterolemia has a much higher risk of coronary vessel disease
- **How can I tell if I have familial hypercholesterolemia?** High cholesterol is asymptomatic. You may have xanthomata, which are cholesterol deposits under the skin, commonly on tendons, elbows, and knees
- **Can the risk of heart attacks be removed or reduced if blood cholesterol can be lowered?** The risk of heart attacks can be decreased by reducing cholesterol
- **What if diet alone is not enough to lower my blood cholesterol to normal?** If a fat-reduced diet fails to control cholesterol levels adequately, there are medications that can be used
- **Is there any proof that lowering cholesterol will help prevent heart attacks?** Yes. There are several clinical trials that show that lowering cholesterol decreases the risk of heart attack
- **Why can't I continue to smoke?** Smoking is a major risk factor for coronary artery disease
- **Can I still drink alcohol?** Yes you can, but in moderation. Alcohol is high in fat and calories, so intake should be limited. Ideally, consume one glass of red wine or equivalent per day
- **Is it safe to exercise?** Yes. Exercise helps burn fat and promote a healthier lipid profile by increasing high-density lipoprotein (HDL) or 'good' cholesterol levels

Health-seeking behavior

- What sort of exercise do you engage in and how often?
- Have you tried modifying your diet to eat less fat?
- Have you tried to stop smoking?
- Have you tried to modify your drinking habits?

MANAGEMENT ISSUES

Goals

- Reduce the risk of atherosclerosis and cardiovascular disease by lowering blood lipid levels
- Dietary modification is the initial step in treatment
- For overweight individuals, weight reduction to ideal body weight is recommended
- Reduction in total calories, cholesterol, and saturated fat is recommended for most individuals
- If there is no improvement in lipid blood levels within 2 months of maximal dietary modification, drug therapy is generally initiated

Management in special circumstances

- Secondary causes of hyperlipidemia (e.g. uncontrolled diabetes mellitus) should be brought under control as much as possible
- Measure lipids again after several weeks to diagnose persisting secondary hyperlipidemia

COEXISTING DISEASE

The following conditions need to be optimally treated to reduce hyperlipidemia, and regular lipid analysis is required:

- Diabetes mellitus
- Hypothyroidism
- Obesity
- Nephrotic syndrome and chronic renal insufficiency
- Biliary obstruction
- Myeloma
- Acute intermittent porphyria

Diabetes:

- Control of insulin-dependent diabetes mellitus with insulin restores lipoprotein lipase activity. Triglyceride levels fall, and any eruptive xanthomas disappear
- Patients with noninsulin-dependent diabetes mellitus are at especially high risk of cardiovascular disease, and some sources recommend managing lipid levels the same as for a patient with known coronary artery disease

Hypothyroidism:

- There is usually a rapid fall in lipid levels in response to treatment with thyroxine.

Chronic renal failure:

- Cardiovascular disease is one of the most frequent complications of hemodialysis, and hyperlipidemia may be an important risk factor in patients receiving this treatment
- Lipoprotein abnormalities often disappear after successful renal transplantation
- Lipoprotein abnormalities often persist if patient's therapy includes remaining on high doses of corticosteroids

Liver disease:

- In many cases changes in lipid levels due to inflammatory liver disease are fully reversible when the cause, such as excessive alcohol consumption, is controlled
- The amount of alcohol required significantly to alter plasma lipid levels varies between individuals

Nephrotic syndrome:

- The diet advised for a patient with nephrotic syndrome and severe hyperlipidemia will need to be specially designed for the individual patient in conjunction with the nephrologist and dietitian
- Drug therapy for a patient with nephrotic syndrome must be adjusted for renal function if excreted by the kidneys, e.g. doses of fibrate drugs must be reduced

COEXISTING MEDICATION

- Some drugs used in treating the hypertension that often accompanies hyperlipidemia may raise plasma lipid levels, including prazosin, calcium antagonists, thiazides, nitrates, and angiotensin-converting enzyme (ACE) inhibitors
- Check lipid levels before starting antihypertensive treatment, or prescribe drugs that do not affect lipid levels
- Steroids or oral contraceptives tend to raise plasma lipid levels

- Advise patients with severe hyperlipidemia against long-term use of these drugs
- Sequestrants and fibric acid-derivatives potentiate the action of warfarin, so prothrombin times need to be monitored
- Estrogen lowers total and LDL cholesterol and increases HDL and triglycerides. Transdermal administration has minimal lipid effects

SPECIAL PATIENT GROUPS

- In women, lipid levels rise in the second half of pregnancy
- Long-term use of combined oral contraceptive preparations is contraindicated in patients with hyperlipidemia
- Preparations of oral contraceptives for short-term use can be designed to minimize their hyperlipidemic effects

PATIENT SATISFACTION/LIFESTYLE PRIORITIES

- Many of the side-effects of drugs prescribed for hyperlipidemia involve the gastrointestinal system
- Embarrassment or inconvenience in patients whose job or lifestyle would conflict with these side-effects must be weighed against the beneficial effects

SUMMARY OF THERAPEUTIC OPTIONS

Choices

- Dietary therapy specific for the type of hyperlipidemia is the initial treatment of choice. Excess body weight may be an important factor and should be addressed prior to any drug therapy
- Physical exercise can be an important ancillary measure
- Contributory disease such as hypothyroidism or diabetes mellitus should be looked for and adequately treated
- The use of drugs should be considered when reasonable attempts have been made to obtain satisfactory results with nonpharmaceutical methods. If the decision ultimately is to use drugs, the patient should be instructed that this does not reduce the importance of adhering to diet
- Cholesterol-lowering drug therapy should take into account coronary risk factors, including age, sex, smoking, hypertension, cardiovascular events, diabetes mellitus, and positive family history of premature coronary artery disease
- The efficacy, safety, and compliance factors for each of the cholesterol-lowering drugs is important when selecting the most appropriate for an individual patient
- The type of drug chosen depends on the type of lipoprotein elevated in the plasma
- There are several choices of medications as listed below, but if there is no response to a drug after 2–3 months of therapy, it should be discontinued
- The main drug groups used in the treatment of hypercholesterolemia include: statins (3-hydroxy-3-methylglutaryl-coenzyme A [HMG-CoA] reductase inhibitors), anion-exchange resins, fibrates, nicotinic acid (niacin)
- Garlic, essential and omega-3 fatty acids, guglipid (*Commiphora molmol*), dietary fiber, and soy protein can help in lowering cholesterol and triglycerides

Guidelines:

- Second report of the Expert Panel on Detection, Evaluation, and Treatment of High Blood Cholesterol in Adults (Adult Treatment Panel II). Circulation 1994;89:1333–445. Available online at the National Guideline Clearinghouse and the National Heart, Lung, and Blood Institute [1]
- Barrie W, Harrison V, Khanderia U, et al. Screening and management of lipids. Ann Arbor (MI): University of Michigan 2000. Guidelines developed by the Lipid Therapy Guideline Team. Available online at the National Guidelines Clearinghouse [2]

Clinical pearl(s)

- Dietary changes may be very difficult to encourage in elderly patients
- Adequate overall nutrition may be more important than optimal control of cholesterol in some elderly patients. It is important to weigh the relative benefit of ensuring adequate nutrition for a person living alone who may not prepare adequate meals with the decreasing benefit of cholesterol control with aging

Never

Adult patients who probably have familial hyperlipidemia and may have narrowing of the coronary arteries without symptoms of heart disease should not be advised to take up sudden vigorous exercise.

DRUGS AND OTHER THERAPIES: DETAILS

Drugs

RESINS

- Cholestyramine and colestipol hydrochloride
- Indicated for elevated total cholesterol and LDL
- Acts by binding bile acids and preventing reabsorption. Increased excretion promotes hepatic conversion of cholesterol into bile acids. Also increases LDL receptor activity in the liver, which increases breakdown of LDL cholesterol

Dose

- Cholestyramine: 4–24g per day, single or divided doses to minimize potential side-effects. Recommended starting dose: 4g 1–2 times per day
- Colestipol hydrochloride: 2–16g per day, single or divided doses, with maximum dose 30g per day. Recommended starting dose: 2g 1–2 times per day. Maximum LDL lowering per unit of drug is seen at lower doses and decreases as the dose is increased
- Adjust dose gradually according to lipid/lipoprotein levels taken 4 weeks after initiation or titration of therapy.

Efficacy

- LDL decreases 15–30%
- HDL increases 3–5%
- Triglycerides usually not affected or may increase

Risks/Benefits

Risks:

- Use caution in pregnancy, breast-feeding, and children
- Use caution if patient is constipated
- Reduces the absorption of many other medications taken concomitantly

Benefits:

- Can lower LDL and decrease risk of coronary atherosclerosis
- Raising HDL levels can help induce regression of vessel disease

Side-effects and adverse reactions

- Gastrointestinal: constipation, nausea, vomiting, abdominal pain, peptic ulceration, bloating and flatulence, indigestion, heartburn, diarrhea
- CNS: dizziness, headache, tinnitus, vertigo
- Musculoskeletal: myalgia
- Skin: rashes
- Hematologic: bleeding

Interactions (other drugs)

- Acarbose ▪ Acetaminophen ▪ Cardiac glycosides ▪ Corticosteroids ▪ Diuretics ▪ Levothyroxine ▪ Methotrexate ▪ Oral anticoagulants ▪ Phenylbutazone ▪ Raloxifene ▪ Valproic acid ▪ Vancomycin

Contraindications

- Biliary obstruction (including primary biliary cirrhosis) ▪ Active liver disease or unexplained elevations of serum transaminases ▪ Significant renal disease ▪ Hypersensitivity ▪ Colestipol is contraindicated in pregnancy and breast-feeding

Evidence

Cholestyramine and colestipol are effective in the treatment of hyperlipidemia:

- They are especially useful for patients with moderately elevated LDL cholesterol, in primary prevention, and for young adult men and premenopausal women when required [1] *Level C*
- Bile acid sequestrants are a suitable alternative to statins for primary prevention treatment [2] *Level C*

Acceptability to patient

The predominantly gastrointestinal side-effects may cause poor compliance.

Follow up plan

- Plasma cholesterol levels should be determined frequently during the first few months of therapy and periodically thereafter
- Plasma triglyceride levels should be measured periodically to detect whether significant changes have occurred
- If the desired therapeutic effect is not obtained at 1–6 doses per day with good compliance and acceptable side-effects, combined therapy or alternate treatment should be considered
- Lifestyle issues of low-fat diet and exercise must be periodically reviewed

Patient and caregiver information

- Sipping or holding the resin suspension in the mouth for prolonged periods may lead to changes in the surface of the teeth, resulting in discoloration, erosion of enamel, or decay. Good oral hygiene should be maintained
- Never take treatment in its dry form
- Report serious side-effects to your doctor, such as black tarry bowel movements, severe stomach pain, severe nausea, vomiting, or constipation
- Patients should take other drugs at least 1h before or 4h after resins to minimize possible interference with their absorption

STATINS

- Some examples include pravastatin, simvastatin, and atorvastatin
- Inhibits cholesterol synthesis by inhibiting HMG-CoA reductase. Also acts to upregulate LDL receptors in liver
- More effective than other classes of drugs in reducing LDL
- Less effective than fibrates for reducing triglycerides and raising HDL
- The drug of choice in patients with a high risk of coronary artery disease, coronary artery bypass surgery, or angioplasty
- Also indicated for patients with other manifestations of vessel disease, such as nonhemorrhagic cerebrovascular accident, transient ischemic attacks, or peripheral vascular disease
- Also indicated for the treatment of heterozygous familial hypercholesterolemia, combined hypercholesterolemia, and common hypercholesterolemia

- The patient should be placed on a standard cholesterol-lowering diet before receiving a statin and should continue on this diet during treatment
- May be used in combination with fibrates or nicotinic acid to reduce a mixed hyperlipidemia, usually under specialist supervision

Dose
- Pravastatin: 10–40mg once daily, starting dose 10, 20 or 40mg
- Simvastatin: 5–80mg per day, usual starting dose is 20mg once a day
- Atorvastatin: 10–80mg once daily, usual starting dose is 10mg once a day
- Statins can be administered in single or divided dose at any time of the day, with or without food
- Adjust dose gradually according to lipid levels taken 4 weeks after initiation or titration of therapy

Efficacy
- Statins reduce total cholesterol, LDL, very-low-density lipoprotein (VLDL), and triglycerides while increasing HDL
- Statins are effective in a wide variety of patient populations with hypercholesterolemia, with and without hypertriglyceridemia
- At highest dosage, LDL decreases 61%
- At highest dosage, HDL increases 5–15%
- At highest dosage, triglycerides decrease 43%
- Therapeutic response is seen within 2 weeks, and maximum response is usually achieved within 4 weeks and maintained during chronic therapy
- HMG-CoA reductase inhibitors are reported to be less effective in patients with rare homozygous familial hypercholesterolemia, possibly because these patients have few functional LDL receptors
- The efficacy of statins has not been evaluated in patients with combined elevated total cholesterol and hypertriglyceridemia (>500mg/dL [>5.7mmol/L]) or in patients with elevated intermediate-density lipoproteins (IDLs) as their primary lipid abnormality

Risks/Benefits

Risks:
- Use caution with past liver disease, alcoholism
- Use caution with severe acute infections, trauma, hypotension, uncontrolled seizure disorders, severe metabolic and electrolyte disorders
- Use caution with children less than 18 years of age

Benefits:
- Marked response seen within 2 weeks of initiation; maximum therapeutic response occurring within 4–6 weeks. Response is maintained during chronic therapy
- Do not need to adjust for renal impairment
- Easy to take in once-daily doses
- Fewer side-effects than resins
- In hypercholesterolemic patients without clinically evident coronary heart disease (CHD), including prior myocardial infarctions (MIs), statins have been demonstrated to reduce the risk of MI, reduce the risk of undergoing myocardial revascularization procedures, and reduce the risk of cardiovascular mortality, stroke, or transient ischemic attack with no increase in death from noncardiovascular causes

Side-effects and adverse reactions
- Gastrointestinal: nausea, vomiting, dyspepsia, flatulence, pancreatitis, abdominal pain, gallstones, liver dysfunction, constipation
- Genitourinary: erectile dysfunction, gallstones

- CNS: dizziness, headache, insomnia, peripheral neuropathy
- Cardiovascular: chest pain
- Hematologic: blood cell disorders
- Musculoskeletal: arthralgia, myalgia, myositis, rhabdomyolysis
- Skin: alopecia, Stevens–Johnson syndrome, pruritus, rash

Interactions (other drugs)

- Azole antifungals ▪ Cholestyramine ▪ Clofibrate ▪ Colestipol ▪ Cyclosporine ▪ Danazol ▪ Digoxin ▪ Fluoxetine ▪ Gemfibrozil (fibric acid derivatives) ▪ Isradipine ▪ Macrolide antibiotics ▪ Nefazodone ▪ Niacin ▪ Oral contraceptives ▪ Warfarin

Contraindications

- Active liver disease ▪ Pregnancy and breast-feeding ▪ Hypersensitivity to statins

Evidence

- In the treatment of hyperlipidemia, statins are effective in lowering cholesterol and preventing cardiovascular disease
- Statins are highly effective in lowering LDL cholesterol [1] *Level C*
- Statins can reduce mortality rate and CHD [2] *Level C*
- Four systematic reviews evaluated statins vs placebo for primary prevention of cardiovascular disorders, for 6 months or longer. All reviews found that after 4–6 years of treatment, major coronary events were decreased, and the cardiovascular mortality rate was decreased with statins [3] *Level M*
- One systematic review of five randomized controlled trials (RCTs) compared statin therapy vs placebo over at least 4 years. The three secondary prevention trials found that statins reduced the CHD mortality rate, cardiovascular mortality rate, and general mortality rate. Major coronary events and mortality rates were also reduced in combined primary and secondary prevention [4] *Level M*
- Several overviews of RCTs showed that a mean total decrease in cholesterol by approximately 21% with statin treatment decreased the relative odds of cerebrovascular accident (CVA) by 24% and reduced the relative odds of CHD by one-third [5] *Level M*

Acceptability to patient

HMG-CoA reductase inhibitors may occasionally cause skeletal muscle pain and gastrointestinal disturbances, which may raise noncompliance issues.

Follow up plan

- Lipid levels should be analyzed within 2–4 weeks and dosage adjusted accordingly
- Aim to achieve a 20–25% reduction in total serum cholesterol concentration in those at high risk of coronary events
- Therapy with lipid-altering agents should be a component of multiple risk factor intervention in individuals at increased risk for atherosclerosis
- Liver function tests should be performed before the initiation of treatment, at 6 and 12 weeks after initiation of therapy or increase in dosage, then every 6 months thereafter
- Patients who develop increased transaminase levels should be monitored with a second liver function assessment to confirm the finding and then frequently thereafter until the abnormality resolves. Should an increase in aspartate aminotransferase (AST) or alanine aminotransferase (ALT) of three times the upper limit of normal or greater persist, the dosage should be decreased or the medication discontinued

Patient and caregiver information

- It is important to continue with dietary modification and exercise programs
- Inform your doctor if you become pregnant because it will be necessary to discontinue the medication for the duration of the pregnancy
- This drug should not be taken by those with liver disease
- Liver function tests will have to be performed periodically

FIBRIC ACID DERIVATIVES

- Stimulates enzymatic breakdown of lipids in lipoproteins
- Drug of choice for treating elevated triglycerides
- Also acts to decrease LDL and raise HDL levels

Dose

Gemfibrozil: recommended dose for adults is 1200mg administered in two divided doses 30min before the morning and evening meals.

Efficacy

- Triglycerides decrease 20–50%
- LDL decreases 10–15%
- HDL increases 10–15%

Risks/Benefits

Risks:

- Treatment of adult patients with very high elevations of plasma triglyceride levels who present a risk of pancreatitis and who do not respond adequately to a determined dietary effort to control them: patients who present such risk typically have plasma triglycerides >2000mg/dL and have elevations of VLDL cholesterol as well as fasting chylomicrons
- Patients with significantly elevated triglycerides should be closely observed when treated with fibric acid derivatives
- In some patients with high triglyceride levels, treatment with fibric acid derivatives is associated with a significant increase in LDL cholesterol

Benefits:

- Most effective drug for lowering triglycerides
- Can be used in combination with other classes to treat mixed hyperlipidemias

Side-effects and adverse reactions

- Cardiovascular: atrial fibrillation
- CNS: fatigue, headache, hypesthesia, paresthesia, vertigo
- Gastrointestinal: abdominal pain, acute appendicitis, constipation, diarrhea, dyspepsia, nausea
- Genitourinary: impotence
- Hematologic: anemia, bone marrow hypoplasia, leukopenia, thrombocytopenia
- Skin: rash, eczema

Interactions (other drugs)

■ HMG-CoA reductase inhibitors (may cause drug-induced myopathy) ■ Glyburide (may cause hypoglycemia) ■ Anticoagulants (dosage of anticoagulant should be reduced to maintain the prothrombin time at appropriate level to prevent bleeding complications)

Contraindications

■ Hepatic or severe renal dysfunction, including primary biliary cirrhosis ■ Pre-existing gallbladder disease ■ Hypersensitivity reactions to a fibrate ■ Nephrotic syndrome

Evidence

In the treatment of hyperlipidemia, fibric acids are effective in lowering cholesterol and preventing cardiovascular disease:

- Fibric acids are effective in lowering triglycerides [1] *Level C*
- Fibric acids may lower LDL and raise HDL levels in certain patients [1] *Level C*
- A review of a RCT of men with CHD and HDL<1mmol/L compared gemfibrozil with placebo. Patients in the treatment group had a lower rate of nonfatal MI and a reduced death rate after a median of 5.1 years [6] *Level P*
- Two RCTs compared bezafibrate with placebo. The larger trial consisted of patients with a previous MI or stable angina, and mortality rate was not reduced in the treatment group. The smaller RCT of young male patients post-MI found that bezafibrate significantly reduced the combined outcome of death, reinfarction, plus revascularization [7] *Level P*
- A RCT of men with CHD and low HDL cholesterol compared gemfibrozil with placebo over approximately 5 years. Gemfibrozil increased HDL, reduced triglycerides, and reduced total cholesterol. Gemfibrozil reduced the incidence of CHD but did not significantly affect stroke [8] *Level P*

Acceptability to patient

Nonspecific complaints such as abdominal discomfort, nausea, and flatulence may lead to noncompliance issues.

Follow up plan

- Aim to decrease cholesterol concentration in the plasma by 20–25%
- When fibric acid derivatives are used in combination with HMG-CoA reductase inhibitors to treat selected cases of hyperlipidemia that are refractory to monotherapy, the result may be increased muscle toxicity that requires extremely careful clinical monitoring

Patient and caregiver information

Patients should be advised to adhere to a low-cholesterol, low-fat diet at the start of treatment with fibric acid derivatives and throughout the treatment period.

NIACIN

- Niacin (nicotinic acid) is a B vitamin that acts by inhibiting lipid synthesis
- Lowers both LDL and triglycerides as well as increasing HDL
- Nicotinic acid is also indicated as adjunctive therapy for the treatment of adult patients with very high plasma triglyceride levels who present a risk of pancreatitis and who do not respond adequately to a determined dietary effort to control them

Dose

- The usual adult dosage of nicotinic acid is 1–2g, two to three times a day
- Doses should be individualized according to the patient's response
- Start with one-half tablet (250mg) as a single daily dose following the evening meal
- The frequency of dosing and total daily dose can be increased every 4–7 days until the desired LDL and/or triglyceride level is achieved or the first-level therapeutic dose of 1.5–2g per day is reached
- If the patient's hyperlipidemia is not adequately controlled after 2 months at this level, the dosage can then be increased at 2–4-week intervals to 3g per day (1g three times per day)
- In patients with marked lipid abnormalities, a higher dose is occasionally required but generally should not exceed 6g per day

Efficacy

At doses ranging from 2–6g per day (1–2g per day of the sustained-release preparation), nicotinic acid can be expected to decrease LDL by 10–25%, increase HDL by 15–35%, and decrease triglycerides by 20–50%.

Risks/Benefits

Risks:

- Cases of severe hepatic toxicity, including fulminant hepatic necrosis, have occurred in patients who have substituted sustained-release (modified-release, timed-release) nicotinic acid products for immediate-release (crystalline) nicotinic acid at equivalent doses
- Nicotinic acid should be used with caution in patients who consume substantial quantities of alcohol and/or have a past history of liver disease
- May exacerbate diabetes by decreasing glucose tolerance

Benefit: may be a useful adjunct when used with other lipid-modifying drugs for severe hyperlipidemia, usually under specialist supervision.

Side-effects and adverse reactions

- Cardiovascular: atrial fibrillation and other cardiac arrhythmias, orthostatic hypotension
- CNS: headache
- Eye: toxic amblyopia, cystoid macular edema
- Gastrointestinal: dyspepsia, vomiting, diarrhea, peptic ulceration, jaundice, abnormal liver function tests
- Metabolic: decreased glucose tolerance, hyperuricemia, gout
- Skin: mild to severe cutaneous flushing, pruritus, hyperpigmentation, acanthosis nigricans, dry skin

Interactions (other drugs)

■ Antihypertensive therapy: nicotinic acid may potentiate the effects of ganglionic blocking agents and vasoactive drugs, resulting in postural hypotension ■ Aspirin: concomitant aspirin may decrease the metabolic clearance of nicotinic acid. The clinical relevance of this finding is unclear ■ Concomitant alcohol or hot drinks may increase the side-effects of flushing and pruritus, and should be avoided at the time of drug ingestion

Contraindications

■ Known hypersensitivity to niacin ■ Significant hepatic dysfunction or unexplained elevation in serum transaminases ■ Active hepatic disease ■ Active peptic ulcer disease ■ Pregnancy or lactation

Evidence

- Total cholesterol and triglycerides are effectively reduced and HDL increased by nicotinic acid [1] *Level C*
- There is evidence that nicotinic acid may reduce the total mortality rate in secondary prevention [1] *Level C*
- Nicotinic acid is of particular use in the treatment of raised cholesterol in patients with low HDL and combined hyperlipidemia [1] *Level C*
- Niacin is a suitable alternative to statins in primary prevention treatment [2] *Level C*

Acceptability to patient

Symptoms related to side-effects of this treatment may cause noncompliance issues.

Follow up plan

- Aim to decrease total plasma cholesterol by 20–25%
- Check that other lifestyle measures to reduce coronary artery disease are being adhered to
- Check blood pressure, liver function tests, and blood glucose
- If the patient is also receiving adjuvant treatment with a statin, question for symptoms of myositis and check muscle enzymes

Patient and caregiver information

Patients should be advised to adhere to a low-cholesterol, low-fat diet throughout the treatment period.

Complementary therapy

GARLIC

Efficacy

Research data has been somewhat conflicting regarding the efficacy of garlic in lowering hyperlipidemia – probably related to the actual preparation used in the studies. Garlic powder and steam-distilled preparations are ineffective, whereas the equivalent of a whole garlic clove daily may reduce cholesterol by up to 9%.

The active ingredient in garlic is allicin, which is unstable in alcohol, water, and oil. Products standardized to 4g/day of garlic are recommended by German Commission E for reduction of cholesterol and triglycerides.

Risks/Benefits

Risks:

- Garlic can produce burning of the oral mucous membranes if chewed as raw cloves
- Some patients may experience gastric irritation and an unusual odor to the breath or sweat when taking large amounts of garlic regularly
- No known risks of garlic therapy

Evidence

- A meta-analysis found that garlic significantly reduced total cholesterol levels compared with placebo [9] *Level M*
- A systematic review found that garlic was superior to placebo for the reduction of total cholesterol levels. The reduction was noted after 1 month of treatment, and persisted for at least 6 months [10] *Level M*

Acceptability to patient

Odor-free preparations are generally more acceptable to patients than plain garlic. Capsules of allicin standardized preparations are generally well tolerated. Whole garlic cloves may be irritating to the oral mucosal or gastrointestinal system in some patients.

Follow up plan

Monitor lipids for therapeutic effectiveness, patient compliance, and side-effects.

ESSENTIAL FATTY ACIDS/OMEGA-3 FATTY ACIDS

Eicosapentaenoic acid (EPA) and docosahexapentaenoic acid (DHA) are the important omega-3 fatty acids. They are prevalent in oily fish (salmon, tuna, mackerel) and some legumes (flax, walnuts), and have antiatherogenic and anti-inflammatory effects. They also inhibit platelet aggregation, and may have a role in managing hyperlipidemia.

Efficacy

Omega-3 fatty acids appear to be particularly useful in lowering triglycerides.

Risks/Benefits

No known risks of the use of n-3 fatty acids.

Evidence

- A systematic review compared cholesterol-lowering agents, and found that statins reduced CHD mortality, and both statins and n-3 fatty acids reduced all-cause mortality [11] *Level M*

- A small RCT compared fish oil (containing low dose omega-3 fatty acids) vs safflower oil (control) for 6 weeks in patients with noninsulin-dependent diabetes mellitus. Fish oil significantly reduced triglyceride levels, and inhibited platelet aggregation and thromboxane A2 production. Fish oil caused a small but significant increase in HBA1c and total cholesterol [12] *Level P*

Acceptability to patient
Highly accepted.

Follow up plan
Monitor lipids for response to therapy.

Patient and caregiver information
Capsules of n-3 fatty acids must be refrigerated for optimal effectiveness. A dose of 1.5g/day is recommended.

GUGULIPID (COMMIPHORA MOLMOL)
Also called Arabian myrrh, Somalian myrrh.

Efficacy
Increases LDL binding sites in the liver.

Risks/Benefits
No recorded adverse drug interactions nor adverse side-effects.

Evidence
A double-blind RCT compared gugulipid with placebo in the treatment of patients with hyperlipidemia. Patients were also on a cholesterol-lowering diet. Gugulipid-treated patients had a reduction in total cholesterol (11.7%), LDL (12.5%), and triglycerides (12%). Patients receiving placebo did not have a change in cholesterol levels [13] *Level P*

Acceptability to patient
Well tolerated.

Follow up plan
Monitor lipid levels for efficacy.

Patient and caregiver information
75mg daily is the recommended dose. Can be found in health food stores in the US.

DIETARY FIBER
The cholesterol-lowering effect of oat bran was noted in 1963, with numerous studies since.

Efficacy
Beta glycan, a soluble fiber, is twice as prevalent in oat bran as in oatmeal. 28g oat bran twice daily has been shown to result in lowering of LDL-C levels. Most significant beneficial effect is seen in older women.

Risks/Benefits
Occasionally patients will note increased flatulence when first introducing fiber into their diet. This effect abates with time.

Evidence
- A meta-analysis found that the incorporation of oat products into the usual diet causes a modest reduction in cholesterol levels [14] *Level M*

- A crossover RCT compared oat bran with wheat cereal (as a supplement to a fat-modified diet) for the reduction of total cholesterol and LDL cholesterol, levels of which were significantly reduced in patients taking oat bran [15] *Level P*

Acceptability to patient

Oat bran is readily available, easy to consume, but has little flavor. Some patients note initial increase in flatulence, but this usually abates over time. Oat bran, as a soluble fiber, also helps keep bowel elimination regular, so it can be of additional benefit to those patients with constipation.

Follow up plan

Monitor lipid levels for efficacy.

SOY PROTEIN

Efficacy

Soy protein in an amount of 25g daily can lower total cholesterol by an average of 6–9%, LDL by 7–13%, and triglycerides by 10% on average.

Risks/Benefits

Some patients have soy allergy, otherwise no known risks.

Evidence

- A meta-analysis found that diets containing soy protein are associated with a lowering of cholesterol levels, compared with control diets. Total cholesterol, LDL cholesterol, and triglycerides were reduced [16] *Level M*
- A crossover RCT compared a soy diet with a carbohydrate control diet in non-hypercholesterolemic, perimenopausal women. A significant reduction in total cholesterol and LDL cholesterol was noted in women on the soy diet [17] *Level P*

Acceptability to patient

Generally well tolerated and readily available.

Follow up plan

Monitor lipid levels for efficacy.

LIFESTYLE

- Dietary adjustments and physical exercise should precede drug treatment for this disease and accompany subsequent drug treatment if the diet and exercise are not sufficient on their own
- The 'Western lifestyle' leads to hyperlipidemia due to overeating, a diet high in saturated fat, obesity, lack of exercise

Diet:

- Calorie control – advise the patient to eat only sufficient calories to maintain lean body weight

Restricted fat intake:

- Advise the patient to reduce the amount of fat eaten. Fats should contribute no more than 30% of an individual's daily calorie intake
- Differentiate between saturated and unsaturated fats
- Only 10% of the fats eaten should be saturated
- Monounsaturated fats are found in olive oil, canola oil, and avocados
- Polyunsaturated fats are found in fish and some vegetable oils
- Use sunflower, safflower, soybean, canola, corn, or olive oil
- Do not use palm or coconut oils
- Check food labels: most food products will have a nutritional breakdown included. This provides a quick reference for amount of fat and cholesterol eaten as well as the type of fat

Meat:

- Choose lean cuts of meat
- Remove the skin before eating chicken or turkey
- Eat more white meat than red because it has less cholesterol
- Foods high in omega-3 oils (cold-water fish, fish oil capsules) can help decrease cholesterol levels
- Be careful with some types of seafood because they can be surprisingly high in cholesterol, e.g. shrimp

Dairy products:

- Limit the amount of butter eaten, and drink skim milk
- Use low-fat yogurt or low-fat cottage cheese instead of sour cream
- Limit full-fat cheeses
- Fruit and vegetables: eat fruits and vegetables daily
- Vegetable proteins have been shown to lower cholesterol levels, whereas animal and milk proteins have been shown to raise them; thus a vegetarian or semivegetarian diet has been shown to be effective

Carbohydrates:

- Avoid processed carbohydrates such as white bread, white rice, and pasta
- Reduce dietary sugar and simple carbohydrates

Vitamins and minerals:

Many supplements are available today, most of which will contain some or all of the following:

- Selenium (200mcg per day) is needed for normal processing of fats
- L-taurine (200mg per day) helps the body excrete extra cholesterol
- Vitamin C (1000mg three times per day) and E (400–800 IU per day) can help cholesterol metabolism
- B complex, especially Bit (1000mcg per day), folic acid (400–800mcg per day), betaine (1000mg per day), and B6 (50–100mg per day) reduce high levels of homocysteine
- Chromium (200mcg one to three times per day) is helpful for patients who have high cholesterol as a complication of diabetes
- Magnesium (200mg two to three times per day) aids metabolism
- Panthenine (500mg three times per day) may help reduce cholesterol

Exercise:

- Patients should be encouraged to adopt a sensible exercise program
- The degree of exertion should be increased gradually, particularly in those who already have CHD
- The exercise should be performed regularly
- A good exercise program should consist of aerobic exercise, which includes any activity that keeps the heart rate up (such as swimming, jogging, walking, and cycling)
- An individual should get 20–30min of aerobic exercise every other day. If the individual has not been exercising, advise starting a new exercise program slowly
- Patients should be advised to stretch before and after exercise
- Many hospitals provide post-MI or coronary artery bypass surgery exercise plans

RISKS/BENEFITS

Risks:

- Make sure the patient is aware of his/her true nutritional requirements – some 'fad' diets can be unbalanced
- Sudden, excessive exercise could precipitate an MI in patients at high risk

Benefits:
- The benefits of a healthy, balanced, low-fat diet are far reaching. Not only can it help lower cholesterol levels, but it will also increase overall health
- Weight loss, improved fitness, increased metabolism, and overall improved health status. May also have beneficial psychologic effects

ACCEPTABILITY TO PATIENT

- The form of exercise should be tailored to the patient because some people may not enjoy all forms of exercise (e.g. jogging, swimming)
- Long-term lifestyle alterations in mature adults may be very difficult to institute and maintain
- Other members of the family may not appreciate a low-fat diet if the meals are shared
- Due to increasing awareness of the prevalence of coronary artery disease and its risk factors, improved diet should be understood if not accepted by most patients

FOLLOW UP PLAN

- Patients should be questioned periodically to ascertain that they are keeping up with the prescribed exercise plan
- Repeat checks of blood lipid levels should be performed
- Take time to question how the dietary therapy is going
- It is important to be receptive to the patient so they feel able to talk to you even if the diet is not going well
- Changing eating habits can be difficult, especially if not highly motivated. Aim always to be encouraging to the patient

PATIENT AND CAREGIVER INFORMATION

- Most patients will accept that exercise is good for them
- Patients with known cardiovascular disease may benefit from the education and monitoring of a structured cardiac rehabilitation program
- Some patients may not be aware of what foods they should be eating. Unless you have time to explain the fundamentals of a good diet, referral to a dietitian is warranted
- For every 1% reduction in cholesterol level, the risk of heart disease is reduced 2%
- Diet therapy is a life-long project but will result in an overall improvement of health
- If lifestyle/diet therapy fails, antihyperlipidemic medication may be added. However, low-fat diet and exercise programs should continue

OUTCOMES

EFFICACY OF THERAPIES

- Coronary heart disease is the major cause of death in the US
- The major risk factors for CHD include smoking, hypertension, hypercholesterolemia, diabetes mellitus, and sedentary lifestyle
- Epidemiologic studies have shown that the risk of cardiovascular disease steadily increases with increasing levels of plasma cholesterol so that it is difficult to define a 'healthy' range
- Many health authorities and organizations have recommended dietary change for the entire population as the first step in reducing the incidence of CHD, and there is strong epidemiologic evidence for the efficacy of this therapy
- There are clinical trials that show that both cardiovascular morbidity and mortality rates are reduced as a result of treating hyperlipidemia
- Dietary therapy is safe and effective. The response to diet should be quantified and goals assessed before drug therapy is considered in the primary prevention of coronary artery disease. Patients with known coronary disease and significantly elevated LDL levels (>130mg/dL) may be considered for earlier drug therapy
- As a general rule, initiation of pharmacologic intervention should be delayed for 6 months after dietary therapy is initiated to see whether dietary therapy alone will work. Exceptions are patients with genetic lipid disorders that cannot be expected to respond to dietary therapy alone and patients with documented atherosclerosis for whom prompt lipid lowering is essential
- Combining a reductase inhibitor and a bile acid sequestrant is attractive because of the synergistic effects of their different mechanisms of action
- The combination of nicotinic acid and colestipol treatment may result in a decrease in LDL
- Combined drug therapy is especially useful for patients with severe hypercholesterolemia and combined hyperlipidemia

Evidence

- The treatment of hypercholesterolemia may reduce the risk of nonfatal MI in people with a high baseline risk. Cardiovascular mortality and overall mortality rates may also be reduced [7] *Level M*
- Cardiovascular risk reduction in patients with hyperlipidemia is related to the baseline cardiovascular risk and the degree of cholesterol lowering rather than to the absolute cholesterol level [3] *Level M*
- Cholesterol reduction in asymptomatic people (primary prevention) may reduce the rate of cardiovascular events, but the overall death rate is not altered for those with a low baseline risk [3] *Level M*
- Combination pharmacologic and dietary therapy reduces cholesterol more than lifestyle interventions alone [3] *Level M*
- In controlled settings, diets that are low in cholesterol and saturated fat can lead to a 10–15% reduction in cholesterol. In the community, these effects are more modest, with 3–5% reduction in cholesterol in general populations and 9% reduction post-MI [18] *Level M*
- Statins are the most effective therapy for cholesterol reduction and cardiovascular risk reduction in primary and secondary prevention [7] *Level M*
- Statins reduce the incidence of stroke in patients with known CHD [5] *Level M*
- Treatment of hyperlipidemia may be beneficial in the symptomatic treatment of lower limb atherosclerosis and in preventing further deterioration of underlying disease [19] *Level M*

Review period

6-monthly review is required.

PROGNOSIS

- For every 1% reduction in cholesterol level, the risk of heart disease is reduced by 2%
- The beneficial effect of cholesterol lowering appears to occur regardless of the means by which lowering is achieved (including dietary changes)
- Drug and diet therapy are likely to continue throughout the life of the affected individual
- Periodic monitoring of blood levels is necessary to determine the response to treatment
- Decreased recurrent cardiac events are seen relatively early after starting lipid-lowering therapy, suggesting that this treatment may play a role in stabilizing plaques and improving endothelial function

Clinical pearl(s)

- Engaging older patients in making life-long changes in diet and exercise is very difficult. Physicians should engage any and all other assistance to make it happen, including physical therapists, dietitians and nutritionists, weight-loss groups, and others
- Participation of family members is critical to success, particularly in making dietary changes

Therapeutic failure

If the first-line of therapy (dietary alterations) does not significantly lower plasma lipid levels, drug therapies can be considered.

Deterioration

For patients refractory to combination drug therapy, referral to a lipidologist is appropriate for consideration of aggressive medical therapies, partial ileal bypass surgery, or plasma exchange with LDL apheresis.

Terminal illness

In the rare homozygous form of familial hypercholesterolemia, drug treatment seldom achieves normal lipid levels and plasma exchange together with combined drug treatment appears to be the therapy of choice: even with treatment, the prognosis is poor and few individuals survive beyond 20 years of age.

COMPLICATIONS

Hyperlipidemias are major risk factors for atherosclerosis, CHD, and stroke.

CONSIDER CONSULT

- Patients refractory to combination drug therapy
- Patients whose primary care provider is uncomfortable following combination drug therapy

PREVENTION

- Screening for hyperlipidemia should be a part of a routine health evaluation for people after 20 years of age along with assessment of other cardiac risk factors
- Patients with 'desirable' cholesterol levels should be rechecked every 5 years

RISK FACTORS

- Lifestyle: sedentary lifestyle is a risk factor for hyperlipidemia
- Diet: a diet high in saturated fats or cholesterol may raise the cholesterol level
- Drugs and alcohol: alcohol abuse can raise lipid levels
- Medical and drug history: cirrhosis, diabetes, hypothyroidism, chronic renal failure, hyperpituitarism, and porphyria may predispose to hyperlipidemia. Certain medications may also raise the cholesterol level
- Genetics: familial history of hyperlipidemia or coronary heart disease

MODIFY RISK FACTORS

Lifestyle and wellness

Lifestyle changes can help reduce cholesterol levels.

TOBACCO

If patients smoke, encourage them to stop. Patients addicted to tobacco may require professional help to quit.

ALCOHOL AND DRUGS

Alcohol abuse is a risk factor for hypercholesterolemia.

DIET

- Qualified dietitians can make recommendations for a low-cholesterol diet
- Read food labels carefully to be alert for 'hidden' fat in prepackaged foods

PHYSICAL ACTIVITY

- Exercise daily: walk for at least 20–30min 3–4 days per week
- Engaging in activities around the house such as house cleaning and yard work have been shown to be beneficial in reducing cardiac risk

FAMILY HISTORY

Patients with a positive family history should have their cholesterol level checked.

SCREENING

- The incidence of CHD in the population is a problem of great severity
- Treatment for hyperlipidemia (one of the major risk factors for CHD) is possible
- Early detection of hyperlipidemia by screening is warranted

CHOLESTEROL

- General practice is the ideal location for initial screening
- All those between 20 and 60 years of age should be screened
- Those >60 years of age may be screened, but identification of hypertension and stroke prevention become more important than cholesterol levels
- For those >75 years of age, the data are less clear about the role of lipid-lowering therapy on the primary prevention of coronary artery disease. However, for patients with known coronary disease, cholesterol as well as all modifiable cardiac risk factors should be treated aggressively
- Both men and women should be screened

PREVENT RECURRENCE

- Compliance with dietary changes and prescribed drug regimen (if any) needs to be readily assessed
- Monitoring of cholesterol and lipid levels must be done periodically

RESOURCES

ASSOCIATIONS

The American Heart Association
National Center
7272 Greenville Avenue
Dallas, TX 75231
Tel: (800) 242-8721
http://www.americanheart.org/

KEY REFERENCES

- Ballantyne SM, Grundy A, Oberman RA, at al. Hyperlipidemia: diagnostic and therapeutic perspectives. J Clin Endocrinol Metab 2000;85:2093–8
- Farmer JA, Gotto AM Jr. Currently available hypolipidaemic drugs and future therapeutic developments. Baillieres Clin Endocrinol Metab 1995;9:825–47
- Peto R, Yusuf S, Collins R. Cholesterol-lowering trial results in their epidemiological context. Circulation 1987;75(Suppl. 2):451
- Braunwald E. Heart disease: a textbook of cardiovascular medicine. Washington, DC: American Sleep Apnea Association, 1997
- Havel RJ, Rapaport E. Management of primary hyperlipidemia. N Engl J Med 1995;332:1491–8
- Scriver CR, Beaudet AL, Sly WS, Valle D. The metabolic basis of inherited disease. New York: McGraw-Hill, 1995
- Oliver MF. Serum cholesterol: the knave of hearts and the joker. Lancet 1981;ii:1090–5
- Van den Hoogen PCW, Fresken SCJ, Nagelkerke NJ, et al. The relation between blood pressure and mortality due to coronary heart disease among men in different parts of the world. N Engl J Med 2000;342:1–8
- Anand SS, Yusuf S, Vuksan V, et al. Differences in risk factors, atherosclerosis, and cardiovascular disease between ethnic groups in Canada: The Study of Health Assessment and Risk in Ethnic Groups (SHARE). The Lancet 2000;35:279–84
- Executive summary of the third report of the National Cholesterol Education Program (NCEP) Expert Panel on Detection, Evaluation, and Treatment of High Blood Cholesterol in Adults (Adult Treatment Panel III). JAMA 2001;285(19):2486–97

Evidence references and guidelines

1. Second report of the Expert Panel on Detection, Evaluation, and Treatment of High Blood Cholesterol in Adults (Adult Treatment Panel II). Circulation 1994;89:1333–445. Available online at the National Guideline Clearinghouse, and the National Heart, Lung, and Blood Institute
2. Barrie W, Harrison V, Khanderia U, et al. Screening and management of lipids. Ann Arbor, MI: University of Michigan, 2000. Guidelines developed by the Lipid Therapy Guideline Team
3. Pignone M. Primary prevention, Cardiovascular disorders. Clinical Evidence 2001;5:63–94
4. Miettinen TA, Pyorala K, Olsson AG, et al. Cholesterol-lowering therapy in women and elderly patients with myocardial infarction or angina pectoris: findings from the Scandinavian Simvastatin Survival Study. Circulation 1997;96:4211–8. Reviewed in: Clinical Evidence 2001;5:95–126
5. Sudlow C. Stroke prevention, Cardiovascular disorders. Clinical Evidence 2001;5:140–57
6. Montagne O, Vedel I, Durand-Zaleski I. Assessment of the impact of fibrates and diet on survival and their cost-effectiveness: evidence from randomized, controlled trials in coronary heart disease and health economic evaluations. Clin Ther 1999;21:2027–2035. Reviewed in: Clinical Evidence 2001;5:95–126
7. Pignone M. Secondary prevention of ischemic cardiac events, Cardiovascular disorders. Clinical Evidence 2001;5:95–126
8. Anonymous. The treatment of cerebrovascular disease with clofibrate. Final Report of the Veteran's Administration Cooperative Study of Atherosclerosis, neurology section. Stroke 1973;4:684–93. Reviewed in: Clinical Evidence 2001;5:140–57
9. Warshafsky S, Kamer RS, Sivak SL. Effect of garlic on total serum cholesterol. A meta-analyisis. Ann Intern Med 1993;119:599–605. Medline
10. Silagy C, Neil A. Garlic as a lipid lowering agent – a meta-analyis. J R Coll Phys Lond 1994;28:39–45. Medline
11. Bucher HC, Griffith LE, Guyatt G. Systematic review of the risk and benefit of different cholesterol-lowering interventions. Arterioscler Thromb Vasc Biol 1999;19:187–95. Reviewed in: Clinical Evidence 2001;6:114–45

12 Axelrod L, Camuso J, Williams E, et al. Effects of a small quantity of omega-3 fatty acids on cardiovascular risk factors in NIDDM. A randomized, prospective, double-blind, controlled study. Diabetes Care 1994;17:37–44. Medline
13 Singh RB, Niaz MA, Ghosh S. Hypolipidemic and antioxidant effects of *Commiphora mukul* as an adjunct to dietary therapy in patients with hypercholesterolemia. Cardiovasc Drugs Ther 1994;8:659–64. Medline
14 Ripsin CM, Keenan JM, Jacobs DR, et al. Oat products and lipid lowering. A meta-analysis. JAMA 1992;267:3317–25. Medline
15 Keenan JM, Wenz JB, Myers S, et al. Randomized, controlled, crossover trial of oat bran in hypercholesterolemic subjects. J Fam Pract 1991;33:600–8. Medline
16 Anderson JW, Johnstone BM, Cook-Newell ME. Meta analysis of the effects of soy protein on serum lipids. N Engl J Med 1995;333:276–82. Medline
17 Washburn S, Burke GL, Morgan T, Anthony MI. Effect of soy protein supplementation on serum lipoproteins, blood pressure and menopausal symptoms in perimenopausal women. Menopause 1999;6:7–13. Medline
18 Ness A, Lonn E. Secondary prevention of ischemic cardiac events, Cardiovascular disorders. Clinical Evidence 2001;5:95–126
19 Leng GC, Price JF, Jepson RG. Lipid-lowering for lower limb atherosclerosis (Cochrane Review). In: The Cochrane Library, 3, 2001. Oxford: Update Software

CONTRIBUTORS

Russell C Jones, MD, MPH
Jane L Murray, MD
John McB Hodgson, MD, FACC, FSCAI
Craig Clark, MD

HYPERTENSION

SUMMARY INFORMATION

DESCRIPTION

- Systolic blood pressure of at least 140mmHg and/or diastolic blood pressure of at least 90mmHg
- About 90% of hypertension has no identifiable cause
- Uncomplicated essential hypertension is asymptomatic
- Hypertension is an important risk factor for subsequent cardiovascular disease

URGENT ACTION

Hypertension should be treated urgently and aggressively in the following emergencies:

- Hypertensive encephalopathy
- Stroke
- Subarachnoid hemorrhage
- Unstable angina
- Acute myocardial infarction

KEY! DON'T MISS!

Pregnancy-induced hypertension is an important cause of fetal loss and maternal death; there may be no warning signs or symptoms. Check the blood pressure of pregnant women at every consultation.

BACKGROUND

ICD9 CODE
- 401.1 Hypertension (malignant)
- 401.1 Hypertension (benign)
- 401.9 Hypertension (unspecified)

SYNONYMS
- Dissecting aortic aneurysm
- Pregnancy-induced hypertension
- Malignant hypertension

CARDINAL FEATURES
- Hypertension is defined as systolic blood pressure of at least 140mmHg and/or diastolic blood pressure of at least 90mmHg
- About 10% of hypertensive patients have an identifiable cause for their hypertension
- In the remaining 90% of patients, hypertension is idiopathic (essential hypertension)
- Uncomplicated essential hypertension is asymptomatic
- Untreated hypertension is a risk factor for development of subsequent cardiovascular disease
- Successful treatment of hypertension reduces the risk of cardiovascular disease

CAUSES
Common causes
About 90% of hypertension has no identifiable cause.

Rare causes
- Renal parenchymal disease
- Renovascular hypertension
- Oral contraceptives
- Primary aldosteronism
- Pheochromocytoma
- Cushing's syndrome
- Coarctation of the aorta

Contributory or predisposing factors
- Increasing age
- Obesity
- Physical inactivity
- Excessive alcohol consumption
- Excessive dietary sodium intake

EPIDEMIOLOGY
Incidence and prevalence
PREVALENCE

Approximately 250 per 1000.

Demographics
AGE
- Prevalence increases with age
- Prevalence is greater than 50% in persons over 60 years old
- Only about 1% of children and adolescents have hypertension

GENDER

- In young and middle-aged persons, hypertension is more common in men than in women
- In women, prevalence of hypertension increases more steeply with age than in men, and elderly women are at least as likely to be hypertensive as elderly men

RACE

More common in African-Americans than in Caucasians.

GENETICS

A family history of hypertension is associated with increased risk of developing the disorder.

SOCIOECONOMIC STATUS

Prevalence of hypertension is greater in lower socioeconomic groups.

DIAGNOSIS

DIFFERENTIAL DIAGNOSIS

Most hypertension is idiopathic; however, it is important to determine whether there is an identifiable secondary cause.

Renal parenchymal disease

FEATURES

- Elevated serum creatinine
- Abnormal urinalysis

Renovascular hypertension

FEATURES

- Onset before age 30 or after age 50 years
- Abrupt onset
- Severe hypertension (diastolic blood pressure >115mmHg)
- Abdominal bruit over renal arteries
- Hypertension refractory to medication

Primary aldosteronism

FEATURES

- Low serum potassium in the absence of diuretics
- High aldosterone levels in 24-h urine

Pheochromocytoma

FEATURES

- Headache
- Palpitations
- Perspiration
- Pallor
- Elevated metanephrines in 24-h urine

Cushing's syndrome

FEATURES

- Truncal obesity
- Purple striae
- Elevated urinary cortisol excretion

Coarctation of the aorta

FEATURES

- Delayed or absent femoral arterial pulses
- Decreased blood pressure in the lower extremities

SIGNS & SYMPTOMS

Signs

Systolic blood pressure at least 140mmHg and/or diastolic blood pressure at least 90mmHg.

Symptoms

Generally there are no symptoms, although some patients with severe hypertension may complain of headache or polyuria. Hypertension often presents with symptoms of underlying vascular disease:

- Impotence
- Claudication
- Angina

KEY! DON'T MISS!

Pregnancy-induced hypertension is an important cause of fetal loss and maternal death, there may be no warning signs or symptoms. Check the blood pressure of pregnant women at every consultation.

CONSIDER CONSULT

- Hypertensive emergencies
- Suspected secondary hypertension
- Renal parenchymal disease
- Renovascular hypertension
- Primary aldosteronism
- Pheochromocytoma
- Cushing's syndrome
- Coarctation of the aorta

INVESTIGATION OF THE PATIENT

Direct questions to patient

- Q **What have previous blood pressure readings been?** A gradual rise in blood pressure with age is normal, but a sudden increase could suggest a secondary cause or malignant hypertension
- Q **Have there been any symptoms or signs of clinically overt cardiovascular disease?** Episodes of weakness or dizziness (cerebrovascular disease), angina pectoris (coronary artery disease), dyspnea due to pulmonary edema (congestive heart failure). This could show that hypertension is already causing target organ damage, and should be treated more aggressively
- Q **Does the patient have diabetes?** Diabetic patients with hypertension are particularly at risk of cardiovascular disease, and should be treated more aggressively than non-diabetic patients
- Q **Have you been experiencing headaches?** Contrary to popular opinion, headache is not a characteristic symptom of hypertension, but may be associated with severe hypertension
- Q **Is there a family history of hypertension or cardiovascular disease?**
- Q **Has your vision been blurred?** May suggest retinal changes

Contributory or predisposing factors

- Q **Alcohol**: excessive alcohol consumption can raise blood pressure
- Q **Diet**: excessive sodium chloride and caffeine consumption can raise blood pressure
- Q **Obesity**: obese patients are at increased risk of hypertension and should be encouraged to lose weight
- Q **Smoking**: smoking increases cardiovascular risk, and a diagnosis of hypertension is a good opportunity for advice on giving up
- Q **Anxiety**: anxiety disorders, especially panic disorder, can result in significant episodic blood pressure elevation

Family history

- Q **Is there a family history of hypertension?** Essential hypertension has a strong genetic component, and the lack of a family history increases the likelihood of a secondary cause
- Q **Is there a family history of other cardiovascular disease?** Patients with a family history of cardiovascular disease are at increased risk of the complications of hypertension

Examination

- Blood pressure should be measured at least twice at each visit
- Blood pressure must be consistently elevated at several visits for a diagnosis of hypertension; the frequency of those visits will be guided by the initial blood pressure: confirmation of a mildly elevated reading (<160/100mmHg) should take place within 2 months, whereas a severely elevated reading (>180/110mmHg) requires confirmation within 1 week
- Measure height and weight to calculate body mass index (BMI) and assess obesity

- Thorough physical examination can help to discover secondary causes of hypertension such as Cushing's syndrome (round facies, truncal obesity, striae), coarctation of the aorta (compare blood pressures in both arms), renovascular hypertension (abdominal bruits may be present)
- Check for evidence of target organ damage
- Examine the cardiovascular system for evidence of heart failure, arterial disease in carotid, renal, and peripheral arteries, and coarctation of the aorta
- Examine the abdomen for bruits, enlarged kidneys, and other masses
- Examine the optic fundi for evidence of hypertensive retinopathy
- Examine the lungs for rales and evidence of bronchospasm

Summary of investigative tests

- Urinalysis is useful to identify renal disease
- Blood chemistry can provide evidence of secondary causes of hypertension
- Electrocardiography (ECG) can help to identify cardiac abnormalities, left ventricular hypertrophy
- Echocardiography is useful in assessing left ventricular hypertrophy and other cardiac abnormalities, if impaired cardiac function is suspected
- Ambulatory monitoring of blood pressure at home has long been used as an adjunct to evaluation

DIAGNOSTIC DECISION

Guidelines

- WHO–ISH Hypertension Guidelines Committee. 1999 World Health Organization–International Society of Hypertension Guidelines for the Management of Hypertension. J Hypertens 1999;17:151–85 [1]

The following guidelines are available:

- The National Heart, Lung, and Blood Institute and the National High Blood Pressure Education Program have developed guidelines. Sixth report of the Joint National Committee on Prevention, Detection, Evaluation, and Treatment of High Blood Pressure. Bethesda (MD): US Department of Health and Human Services, Public Health Service, National Institutes of Health, National Heart, Lung, and Blood Institute, 1997 [2]
- Institute for Clinical Systems Improvement. Hypertension diagnosis and treatment. Bloomington (MN): ICSI, 2000 [3]
- Veterans Health Administration. Diagnosis and management of hypertension in the primary care setting. The Hypertension Working Group. Washington (DC): Department of Veterans Affairs, 1999 [4]

The following points should be borne in mind:

- Hypertension should be diagnosed only after elevated blood pressure has been confirmed on the initial visit and two subsequent follow-up visits in which two readings should be made at each visit
- The minimum blood pressure for a diagnosis of hypertension is a systolic pressure of 140mmHg and/or diastolic pressure of 90mmHg
- Essential hypertension is diagnosed if no identifiable cause is found for the elevated blood pressure (about 90% of hypertensive patients)
- Secondary hypertension is diagnosed if investigations reveal a cause, such as renal disease
- Malignant hypertension is diagnosed if blood pressure has increased rapidly and grade 3 or 4 retinopathy is present

CLINICAL PEARL(S)

- 'White coat' hypertension – in which the blood pressure is higher in the office than if the patient takes it at home – is common. However, it may not be as benign as previously believed. All studies have been based on blood pressures taken in doctors' offices
- Current trials confirm that treatment of hypertension results in a reduction in risk of stroke, renal failure, and other complications
- Although 5–10% of patients have a 'secondary' cause of hypertension, such as renal artery stenosis, unfortunately specific treatment of the stenosis does not always improve blood pressure. Thus, empiric treatment is still the cornerstone of treatment

THE TESTS

Body fluids

URINALYSIS

Description

Urine.

Advantages/Disadvantages

Advantages:

- Specimen easily obtained
- Inexpensive, routine laboratory test

Disadvantages: Provides information only about some types of secondary renal damage due to hypertension.

Abnormal

- Presence of blood, protein, or glucose
- Keep in mind the possibility of a false-positive result (e.g. caused by a urinary tract infection) or a falsely abnormal result

Cause of abnormal result

- Renal disease
- Noninsulin-dependent diabetes mellitus

Drugs, disorders, and other factors that may alter results

- Menstruation – blood is often found in urine samples taken from menstruating women
- Urinary tract infection

BLOOD CHEMISTRY

Description

Venous blood.

Advantages/Disadvantages

Advantages:

- Sample easily obtained
- Routine laboratory test

Disadvantages:

Provides information only about some types of secondary hypertension.

Normal
- Potassium: 3.5–5.0meq/L (3.5–5.0mmol/L)
- Creatinine: 0.6–1.3mg/dL (53–115mcmol/L)
- Glucose: 70–115mg/dL (3.9–6.4mmol/L)
- Total cholesterol: <200mg/dL desirable (<5.20mmol/L, 200–239mg/dL borderline (5.2–6.18mmol/L), >240mg/dL high (>6.21mmol/L)
- HDL cholesterol > 35mg/dL (>0.9mmol/L) desirable, <35mg/dL (<0.9mmol/L) low
- LDL cholesterol <130mg/dL desirable, 130–159mg/dL borderline, >160mg/dL high (in patients with documented coronary artery disease, desirable is <100mg/dL)
- Triglycerides <160mg/dL (<1.8mmol/L)
- Each laboratory will define the normal range for each of the above parameters, and these ranges may differ depending on the analytic techniques employed

Abnormal
- Values outside the normal ranges
- Keep in mind the possibility of a falsely abnormal result

Cause of abnormal result
- Low potassium could suggest primary aldosteronism
- High creatinine could suggest renal disease
- High glucose could suggest diabetes, which can affect the overall cardiovascular risk of the patient
- High cholesterol, HDL cholesterol, or triglycerides increase cardiovascular risk

Imaging
ECHOCARDIOGRAPHY

Advantages/Disadvantages

Advantages:
- Noninvasive
- Provides detailed information about cardiac anatomy and function

Disadvantages:
- Unlikely to be available in primary care office; requires referral
- Interpretation requires experience

Abnormal

Left ventricular hypertrophy.

Cause of abnormal result
- Abnormalities of cardiac anatomy (e.g. left ventricular hypertrophy)
- Impaired left ventricular systolic function
- Impaired left ventricular diastolic function
- Valvular defects
- Keep in mind the possibility of a falsely abnormal result

Other tests
ELECTROCARDIOGRAPHY (ECG)

Advantages/Disadvantages

Advantages:
- Relatively easy to perform
- Noninvasive
- Provides useful information about cardiac function

Abnormal

- Left ventricular hypertrophy
- ST-segment depression or T-wave inversion
- Arrhythmias

Cause of abnormal result

- Cardiac arrythmias (e.g. atrial fibrillation)
- Abnormalities of the cardiac conducting system (e.g. AV block)
- Previous myocardial infarction
- Abnormalities of cardiac anatomy (e.g. left ventricular hypertrophy)
- Myocardial ischemia
- Keep in mind the possibility of a falsely abnormal result

AMBULATORY BLOOD PRESSURE MONITORING

Description

Monitoring of blood pressures at home has long been used as an adjunct to evaluation. This could be with either a standard blood pressure cuff performed by a trained person, or with an automated blood pressure device, or with at 24-h ambulatory monitor.

Advantages/Disadvantages

Advantages:

- Elimination of 'white coat' effect
- Increased amount of blood pressure data for evaluation
- Can monitor blood pressure more closely
- Improves patient awareness and potentially compliance

Disadvantages:

- Limited prognostic data available
- Blood pressure readings may be misread by the patient

Abnormal

Same as for standard blood pressure: blood pressure >140/90mmHg over a 3-month period indicates hypertension.

TREATMENT

CONSIDER CONSULT

- Refer all patients whose blood pressure is not adequately controlled despite adequate lifestyle measures and three antihypertensive medications
- Consider referring patients whose blood pressure is not adequately controlled despite adequate lifestyle measures and two antihypertensive medications

IMMEDIATE ACTION

Hypertension should be treated urgently and aggressively in the following emergencies:

- Hypertensive encephalopathy
- Intracranial hemorrhage
- Unstable angina
- Acute myocardial infarction
- Acute left ventricular failure with pulmonary edema
- Dissecting aortic aneurysm
- Pregnancy-induced hypertension
- Malignant hypertension

Blood pressure should be lowered within hours in hypertensive urgencies such as:

- Very high blood pressure
- Hypertension with optic disk edema
- Uncomplicated malignant hypertension
- Progressive target organ complications
- Severe perioperative hypertension

MANAGEMENT ISSUES

Goals

- The main aim of treatment is to reduce the risk of clinically overt cardiovascular disease
- Blood pressure should be reduced to less than 140/90mmHg (and ideally to 120/80mmHg)
- Blood pressure should not be viewed in isolation; rather, the whole cardiovascular risk profile (e.g. smoking, dyslipidemia, obesity, diabetes) of the patient should be considered

Management in special circumstances

- It is important to consider the patient's overall cardiovascular risk profile, and not to focus on blood pressure alone
- The important determinant of thresholds for intervention is overall cardiovascular risk

COEXISTING DISEASE

- Patients with diabetes mellitus type 1 or type 2 are at increased cardiovascular risk, so hypertension should be treated more aggressively in these patients, with a target blood pressure of 130/80–85mmHg
- Patients with dyslipidemia are at increased cardiovascular risk, so hypertension should be treated more aggressively
- Patients with clinically overt cardiovascular disease (e.g. angina, previous myocardial infarction, heart failure) are at increased risk of further cardiovascular events, so hypertension should be treated more aggressively in these patients
- Patients with angina and hypertension may benefit from calcium channel blockers or beta-blockers
- Patients with heart failure and hypertension may benefit from angiotensin-converting enzyme (ACE) inhibitors and diuretics

COEXISTING MEDICATION

- Many drugs can increase blood pressure (e.g. oral contraceptives), so it is important to take a full drug history in patients with elevated blood pressure
- Hypertensive women taking oral contraceptives should be advised to discontinue them if feasible; this may result in blood pressure returning to normal levels within a few months
- For hypertensive women who are unwilling to discontinue oral contraceptives, antihypertensive medication may be necessary

SPECIAL PATIENT GROUPS

Ethnic minorities

- African-American patients and those of south Asian descent are at increased risk of cardiovascular disease compared with Caucasians, and it is therefore particularly important that they receive adequate antihypertensive treatment
- African-American patients may not respond well to beta-blockers

Pregnant women

- Pregnancy-induced hypertension is an important cause of fetal loss and maternal death; there may be no warning signs or symptoms. Check the blood pressure of pregnant women at every consultation. Specialist referral for the management of hypertension in pregnancy is usually required
- ACE inhibitors and angiotensin II antagonists are contraindicated in pregnancy because of the risk of fetal malformations
- Women previously diagnosed as hypertensive before becoming pregnant can continue previous antihypertensive therapy (except ACE inhibitors or angiotensin II antagonists) during pregnancy
- Beta-blockers such as atenolol may produce poor fetal growth and should be avoided. Labetolol, however, does appear to be safe
- The most useful non-pharmacologic measure for treating hypertension in pregnancy is rest, or at least a reduction in activities
- Methyldopa is the drug of choice for women whose hypertension is first diagnosed during pregnancy, if drug treatment is indicated

Women of childbearing potential

- ACE inhibitors and angiotensin II antagonists should be avoided in women who may become pregnant

Children and adolescents

- Hypertension is defined in children as systolic or diastolic blood pressure consistently above the 95th centile for the child's age and height
- In children with blood pressure far above the 95th centile, a secondary cause is likely, and appropriate investigations are necessary
- Non-pharmacologic measures (weight loss, exercise, and diet) are the first-line treatment of hypertension in children
- Drug treatment may be indicated in children with blood pressure consistently above the 95th centile despite adequate non-pharmacologic measures. These patients should be referred promptly for specialist care

Very elderly patients

- Randomized controlled trials (RCTs) have shown clear benefits of antihypertensive treatment in patients up to about 80 years of age
- Patients aged over 80 years previously diagnosed with hypertension should continue any existing medication
- In patients aged over 80 years who are newly diagnosed with hypertension, there is limited evidence to guide treatment decisions. Treatment should be initiated, but side-effects should

be monitored closely and careful selection of antihypertensive medications is appropriate to avoid adverse events and side-effects that may negate any putative long-term benefit of treatment
- First-line antihypertensive drugs for elderly patients are low-dose thiazides

PATIENT SATISFACTION/LIFESTYLE PRIORITIES
- Patients may find it difficult to make necessary lifestyle modifications, and require support and encouragement
- It is important that drugs be as well tolerated as possible, as patients are unlikely to comply with long-term medication for a condition with no symptoms if the medication is troublesome

SUMMARY OF THERAPEUTIC OPTIONS

Choices

Guidelines

- WHO–ISH Hypertension Guidelines Committee. 1999 World Health Organization–International Society of Hypertension Guidelines for the Management of Hypertension. J Hypertens 1999;17:151–85 [1]

The following guidelines are available:
- National Heart, Lung, and Blood Institute and the National High Blood Pressure Education Program have developed guidelines. Sixth report of the Joint National Committee on Prevention, Detection, Evaluation, and Treatment of High Blood Pressure. Bethesda (MD): US Department of Health and Human Services, Public Health Service, National Institutes of Health, National Heart, Lung, and Blood Institute, 1997 [2]
- Institute for Clinical Systems Improvement. Hypertension diagnosis and treatment. Bloomington (MN): ICSI, 2000 [3]
- Veterans Health Administration. Diagnosis and management of hypertension in the primary care setting. The Hypertension Working Group. Washington (DC): Department of Veterans Affairs, 1999 [4]

The following points should be borne in mind:
- Therapy should be dictated by the patient's overall cardiovascular risk, not by blood pressure alone
- Lifestyle modifications are indicated in all hypertensive patients; in those with relatively low cardiovascular risk, they may be all that is required
- Choices about drug treatment should take into account any coexisting disease, as this may favor or limit the use of particular drugs (e.g. calcium channel blockers or beta-blockers may be preferred in patients with angina)
- If initial treatment is insufficient, combining drugs from different classes frequently provides better control of blood pressure with fewer side-effects than increasing the dose of a single drug

The main pharmacotherapeutic options are:
- Diuretics or beta-blockers are first-line drug treatments, unless there are specific indications for another class of drug, as they are effective in reducing blood pressure and have been shown to reduce morbidity and mortality in RCTs
- ACE inhibitors are safe and effective in lowering blood pressure, and are particularly suitable for patients with heart failure, diabetes, or proteinuria
- Calcium channel blockers are effective and well tolerated in lowering blood pressure, and are of particular benefit in preventing stroke in elderly patients with systolic hypertension
- Angiotensin II antagonists have much in common with ACE inhibitors, including some benefits in patients with heart failure; however, they are a relatively new class of agent, and long-term data on their effects on cardiovascular risk are lacking, so they should be considered primarily for patients who are unable to tolerate ACE inhibitors

- Alpha-blockers are safe and effective in lowering blood pressure, although their long-term effects on cardiovascular risk are unknown; they may be suitable for patients with coexisting benign prostatic hyperplasia
- Methyldopa has an important place in the management of hypertension in pregnancy
- Minoxidil is a centrally acting antihypertensive drug, which may have a role when standard medications have failed to control blood pressure. It can be used in combination with a beta-blocker and a diuretic in severe hypertension resistant to other drugs
- Hydralazine can be used in combination with other drugs in moderate to severe hypertension, but its side-effect profile makes it generally unsuitable as monotherapy
- Clonidine is a centrally acting $alpha_2$ agonist; it is a potent antihypertensive drug, and useful in patients resistant to other therapies
- Sodium nitroprusside is used intravenously for rapid reduction in blood pressure in hypertensive emergencies; it would not usually be used in primary care

Clinical pearl(s)

- Don't forget about diuretics. This class of drugs is clinically proven to reduce mortality and diuretics frequently overlooked
- Diuretics can frequently improve the blood pressure control achieved with vasodilators, and help reduce fluid retention associated with vasodilators
- If a patient requires three or more drugs, screen for secondary causes of hypertension (e.g. renal artery stenosis) and consider noncompliance. Use of once a day medications improves compliance
- Data from a recent large trial show dramatic clinical cardiac event reductions with ACE inhibitors, thus this class represents a good first- or second-line drug choice
- Talk to your patient about good compliance

Never

- ACE inhibitors or angiotensin II antagonists must not be used in pregnant women, and should be avoided in women of childbearing potential and in patients with bilateral renal artery stenosis
- Never ignore hypertension in a pregnant woman. Pregnancy-induced hypertension may be rapidly fatal

FOLLOW UP

Plan for review

- After an elevated blood pressure is first detected, patients should return for several visits to confirm the diagnosis of hypertension; the frequency of visits will be guided by the initial blood pressure: confirmation of a mildly elevated reading (<160/100mmHg) should take place within 2 months, whereas a severely elevated reading (>180/110mmHg) requires confirmation within 1 week
- Patients who are advised about lifestyle measures and not prescribed drug treatment should be seen at frequent intervals over the first few months to assess the effect on blood pressure
- The length of time for which lifestyle measures are tried before drug treatment is started, if blood pressure does not normalize, will depend on the patient's overall cardiovascular risk; up to 1 year may be appropriate for patients at low risk
- Most patients should be seen within 1–2 months after starting drug treatment to assess efficacy in controlling blood pressure and adverse effects
- If initial drug treatment does not lower blood pressure adequately, it is usually preferable to add another drug from a different class, rather than to increase the dose of the first drug
- If initial drug treatment fails to lower blood pressure at all, or is poorly tolerated, a switch to a drug in an alternative class is indicated
- If blood pressure is still high despite adequate lifestyle measures and treatment with two drugs, consider referral to a hypertension specialist

- Frequent visits should continue until blood pressure is well controlled. Once blood pressure is stabilized, patients should be seen every 3–6 months, depending on cardiovascular risk and complexity of treatment regimen, to ensure continued blood pressure control and to detect any complications

Information for patient or caregiver

- The importance of lifestyle measures, particularly giving up smoking, for reducing cardiovascular risk should be stressed
- Patients should be counseled about the need for compliance with treatment, despite their lack of symptoms from hypertension

DRUGS AND OTHER THERAPIES: DETAILS

Drugs

DIURETICS

- Diuretics should be considered as first-line treatment for uncomplicated hypertension
- In addition to being effective in reducing blood pressure, they have been shown to reduce morbidity and mortality in RCTs
- Doses should be given in the morning so that diuresis does not interfere with sleep

Dose

Thiazide diuretics:

- Bendrofluazide: 2.5mg once daily
- Chlorothiazide: 250–500mg once daily
- Chlorthalidone: 25–50mg once daily
- Cyclopenthiazide: 250–500mcg once daily
- Hydrochlorothiazide: 25–50mg once daily
- Indapamide: 2.5mg once daily
- Mefruside:25–50mg once daily
- Metolazone: 5mg once daily
- Polythiazide: 0.5–4mg once daily
- Xipamide: 20mg once daily

Loop diuretics:

- Furosemide: 20–80mg once daily
- Torasemide: 2.5–5mg once daily

Efficacy

- Long-term use of diuretics in hypertensive patients reduces the risk of cardiovascular complications
- Diuretics are usually effective in reducing blood pressure
- Antihypertensive response to diuretics is variable, and not all patients will have blood pressure within the target range on diuretics alone
- If blood pressure is not satisfactorily controlled within 1–2 months of starting treatment, consider adding a drug from a different class or increasing the dose of diuretic

Risks/Benefits

- Treatment with diuretics can occasionally lead to hypokalemia, although the risk is small with low doses
- The benefits of reductions in cardiovascular morbidity and mortality have been well established in RCTs

Thiazide diuretics:
- Use caution in fluid or electrolyte imbalances
- Use caution in patients with high cholesterol levels or elevated triglyceride levels
- Avoid exposure to sunlight

Loop diuretics:
- Use caution in the elderly
- Use caution in fluid/electrolyte imbalances
- Use caution in gastrointestinal disease
- Use caution in renal impairment
- Use caution in gout
- Use caution in diabetes mellitus
- Avoid exposure to sunlight

Side-effects and adverse reactions
Thiazide diurectics:
- Gastrointestinal: nausea, vomiting, diarrhea, abdominal pain, anorexia, constipation, jaundice, hepatitis, pancreatitis, dry mouth
- Metabolic: hyperglycemia, hyperuricemia, glycosuria, electrolye imbalance
- Cardiovascular: hypotension, orthostatic hypotension, palpitations
- Genitourinary: nocturia, change in libido, impotence, interstitial nephritis, renal failure
- CNS: headache, dizziness, vertigo, parasthesias, weakness, insomnia, anxiety
- Hematologic: anemia, thrombocytopenia, leukopenia, agranulocytosis
- Skin: rash, urticaria, purpura, photosensitivity, vasculitis

Loop diuretics:
- Gastrointestinal: nausea, vomiting, pancreatitis
- Metabolic: hypercholesterolemia, hypertriglyceridemia, hypokalemia, hypomagnesemia, hyperglycemia
- Genitourinary: polyuria
- Cardiovascular: orthostatic hypotension, ECG abnormalities, chest pain, thrombophlebitis
- EENT: tinnitus, deafness
- Hematologic: bone marrow depression
- Skin: photosensitivity, rashes

Interactions (other drugs)
Thiazide diuretics:
▪ ACE inhibitors ▪ Allopurinol ▪ Amphotericin B ▪ Anesthetics ▪ Anticholinergics ▪ Anticoagulants ▪ Antidiabetics ▪ Antidysrhythmics (cardiac glycosides, amiodarone, disopyramide, flecainide, mexiletine, quinidine, sotalol) ▪ Antineoplastics ▪ $Beta_2$ agonists ▪ Calcium salts ▪ Carbenoxolone ▪ Cholestyramine, colestipol ▪ Corticosteroids ▪ Diazoxide ▪ Lidocaine ▪ Lithium ▪ Loop diuretics, acetazolamide ▪ Methenamines ▪ Methyldopa ▪ Nondepolarizing muscle relaxants ▪ NSAIDs ▪ Pimozide ▪ Reboxetine ▪ Toremifene ▪ Vitamin D

Loop diuretics:
▪ ACE inhibitors ▪ Aminoglycosides, cephalosporins, polymyxins, vancomycin ▪ Amphotericin B ▪ Anticoagulants ▪ Antidiabetics ▪ Antidysrhythmics (amiodarone, cardiac glycosides, disopyramide, flecainide, mexiletine, quinidine) ▪ Beta-blockers ▪ $Beta_2$ agonists ▪ Carbenoxolone ▪ Charcoal ▪ Chloral hydrate ▪ Cisplatin ▪ Clofibrate ▪ Ethanol ▪ Hydantoins ▪ Lithium ▪ Nondepolarizing muscle relaxants ▪ NSAIDs ▪ Probenecid ▪ Reboxetine ▪ Salicylates ▪ Theophyllines ▪ Thiazide diuretics, acetazolamide

Contraindications
- Anuria
- Renal impairment
- Hepatic coma

Evidence
- Beta-blockers and diuretics are recommended first-line antihypertensives for uncomplicated hypertension, due to their proven efficacy in reduction of morbidity and mortality. Diuretics are particularly useful for elderly patients with systolic hypertension [2–4] *Level C*
- A systematic review found that the treatment of hypertension in healthy elderly people with diuretics and beta-blockers is clearly beneficial [5] *Level M*
- An overview of RCTs assessing therapies (usually diuretics, beta-blockers or both) for people with hypertension (most without a history of vascular disease) found that a reduction in blood pressure over 2–3 years reduced the risk of stroke [6] *Level P*
- A systematic review (consisting mainly of RCTs comparing diuretics or beta-blockers with placebo) found that antihypertensive medications produced variable reductions in systolic/diastolic blood pressure (average 12–16/5–10mmHg). Benefit was noted in terms of total death rate, cardiovascular death rate, stroke, major coronary events, and congestive heart failure in treated patients [7] *Level M*
- Two systematic reviews compared diuretics and beta-blockers as first-line agents in the treatment of hypertension. No significant difference was found between the drugs for the lowering of blood pressure [8] *Level M*

Acceptability to patient
- Diuretics are generally well tolerated
- However, any tolerability problems may lead to poor compliance, as patients may be unwilling to accept side-effects when treating an asymptomatic condition

Follow up plan
Patients should be reviewed regularly to ensure that blood pressure is maintained within the target range.

Patient and caregiver information
Patients must be educated about the importance of continuing to take their medication, even though they do not feel unwell.

BETA-BLOCKERS
Beta-blockers should be considered as first-line treatment for uncomplicated hypertension. As well as being effective in reducing blood pressure, they have been shown to reduce morbidity and mortality in RCTs.

Dose
- Propranolol hydrochloride: 40–160mg twice daily
- Atenolol: 50–100mg once daily
- Betaxolol hydrochloride: 10–20mg once daily
- Bisoprolol fumarate: 5–20mg once daily
- Carvedilol: initially 6.25mg twice daily initially, increased after 7–14 days as tolerated, up to 25mg twice daily
- Labetolol hydrochloride: 100–400mg twice daily
- Metoprolol tartrate: 50–200mg once daily
- Nadolol: 40–320mg once daily
- Timolol maleate: 10–20mg twice daily

Efficacy

- Long-term use of beta-blockers in hypertensive patients reduces the risk of cardiovascular complications
- Beta-blockers are usually effective in reducing blood pressure
- Antihypertensive response to beta-blockers is variable, and not all patients will have blood pressure within the target range on beta-blockers alone
- If blood pressure is not satisfactorily controlled within 1–2 months of starting treatment, consider adding a drug from a different class or increasing the dose of beta-blocker

Risks/Benefits

- Generally few risks
- The benefits of reductions in cardiovascular morbidity and mortality have been well established in RCTs
- Use caution in pregnancy and breast-feeding
- Use caution in diabetes mellitus
- Use caution in liver and renal impairment
- Use caution in AV block
- Use caution in myasthenia gravis
- Do not withdraw abruptly in angina

Side-effects and adverse reactions

- Gastrointestinal: nausea, vomiting
- Cardiovascular: hypotension, bradycardia, conduction abnormalities, heart failure, peripheral vasoconstriction
- CNS: fatigue, sleep disturbances
- Respiratory: bronchospasm
- Genitourinary: sexual dysfunction
- EENT: dry eyes
- Skin: rashes, exacerbation of psoriasis

Interactions (other drugs)

■ ACE inhibitors ■ Adrenergic neurone blockers ■ Alcohol ■ Alpha-blockers ■ Alprostadil ■ Anesthetics, general ■ Angiotensin II receptor antagonists ■ Antiarrhythmics (especially amiodarone) ■ Antidiabetics ■ Antihypertensives (clonidine, diazoxide, hydralazine, methyldopa, minoxidil, nitroprusside) ■ Anxiolytics/Hypnotics ■ Baclofen, tizanidine ■ Calcium channel blockers (especially verapamil) ■ Cardiac glycosides ■ Corticosteroids ■ Diuretics ■ Dobutamine ■ Epinephrine, norepinephrine ■ Estrogens ■ Levodopa ■ MAOIs ■ Mefloquine ■ NSAIDs ■ Nitrates ■ Phenothiazines ■ Pilocarpine ■ Theophylline

Contraindications

■ Second- or third degree heart block ■ Asthma ■ Chronic obstructive airways disease ■ Class III/IV congestive heart failure ■ Pheochromocytoma ■ Metabolic acidosis ■ Sick sinus syndrome, marked bradycardia, hypotension, cardiogenic shock, peripheral arterial disease, Prinzmetal's angina

Evidence

- Beta-blockers and diuretics are recommended first-line antihypertensives for uncomplicated hypertension, due to their proven efficacy in reduction of morbidity and mortality [2–4] *Level C*
- A systematic review found that the treatment of hypertension in healthy elderly people with diuretics and beta-blockers was clearly beneficial [5] *Level M*

- An overview of RCTs assessing therapies (usually diuretics, beta-blockers or both) for people with hypertension (most without a history of vascular disease) found that a reduction in blood pressure over 2–3 years reduced the risk of stroke [6] *Level P*
- A systematic review (consisting mainly of RCTs comparing diuretics or beta-blockers with placebo) found that antihypertensive medications produced variable reductions in systolic/diastolic blood pressure (average 12–16/5–10mmHg). Benefit was noted in terms of total death rate, cardiovascular death rate, stroke, major coronary events, and congestive heart failure in treated patients [7] *Level M*
- Two systematic reviews compared diuretics and beta-blockers as first-line agents in the treatment of hypertension. No significant difference was found between the drugs for the lowering of blood pressure [8] *Level M*

Acceptability to patient
Side-effects may limit compliance when treating an asymptomatic condition.

Follow up plan
Patients should be reviewed regularly to ensure that blood pressure is maintained within the target range.

Patient and caregiver information
Patients must be educated about the importance of continuing to take their medication. The physician should be promptly notified if the patient is planning to discontinue the medication.

CALCIUM CHANNEL BLOCKERS
The long-term benefits of calcium channel blockers are less well established than those of diuretics and beta-blockers, so the latter drugs should be preferred to calcium channel blockers as first-line therapy for uncomplicated hypertension.

However, calcium channel blockers are effective in reducing blood pressure, and are useful in the following circumstances:
- In patients who do not respond to or do not tolerate diuretics or beta-blockers
- In combination with selected beta-blockers in patients not adequately controlled on beta-blockers alone
- In elderly patients with isolated systolic hypertension
- In patients with coexisting angina

Dose
- Amlodipine besylate: 5–10mg once daily
- Diltiazem hydrochloride: 30mg four times a day, up to 360mg/day divided three/four times a day, immediate release
- Felodipine: 5–10mg once daily
- Isradipine: 2.5–10mg twice daily
- Nicardipine hydrochloride: 20–30mg three times daily
- Nifedipine: immediate-release nifedipine should not be used for the treatment of hypertension; 30–90mg of extended-release forms
- Nisoldipine: 20–60mg once daily
- Verapamil hydrochloride: 80–240mg twice daily or 180–360mg once daily with sustained-release preparations

Efficacy

- Calcium channel blockers are usually effective in reducing blood pressure
- Calcium channel blockers have been shown to reduce the risk of stroke in elderly patients with isolated systolic hypertension
- Antihypertensive response to calcium channel blockers is variable, and not all patients will have blood pressure within the target range on calcium channel blockers alone
- If blood pressure is not satisfactorily controlled within 1–2 months of starting treatment, consider adding a drug from a different class or increasing the dose of calcium channel blocker

Risks/Benefits

- Immediate-release nifedipine can precipitate ischemic events, and should not be prescribed for hypertensive patients
- Other calcium channel blockers (and extended-release formulations of nifedipine) are not associated with important risks
- Calcium channel blockers reduce the incidence of stroke in elderly patients with isolated systolic hypertension
- In other patient groups, although calcium channel blockers are effective in reducing blood pressure, the long-term benefits are not well established
- Diltiazem should not be used in patients with congestive heart failure or left ventricular dysfunction because it increased mortality in one large study
- Use caution in hepatic impairment
- Use caution in edema

Side-effects and adverse reactions

- Gastrointestinal: nausea, vomiting, diarrhea, constipation, hepatitis, abdominal pain, dry mouth, flatulence
- Cardiovascular: hypotension, peripheral edema, palpitations, AV block, bradycardia, tachycardia, congestive heart failure, myocardial infarction, angina
- CNS: headache, dizziness, tremor, weakness, somnolence, insomnia, paresthesias, nervousness
- Respiratory: dyspnea, cough, respiratory infection
- Genitourinary: sexual dysfunction, urinary disorders
- Musculoskeletal: cramps, myalgia
- Skin: sweating, flushing, dermatitis, rash, pruritus, urticaria

Interactions (other drugs)

▪ ACE inhibitors ▪ Adrenergic neurone blockers ▪ Alcohol ▪ Alpha-blockers ▪ Alprostadil ▪ Anesthetics ▪ Angiotensin II receptor antagonists ▪ Antiarrhythmics ▪ Antihypertensives (beta-blockers, clonidine, diazoxide, hydralazine, methyldopa, minoxidil, nitrates, nitroprusside) ▪ Antipsychotics ▪ Anxiolytics and hypnotics ▪ Baclofen, tizanidine ▪ Cimetidine ▪ Corticosteroids ▪ Diuretics ▪ Estrogens ▪ Levodopa ▪ NSAIDs ▪ Ritonavir ▪ Theophylline

Contraindications

▪ Sick sinus syndrome or second- or third-degree AV block except with a functioning pacemaker, hypotension <90mmHg systolic (diltiazem and verapamil) ▪ Acute myocardial infarction and pulmonary congestion (diltiazem) ▪ Severe left ventricular dysfunction; cardiogenic shock and severe congestive heart failure, unless secondary to a supraventricular tachycardia amenable to verapamil therapy and in patients with atrial flutter or atrial fibrillation and an accessory bypass tract (verapamil) ▪ Do not administer intravenous verapamil concomitantly with intravenous beta-adrenergic blocking agents (within a few hours) ▪ Ventricular tachycardia (verapamil) ▪ Advanced aortic stenosis (nicardipine)

Evidence

- Calcium channel blockers are effective for blood pressure reduction. They are particularly recommended for elderly patients with systolic hypertension. Long-acting calcium channel antagonists are preferred, and short-acting antagonists should be avoided [1] *Level C*
- A RCT compared nitrendipine with placebo in the management of elderly patients with systolic hypertension. Blood pressure reduction over 2 years with the calcium channel antagonist reduced the risk of stroke [9] *Level P*
- Short- and intermediate-acting dihydropyridine calcium channel blockers may increase cardiovascular morbidity and mortality [8]

Acceptability to patient

Side-effects may limit compliance when treating an asymptomatic condition.

Follow up plan

Patients should be reviewed regularly to ensure that blood pressure is maintained within the target range.

Patient and caregiver information

Patients must be educated about the importance of continuing to take their medication, even though they do not feel unwell.

ACE INHIBITORS

ACE inhibitors are effective in reducing blood pressure, and are particularly useful in the following circumstances:

- In patients who do not respond to or do not tolerate diuretics or beta-blockers
- In combination with diuretics in patients not adequately controlled on diuretics alone
- In patients with coexisting heart failure
- In patients with diabetes and in any patient with proteinuria

Dose

NB: lower doses than those given below should be used if ACE inhibitors are given in combination with diuretics

- Captopril: 12.5–50mg two or three times daily
- Enalapril maleate: 5–20mg once or twice daily
- Fosinopril: 10–40mg once daily
- Lisinopril: 10–40mg daily
- Moexipril hydrochloride: 7.5–30mg once daily
- Quinapril: 10–40mg once daily
- Ramipril: 2.5–20mg once daily
- Trandolapril: 0.5–4mg once daily

Efficacy

- ACE inhibitors are usually effective in reducing blood pressure
- ACE inhibitors have been shown to reduce morbidity and mortality in patients with heart failure, and to delay the progression of renal disease in patients with diabetes
- Antihypertensive response to ACE inhibitors is variable, and not all patients will have blood pressure within the target range on ACE inhibitors alone
- If blood pressure is not satisfactorily controlled within 1–2 months of starting treatment, consider adding a drug from a different class or increasing the dose of ACE inhibitor

Risks/Benefits

- In rare cases, ACE inhibitors may cause life-threatening angioedema
- ACE inhibitors reduce morbidity and mortality in patients with heart failure
- ACE inhibitors delay the progression of renal disease in patients with diabetes

- Use caution in patients receiving diuretics
- First dose may cause hypotension in those on diuretics, a low sodium diet or dialysis, those who are dehydrated or have heart failure
- Use caution in atherosclerosis
- Use caution in renal impairment
- Use caution in breast-feeding
- Use caution in angioedema

Side-effects and adverse reactions

- Gastrointestinal: nausea, vomiting, diarrhea, constipation, dyspepsia, hepatitis, altered liver function tests, cholestatic jaundice, pancreatitis
- Cardiovascular: hypotension, angioedema, vasculitis
- Genitourinary: renal impairment
- CNS: headache, dizziness, fatigue, paresthesias, fever, malaise
- Hematologic: blood cell dyscrasias
- Respiratory: dry cough, upper respiratory tract infections
- Musculoskeletal: myalgia, arthralgia
- Skin: rash, photosensitivity

Interactions (other drugs)

■ Adrenergic neurone blockers ■ Alcohol ■ Alpha-blockers ■ Alprostadil ■ Angiotensin II receptor antagonists ■ Antacids ■ Antidiabetics (insulin, metformin, sulfonylureas) ■ Antihypertensives (beta-blockers, clonidine, diazoxide, hydralazine, methyldopa, minoxidil, nitrates, nitroprusside) ■ Anxiolytics and hypnotics ■ Baclofen, tizanidine ■ Calcium channel blockers ■ Cyclosporine ■ Corticosteroids ■ Diuretics ■ Estrogens ■ Heparins ■ Levodopa ■ Lithium ■ NSAIDs ■ Phenothiazines ■ Potassium salts

Contraindications

■ Pregnancy ■ Bilateral renal artery stenosis ■ Aortic stenosis ■ Renovascular disease

Evidence

- ACE inhibitors are effective for the treatment of hypertension [1] *Level C*
- A systematic review found no significant difference in outcomes when beta-blockers, diuretics, and ACE inhibitors were compared for the initial treatment of hypertension [10] *Level M*

Acceptability to patient

Side-effects may limit compliance when treating an asymptomatic condition.

Follow up plan

Patients should be reviewed regularly to ensure that blood pressure is maintained within the target range.

Patient and caregiver information

Patients must be educated about the importance of continuing to take their medication, even though they do not feel unwell.

ANGIOTENSIN II ANTAGONISTS

- Angiotensin II antagonists have much in common with ACE inhibitors, including beneficial effects in patients with heart failure
- However, angiotensin II antagonists are a relatively new class of drug and their long-term effects are less well established than those of ACE inhibitors
- The main place of angiotensin II antagonists is for patients for whom ACE inhibitors are indicated but who are unable to tolerate them

- Angiotensin II antagonists generally have fewer side-effects than ACE inhibitors; in particular, they lack the propensity of ACE inhibitors to cause dry cough

Dose
- Candesartan cilexetil: 8–32mg once daily
- Irbesartan: 150–300mg once daily
- Losartan potassium: 25–100mg once daily
- Valsartan: 80–320mg once daily

Efficacy
- Angiotensin II antagonists are usually effective in reducing blood pressure
- The long-term effects of angiotensin II antagonists on cardiovascular outcomes are largely unknown
- Antihypertensive response to angiotensin II antagonists is variable, and not all patients will have blood pressure within the target range on angiotensin II antagonists alone
- If blood pressure is not satisfactorily controlled within 1–2 months of starting treatment, consider adding a drug from a different class or increasing the dose of angiotensin II antagonist

Risks/Benefits
- Generally few risks
- Long-term benefit remains to be established
- Use caution in renal artery stenosis
- Use caution in aortic or mitral valve stenosis
- Use caution in obstructive hypertrophic cardiomyopathy
- Use caution in renal and hepatic impairment

Side-effects and adverse reactions
- Gastrointestinal: nausea, vomiting, diarrhea, hepatitis, altered liver function tests, taste disturbance
- Cardiovascular: hypotension, angioedema
- Metabolic: hyperkalemia
- CNS: dizziness, migraine
- Hematologic: anemia
- Musculoskeletal: myalgia
- Skin: rash, urticaria, pruritus

Interactions (other drugs)
▪ ACE inhibitors ▪ Adrenergic neurone blockers ▪ Alcohol ▪ Alpha-blockers ▪ Alprostadil ▪ Anesthetics ▪ Antihypertensives (beta-blockers, clonidine, diazoxide, hydralazine, methyldopa, minoxidil, nitrates, nitroprusside) ▪ Anxiolytics and hypnotics ▪ Baclofen, tizanidine ▪ Calcium channel blockers ▪ Cyclosporine ▪ Corticosteroids ▪ Diuretics ▪ Estrogens ▪ Heparins ▪ Levodopa ▪ Lithium ▪ NSAIDs ▪ Phenothiazines ▪ Potassium salts

Contraindications
▪ Pregnancy ▪ Breast-feeding ▪ Severe hepatic impairment

Acceptability to patient
Side-effects may limit compliance when treating an asymptomatic condition.

Follow up plan

Patients should be reviewed regularly to ensure that blood pressure is maintained within the target range.

Patient and caregiver information

Patients must be educated about the importance of continuing to take their medication, even though they do not feel unwell.

ALPHA-BLOCKERS

The long-term benefits of alpha-blockers are less well established than those of diuretics and beta-blockers, so the latter drugs should be preferred to alpha-blockers as first-line therapy for uncomplicated hypertension.

However, alpha-blockers are effective in reducing blood pressure, and are useful in the following circumstances:

- In patients who do not respond to or do not tolerate diuretics or beta-blockers
- In combination with beta-blockers in patients not adequately controlled on beta-blockers alone
- In patients with coexisting benign prostatic hyperplasia

Dose

- Doxazosin: 1–16mg once daily
- Prazosin: initially 500mcg two to three times daily, increased to 1mg two to three times daily after 3–7 days; further increased if necessary to maximum daily dose of 20mg
- Terazosin: 1–10mg once daily

Efficacy

- Alpha-blockers are usually effective in reducing blood pressure
- Antihypertensive response to alpha-blockers is variable, and not all patients will have blood pressure within the target range on alpha-blockers alone
- If blood pressure is not satisfactorily controlled within 1–2 months of starting treatment, consider adding a drug from a different class or increasing the dose of alpha-blocker

Risks/Benefits

- Generally few risks
- Alpha-blockers may be of benefit beyond their blood pressure-lowering effects in patients with benign prostatic hyperplasia
- Alpha-blockers may also be of particular benefit in patients with glucose intolerance or dyslipidemia
- Long-term benefits on cardiovascular risk are unknown
- Use caution with first dose as this may cause postural hypotension
- Use caution in hepatic impairment
- Use caution in pregnancy and breast-feeding

Side-effects and adverse reactions

- Gastrointestinal: nausea, vomiting, diarrhea, abdominal pain, jaundice, hepatitis, cholestasis
- Cardiovascular: postural hypotension, edema, tachycardia, palpitations
- CNS: headache, drowsiness, dizziness, somnolence, fatigue, vertigo, tremor, agitation, asthenia, depression
- Genitourinary: urinary incontinence, hematuria, sexual dysfunction
- EENT: epistaxis, rhinitis, blurred vision, dry mouth
- Hematologic: thrombocytopenia, leukopenia, purpura
- Skin: rash, pruritus

Interactions (other drugs)

- ACE inhibitors ▪ Adrenergic neurone blockers ▪ Alcohol ▪ Alprostadil ▪ Anesthetics ▪ Angiotensin II receptor antagonists ▪ Antihypertensives (beta-blockers, clonidine, diazoxide, hydralazine, methyldopa, minoxidil, nitrates, nitroprusside) ▪ Antipsychotics ▪ Anxiolytics and hypnotics ▪ Baclofen, tizanidine ▪ Calcium channel blockers ▪ Cyclosporine ▪ Corticosteroids ▪ Diuretics ▪ Estrogens ▪ Levodopa ▪ Lithium ▪ NSAIDs

Contraindications

- Urinary incontinence ▪ History of orthostatic hypotension or micturition syncope ▪ Heart failure

Evidence

- Alpha-blockers are effective and safe for lowering blood pressure; however, there is no evidence about their effects on cardiovascular risk in hypertensive patients [1] *Level C*
- Doxazosin was compared with chlorthalidone in a RCT. No differences were found between the groups for coronary heart disease outcomes. Doxazosin-treated patients had an increased number of cardiovascular events, particularly congestive cardiac failure [11] *Level P*

Acceptability to patient

Side-effects may limit compliance when treating an asymptomatic condition.

Follow up plan

Patients should be reviewed regularly to ensure that blood pressure is maintained within the target range.

Patient and caregiver information

Patients must be educated about the importance of continuing to take their medication, even though they do not feel unwell. The physician should be notified promptly if the patient is planning on discontinuing the medication.

METHYLDOPA

- Centrally acting antihypertensive agent
- Used in the management of moderate to severe hypertension
- Particularly useful in the management of hypertension in pregnancy

Dose

- 250mg by mouth two or three times daily
- Can be gradually increased at intervals of 2 days or longer to usual dose of 1000–1500mg/day in two or three divided doses
- Maximum dose 3000mg/day

Efficacy

Effective at reducing hypertension.

Risks/Benefits

- Has been widely used in pregnancy without reported adverse effects
- Compatible with breast-feeding
- Use caution in liver and renal impairment
- Use caution in pheochromocytoma

Side-effects and adverse reactions

- Gastrointestinal: nausea, vomiting, diarrhea, constipation, hepatitis, pancreatitis, colitis
- Cardiovascular: postural hypotension, bradycardia, edema
- Hematologic: blood cell disorders
- CNS: headache, sedation, dizziness, weakness, paresthesias
- Skin: rash
- Genitourinary: amenorrhea, breast tenderness and enlargement

Interactions (other drugs)

- Antihypertensives ■ Entacapone ■ Iron ■ Levodopa ■ Lithium
- MOAIs and tricyclic antidepressants ■ Sympathomimetics ■ Tolbutamide

Contraindications

- Liver disease.

Acceptability to patient

Generally good.

Follow up plan

Patients should be reviewed regularly to ensure that blood pressure is maintained within the target range.

MINOXIDIL

- Centrally acting antihypertensive agent
- Used when standard medications have failed to control blood pressure
- Can be used in combination with a diuretic and a beta-blocker

Dose

- 2.5–5mg/day in one or two divided doses initially, increased by 5–10mg/day at intervals of 3 days or longer to usual dose of 10–40mg/day
- Maximum dose 100mg/day

Efficacy

Effective at reducing severely raised blood pressure in combination with a diuretic and a beta-blocker.

Risks/Benefits

- Use caution in pregnancy and breast-feeding
- Use caution in cardiac and cerebrovascular disease
- Use caution in angina, congestive heart failure
- Use caution in renal disease
- Use caution in pulmonary hypertension

Side-effects and adverse reactions

- Gastrointestinal: nausea, vomiting,
- Cardiovascular: edema, hypotension, cardiac lesions, cardiac tamponade, pericardial effusion, reflux and sinus tachycardia, angina
- Genitourinary: sodium and water retention, mastalgia
- CNS: headache
- Skin: hypertrichosis, rash, Stevens–Johnson syndrome

Interactions (other drugs)

- Antihypertensive agents ■ Estrogens ■ NSAIDs ■ Sympathomimetics

Contraindications

- Recent MI
- Pheochromocytoma
- Dissecting aortic aneurysm

Acceptability to patient

Generally good.

Follow up plan

Patients should be reviewed regularly to ensure that blood pressure is maintained within the target range.

HYDRALAZINE

- Vasodilator antihypertensive agent
- Used in combination with other drugs in moderate to severe hypertension

Dose

10mg four times daily, increased by 10–25mg at intervals of 2–5 days as needed up to maximum dose of 300mg/day.

Efficacy

Can be a useful adjunctive therapy in moderate to severe hypertension that is not controlled adequately on other treatment.

Risks/Benefits

- Use caution in renal disease or 'slow acetylation' phenotype
- Use caution in systemic lupus erythromatosus (patients should be instructed to report adverse symptoms of joint pain, angina, fever or continued weakness to their physician)
- Use caution in pregnancy (however, widely used in pre-eclampsia)
- Use caution in children or elderly patients
- Use caution in sulfite or tartrazine dye hypersensitivity

Side-effects and adverse reactions

- Gastrointestinal: nausea, vomiting, diarrhea, anorexia, constipation, weight gain
- Cardiovascular: angina, palpitations, sinus tachycardia, orthostatic hypotension, sodium and water retention, edema
- Genitourinary: glomerulonephritis
- CNS: headache, dizziness, peripheral neuritis, paresthesias
- Hematologic: blood dyscrasias
- Skin: lupus-like symptoms, rash

Interactions (other drugs)

- Antihypertensive agents
- Estrogens
- MAOIs
- NSAIDs
- Sympathomimetics

Contraindications

- Coronary artery disease
- Mitral valvular rheumatic heart disease

Acceptability to patient

Side-effect profile limits acceptability.

Follow up plan

Patients should be reviewed regularly to ensure that blood pressure is maintained within the target range.

Patient and caregiver information

Patients should be instructed to report adverse symptoms of joint pain, angina, fever or continued weakness to their physician.

CLONIDINE

Centrally acting $alpha_2$ agonist.

Dose

- 0.1mg twice daily, increased by 0.1–0.2mg/day as necessary up to a maximum dose of 2.4mg/day
- Sedation can be minimized by giving the major part of the daily dose at bedtime

Efficacy

Potent antihypertensive drug that is useful in patients whose hypertension is resistant to other treatments.

Risks/Benefits

- Sudden withdrawal may provoke a hypertensive crisis
- Use caution with severe coronary insufficuency, recent MI or cerebrovascular disease
- Use caution with renal disease

Side-effects and adverse reactions

- Gastrointestinal: constipation, dry mouth, nausea
- Genitourinary: impotence, loss of libido
- CNS: depression, dizziness, drowsiness, sedation, headache
- Cardiovascular: congestive heart failure, dysrhthymias, orthostatic hypotension, Raynaud's phenomenon, rebound hypertension
- Metabolic: gynecomastia
- Skin: rash

Interactions (other drugs)

▪ ACE inhibitors ▪ Adrenergic neurone blockers ▪ Alcohol ▪ Aldesleukin ▪ Alprostadil ▪ Angiotensin II receptor antagonists ▪ Antidepressants ▪ Anxiolytics and hypnotics ▪ Baclofen ▪ Beta-blockers ▪ Calcium-channel blockers ▪ Carbenoxolone ▪ Corticosteroids ▪ Diazoxide ▪ Diuretics ▪ General anesthetics ▪ Hydralazine ▪ Levodopa ▪ Methyldopa ▪ MAOIs ▪ Minoxidil ▪ Moxonidine ▪ NSAIDs ▪ Nitrates ▪ Nitroprusside ▪ Estrogens ▪ Phenothiazines ▪ Tizanidine

Contraindications

▪ Severe bradyarhythmias ▪ Second- or third-degree AV block

Acceptability to patient

Reasonable.

Follow up plan

Patients should be reviewed regularly to ensure that blood pressure is maintained within the target range.

Patient and caregiver information

Patients must be warned not to stop clonidine suddenly.

LIFESTYLE

All patients with hypertension should be encouraged to take the following lifestyle measures:

- Give up smoking
- Lose weight if overweight
- Take regular aerobic exercise
- Limit alcohol intake to no more than 30mL (men) or 15mL (women) ethanol per day
- Reduce dietary sodium intake

RISKS/BENEFITS

- Patients with pre-existing cardiac disease may be at risk of precipitating cardiac events if too vigorous an exercise program is started
- There are no other risks associated with these measures
- These measures, particularly smoking cessation, will have general benefits for health in addition to their effects on blood pressure

ACCEPTABILITY TO PATIENT

- Many smokers find it very difficult to give up, and should be offered appropriate encouragement and support
- Similarly, many patients find weight loss difficult, and require support
- Patients used to adding salt to food may find that it tastes bland without it

FOLLOW UP PLAN

Patients should be reviewed regularly when lifestyle advice is first given to assess compliance with lifestyle measures and monitor the effects on blood pressure.

PATIENT AND CAREGIVER INFORMATION

- All patients who smoke should be made aware of the great risks attached to smoking, and the benefits to blood pressure and general health that will result from giving up
- Patients should be advised about suitable exercise programs for their existing levels of fitness; overambitious targets can be demoralizing, and even dangerous in patients with pre-existing cardiovascular disease
- Patients who find it difficult to cut down on salt added to food should be encouraged to use alternative ways of flavoring food (e.g. pepper, garlic, chilli) and reassured that most people soon get used to unsalted food

OUTCOMES

EFFICACY OF THERAPIES

- Response to antihypertensive medication is variable: while some patients will have their blood pressure normalized quickly after starting treatment, others will take many months and possibly several medication regimens before blood pressure stabilizes at an acceptable level
- Long-term treatment with diuretics or beta-blockers reduces the risk of cardiovascular events in hypertensive patients

Evidence

- A systematic review found that treatment of systolic hypertension (>160mmHg) in people over 60 years of age reduced total mortality and fatal and nonfatal cardiovascular events [12] *Level M*
- Treatment of hypertension lowers the risk of cardiovascular morbidity and mortality in women 55 years or older, and in African-American women of any age [13] *Level M*
- The treatment of hypertension in healthy elderly people with diuretics and beta-blockers is clearly beneficial [5] *Level M*
- An overview of randomized cotrolled trials (RCTs) assessing antihypertensive therapy (usually diuretics, beta-blockers or both) in people with hypertension (most without a history of vascular disease) found that a reduction in blood pressure over 2–3 years reduced the risk of stroke [6] *Level P*
- A systematic review (consisting mainly of RCTs comparing diuretics or beta-blockers with placebo) found that antihypertensive medications produced variable reductions in systolic/diastolic blood pressure (average 12–16/5–10mmHg). Benefit was noted in terms of total death rate, cardiovascular death rate, stroke, major coronary events, and congestive heart failure in treated patients [7] *Level M*
- Blood pressure reduction over 2 years with nitrendipine has been shown to reduce the risk of stroke compared with placebo in elderly patients with systolic hypertension [9] *Level P*
- Short- and intermediate-acting dihydropyridine calcium channel blockers may increase cardiovascular morbidity and mortality [8]
- A systematic review found no significant difference in outcomes when beta-blockers, diuretics, and angiotensin-converting enzyme (ACE) inhibitors were compared for the initial treatment of hypertension. However, beta-blockers and diuretics were found to decrease coronary events compared with calcium channel antagonists, and increase stroke rate, although there was no significant difference in all-cause mortality. Stroke rate and all-cause mortality were not significantly altered by ACE inhibitors compared with calcium channel blockers, but ACE inhibitors decreased coronary events [10] *Level M*
- A systematic review found that weight-reducing diets for overweight hypertensive patients are effective in achieving modest weight reduction, and are probably associated with modest reductions in blood pressure. Weight-reducing diets may allow a decrease in the required dose of antihypertensive medications [14] *Level M*
- Lifestyle interventions (aerobic exercise, low fat, high fruit and vegetable diet, dietary salt restriction) have been shown to be effective in the reduction of high blood pressure, but there is insufficient evidence that these interventions reduce mortality and morbidity [8] *Level M*

PROGNOSIS

- Some forms of secondary hypertension may be curable
- Essential hypertension, once established, persists throughout the patient's life, and blood pressure generally increases with age
- Patients who require medication to treat hypertension will generally have to continue taking medication for life
- Untreated hypertension is associated with increased risk of stroke, coronary heart disease, and heart failure
- Successful treatment of hypertension with diuretics or beta-blockers reduces the risk of those events

Clinical pearl(s)
Good control of blood pressure is critical to improving cardiac outcomes.

Therapeutic failure
- The most useful treatment for hypertension that does not respond to initial drug treatment is combination treatment with drugs from two different classes
- Patients whose blood pressure is not adequately controlled after several months and adequate trials of combined medications should be considered for referral
- Regular review is important

Deterioration
- Therapeutic options for deterioration are similar to those for therapeutic failure
- Sudden deterioration in a patient with previously well controlled blood pressure could suggest a secondary cause for hypertension or onset of malignant hypertension, which should be investigated appropriately

COMPLICATIONS
- Patients with hypertension are at risk of developing cardiovascular complications, such as stroke, myocardial infarction, angina, or heart failure
- Essential hypertension may progress to malignant hypertension

CONSIDER CONSULT
- A sudden deterioration could suggest a secondary cause for hypertension, which may require referral for diagnosis
- A patient whose blood pressure can no longer be controlled despite adequate trials of appropriate combination drug treatment should be considered for referral

PREVENTION

- Because of the huge burden of hypertension, small individual advantages from primary prevention can translate into large population gains in morbidity, mortality, and treatment costs
- Lifestyle measures for treating hypertension are also appropriate for prevention of hypertension, and can be introduced at low cost and with few health risks

Measures for preventing hypertension are therefore important for everyone, but particularly for persons at risk of developing hypertension (e.g. those with a family history)

RISK FACTORS

- **Obesity**: persons with a body mass index above 27kg/m^2 are more likely to become hypertensive and suffer cardiovascular complications as a result, and should be advised to lose weight by a combination of appropriate diet and physical activity
- **Alcohol**: excessive alcohol consumption increases the risk of hypertension and stroke
- **Physical activity**: sedentary individuals are at increased risk of hypertension and subsequent cardiovascular disease compared with those who are physically active
- **Dietary sodium**: high levels of dietary sodium intake are associated with increased blood pressure, particularly in African-Americans, diabetics, and the elderly
- **Smoking**: smoking has moderate effects on blood pressure, but greatly increases the risk of subsequent cardiovascular disease

MODIFY RISK FACTORS

Lifestyle and wellness

TOBACCO

- Visits from smokers to healthcare providers for whatever reason should be seen as an opportunity to provide advice on the benefits of giving up
- Smoking cessation is important for all smokers, but particularly so for those at risk of hypertension or other cardiovascular disease
- Many smokers would like to give up but find it very difficult to do so
- Smokers attempting to give up require support, which may include prescription of nicotine replacement products or bupropion

ALCOHOL AND DRUGS

- Excessive alcohol consumption is associated with hypertension
- To reduce the risk of developing hypertension, alcohol consumption should be limited to the equivalent of 30mL (men) or 15mL (women) of ethanol per day
- Moderate alcohol consumption reduces the risk of cardiovascular disease, so there is no rationale for advising complete abstinence
- The cardiovascular benefits of alcohol may be greater for red wine than for other alcoholic drinks, although this has not yet been proved beyond reasonable doubt

DIET

- Obese and overweight persons should be advised to lose weight by restricting caloric intake
- Sodium intake should be limited to no more than 100mmol per day (approximately 6g sodium chloride or 2.4g sodium)
- Adequate potassium intake should be maintained, preferably from food sources such as fresh fruit and vegetables; supplements are rarely necessary
- Although moderating intake of saturated fat has general benefits for cardiovascular health, it is unlikely to affect blood pressure

PHYSICAL ACTIVITY

- Physical activity should be encouraged in everyone
- Strenuous exercise is not necessary to reduce cardiovascular risk
- Approximately 30–45min of brisk walking most days of the week is enough to have important benefits on the risk of blood pressure and other cardiovascular disease
- Patients with pre-existing cardiac disease should not undertake an exercise program without proper medical assessment

SCREENING

- Screening is the primary method of detecting hypertension
- All visits to a healthcare provider for whatever reason can be regarded as an opportunity to measure blood pressure
- Periodic screening for hypertension is recommended for all persons aged 21 years or older. The optimal interval for blood pressure screening has not been determined and is left to clinical discretion
- Those with high normal pressures (>130/80mmHg but not fulfilling criteria for hypertension) should have their blood pressure measured annually or sooner

CHOLESTEROL

Although lipid levels do not affect blood pressure, it is sensible to measure lipid levels in hypertensive patients as they affect overall cardiovascular risk, which should determine the intensity of antihypertensive therapy.

RESOURCES

ASSOCIATIONS

American Heart Association
National Center
7272 Greenville Avenue
Dallas, Texas 75231
Web: http://www.americanheart.org

American College of Cardiology
Heart House
9111 Old Georgetown Road
Bethesda, MD 20814-1699
Phone: (800) 253-4636 or (301) 897-5400
Fax: (301) 897-9745
Web: http://www.acc.org

Hypertension Education Foundation
13 Murray Hill Road
Scarsdale, NY 10583
Web: http://www.hypertensionfoundation.org

KEY REFERENCES

- Ramsay LE, Williams B, Johnston GD, et al. British Hypertension Society guidelines for hypertension management 1999: summary. BMJ 1999;319:630–5
- Magee LA, Ornstein MP, von Dadelszen P. Management of hypertension in pregnancy. BMJ 1999;318:1332–6
- National High Blood Pressure Education Program. Working group report on high blood pressure in pregnancy. National Institutes of Health Publication No. 91-3029, August 1991
- Update on the task force report (1987) on high blood pressure in children and adolescents: a working group report from the National High Blood Pressure Education Program. National Institutes of Health Publication No. 96-3790, September 1996
- Kitiyakara C, Guzman NJ. Malignant hypertension and hypertensive emergencies. J Am Soc Nephrol 1998;9:133–42
- Adamson H, Jacobs A, Warrington SJ. Reference ranges for laboratory safety tests in young healthy subjects. Int J Pharm Med 1998;12:293–6

Evidence references and guidelines

1 WHO–ISH Hypertension Guidelines Committee. 1999 World Health Organization–International Society of Hypertension Guidelines for the Management of Hypertension. J Hypertens 1999;17:151–185

2 National Heart, Lung, and Blood Institute and National High Blood Pressure Education Program. Sixth report of the Joint National Committee on Prevention, Detection, Evaluation, and Treatment of High Blood Pressure. Bethesda (MD): US Department of Health and Human Services, Public Health Service, National Institutes of Health, National Heart, Lung, and Blood Institute, 1997

3 Institute for Clinical Systems Improvement. Hypertension diagnosis and treatment. Bloomington (MN): ICSI, 2000

4 Veterans Health Administration. Diagnosis and management of hypertension in the primary care setting. The Hypertension Working Group. Washington (DC): Department of Veterans Affairs, 1999

5 Mulrow C, Lau J, Brand M. Pharmacotherapy for hypertension in the elderly (Cochrane Review). In: The Cochrane Library, 1, 2002. Oxford: Update Software

6 Collins R, MacMahon S. Blood pressure, antihypertensive drug treatment and the risks of stroke and of coronary heart disease. Br Med Bull 1994;50:272–98. Reviewed in: Clinical Evidence 2001;6:160–77

7 Gueyffier F, Froment A, Gouton M. New meta-analysis of treatment trials of hypertension: improving the estimate of therapeutic benefit. J Hum Hypertens 1996;10:1–8. Reviewed in: Clinical evidence 2001;6:82–113

8 Mulrow C. Primary prevention: cardiovascular disorders. In: Clinical Evidence 2001;6:82–113. London: BMJ Publishing Group

9 Staessen JA, Fagard R, Thijs L, et al for the Systolic Hypertension in Europe (Syst-Eur) Trial Investigators. Randomised double-blind comparison of placebo and active treatment for older patients with isolated systolic hypertension. Lancet 1997;350:757–64. Reviewed in: Clinical Evidence 2001;6:160–77

10 Blood Pressure Lowering Treatment Trialists' Collaboration. Effects of ACE inhibitors, calcium antagonists, and other blood-pressure-lowering drugs: results of prospectively designed overviews of trials. Lancet 2000;356:1955–64. Reviewed in: Clinical Evidence 2001;6:82–113
11 The ALLHAT Officers and Coordinators for the ALLHAT Collaborative Research Group. Major cardiovascular events in hypertensive patients randomized to doxazosin vs chlorthalidone: the antihypertensive and lipid-lowering treatment to prevent heart attack trial (ALLHAT). JAMA 2000;283:1967–75. Reviewed in: Clinical Evidence 2001;6:82–113
12 Staessen JA, Gasowski J, Wang JG, et al. Risks of untreated and treated isolated systolic hypertension in the elderly: meta-analysis of outcome trials. Lancet 2000;355:865–72. Reviewed in: Clinical Evidence 2001;6:82–113
13 Quan A, Kerlikowske K, Gueyffier F, Boissel JP, INDIANA investigators. Pharmacotherapy for hypertension in women of difference races (Cochrane Review). In: The Cochrane Library, 1, 2002. Oxford: Update Software
14 Mulrow CD, Chiquette E, Angel L, et al. Dieting to reduce body weight for controlling hypertension in adults (Cochrane Review). In: The Cochrane Library, 1, 2002. Oxford: Update Software

CONTRIBUTORS

Fred F Ferri, MD, FACP
Christopher P Cannon, MD
James Orford, MD

MITRAL STENOSIS

SUMMARY INFORMATION

DESCRIPTION

- Narrowing of the mitral valve, causing obstruction to blood flow into the left ventricle during diastole
- Most common cause is rheumatic heart disease
- Latent period of 20–40 years before symptoms of left-sided heart failure occur
- Valvular changes include thickening of the valve leaflets, calcification, commissural fusion, and fusion of the chordae
- May present with atrial fibrillation and systemic embolism
- If untreated, mitral stenosis can lead to pulmonary hypertension and death

URGENT ACTION

Need to establish whether the patient is, or wishes to become, pregnant. Pregnancy in a patient with mitral stenosis has a high fetal and maternal rate of complications, including death.

KEY! DON'T MISS!

Patients with signs and symptoms of systemic embolism require anticoagulation.

ICD9 CODE
394.0 Mitral stenosis.

CARDINAL FEATURES
- Progressive disease most common between the ages of 40 and 70 years and in women (ratio 2:1)
- Initially asymptomatic
- Progresses to produce signs, symptoms, and sequelae of congestive heart failure, pulmonary hypertension, systemic thromboembolism, and atrial fibrillation
- Symptoms: dyspnea on exertion, paroxysmal nocturnal dyspnea, palpitation, hemoptysis, and stroke
- Signs: mitral facies, prominent *a* wave in the jugular venous pulse, enlarged right ventricle leading to a right ventricular heave, peripheral edema (in late stages)
- Auscultation: loud S1, opening snap, apical early diastolic rumbling murmur, which fades in mid-diastole and then may exhibit presystolic accentuation. It should be noted that the murmur is variable in severe stenosis; when the valve is mobile and not calcified, the murmur persists throughout diastole, and S1 and the opening snap remain loud; when the valve is heavily calcified, the murmur is often difficult to hear, and S1 and the opening snap become soft and may be absent

CAUSES
Common causes
The most common cause is rheumatic heart disease. The mitral valve is the valve most commonly affected by rheumatic heart disease.

Rare causes
- Congenital (parachute valve)
- Malignant carcinoid
- Systemic lupus erythematosus
- Rheumatoid arthritis
- Methysergide therapy
- Left atrial myxoma

Contributory or predisposing factors
Rheumatic heart disease: higher incidence of rheumatic heart disease in developing countries due to poorer recognition and treatment of streptococcal infections.

EPIDEMIOLOGY
Incidence and prevalence
Incidence of acquired mitral stenosis has decreased in the US and worldwide because of a decreased incidence of rheumatic heart disease.

INCIDENCE
- Closely related to rheumatic fever
- The incidence of rheumatic fever is very low in the West (e.g. in Scotland, 6 per million population per year; in the US, <0.02/1000). In developing countries it may exceed 1/1000

FREQUENCY
Congenital mitral stenosis is rare; occurs in 0.42% of children with congenital heart disease.

Demographics

AGE

- Congenital mitral stenosis presents in infancy
- In developed countries, symptomatic disease usually presents late, at 40–70 years of age
- In developing countries, symptoms often develop in early adulthood and may be evident as soon as 2 years after an episode of rheumatic fever

GENDER

Two-thirds of mitral stenosis cases occur in women.

GENETICS

A familial incidence of rheumatic fever has been documented and appears to be related to the presence of specific alloantigens that cross-react with antibodies against some components of the streptococcus.

GEOGRAPHY

- Higher incidence in developing countries
- More rapid progression of disease in tropical climates, with disease sometimes presenting in adolescence

SOCIOECONOMIC STATUS

Crowded conditions favor the spread of streptococcal infection.

DIAGNOSIS

DIFFERENTIAL DIAGNOSIS

Infective endocarditis

Infective endocarditis is an infection of the heart valves and/or myocardium.

FEATURES

- Mitral valvular vegetations (accretions of bacteria, fibrin, and platelets) on rare occasion can be large enough to impede blood flow, mimicking mitral stenosis
- Rheumatic heart disease is a predisposing factor
- Presenting signs and symptoms: dyspnea, congestive cardiac failure, variable murmurs, palpitations, systemic embolism, and a low-grade fever

Increased flow through normal valve

Increased flow sufficient to cause a murmur across a normal mitral valve can occur in anemia, hyperthyroidism, pregnancy, and significant mitral regurgitation.

Left atrial myxoma

The features of left atrial myxoma are as follows.

FEATURES

- Benign primary cardiac tumor
- Comprises roughly 30% of all tumors of the heart (of an overall incidence of 0.28%)
- >85% occur in the left atrium
- Mechanical obstruction of the mitral valve causes dyspnea on exertion and fatigue; low-grade fever, systemic embolism, and syncopal attacks may be presenting features

Cor triatriatum

The features of cor triatriatum are as follows.

FEATURES

- A rare congenital abnormality
- The atrium has two chambers
- Blood flow may be impeded by the membrane between the more posterior chamber and the chamber adjacent to the mitral valve

SIGNS & SYMPTOMS

Signs

- Pulse may be irregular (30–40% of patients with symptomatic mitral stenosis develop atrial fibrillation)
- Prominent *a* wave in the jugular venous pulse
- Displaced apex beat due to the enlarged right ventricle and often with a right ventricular heave
- Basal crepitations on pulmonary auscultation
- In late stage: signs of peripheral edema, enlarged liver, ascites
- 'Mitral facies' – a florid appearance with cyanosed cheeks (if pulmonary hypertension has developed)
- Signs of systemic embolization – highest risk in patients >35 years of age with atrial fibrillation
- Auscultation: loud S1, opening snap, apical early diastolic, rumbling murmur, which fades in mid-diastole and then may exhibit presystolic accentuation. In severe stenosis the murmur is variable; when the valve is mobile and not calcified, the murmur persists throughout diastole, and S1 and the opening snap remain loud; when the valve is heavily calcified, the murmur is often difficult to hear, and S1 and the opening snap become soft and may be absent

Symptoms

- In most cases, it develops 20–40 years after an episode of rheumatic fever but may occur as early as a few years afterwards
- May progress rapidly to congestive heart failure after complications begin (e.g. atrial fibrillation, pregnancy, or pulmonary hypertension)
- Symptoms of congestive heart failure: dyspnea on exertion, orthopnea, paroxysmal nocturnal dyspnea, edema
- Symptoms of atrial fibrillation: sudden worsening of left heart failure, palpitations, syncope, systemic embolism
- Other symptoms: hemoptysis, chest pain, weight loss, signs of right heart failure, hoarseness from left atrial enlargement and pressure on recurrent laryngeal nerve, fatigue secondary to decreased cardiac output

ASSOCIATED DISORDERS

Common:

- Mitral regurgitation (40% of all patients with rheumatic heart disease have combined mitral stenosis and mitral regurgitation)
- Coexisting coronary artery disease: present in approx. one-third of patients >40 years of age

Rare:

- Atrial septal defect (Lutembacher's syndrome)
- Malignant carcinoid
- Systemic lupus erythematosus
- Rheumatoid arthritis
- Mucopolysaccharidoses of the Hunter–Hurler phenotype
- Amyloidosis
- Giant left atrial thrombus causing further obstruction of the valve

KEY! DON'T MISS!

Patients with signs and symptoms of systemic embolism require anticoagulation.

CONSIDER CONSULT

- Refer all cases of suspected mitral stenosis for baseline echocardiographic evaluation
- Refer all symptomatic patients where an intervention to reduce the stenosis is appropriate
- Refer all pregnant patients with more than mild stenosis

INVESTIGATION OF THE PATIENT

Direct questions to patient

- Q **Have you ever had rheumatic fever?** Rheumatic fever is the most common cause of mitral stenosis
- Q **Do you get unusually breathless with exertion (such as when going up a flight of steps)?** Breathlessness is a common symptom of mitral stenosis
- Q **Do you get breathless when lying down?** Orthopnea and paroxysmal nocturnal dyspnea may both occur in mitral stenosis
- Q **Have you ever coughed up blood or pink sputum?** Hemoptysis may indicate pulmonary embolus or pulmonary hypertension. Pink sputum may be an indication of acute pulmonary edema
- Q **Do you suffer from palpitations or a sensation that your heart skips a beat at times?** Atrial fibrillation is commonly associated with mitral stenosis
- Q **Have you had any fainting episodes?**
- Q **Do you suffer from chest pains?** May be a symptom of mitral stenosis, pulmonary embolism, or coexistent cardiac disease
- Q **In which other countries have you lived and when?** Rheumatic fever is more common in developing countries

Contributory or predisposing factors

Q **Have you ever used migraine drugs before, and, if so, what were they?** Methysergide exposure is rarely associated with the development of mitral stenosis

Q **Have you ever been diagnosed with a connective tissue disease?** Connective tissue diseases are occasionally associated with mitral stenosis

Family history

Q **Is there anyone in your family with a history of mitral stenosis?** Siblings may also have evidence of mitral stenosis or a history of rheumatic fever

Examination

- General inspection may show mitral facies and tachypnea
- Heart rate may be irregularly irregular if in atrial fibrillation
- Jugular venous pulsation may show prominent jugular *a* wave
- Chest wall palpation may demonstrate a displaced apex beat due to right ventricular enlargement and a right ventricular heave
- Cardiac auscultation: loud S1, opening snap, apical early diastolic, rumbling murmur, which fades in mid-diastole and then may exhibit presystolic accentuation. It should be noted that the murmur is variable in severe stenosis; when the valve is mobile and not calcified, the murmur persists throughout diastole, and S1 and the opening snap remain loud; when the valve is heavily calcified, the murmur is often difficult to hear, and S1 and the opening snap become soft and may be absent
- Pulmonary auscultation may reveal basal crepitations
- Abdominal examination may reveal hepatomegaly or ascites (late signs)
- Inspection of the legs may show signs of peripheral edema (in later stages)

Summary of investigative tests

- ECG can provide evidence of electrocardiographic features associated with mitral stenosis, specifically atrial fibrillation, left atrial enlargement, or right ventricular hypertrophy
- Chest X-ray may show features that are suggestive of mitral stenosis and signs of interstitial edema
- Echocardiography is the test of choice to diagnose mitral stenosis and confirm the degree of stenosis
- Cardiac catheterization is usually reserved for those patients for whom an intervention is planned. It can help clarify the severity of stenosis when there is a discrepancy between the symptoms and the echocardiographic findings. It is performed by a specialist

DIAGNOSTIC DECISION

- A history of rheumatic fever, typical current symptoms, and positive findings on auscultation strongly suggest mitral stenosis. The diagnostic test of choice is echocardiography
- The American Academy of Family Physicians has published material containing information on mitral stenosis. Shipton B, Wahba H. Valvular heart disease: Review and update

CLINICAL PEARL(S)

- A loud S1 is often the clue to the presence of mitral stenosis
- Auscultation may be difficult in some patients, so echocardiography should be performed whenever the signs and symptoms are consistent with mitral stenosis
- Pregnancy can result in rather abrupt onset of symptoms in previously asymptomatic patients

THE TESTS

Tests of function

ECG

Advantages/Disadvantages

Advantages:

- Noninvasive
- Relatively inexpensive
- Gives immediate results
- Easily interpreted

Disadvantages:

- Nonspecific, insensitive test (many false-positives and false-negatives)
- Findings resemble those associated with any cause of pulmonary hypertension, enlarged left atrium, or right heart strain

Abnormal

- Atrial fibrillation may be present
- Right ventricular hypertrophy
- Right axis deviation
- Left atrial enlargement shown by broad notched P waves in the limb leads and a large negative deflection in V1
- Keep in mind the possibility of a false-positive result

Cause of abnormal result

- Right axis deviation is a result of pulmonary hypertension
- An abnormal P wave is secondary to the increased left atrial size and left atrial hypertrophy

Imaging

ECHOCARDIOGRAPHY

Advantages/Disadvantages

Advantages:

- Noninvasive, relatively inexpensive
- Is the gold standard investigation and will confirm the diagnosis, evaluate the degree of valvular abnormality, determine the valve area, assess the pulmonary arterial pressure, and identify associated lesions
- Left atrium can be examined and risk of clot established
- Left ventricular function can be determined – bear in mind that mitral stenosis 'protects' the left ventricle and may lead to falsely reassuring estimates of left ventricular function
- Transesophageal echocardiography is very sensitive for detecting atrial thrombus

Disadvantages:

- May not be available in all centers or the center has had little experience in studying patients with mitral stenosis
- Requires expertise in both the performance and interpretation

Abnormal

- Thickening and/or calcification of valve cusps
- Fusion of the valve commissures, causing restricted motion
- Diminished E to F slope of the anterior mitral valve leaflet during diastole
- Anterior movement of the posterior mitral valve leaflet during diastole
- Occasionally clot can be demonstrated in the left atrium
- High transmitral pressure gradient
- Decreased valve area

CHEST X-RAY

Advantages/Disadvantages

- Advantage: noninvasive, minimal radiation exposure, relatively inexpensive
- Disadvantage: findings are nonspecific

Abnormal

- Straightening of the curve of the left cardiac border, which is caused by a dilated left atrial appendage
- Left atrial enlargement
- Prominent pulmonary arteries
- Pulmonary congestion
- Keep in mind the possibility of a false-positive result

TREATMENT

CONSIDER CONSULT

All symptomatic patients should be considered for an intervention to improve cardiac output by increasing the mitral valve area. Urgent assessment is indicated if a patient with known or suspected mitral stenosis presents with any of the following:

- Signs and symptoms of congestive heart failure
- Signs and symptoms suggestive of pulmonary hypertension
- Hemoptysis
- Abnormal heart rhythm, especially if of recent or unknown onset or if associated with symptoms
- Signs or symptoms suggestive of systemic embolization, indicating the possibility of left atrial thrombus
- Signs and symptoms suggestive of bacterial endocarditis
- Any symptoms during pregnancy

IMMEDIATE ACTION

- Patients in sustained atrial fibrillation that is compromising cardiac output and/or leading to severe symptoms of pulmonary congestion may need hospitalization and urgent cardioversion
- Patients with new-onset or recently exacerbated congestive cardiac failure may require hospitalization and treatment
- Patients with bacterial endocarditis require immediate evaluation, including blood cultures and echocardiogram, and institution of appropriate antimicrobial therapy
- Refer if any symptoms during the second or third trimester of pregnancy

PATIENT AND CAREGIVER ISSUES

Patient or caregiver request

- Diagnosis of a 'heart murmur' can be very frightening. Reassurance is important if there is no echocardiographic evidence of stenosis or the stenosis is very mild (valve area >$2.0cm^2$)
- Patients with definite mitral stenosis should be informed of the natural history of the disease so as to understand the importance of continued care
- Explain the significance of rheumatic fever and differentiate it from 'rheumatism'
- Patients needs to be counseled regarding exercise. A moderate amount is desirable to maintain some degree of cardiovascular fitness, but exercise that is more strenuous than usual for the patient should be avoided

MANAGEMENT ISSUES

Goals

- Control symptoms of congestive heart failure
- Control atrial fibrillation if present
- Monitor disease progression
- Endocarditis prophylaxis for dental procedures and other indicated surgical procedures
- Antithrombotic therapy for prevention of stroke and systemic embolism
- Prevention of rheumatic fever recurrences

Management in special circumstances

COEXISTING DISEASE

- Any dental or surgical procedure likely to result in bacteremia must be accompanied by appropriate prophylaxis. Guidelines for the prevention of endocarditis have been issued by the American Heart Association
- Hyperthyroidism will increase mitral valve flow and may cause sudden deterioration
- Tachyarrhythmias will shorten diastolic time for ventricular filling and result in decreased cardiac output

SPECIAL PATIENT GROUPS

Pregnancy:

The increased metabolic demands during the second and third trimesters can lead to sudden and life-threatening deterioration in previously asymptomatic patients.

Older patients:

- Heavy calcification and fibrosis of the mitral valve leaflets with significant subvalvular fusion are more common with increasing age
- The success rate of percutaneous valvotomy is lower than in younger patients, with an increased risk of complications

PATIENT SATISFACTION/LIFESTYLE PRIORITIES

- Diuretics: may cause increased urination and erectile dysfunction
- Anticoagulation: can affect the safety of certain physical activities and has significant interactions with over-the-counter and prescription medications

SUMMARY OF THERAPEUTIC OPTIONS

Choices

Medical therapy is directed toward the control of the hemodynamic consequences of mitral stenosis but is not curative and is not universally used.

The definitive treatment of mitral stenosis is enlargement of the mitral orifice:

- Percutaneous mitral balloon valvotomy often gives good results, especially in young and middle-aged patients
- Surgical mitral commissurotomy is performed with cardiopulmonary bypass and enables thrombi to be removed from the left atrium, fused chordae to be separated, and valve leaflets to be débrided of calcium, and mild or moderate mitral regurgitation to be corrected
- Mitral valve replacement is required with heavily calcified valves or when the concomitant mitral regurgitation is marked. Valve replacement is eventually necessary in symptomatic patients with recurrent stenosis after a prior procedure

In addition:

- Management of conditions associated with mitral stenosis, such as congestive heart failure and atrial fibrillation (including prophylaxis of embolism and antibiotic prophylaxis for surgical and dental procedures), should be undertaken as appropriate
- Long-term secondary prevention of rheumatic fever should be considered
- Maintaining a low-sodium diet is important
- Patients requiring chronic anticoagulation will need to have a fairly constant intake of leafy vegetables rich in vitamin K1

Guidelines

- The American College of Cardiology and the American Heart Association have produced guidelines containing information on mitral stenosis. Bonow RO, Carabello B, de Leon AC Jr, et al. Management of patients with valvular heart disease. J Am Coll Cardiol 1998; 32:1486–588. Also available online at the National Guideline Clearinghouse [1]

Clinical pearl(s)

- Always consider a patient for possible intervention with the onset of symptoms; medical therapy can be of modest benefit but does not result in any long-term relief
- Refer to a center experienced in balloon valvotomy

- Transthoracic echocardiography may sometimes underestimate the severity of mitral regurgitation, in which case transesophageal echocardiography may be indicated to obtain an accurate estimate of the regurgitation
- Patients with symptoms that seem out of proportion to the resting echocardiographic assessment should undergo either exercise echocardiography or right heart catheterization during stress

Never

Never attempt to convert a patient from atrial fibrillation to sinus rhythm without having ruled out the presence of atrial thrombus and initiated anticoagulation therapy. Return of sinus rhythm may otherwise precipitate embolization.

FOLLOW UP

Ascertain the valve gradient and pulmonary arterial pressure. Follow up will depend on the severity of the mitral stenosis and the patient's symptoms.

Plan for review

- Asymptomatic patients: annual history and examination; other tests can be deferred
- Echocardiogram in those patients with changes in symptoms or signs
- Symptomatic patients are reviewed according to individual therapy, symptoms, and signs

Information for patient or caregiver

- Long-term secondary prevention of rheumatic fever should be considered
- Any dental or surgical procedure likely to result in bacteremia must be accompanied by appropriate prophylaxis. Guidelines for the prevention of endocarditis have been issued by the American Heart Association

DRUGS AND OTHER THERAPIES: DETAILS

Surgical therapy

Surgical treatment of mitral stenosis consists of some form of mechanical dilation of the valve orifice or valve replacement.

PERCUTANEOUS MITRAL BALLOON VALVOTOMY

Efficacy

Applicable to most younger patients since calcification and extensive fibrosis of the valve apparatus is uncommon in those <50 years of age.

- Typically increases valve area from 1.0–2.0cm^2
- Symptomatic improvement in most patients, with young and middle-aged patients having significantly better results
- Outcomes are dependent on the experience of the operators
- Immediate results of percutaneous mitral valvotomy are similar to those of commissurotomy
- Overall, 80–95% may have a successful procedure

Risks/Benefits

Risks:

- Mortality rate is 1–3%
- Severe regurgitation occurs in 0.3–5% of cases
- Other complications include cardiac perforation, iatrogenic atrial septal defect, and systemic embolization

Benefits:
- Less expensive than other surgical methods
- Restenosis rates range from 2 to 60%; after balloon valvuloplasty, restenosis occurs in <15% of cases within 3–7 years
- Symptomatic improvement in 86%
- Five-year survival rates are 90–96%

Evidence

Balloon mitral valvotomy or commissurotomy can be effective in the management of mitral valve prolapse. The underlying mitral valve morphology will determine the outcome.
- Randomized controlled trials (RCTs) have shown no significant difference in short-term hemodynamic outcomes, clinical improvement, or complication rates between percutaneous balloon valvotomy and open or closed commissurotomy. Long-term follow up at 3–7 years does, however, indicate a benefit with balloon and open procedures [2] *Level C*
- Overall, 80–95% of patients with mitral stenosis may have a successful procedure with balloon valvotomy, and overall event-free survival is 50–65% over 3–5 years. Event-free survival is 80–90% for patients with favorable valve morphology [2] *Level C*
- A nonblinded RCT compared open (OMC), closed (CMC), and percutaneous balloon (BMC) mitral commissurotomy in the management of rheumatic mitral stenosis. Early subjective improvements in hemodynamic functioning were higher in patients treated with OMC and BMC. At 7-year follow up, OMC and BMC patients had less need for reintervention and less restenosis or residual stenosis [3] *Level P*

Acceptability to patient

The absence of any type of thoracotomy allows the patient to return to normal activities shortly after the procedure.

Follow up plan
- Management after successful percutaneous mitral balloon valvotomy or surgical commissurotomy is similar to that of the asymptomatic patient with mitral stenosis
- Echocardiogram should be performed after the procedure
- Annual history, physical examination, chest X-ray, and ECG in asymptomatic patients
- Prophylaxis against infective endocarditis and recurrence of rheumatic fever

Patient and caregiver information
- This procedure is performed according to the individual patient's preoperative and postoperative condition
- This procedure is not applicable to patients whose valve is heavily calcified and/or scarred, or when there is a blood clot is in the left atrium

SURGICAL MITRAL COMMISSUROTOMY
- Performed with cardiopulmonary bypass
- Thrombi can be removed from the left atrium, fused chordae can be separated, and valve leaflets can be débrided of calcium, and mild or moderate mitral regurgitation may be corrected

Efficacy
- Similar or improved survival and restenosis rates to closed procedures
- Better hemodynamic relief with open valve procedures than with closed procedures

Risks/Benefits

Benefits:

- Mortality rate is 1–3% after open or closed valvotomy
- Five-year survival rates are 90–96%
- Event-free 5-year survival rates are 72–94%

Evidence

There is evidence that open surgical commissurotomy is more effective than the closed procedure in the management of mitral stenosis.

- A nonblinded RCT compared open (OMC), closed (CMC), and percutaneous balloon (BMC) mitral commissurotomy in the management of rheumatic mitral stenosis. Early subjective improvements in hemodynamic functioning were higher in patients treated with OMC and BMC. At 7-year follow up, OMC and BMC patients had less need for reintervention and less restenosis or residual stenosis [3] *Level P*
- An RCT compared OMC with CMC in patients with severe, noncalcified mitral stenosis. The open technique resulted in better hemodynamic values at rest and exercise [4] *Level P*

Acceptability to patient

- Major surgery with significant expense, significant recovery period, and significant morbidity may be daunting
- Chronic anticoagulation is avoided unless atrial fibrillation is present

Follow up plan

Regular follow up by surgeon and primary care physician in the postoperative period.

Patient and caregiver information

- The procedure is generally performed when balloon valvotomy is unlikely to be beneficial
- Some valves cannot be adequately treated even by OMC, and the surgeon may need to replace the valve

MITRAL VALVE REPLACEMENT

- Surgery and mitral valve replacement with a prosthetic valve is necessary in patients with severe stenosis and a heavily calcified and/or markedly fibrotic valve
- Patients with prior valve procedures may also require valve replacement when restenosis develops

Efficacy

- Prosthetic valves have an area that is less than the normal valve area; therefore severe stenosis is converted to mild stenosis
- Current mechanical prostheses have an exceedingly low rate of mechanical failure
- An adjunct procedure called the Maze operation may restore sinus rhythm in patients with recurrent or sustained atrial fibrillation

Risks/Benefits

Risks:

- Operative mortality-rate 3–8%
- Life-long anticoagulant treatment in patients with mechanical prostheses is usually necessary to avoid chronic hemolysis
- Tissue prosthetic valves have a high rate of degeneration in younger patients so are usually reserved for patients >70 years of age

Benefit: Significant clinical improvement occurs in most patients, and long-term survival is improved.

Evidence

- Mitral valve replacement is recommended for patients with symptomatic moderate to severe mitral stenosis who are not suitable candidates for balloon valvotomy or valve repair [1] *Level C*
- Patients with symptomatic severe mitral stenosis and severe pulmonary hypertension may be recommended for valve replacement rather than balloon valvotomy or repair [1] *Level C*

Acceptability to patient

- Significant clinical improvement can be anticipated
- Major surgery with significant expense, significant recovery period, and significant morbidity may be daunting
- Patients with a mechanical valve will need lifetime monitoring of anticoagulation therapy

Follow up plan

- Regular follow-up by surgeon and primary care physician in the postoperative period
- Careful monitoring of anticoagulation therapy is essential in all patients with a mechanical valve and in those with atrial fibrillation
- Echocardiography should be performed after recovery from surgery to establish a baseline related to the prosthetic valve function

Patient and caregiver information

- Women wishing to become pregnant should discuss the various options regarding valve surgery with a cardiac surgeon and cardiologist
- Patients may be able to hear the closing sound of a mechanical valve
- Maximum improvement in cardiac symptoms may take up to 1 year after surgery
- Current mechanical prosthetic valves have a very low risk of mechanical failure

LIFESTYLE

- Low-sodium diet: avoid salty foods; do not use salt in cooking
- Patients requiring chronic anticoagulation will need to have a fairly constant intake of leafy vegetables rich in vitamin K1 in order to avoid frequent adjustments in the dosage of the anticoagulant

ACCEPTABILITY TO PATIENT

It may be difficult initially, but usually the patient habituates.

FOLLOW UP PLAN

Dietitian follow up may be useful.

PATIENT AND CAREGIVER INFORMATION

Patients should be advised that perseverance will usually result in food being more acceptable due to adjustment of taste threshold.

OUTCOMES

EFFICACY OF THERAPIES

There are no known medical therapies that can prevent worsening stenosis except the prevention of recurrent rheumatic fever.

Prognosis for patients undergoing surgical correction of mitral stenosis is good, provided that patients have not developed significant pulmonary hypertension.

More than 90% of patients free of events remain in New York Heart Association (NYHA) functional class I or II after percutaneous mitral valvotomy. Trials comparing percutaneous balloon valvotomy with both closed and open surgical commissurotomy showed no significant difference in complication rate between percutaneous mitral valvotomy and surgery. Early follow up data indicate no differences in measured parameters, but longer-term follow up studies at 3–7 years indicate more favorable hemodynamic and symptomatic results with percutaneous balloon valvotomy than with closed commissurotomy, and results equivalent to those of open commissurotomy.

Evidence

- In the management of rheumatic mitral stenosis, patients treated with open mitral commissurotomy (OMC) and balloon mitral commissurotomy may have less need for reintervention and less restenosis or residual stenosis than patients managed with the closed procedure in the long term [3] *Level P*
- OMC may result in better hemodynamic values at rest and exercise than the closed technique for patients with severe, noncalcified mitral stenosis [4] *Level P*

PROGNOSIS

- The severity of mitral stenosis progresses over time in almost all patients. There are no known medical therapies, apart from prevention of recurrent rheumatic fever, that alter this natural history. When symptoms develop, balloon valvotomy, OMC or closed commissurotomy provides effective means of reducing stenosis but is not curative. Restenosis sometimes occurs and can be early (<5 years) or late (>20 years)
- Appropriate medical treatment can delay necessity for surgery for patients, and surgical treatment prolongs survival substantially in patients with mitral stenosis

Clinical pearl(s)

- Progression of mitral stenosis can be very slow and insidious so that the patient accepts his or her increasing limitations as 'normal aging'. Periodic objective evaluation by X-ray and echocardiography is essential to ensure timely intervention
- Concomitant mitral regurgitation may worsen symptoms

COMPLICATIONS

- Left heart failure
- Atrial fibrillation
- Systemic embolization
- Bacterial endocarditis
- Pulmonary hypertension
- Right heart failure

CONSIDER CONSULT

- The low prevalence of mitral stenosis in developed countries means that few primary care physicians will have had any experience of caring for such patients. Therefore periodic follow up with a cardiologist can be helpful

PREVENTION

Prevention of rheumatic fever will largely prevent mitral stenosis.

RISK FACTORS

Streptococcal pharyngitis: young people in close proximity to other youngsters are at increased risk of streptococcal pharyngitis.

MODIFY RISK FACTORS

Lifestyle and wellness

FAMILY HISTORY

A family history of rheumatic fever probably increases the risk in offspring.

CHEMOPROPHYLAXIS

Treatment of streptococcal pharyngitis prevents rheumatic fever. If the patient has had rheumatic fever, prophylaxis for recurrent rheumatic fever is useful in preventing mitral stenosis.

RESOURCES

ASSOCIATIONS

American College of Cardiology
Heart House
9111 Old Georgetown Road
Bethesda, MD 20814-1699
Phone: (800) 253-4636 or (301) 897-5400
Fax: (301) 897-9745
www.acc.org

American Heart Association
National Center Mailing Address
American Heart Association
National Center
7272 Greenville Avenue
Dallas, TX 75231
http://www.americanheart.org

KEY REFERENCES

- Carroll JD, Feldman T. Percutaneous mitral balloon valvotomy and the new demographics of mitral stenosis. JAMA 1993;270:1731–6
- Feldman T. Rheumatic mitral stenosis: on the rise again. Postgrad Med 1993;93:93–104
- Carabello BA. Indications for valve surgery in asymptomatic patients with aortic and mitral stenosis. Chest 1995;108:1678–82
- Braunwald E. Heart disease: a textbook of cardiovascular medicine, 6th edn. Philadelphia: WB Saunders, 2001.
- ACC/AHA Guidelines for the management of patients with valvular heart disease. A Report of the American College of Cardiology/American Heart Association Task Force on Practice Guidelines (Committee on Management of Patients with Valvular Heart Disease). J Am Coll Cardiol 1998;32:1486–588
- Sixth American College of Chest Physicians consensus conference on antithrombotic therapy http://www.chestnet.org
- Dajani AS, Taubert KA, Wilson W, et al. Prevention of bacterial endocarditis: recommendations by the American Heart Association. Circulation 1997;96:358–366

Evidence references and guidelines

1 ACC/AHA guidelines for the management of patients with valvular heart disease. A Report of the American College of Cardiology/American Heart Association Task Force on Practice Guidelines (Committee on Management of Patients with Valvular Heart Disease). J Am Coll Cardiol 1998;32:1486–588

2 ACC/AHA guidelines for the management of patients with valvular heart disease: executive summary. A Report of the American College of Cardiology/American Heart Association Task Force on Practice Guidelines (Committee on Management of Patients With Valvular Heart Disease). Circulation 1998;98(18):1949–84

3 Ben Farhat M, Ayari M, Maatouk F, et al. Percutaneous balloon versus surgical closed and open mitral commissurotomy: seven-year follow-up results of a randomized trial. Circulation 1998;97:245–50. Medline

4 Ben Farhat M, Boussadia H, Gandjbakhch I, et al. Closed versus open mitral commissurotomy in pure noncalcific mitral stenosis: hemodynamic studies before and after operation. J Thorac Cardiovasc Surg 1990;99:639–44. Medline

FAQS

Question 1

The patient has mitral stenosis and is, or wishes to become, pregnant. What do you advise?

ANSWER 1

The severity of stenosis must be accurately assessed by an experienced echocardiography laboratory. If the stenosis is mild, an uncomplicated and successful pregnancy is anticipated. When the stenosis is moderate or severe, a balloon valvotomy should be performed.

Question 2
The patient has exertional dyspnea, but I am uncertain whether it is due to the mitral stenosis, obesity, or continued smoking and the associated pulmonary disease. How should this patient be evaluated?

ANSWER 2
An accurate echocardiogram will help quantitate the severity of mitral stenosis and determine the pulmonary arterial pressure. If the mitral stenosis does not appear to be of sufficient severity to account for the symptoms, the patient should undergo an assessment of the valve gradient during exercise by either exercise echocardiography or a right heart catheterization with hemodynamic monitoring during exercise.

Question 3
When should this patient with moderate mitral stenosis undergo an intervention to reduce the stenosis?

ANSWER 3
Limiting symptoms are the primary indication for intervention. However, if there is evidence of worsening pulmonary hypertension and/or right ventricular dysfunction, intervention is warranted. Inactive patients may remain nearly asymptomatic and then present at a later date with heart failure. Periodic objective evaluation is important.

Question 4
To where should I refer the patient for intervention?

ANSWER 4
Select a center with substantial experience in both percutaneous valvotomy and surgical repair. If the echocardiographic data indicate that mitral valve replacement is required, almost all centers will be experienced in this procedure.

CONTRIBUTORS
Dennis F Saver, MD
John McB Hodgson, MD, FACC, FSCAI
Gail A Van Norman, MD

MITRAL VALVE PROLAPSE

SUMMARY INFORMATION

DESCRIPTION

- Abnormality of the mitral valve in which one or both of the valve's leaflets bulge into the left atrium during systole. In most instances, the condition is benign and not progressive
- Hallmark auscultatory feature is a mid-systolic click, commonly accompanied by a late-systolic murmur
- A subset of patients with mitral valve prolapse have mitral valve prolapse syndrome, in which the mitral valve abnormality occurs in conjunction with atypical chest pain, palpitations, and/or autonomic dysfunction
- Endocarditis prophylaxis prior to dental, oral, respiratory tract, or esophageal procedures is indicated for patients with mitral valve prolapse accompanied by mitral regurgitation or thickened leaflets

URGENT ACTION

Urgent action is seldom called for, but complications of this condition, including infective endocarditis and ruptured chordae tendineae, may require immediate referral and aggressive treatment.

KEY! DON'T MISS!

A rare, but particularly important, complication of mitral valve prolapse is infective endocarditis. This should be considered when evaluating a patient with known mitral valve prolapse and a febrile illness.

ICD9 CODE

424.0 Mitral valve prolapse.

SYNONYMS

- Click-murmur syndrome
- Barlow's syndrome
- Balloon mitral valve
- Floppy valve syndrome
- Da Costa syndrome
- Soldier heart syndrome
- Billowing mitral cusp syndrome
- Myxomatous mitral valve
- Redundant cusp syndrome

CARDINAL FEATURES

- Prolapse of the mitral valve leaflets into the left atrium during systole
- Typically produces a midsystolic click or clicks that can be altered by maneuvers that affect left ventricular volume (such as the Valsalva maneuver). A late systolic murmur of mitral regurgitation may also be present
- Thickening and redundancy of the mitral valve leaflets is present in some patients and identifies a subset of patients at increased risk of progressive mitral regurgitation

CAUSES

Common causes

Primary disorder involving myxomatous degeneration of the mitral valve.

Rare causes

- Hereditary connective tissue disorders, including Marfan syndrome, Ehlers–Danlos syndrome, and osteogenesis imperfecta
- Postinflammatory changes to the heart including those following rheumatic fever
- Congenital malformations such as Ebstein's anomaly of the tricuspid valve, as well as large atrial septal defect
- Collagen vascular disease
- Coronary artery disease
- Cardiomyopathies, including hypertrophic cardiomyopathy

EPIDEMIOLOGY

Incidence and prevalence

PREVALENCE

20–60 per 1000. The reported prevalence of this abnormality is dependent on the diagnostic criteria used to define the condition.

Demographics

AGE

- Can occur at any age
- Patients above 45 years of age face a greater likelihood of complications

GENDER

- Prevalence is greater in females and most commonly diagnosed in females aged 20–30
- Males above age 50 are at the highest risk of complications

GENETICS

May be inherited as an autosomal-dominant trait, but with variable phenotypic expression.

DIAGNOSIS

DIFFERENTIAL DIAGNOSIS

Aortic stenosis

Obstruction of blood flow from left ventricle into aorta due to narrowing of aortic valve. The main features of aortic stenosis are as follows.

FEATURES

- Causes a diamond-shaped, harsh systolic murmur with peak intensity in midsystole
- If the aortic valve is heavily calcified, A2 may be soft or inaudible

Aortic sclerosis

Obstruction of blood flow from left ventricle into aorta due to stiffening of the aortic valve.

FEATURES

- An ejection systolic murmur that peaks early in systole
- Murmur has a quality similar to that of aortic stenosis but is of shorter duration and A2 is preserved

Mitral insufficiency

Mitral insufficiency can be caused by a variety of pathologies that affect either the valve leaflets or the left ventricle. Examples are rheumatic mitral valve disease, ruptured chordae tendineae, a dilated mitral annulus, papillary muscle dysfunction secondary to ischemic heart disease, cardiomyopathy, and hypertrophic obstructive cardiomyopathy.

FEATURES

- Typically produces a high-pitched, pansystolic murmur, heard best near the left ventricular apex
- Some murmurs are late-systolic or mid-systolic

Papillary muscle dysfunction

May occur as a complication of myocardial infarction.

FEATURES

Potential cause of mitral valve regurgitation and attendant murmur.

Constrictive pericarditis

In constrictive pericarditis diastolic filling is impaired by a thick fibrotic pericardium.

FEATURES

- May cause a pericardial knock resembling the click heard in mitral valve prolapse
- Elevation of jugular venous pressure is a key diagnostic feature

Innocent vibratory systolic murmur

Rarely heard above the teen years.

FEATURES

Murmur decreases greatly with standing, but unaffected by squatting.

SIGNS & SYMPTOMS

Signs

- Typically, a systolic click (or clicks) that is most pronounced at apex, occurs at least 0.14s after S1, and is affected by maneuvers that change left ventricular volume
- Late-systolic murmur is commonly present, signaling mitral regurgitation

- Patients may have low body weight, low blood pressure
- Skeletal abnormalities may be present, including straight-back syndrome, scoliosis, and pectus excavatum

Symptoms

- Asymptomatic in most instances
- Palpitations, atypical chest pain, syncope/presyncope, and dyspnea have been attributed to mitral valve prolapse, but in most cases other etiologies can be identified to explain the symptoms. Population surveys have found that these symptoms have a similar prevalence in subjects without mitral valve prolapse

ASSOCIATED DISORDERS

- Tricuspid valve prolapse (rare)
- Autonomic dysfunction, including orthostatic hypotension
- Skeletal abnormalities, including straight-back syndrome, scoliosis, and pectus excavatum
- Marfan syndrome

KEY! DON'T MISS!

A rare, but particularly important, complication of mitral valve prolapse is infective endocarditis. This should be considered when evaluating a patient with known mitral valve prolapse and a febrile illness.

CONSIDER CONSULT

- Infective endocarditis
- Progressive or significant mitral regurgitation
- Significant arrhythmias
- Family history of sudden death caused by mitral valve prolapse

INVESTIGATION OF THE PATIENT

Direct questions to patient

Q Do you experience palpitations, chest pain, or faintness? These symptoms are fairly common among all types of patients and may be somewhat more common with mitral valve prolapse and significant mitral insufficiency. In some instances, chest pain or palpitations may require treatment with beta-blockers, diltiazem, or verapamil.

Q Do you become short of breath with exertion? Possible symptom of important mitral regurgitation

Q Are you anxious or concerned about having this condition? Patient may require assurance that mitral valve prolapse is benign and nonprogressive in the majority of cases

Family history

Q Do you have family members with the same condition? Mitral valve prolapse may be inherited as an autosomal-dominant trait with variable penetrance

Q Have any family members died suddenly as a result of mitral valve prolapse? Affirmative answer provides cause to refer to a specialist

Examination

Auscultation:

- The click of mitral valve prolapse is a brief, high-pitched sound that occurs at least 0.14s after S1. Unlike a systolic ejection click, it can be detected after the beginning of the upstroke of the carotid pulse. Multiple clicks may be heard, possibly corresponding to the tensing of chordae tendineae and prolapsing leaflets
- The mid-systolic click may be followed by a mid to late crescendo systolic murmur. Regurgitation is usually not severe if the murmur is limited to the latter part of systole. A holosystolic murmur suggests more severe regurgitation

- Some patients with mitral valve prolapse have only a click or only a murmur, and others may have no abnormality that is evident with auscultation

Dynamic auscultation:

- Sudden standing causes both the click and the beginning of the murmur to occur earlier in systole. The murmur may become longer
- Changing from a standing to a supine position delays the click and the onset of the murmur
- Squatting delays the click and shortens the murmur

Summary of investigative tests

- Echocardiography: preferred diagnostic modality for confirming mitral valve prolapse and determining whether there is any thickening of the mitral leaflets (typically performed by a specialist)
- Electrocardiography: generally not helpful in the diagnosis but may be useful for other causes of mitral regurgitation
- Holter monitoring or an ECG event recorder: used to evaluate arrhythmias in patients with palpitations
- Graded exercise stress test: detects the rare individual with exercise-induced arrhythmias and quantitates exercise tolerance (normally performed by a specialist)
- Stress echocardiogram: may be helpful when there is a suspicion of underlying ischemic heart disease or when there is uncertainty regarding the severity of mitral regurgitation (normally performed by a specialist)
- Cardiac catheterization and angiography (always performed by a specialist): should be reserved for patients being evaluated for mitral valve surgery
- Tilt-table testing (normally performed by a specialist): may be useful to evaluate symptoms suggesting autonomic dysfunction

DIAGNOSTIC DECISION

- The diagnostic criteria for mitral valve prolapse have been well established. Echocardiography is recommended for diagnosing mitral valve prolapse, evaluating hemodynamic severity of mitral regurgitation, and assessing leaflet morphology and ventricular compensation in patients with physical signs of mitral valve prolapse
- According to above guidelines, mitral valve prolapse is evident if M-mode echocardiography reveals leaflet posterior displacement greater than or equal to 2mm, or holosystolic posterior 'hammocking' greater than 3mm. Leaflet thickness greater than 5mm increases the certainty of the diagnosis

Guidelines

- Bonow R, Carabello B, de Leon AC Jr, et al. ACC/AHA guidelines for the management of patients with valvular heart disease: a report of the American College of Cardiology/American Heart Association Task Force on Practice Guidelines (Committee on Management of Patients with Valvular Heart Disease). J Am Coll Cardiol 1998;32:1486–588. Also available online at the National Guideline Clearinghouse [1]
- Cheitlin MD, Alpert JS, Armstrong WF, et al. ACC/AHA guidelines for the clinical application of echocardiography: a report of the American College of Cardiology/American Heart Association Task Force on Practice Guidelines (Committee on Clinical Application of Echocardiography). Circulation 1997;95(6):1686–744. Available online at the National Guideline Clearinghouse [2]

CLINICAL PEARL(S)

- Inexperienced echocardiography laboratories may overestimate the severity of mitral regurgitation by assuming the regurgitation seen by color Doppler in late systole is occurring throughout systole
- Many patients have been told they have mitral valve prolapse based on outdated echocardiographic criteria. More than half of the patients referred to an echocardiography laboratory to evaluate mitral valve prolapse do not prove to have it

- Always be hesitant in attributing nonspecific cardiovascular symptoms to mitral valve prolapse
- In most patients the coexistence of symptoms such as chest pain, palpitations, and mitral valve prolapse is only coincidental and not causal

THE TESTS

Imaging

ECHOCARDIOGRAPHY

Description

- Uses ultrasound to create a dynamic picture of the heart and its chambers and valves
- Two-dimensional images of the long axis of the heart are used to establish the diagnosis

Advantages/Disadvantages

Advantages:

- Noninvasive, painfree, and quick
- Will define the degree of leaflet prolapse, leaflet thickening, and valvular regurgitation
- May exclude alternative etiologies of mitral valve disease
- May identify associated cardiac abnormalities, including cardiomyopathy, endocarditis, or other valvular abnormalities not detected by clinical examination

Disadvantages:

- Typically performed and interpreted by a specialist
- Operator-dependent

Abnormal

- A definite diagnosis of mitral valve prolapse is established when a mitral leaflet(s) prolapses 2mm or more into the left atrium
- Lesser degrees of prolapse can occur but may be normal if the leaflets are normal in appearance
- The M-mode echocardiographic definition of mitral valve prolapse includes 2mm or more posterior displacement of one or both leaflets, or holosystolic 'hammocking' of more than 3mm
- Leaflet thickening over 5mm during ventricular diastole identifies a subpopulation with a much higher probability of future complications
- Leaflet redundancy and elongated chordae tendineae can be seen with the two-dimensional imaging

Cause of abnormal result

Mitral valve prolapse.

Other tests

ELECTROCARDIOGRAPHY

Description

- 12-lead ECG
- Creates an electrical picture of the heart

Advantages/Disadvantages

Advantages:

- Noninvasive procedure, quick, and cheap
- May indicate conduction disturbance, arrhythmias, and hypertrophic changes
- Highly useful as a later reference

Disadvantage:

- Has no diagnostic value for mitral valve prolapse

Abnormal

- In many symptomatic patients and some asymptomatic patients, ECG reveals inverted or biphasic T waves and nonspecific ST-segment alterations in leads II, III, and aVF. Occasionally, changes may also be seen in anterolateral leads. Similar nonspecific changes can be seen in patients without mitral valve prolapse
- Arrhythmia may be seen, including premature atrial and ventricular complexes, supraventricular tachycardias, and, rarely, ventricular tachycardia

Cause of abnormal result

- May be related to increased tension on the papillary muscles
- In rare instances, may reflect an underlying cardiomyopathy

24-H HOLTER MONITORING/ECG EVENT RECORDER

Description

- The Holter monitor is a continuous 24-h recording of the heart rhythm using a small battery-powered recorder
- Several recording electrodes are applied to the patient's chest wall
- The event recorder is a similar device that continuously records the heart rhythm but stores the recording only when the patient activates the device. The advantage of this approach is that there is a clear temporal relation between the patient's symptoms and the heart rhythm; this device can be carried for several weeks by patients with intermittent symptoms

Advantages/Disadvantages

Advantage:

- May reveal serious ventricular or supraventricular arrhythmias

Disadvantages:

- Not recommended for patients without palpitations
- The 24-h Holter monitor is not recommended for patients with symptoms occurring less than daily. An event monitor should be used in these cases

Abnormal

- Ventricular tachycardia
- Paroxysmal supraventricular tachycardia

Cause of abnormal result

- Ventricular tachycardia occurs with myocardial disease and ischemia, and so is rare in mitral valve prolapse
- Supraventricular arrhythmias are common in patients with and without mitral valve prolapse and may be the consequence of abnormal electrical pathways in the atrioventricular junction

TREATMENT

IMMEDIATE ACTION

Infective endocarditis may complicate mitral valve prolapse and requires immediate referral and aggressive treatment.

MANAGEMENT ISSUES

Goals

- Evaluate the status of the mitral valve with echocardiography. Refer to specialist if mitral regurgitation is significant or progressive
- Educate appropriate patients (those who have mitral valve prolapse with mitral regurgitation and/or thickened leaflets) about the need for prophylaxis prior to undergoing dental, oral, respiratory tract, or esophageal procedures
- Initiate therapy as needed to prevent cerebrovascular accidents and life-threatening arrhythmias
- Help symptomatic patients minimize palpitations, chest pain, fatigue, or autonomic dysfunction
- For patients with undue anxiety, provide reassurance about the benign prognosis of the condition in the large majority of cases

Management in special circumstances

COEXISTING DISEASE

Patients who have both mitral regurgitation and hypertension should be followed closely, based on concern that elevated blood pressure may increase the likelihood of chordal rupture and progressive mitral regurgitation.

SPECIAL PATIENT GROUPS

- Most patients with mitral valve prolapse can safely engage in any sport or exercise
- Those with serious arrhythmias, significant mitral regurgitation, a prolonged QT interval, unexplained syncope, aortic root enlargement, or a family history of sudden death due to mitral valve prolapse should avoid high-intensity, competitive sports
- Those with moderate-to-severe mitral regurgitation should avoid weight-lifting, which might increase blood pressure and worsen regurgitation

PATIENT SATISFACTION/LIFESTYLE PRIORITIES

- Athletes with serious arrhythmias, significant mitral regurgitation, prolonged QT interval, unexplained syncope, aortic root enlargement, or family history of sudden death due to mitral valve prolapse should be informed of the serious risks of high-intensity activities. They may find it problematic to avoid high-intensity competitive sports but need to be clearly aware of the risks
- Those who have a history of focal neurologic events and who are in sinus rhythm but lack atrial thrombi should refrain from smoking cigarettes and should not take oral contraceptives

SUMMARY OF THERAPEUTIC OPTIONS

Choices

- Certain lifestyle changes benefit many patients with mitral valve prolapse; the changes to be recommended depend on each patient's circumstances
- In most instances no drugs or other therapies are needed other than endocarditis prophylaxis before dental, oral, respiratory tract, or esophageal procedures. This is necessary for patients with mitral valve prolapse accompanied by a regurgitant murmur and/or thickened leaflets
- Daily aspirin therapy is recommended for patients with a history of focal neurologic events and who are in sinus rhythm but do not have atrial thrombi; and for patients with atrial fibrillation who are younger than 65 and who lack a history of hypertension or heart failure. Many physicians recommend aspirin therapy for patients with high-risk echocardiographic findings

- Warfarin is recommended for patients with a prior systemic embolic event and for patients with atrial fibrillation who are 65 or older or have a history of hypertension or heart failure
- Beta-blockers may benefit patients with palpitations due to mild tachyarrhythmias. They may also help patients with adrenergic symptoms, chest pain, or fatigue
- Referral for valvular surgery (performed by a specialist) may be needed for patients whose symptoms are severe or progressive. Surgery is indicated for mitral valve prolapse patients with a flail mitral leaflet resulting from the rupture or elongation of chordae tendineae. Operation may involve valve repair, or replacement of valve with a prosthetic valve. Valve repair is associated with lower operative mortality and has a lower risk of thrombosis and endocarditis. The surgery may correct mitral regurgitation, repair ruptured chordae tendineae, and preserve left ventricular function. Mortality is low in reported surgical series. However, this open-heart surgery may be complicated by morbid events that include bleeding, infection, and atrial arrhythmias

Guidelines

- Bonow R, Carabello B, de Leon AC Jr, et al. ACC/AHA guidelines for the management of patients with valvular heart disease: a report of the American College of Cardiology/American Heart Association Task Force on Practice Guidelines (Committee on Management of Patients with Valvular Heart Disease). J Am Coll Cardiol 1998;32:1486–588 [1]
- AHA Scientific Statements: Prevention of Bacterial Endocarditis (Summary of recommendations published in JAMA 1997;277:1794). Available online at http://www.sc-ds.org/aha.htm/ [3]

FOLLOW UP

- Asymptomatic patients with mild or no mitral regurgitation require only routine health-maintenance care that includes a periodic physical examination
- High-risk patients should be examined yearly
- Repeated echocardiograms are necessary only in the following circumstances: development of cardiovascular symptoms, physical findings suggestive of progression of mitral regurgitation, or high-risk characteristics evident on initial echocardiogram

Information for patient or caregiver

- In most instances, mitral valve prolapse is a benign condition that does not worsen over time
- Some people with mitral valve prolapse are at higher than average risk of developing a heart-valve infection following dental work or certain medical procedures. Your doctor may advise you to take antibiotics in advance of such procedures
- A very small minority of people with mitral valve prolapse experience heart palpitations, chest pain that differs from the pain of angina, and light-headedness upon standing up suddenly. These conditions are usually not serious, but you should report them to your doctor if they occur. You should also inform your doctor if you feel short of breath when you exercise
- Rarely, the valve associated with mitral valve prolapse becomes seriously impaired and needs to be surgically repaired or replaced. A noninvasive test called echocardiography can reveal the health of the valve. Doctors commonly order an echocardiogram when they first detect mitral valve prolapse in a patient. If the patient has any characteristics that might be associated with the possible declining function of the valve, the doctor may order repeated echocardiograms to be performed at intervals of 1–3 years

DRUGS AND OTHER THERAPIES: DETAILS

Drugs

ASPIRIN

- Off-label indication
- Inhibits platelet aggregation

Dose
81–325mg/day.

Efficacy
The risk of primary stroke is approximately 3.2% in patients with atrial fibrillation on aspirin therapy – a risk reduction of 20–49% compared to untreated patients.

Risks/Benefits
The benefits of stroke and myocardial risk reduction far outweigh the risks in most patients.

Risks:
- Use caution in anemia, Hodgkin's disease, gout, hepatic and renal disease, asthma, nasal polyps, and nasal allergies
- Use caution with children and teenagers (Reye's syndrome)

Benefits:
- Simple dosing regimen allows for better patient compliance
- Easy to take
- Widely available
- Effective in low doses

Side-effects and adverse reactions
- Gastrointestinal: abdominal pain, nausea, dyspepsia, hepatotoxicity, gastrointestinal bleeding
- EENT: hearing loss and tinnitus
- Hematologic: bleeding disorders, thrombocytopenia
- Respiratory: hyperpnea, asthma
- Skin: angioedema, bruising, rash, urticaria
- CNS: dizziness, headache

Interactions (other drugs)
- ACE inhibitors
- Acetazolamide
- Antacids
- Corticosteroids
- Diltiazem
- Ethanol
- Griseofulvin
- Methotrexate
- Oral anticoagulants
- Antigout medicines
- Warfarin (enhanced hypoprothrombinemic effect of warfarin)

Contraindications
- Gastrointestinal bleeding
- Bleeding disorders
- Bone marrow suppression
- Hypersensitivity to salicylates, NSAIDs, or tartrazine

Evidence
- Treatment with aspirin is recommended for patients with mitral valve prolapse who have experienced cerebral transient ischemic attacks [1] *Level C*
- Aspirin therapy is recommended for patients aged less than 65 years with mitral valve prolapse, atrial fibrillation without history of mitral regurgitation, hypertension, or heart failure [1] *Level C*

Acceptability to patient
Highly acceptable.

Patient and caregiver information
Patients should understand the reasons for aspirin therapy.

WARFARIN

- Oral anticoagulant
- Antagonizes vitamin K pathway
- Takes 48–72h before effective anticoagulation

Dose

Dosage should be adjusted individually to maintain an international normalized ratio (INR) between 2 and 3.

Efficacy

- For patients with atrial fibrillation, warfarin treatment in the therapeutic range reduces stroke risk by approximately 60% compared to untreated patients
- Risk of stroke on warfarin is approximately 0.8–2.3%

Risks/Benefits

Risks:

- Use caution with infection and trauma, diverticulitis, renal and hepatic disease, hypertension, congestive heart failure, tuberculosis, thyroid disease, diabetes mellitus, protein C deficiency, polyarteritis, and vasculitis
- Use caution in the elderly, children, and nursing mothers

Benefits:

- Reduces the risk of ischemic stroke
- Has many dietary and lifestyle implications
- Requires ongoing monitoring of INR

Side-effects and adverse reactions

- Gastrointestinal: cramps, diarrhea, vomiting
- CNS: fatigue, headache
- Genitourinary: gonadal dysfunction
- EENT: blurred vision
- Skin: contact dermatitis
- Metabolic: altered thyroid, pituitary, and adrenal hormones
- Musculoskeletal: weakness

Interactions (other drugs)

■ Acetaminophen ■ Allopurinol ■ Aminoglutethimide ■ Amiodarone ■ Aspirin (increased risk of bleeding) ■ Azathioprine ■ Barbiturates ■ Bile acid-binding resins ■ Carbamazepine ■ Cephalosporins ■ Chloral hydrate ■ Chloramphenicol ■ Clofibrate ■ Co-trimoxazole ■ Danazole ■ Dextrothyroxine ■ Disulfiram ■ Ethanol ■ Ethchlorvynol ■ Fluconazole ■ Fluorouracil ■ Gemfibrozil ■ Glutethimide ■ Griseofulvin ■ Glucagon ■ Heparin ■ Isoniazid ■ Metronidazole ■ Nalidixic acid ■ Neomycin ■ NSAIDs ■ Oral contraceptives ■ Phenytoin ■ Propafenones ■ Propoxyphene ■ Quinidines ■ Quinolones ■ Rifampin ■ Salicylates ■ Sertraline ■ Sulfonamides ■ Sulfonylureas ■ Testosterone derivatives

Contraindications

■ Active bleeding ■ Bacterial endocarditis ■ Cerebral hemorrhage ■ Eclampsia ■ Gastrointestinal ulceration ■ Hemorrhagic blood dyscrasias ■ Hemorrhagic tendencies ■ Hypertension ■ Pericarditis ■ Pregnancy and threatened abortion ■ Recent surgery presenting heightened risk of bleeding ■ Ulcerative colitis ■ Visceral carcinoma

Evidence

- Treatment with warfarin is recommended for patients with mitral valve prolapse, aged 65 or older, who have atrial fibrillation with hypertension, murmur of mitral regurgitation, or history of heart failure [1] *Level C*
- Warfarin therapy is recommended for mitral valve prolapse patients who have had a stroke, or for those with recurrent transient ischemic attacks while on aspirin [1] *Level C*

Acceptability to patient

- Elderly, psychotic, and alcoholic patients present significant noncompliance problems
- Patients may not like the dietary and lifestyle restrictions
- Patients may find ongoing monitoring of INR difficult

Follow up plan

Prothrombin time should be assessed daily until correct maintenance dose is established.

Patient and caregiver information

Patients should be informed of the risk of bleeding and of the impact of diet and other factors on prothrombin time.

BETA-ADRENERGIC BLOCKERS

Dose

- Varies with individual drug
- The selective $beta_1$ antagonists are commonly prescribed
- Metoprolol: 25–100mg twice daily
- Atenolol: 25–50mg once daily

Efficacy

- Slows heart rate
- Reduces hypertension in patients <65 years of age
- Helps prevent arrhythmias
- Reduces chest pain

Risks/Benefits

Risks:

- Use caution in pregnancy and breast-feeding
- Use caution in diabetes mellitus
- Use caution in liver and renal impairment
- Use caution in AV block
- Use caution in myasthenia gravis
- Do not withdraw abruptly in angina

Benefit: Slows heart rate, may prevent arrhythmias, lowers blood pressure, and may reduce or eliminate chest pain.

Side-effects and adverse reactions

- Cardiovascular: hypotension, bradycardia, conduction abnormalities, heart failure, peripheral vasoconstriction
- CNS: fatigue, sleep disturbances
- EENT: dry eyes
- Gastrointestinal: nausea, vomiting
- Respiratory: bronchospasm
- Skin: rashes, exacerbation of psoriasis

Interactions (other drugs)

■ Adenosine (may cause bradycardia) ■ Amoxicillin (reduced atenolol availability) ■ Antacids (reduced atenolol availability) ■ Calcium channel blockers (see dihydropyridine and verapamil) ■ Clonidine (exacerbation of rebound hypertension upon discontinuation of clonidine) ■ Digoxin (concomitant slowing of AV node conduction) ■ Dihydropyridines (additive hemodynamic effects; increased serum concentration of atenolol) ■ Lidocaine (increased serum lidocaine possible) ■ Neostigmine (may cause bradycardia) ■ NSAIDs (reduced antihypertensive effects of atenolol) ■ Physostigmine (bradycardia aggravated) ■ Prazosin (first-dose response to prazosin may be enhanced by beta-blockade) ■ Tacrine (may cause bradycardia) ■ Theophylline (antagonistic pharmacodynamic effects) ■ Verapamil (enhanced effects of both drugs)

Contraindications

■ Pheochromocytoma ■ Metabolic acidosis ■ Asthma ■ Second- or third-degree AV block, sick sinus syndrome, marked bradycardia, hypotension, cardiogenic shock, peripheral arterial disease, uncontrolled heart failure, Prinzmetal's angina

Evidence

Patients with mitral valve prolapse who experience 'palpitations associated with mild tachyarrhythmias or increased adrenergic symptoms, and those with chest pain, anxiety, or fatigue' are frequently responsive to beta-blocker therapy [1] *Level C*

Acceptability to patient

- The afore-mentioned side-effects may limit patient compliance
- Impotence is also a common reason for discontinuation of this class of drug

Patient and caregiver information

- Patients should learn to monitor their pulse rate and report irregularities to their physician
- Patients should be educated about the importance of taking the drug at regular intervals without changing or skipping doses
- If a decision is made to discontinue the treatment, the dosage should be gradually tapered rather than abruptly withdrawn

LIFESTYLE

- Patients with palpitations may benefit from avoiding caffeine, alcohol, and cigarettes
- Weight loss should be encouraged in overweight patients
- Those with hypotension should increase salt and fluid intake
- Patients with a history of focal neurologic events and who are in sinus rhythm should avoid smoking cigarettes and taking oral contraceptives
- Nearly all patients should be encouraged to exercise; however, those with serious arrhythmias, significant mitral regurgitation, prolonged QT interval, unexplained syncope, aortic root enlargement, or family history of sudden death due to mitral valve prolapse should avoid high-intensity competitive sports

RISKS/BENEFITS

Benefits: these lifestyle changes may help to reduce symptoms and avert serious complications.

ACCEPTABILITY TO PATIENT

- Some patients may be reluctant to avoid caffeine, cigarettes
- Others may wish to compete in high-intensity sports
- Weight loss may also be difficult

PATIENT AND CAREGIVER INFORMATION

Patients should understand the reasons for making lifestyle changes.

OUTCOMES

EFFICACY OF THERAPIES

Therapy may reduce symptoms associated with mitral valve prolapse, but this condition will persist unless it is surgically corrected.

Evidence

PDxMD are unable to cite evidence that meets our criteria for evidence.

PROGNOSIS

- 75% of patients have no increase in morbidity or mortality and do not require medical treatment
- Up to 25% of patients may need valvular surgery after the age of 50
- Several studies show that mitral valve prolapse has a complication rate of less than 2% each year

Clinical pearl(s)

- Excessive patient anxiety is often a problem in patients with mitral valve prolapse
- Women with no echocardiographic evidence of valve thickening have an excellent prognosis
- Men with leaflet thickening by echocardiography are at highest risk of complications

COMPLICATIONS

- Progressive mitral regurgitation
- Bacterial endocarditis
- Serious arrhythmias
- Cerebrovascular accidents

PREVENTION

There are no behaviors for preventing mitral valve prolapse.

RESOURCES

ASSOCIATIONS

American Heart Association
7272 Greenville Ave.
Dallas, TX 75231-4596
Phone, toll-free: (800) 242-8721
http://www.americanheart.org

KEY REFERENCES

- Braunwald E. Heart disease: a textbook of cardiovascular medicine, 6th edn. Philadelphia: WB Saunders, 2001
- Goldman L, Braunwald E. Primary cardiology. Philadelphia: WB Saunders, 1998
- Bouknight DP, O' Rourke RA. Current management of mitral valve prolapse. Am Fam Physician 2000;61(11):3343
- Joy E. Mitral valve prolapse in active patients: Recognition, treatment, and exercise recommendations. Physician Sportsmed 1996;24(7):78

Guidelines

1 Bonow R, Carabello B, de Leon AC Jr, et al. ACC/AHA guidelines for the management of patients with valvular heart disease: a report of the American College of Cardiology/American Heart Association Task Force on Practice Guidelines (Committee on Management of Patients With Valvular Heart Disease). J Am Coll Cardiol 1998;32:1486–588

2 ACC/AHA guidelines for the clinical application of echocardiography: a report of the American College of Cardiology/American Heart Association Task Force on Practice Guidelines (Committee on Clinical Application of Echocardiograph). Circulation 1997;95(6):1686–744

3 AHA Scientific Statements: Prevention of Bacterial Endocarditis (Summary of recommendations published in JAMA 1997;277:1794). Available online at: http://www.sc-ds.org/aha.htm

FAQS

Question 1

What are the characteristic auscultatory findings in a patient with mitral valve prolapse?

ANSWER 1

A mid-systolic click that may be followed by a late-systolic murmur of mitral regurgitation, if present.

Question 2

What are the characteristic clinical features of the mitral valve prolapse syndrome?

ANSWER 2

The vast majority of patients with mitral valve prolapse are asymptomatic. In those patients with atypical chest pain, palpitations, and/or autonomic dysfunction, the clinician often searches for an explanation, and if mitral valve prolapse is detected, the symptoms become linked to mitral valve prolapse. This linkage is appropriate in an occasional case but often only increases the patient's concern about the symptoms.

Question 3

Which patients with mitral valve prolapse should receive endocarditis prophylaxis?

ANSWER 3

Patients with a murmur of mitral regurgitation, evidence of mitral regurgitation by Doppler echocardiographic studies, or markedly thickened and redundant mitral valve leaflets should receive endocarditis prophylaxis.

Question 4

What are the most common electrocardiographic abnormalities associated with mitral valve prolapse?

ANSWER 4

ST–T-wave abnormalities, including ST-segment depression and T-wave inversion, are seen in patients with mitral valve prolapse, but these changes are not specific for mitral valve prolapse. The nonspecific ST–T changes may represent inferior wall ischemia secondary to traction on the posteromedial papillary muscle by the prolapsing mitral valve leaflets, but the mechanism(s) is not fully understood. The need to exclude coronary insufficiency should be guided by clinical correlation.

Question 5

Which test is best to determine whether chest pain in a patient with mitral valve prolapse is due to myocardial ischemia secondary to associated coronary artery disease?

ANSWER 5

An exercise stress test using only the electrocardiogram to detect ischemia is not appropriate in women because of their high prevalence of nonspecific ST changes with stress. Exercise stress echocardiography is preferred in that both mitral insufficiency and myocardial ischemia can be evaluated. Nuclear stress imaging is less specific in women, since breast tissue can attenuate radioactivity and produce a false-positive scan.

CONTRIBUTORS

Russell C Jones, MD, MPH
John McB Hodgson, MD, FACC, FSCAI
James Orford, MD

MYOCARDIAL INFARCTION

SUMMARY INFORMATION

DESCRIPTION

- Myocardial infarction (MI) is a disorder in which necrosis of the heart muscle (myocardium) occurs owing to an inadequate supply of oxygen. The syndrome is usually caused by a sudden and complete, or nearly complete, blockade of at least one major epicardial coronary artery
- Unless death occurs within minutes (e.g. from arrhythmia), myocardial necrosis is always evident
- Treatment of choice is restoration of blood flow to the myocardium in the shortest possible period of time, either pharmacologically (i.e. by thrombolysis) or by mechanical means (e.g. primary angioplasty)

URGENT ACTION

- Time is critical – approx. half of all deaths from MI occur within 1h of the onset of symptoms
- If the patient becomes unconscious, administer CPR
- Administration of aspirin – patient should chew on 325mg nonenteric-coated tablet
- Administration of oxygen
- Connection to ECG monitor
- Support of circulation and respiration
- Make arrangements to institute reperfusion therapy (thrombolysis or primary angioplasty) as soon as possible in the case of ST-segment elevation MI
- Rarely, emergency coronary artery bypass surgery

KEY! DON'T MISS!

- Take immediate action if MI is suspected
- A 12-lead ECG should be obtained as soon as possible
- Up to one-third of patients do not experience classic substernal chest pain – this is especially true of older patients, females, and diabetics
- MI in the elderly may present in atypical fashion. A high index of suspicion is needed for any patient with dypsnea, discomfort, syncope, or undue fatigue
- In patients presenting with classic symptoms but no obvious ECG changes, reverse the leads and perform a right-sided ECG. This will more sensitively screen for the easily missed posterior wall MI (will enhance evidence of ischemia in lead V1)

BACKGROUND

ICD9 CODE
410.9 Myocardial infarction

SYNONYMS
- Heart attack
- MI
- AMI (acute myocardial infarction)

CARDINAL FEATURES
- Classically, acute onset of squeezing substernal chest pain or pressure, often radiating to one or both upper extremities, to the neck or jaw, or through to the back
- Difficulty in breathing or shortness of breath
- Nausea
- Light-headedness
- Weakness
- Feeling of impending doom
- ECG shows classic evolving changes. For a transmural infarction: ST-segment elevation and T-wave inversion in the leads overlying the infarcted area evolving into a Q-wave pattern in the same areas; ST depression may be present in reciprocal leads. In nontransmural infarction (usually subendocardial): ST-segment depression in the leads overlying the affected area with nonspecific T-wave abnormalities may be the only changes noted. In patients presenting with classic symptoms, but no obvious ECG changes, reverse the leads to screen more carefully for a possible posterior wall MI (especially helpful in patients with known history of right bundle branch block or right axis deviation)
- Arrhythmias triggered by ischemia may appear. The most serious arrhythmias are ventricular tachycardia and ventricular fibrillation leading to death. Sinus bradycardia and/or AV block may be present, especially in the case of inferior MI
- Infarction of a significant portion of functioning myocardium can lead to acute congestive heart failure. Infarction of >40% of myocardium generally leads to cardiogenic shock

CAUSES
Common causes
Most common cause is coronary thrombosis (blood clot), usually occurring on an atherosclerotic plaque (which often shows evidence of recent plaque rupture). Involved plaques are usually not severe (i.e. <50% diameter stenosis) prior to rupture and thrombus activation.

Rare causes
- Embolization of material into a coronary artery (e.g. from a valvular endocarditis, mural thrombosis, paradoxical emboli)
- Trauma causing coronary artery laceration or dissection (including iatrogenic during angioplasty)
- Vasculitis (e.g. systemic lupus erythematosus and other collagen vascular diseases)
- Vasospasm (e.g. with cocaine or amphetamine use and/or variant [Prinzmetal's] angina)
- Proximal extension of an aortic aneurysm into a coronary artery ostium
- Degenerative or infiltrative coronary artery disease (e.g. amyloidosis)
- Congenital abnormalities (e.g. anomalous origin of left coronary artery)
- Conditions that suddenly increase myocardial oxygen requirements or decrease supply (e.g. shock, carbon monoxide poisoning)

Contributory or predisposing factors

- Smoking
- Dyslipidemias (especially elevation of low-density lipoprotein cholesterol and/or reduction of high-density lipoprotein cholesterol)
- Hypertension
- Diabetes mellitus
- Obesity
- Physical inactivity
- Male gender
- Strong family history
- Acute triggering events, such as sudden intense emotion or extreme physical exertion, may contribute to the onset of infarction

EPIDEMIOLOGY

Incidence and prevalence

INCIDENCE

- >900,000 cases/year in the US
- Approx. 225,000 deaths/year in the US

PREVALENCE

>5 cases/1000 population.

Demographics

AGE

- Most common after 40 years of age
- Peak occurrence between 50 and 70 years of age

GENDER

- Between the ages of 40 and 65, most common in males
- Over 65 years of age, no difference between males and females

GENETICS

Genetic predisposition. Tends to run in families.

GEOGRAPHY

Worldwide, but much more common in 'developed' countries.

SOCIOECONOMIC STATUS

- Cuts across socioeconomic groups
- More common in groups with higher socioeconomic status since incidence increases with age
- Risk factors (especially obesity, dyslipidemias, and diabetes) more common as socioeconomic status increases

DIFFERENTIAL DIAGNOSIS

Pericarditis

Pericarditis is an inflammation of the pericardium, the sac that surrounds the heart. It may be caused by a virus or bacterial infection, such as tuberculosis, or by an injury. It often occurs after a respiratory infection.

FEATURES

- Pain of acute myocardial infarction (MI) may simulate and be simulated by acute pericarditis
- Usually aggravated by respiratory movements and coughing, and relieved by sitting up in a forward position
- Characteristic ECG changes include saddle-shaped elevated ST segments in all leads except a PR. Depression of the PR segment is quite specific

Pleural pain

Pain related to the covering of the lung.

FEATURES

Usually knife-like, sharp, aggravated by breathing, radiates to the shoulder but not down the arm.

Pulmonary embolism

Pulmonary embolism is not a disease in and of itself but rather an often fatal complication of underlying venous thrombosis.

FEATURES

- Pulmonary embolism produces pain laterally in the chest – often pleuritic in nature. Acute embolism may mimic the dull pain of ischemia
- Dyspnea and sinus tachycardia are common. Cardiovascular collapse possible in large emboli obstructing the major pulmonary arteries
- Predisposing factors such as recent trauma, surgery, inactivity, pregnancy, estrogen use
- Hypoxia is out of proportion to pulmonary distress

Aortic dissection

Aortic dissection is dissection of the thoracic aorta.

FEATURES

- Produces a 'ripping' or 'tearing' pain localized in center of chest or back. It is extremely severe and persists relatively unchanged for hours or may migrate downward as dissection advances
- The right coronary artery is most commonly affected by dissection
- Aortic insufficiency is common in ascending involvement

Costochondritis and chondrosternal inflammation

Costochondritis is an inflammatory process of the costochondral or costosternal joints that causes localized pain and tenderness.

FEATURES

- Pain usually sharp, localized, and darting in costochondritis
- Look for associated localized swelling and redness
- Often there is point tenderness or pain on palpation along the sternum

Cholecystitis

Cholecystitis is inflammation of the gall bladder.

FEATURES
- Upper abdominal pain, often radiating towards back and/or right shoulder
- Nausea and vomiting usually prominent in cholecystitis
- Most common in obese females >40 years

Peptic ulcer disease
Peptic ulcer disease refers to a discrete mucosal defect in the portions of the gastrointestinal tract (gastric or duodenal) exposed to acid and pepsin secretion.

FEATURES
- Burning-type epigastric pain is seen
- May be accompanied by evidence of upper gastrointestinal bleeding

Esophagitis
Inflammation of the lining of the esophagus often due to gastrointestinal reflux.

FEATURES
- Burning-type epigastric pain
- Reflux of acid may be noted
- Gastrointestinal sources are the most common cause of chest pain in patients presenting to the emergency room

SIGNS & SYMPTOMS
Signs
- Diaphoretic skin, pallor, cool skin, or other signs of vasoconstriction
- Hypertension (initially due to pain and adrenergic discharge) may be followed by hypotension in larger infarcts or inferior wall infarction
- Restlessness
- Apical systolic murmur, caused by mitral regurgitation secondary to papillary muscle dysfunction may be present
- Tachycardia (sinus or tachyarrhythmia) or bradycardia (sinus or secondary to heart block – especially in inferior infarctions as a manifestation of the Bezold–Jarish reflex)
- Irregular rhythm (premature auricular contractions [PACs] and premature ventricular contractions [PVCs], Wenkebach, other arrhythmias)
- Signs of left ventricular failure and/or right ventricular dysfunction/failure in large infarcts
- Rales, other evidence of pulmonary congestion
- Signs of low cardiac output, e.g. hypotension, poor carotid pulses, and pulsus alternans
- Confusion, especially in elderly patients
- Apical systolic murmur, S3 or S4 may be present
- Conduction disturbances on ECG
- 'Nonspecific' repolarization abnormalities useful in identifying MI if classic ST-segment elevation/T-wave inversion is not present
- ST-segment depression, isolated T-wave inversion, and new-onset bundle branch block are less specific but may be supportive of a diagnosis of MI
- Exclude pulmonary embolism, aortic dissection, spontaneous pneumothorax, pericarditis, and cholecystitis

Symptoms
- Main symptom is chest pain
- Crushing or squeezing in nature
- Most often retrosternal
- May be epigastric or upper back
- Radiation is often present: inner aspect of arms (L>R), shoulders, neck, teeth, jaw
- Lasts at least 30min, unresponsive (or only partially so) to nitroglycerin

Up to one-third of patients do not experience classic substernal chest pain – this is especially true of older patients, females, and diabetics.

Other symptoms are:
- Weakness
- Fatigue
- Restlessness, feeling of impending doom
- Diaphoresis
- Palpitation, presyncope
- Nausea, vomiting, hiccuping
- Shortness of breath, difficulty breathing
- Anxiety
- Abdominal pain, possibly described as indigestion, but severe
- Dry mouth

ASSOCIATED DISORDERS
- Peripheral vascular disease
- Atrial fibrillation or other arrhythmias
- Congestive heart failure
- Aortic aneurysm/dissection
- Pericarditis
- Pulmonary embolism
- Stroke
- Anxiety/depression

KEY! DON'T MISS!
- Take immediate action if MI is suspected
- A 12-lead ECG should be obtained as soon as possible
- Up to one-third of patients do not experience classic substernal chest pain – this is especially true of older patients, females, and diabetics
- MI in the elderly may present in atypical fashion. A high index of suspicion is needed for any patient with dypsnea, discomfort, syncope, or undue fatigue
- In patients presenting with classic symptoms but no obvious ECG changes, reverse the leads and perform a right-sided ECG. This will more sensitively screen for the easily missed posterior wall MI (will enhance evidence of ischemia in lead V1)

CONSIDER CONSULT
- All patients with a diagnosis of acute MI should be referred to a cardiologist
- Refer as soon as possible after MI is suspected

INVESTIGATION OF THE PATIENT
Direct questions to patient

Q Have you had recent chest pain? What was the nature of the pain? Did anything seem to bring the pain on or make it get better? History of recent episodes of 'pressure in the chest,' especially if brought on by exercise and relieved by rest, or triggered by severe emotional stress, strongly points to ischemic heart disease. Note that new onset of such symptoms, or episodes of such pain occurring at rest, constitutes unstable angina by definition

Q Did the pain radiate to your neck, through to your back, or travel down your arms? Radiation of pain into the neck or jaw, or into the arms, especially the ulnar distribution of the left arm, is characteristic of MI. Pain radiating through to the back may be suggestive of aortic dissection

Q What were you doing when the current episode started? Identify 'trigger factors' such as emotional stress

- **Q Did you take any nitroglycerin (NTG) after the pain started? How many? For how long did the pain continue after you took the NTG?** Pain of MI (as opposed to myocardial ischemia or angina) is almost never totally and promptly relieved by nitrate administration
- **Q What does/did the pain feel like?** The patient's own description of the pain is extremely important. A patient who spontaneously describes squeezing pain or pressure in the chest using a clenched fist over the precordium to illustrate the type of pain is almost always describing ischemic chest pain. Conversely, description of a sharp pain, the exact location of which the patient indicates by pointing with a single finger, only very rarely describes the pain of myocardial ischemia or infarction. Tearing or ripping pain felt in the chest, particularly if it radiates to the back, may be indicative of aortic dissection
- **Q Have you felt any palpitations?** Attempt to elicit possible symptoms of associated arrhythmia
- **Q Were you dizzy or did you pass out?** May indicate a potentially lethal arrhythmia (e.g.ventricular tachycardia) – but can occur in its absence

Contributory or predisposing factors

- **Q Have you ever been told you had a 'heart problem'?** Identify risk factor
- **Q Do you have high blood pressure?** Hypertension is a risk factor for ischemic heart disease
- **Q Do you have hypercholesterolemia or other dyslipidemia?** Identify risk factor
- **Q Have you ever smoked? How many packs? For how long?** Identify risk factor
- **Q Do you have diabetes?** Diabetes is a cardiac disease equivalent risk factor
- **Q What medications are you taking?** Identify risk factor and current diagnoses

Family history

- **Q Have any of your close relatives (brother, sister, mother, father) ever had a heart attack?** Identify risk factor – reliable history of a MI in a first-degree relative, particularly at a young age, is especially relevant
- **Q Has any family member ever died unexpectedly from no obvious cause?** Many sudden unobserved deaths are due to myocardial ischemia/infarction

Examination

- **Record the vital signs.** In patients with MI, vital signs are affected by a great many factors and may vary widely. For example, a sinus tachycardia may be the result of simple anxiety, or may represent a secondary compensatory response to an inadequate stroke volume in a large infarct. Hypotension may be due to inadequate cardiac output, to bradycardia secondary to ischemia of the SA or AV node, or to inadequate hydration. No one constellation of vital signs is pathognomonic or even characteristic of MI
- **Assess the peripheral perfusion.** Signs of decreased peripheral perfusion include cold clammy skin, thready peripheral pulses, and confusion. A poor carotid pulse upstroke is consistent with diminished cardiac output
- **Assess left ventricular function.** In addition to poor peripheral perfusion, rales may indicate increased left ventricular end-diastolic pressure with early pulmonary edema. An S4 gallop may simply indicate an acute change in ventricular compliance, while a new S3 gallop usually indicates frank failure. Precordial impulse is frequently diffuse or dyssynergic. S1 and S2 may be soft because of decreased contractility. The second heart sound may be single or paradoxically split in severe failure. The Killup classification defines: class I, no rales or S3; class II, rales involving <50% of lung fields, no S3; class III, rales involving >50% of lung fields, S3 present; class IV, cardiogenic shock
- **Assess for signs of acutely diminished right ventricular function.** These include elevated jugular venous pressure, prominent a-wave in the venous pulse and/or Kussmaul's sign (increase in the venous pressure with inspiration). Right ventricular dysfunction in acute myocardial infarction is usually secondary to significant left ventricular dysfunction. However, when prominent, particularly in an inferior MI, it may indicate significant right ventricular infarction

- **Examine for the presence of arrythmias.** Arterial pulses will be consistent with the specific arrhythmia. Giant a-waves in the venous pulse suggest premature ventricular contractions (PVCs) or atrioventricular (AV) dissociation
- **Assess for signs of mitral valvular dysfunction.** Listen for new or changing systolic murmurs
- **Examine for the presence of ventricular septal defect (VSD).** Loud holosystolic murmur in the presence of shock is consistent
- **Examine for the presence of a pericardial friction rub.** Pericarditis can cause chest pain which may be mistaken for myocardial ischemia. In addition, MI can cause Dressler's syndrome, or postinfarction pericarditis; however, this occurs several days to weeks after the acute event

Summary of investigative tests

- Blood tests to measure white blood cell count and levels of blood sugar, plasma urea (BUN), creatinine, LDL cholesterol, and HDL cholesterol, should be performed in the hospital during the acute stage, and by the primary care physician during follow up. Potassium should be measured when arrhythmias are present
- Serum creatine kinase enzyme studies to measure creatine kinase and myocardial creatine kinase isoenzyme (CK-MB)
- Cardiac troponin levels (cTnl and cTnT). Allows for specific diagnosis of myocardial necrosis
- 12-lead ECG. Examine for ST-segment elevation and Q-wave infarction or non-Q-wave infarction. ECG is the most useful initial investigation
- Chest radiography is performed to evaluate pulmonary congestion and/or cardiomegaly and to exclude pneumonia, pneumothorax, and mediastinal widening. This examination would be performed in hospital in the acute stage, or later to evaluate for complications
- Myocardial perfusion imaging with thallium or other radiopharmaceutic agent for postinfarct risk stratification
- Radionuclide blood pool imaging for ventricular function assessment after the acute stage
- Standard echocardiography to evaluate wall motion abnormalities, mural thrombus, mitral regurgitation, VSD, and other infarct complications
- Transesophageal echocardiography (TEE) may be particularly useful to evaluate left atrial thrombus and aortic dissection (normally performed by a specialist)
- Coronary arteriography (normally performed by a specialist) is useful for a definitive diagnosis and to aid in the potential treatment of significant coronary artery blockade. It is the only test that provides a direct and detailed visualization of the coronary anatomy to locate specific areas of impaired blood flow. It is indicated and useful for ST-segment elevation MI and for medically refractory patients with unstable angina or non-ST-segment infarctions. It is also useful in patients with postinfarction angina at rest or with minimal exertion, those with persistent hemodynamic instability, and individuals who will be undergoing definitive repair of a mechanical complication of infarction (e.g. mitral regurgitation, VSD)

DIAGNOSTIC DECISION

- Clinical history of ischemic-type chest discomfort
- Serial electrocardiographic tracings indicative of MI
- A rise and fall in serum cardiac markers
- Initial ECG is abnormal and followed by definitive serial changes
- CK-MB and troponin elevated in the initial or subsequent plasma samples with typical and sequential changes
- Critical differential diagnosis is aortic dissection. It should be suspected whenever pain is localized to the back or radiates to the lower extremities, rapidly becomes extremely severe and lasts with little change for hours, is described as tearing or ripping, is not associated with ECG changes typical of infarction, and when one or more major arterial pulses are absent. Note that aortic root dissection that extends proximally to the coronaries may produce ST-segment elevation; most commonly this involves the right coronary artery

Guidelines

A Consensus Document of the Joint European Society of Cardiology/American College of Cardiology Committee for the Redefinition of Myocardial Infarction has been developed. Alpert, Thygesen K, Alpert JS, Antman E, Bassand JP. Myocardial infarction redefined. J Am Coll Cardiol 2000;36(3):959–69. In this guideline, the diagnosis of acute, recent, or evolving MI is established by a typical rise and gradual fall (troponin) or more rapid rise and fall (CPK-MB) of biochemical markers of myocardial necrosis with at least one of the following:

- Ischemic symptoms
- Development of pathologic Q waves on ECG
- ECG changes indicative of ischemia (ST-segment elevation or depression)
- Coronary artery intervention (e.g. angioplasty)
- Pathology findings of an acute MI

The diagnosis of established MI is made when any one of the following criteria is met:

- Development of new pathologic Q waves on serial ECGs, with or without previous symptoms. Biochemical markers may have normalized, depending on the amount of time that has passed since the infarction
- Pathology findings of a healed or healing MI

CLINICAL PEARL(S)

- Time to diagnosis is critical. An ECG should be obtained as soon as possible. If it shows ST elevation, immediate consultation with a cardiologist is needed to allow definitive therapy aimed at myocardial preservation
- A very high index of suspicion is needed in people with diabetes and the elderly. Females also commonly present with atypical vs classic symptoms
- Decision to admit the patient for a 'rule out MI' is made primarily on the history. Laboratory tests only confirm the clinical suspicion

THE TESTS

Body fluids

BLOOD TESTS

Description

Venous blood for measurement of white blood cell count, blood sugar level, plasma urea (BUN), creatinine, LDL cholesterol, and HDL cholesterol. Potassium should be measured when arrhythmias are present.

Advantages/Disadvantages

Advantages:

- Relatively easy collection
- Standard laboratory tests

Normal

- White blood cell count: 4–10.5x10^9/L
- Blood sugar: 30–60mg/dL
- Plasma urea (BUN): 8–18mg/dL
- Creatinine: 0.6–1.2mg/dL
- LDL cholesterol: 50–130mg/dL
- HDL cholesterol: males 45–70mg/dL; females 45–90mg/dL
- Potassium: 3.5–5.0mEq/L

Abnormal

- Values outside normal range
- Keep in mind the possibility of a false-positive result

Cause of abnormal result

- White blood cell count: elevation frequently occurs in MI, but is of limited usefulness due to lack of specificity
- Blood sugar: MI may raise blood sugar during the acute phase, and should be measured after the acute phase to assess for diabetes mellitus
- Plasma urea (BUN) and creatinine: plasma urea and creatinine concentrations are normal in acute MI (AMI), except in patients with severe heart failure for whom reduced renal perfusion and glomerular filtration may result in azotemia. In such cases, BUN is usually elevated more than creatinine
- Hypercholesterolemia may be detected

Drugs, disorders, and other factors that may alter results

- White blood cell count: infection
- Blood sugar: sulfonylureas, metformin
- Plasma urea (BUN)/creatinine: renal disease, liver disease, urinary tract infection, congestive heart failure, dehydration, gastrointestinal bleeding
- Acidosis (metabolic or respiratory) may cause hyperkalemia

SERUM CREATINE KINASE ENZYME STUDIES

Description

Measurement of creatine kinase (CK) and myocardial creatine kinase isoenzyme (CK-MB) in a blood sample.

Advantages/Disadvantages

Advantages:

- CK is sensitive but not specific
- CK-MB is more specific than undifferentiated CK for MI
- Allows 'late' diagnosis or confirmation of infarction
- May be elevated with chronic skeletal muscle injury

Normal

- CK: 0–130U/L
- CK-MB: <5% of total CK

Abnormal

- CK: >130U/L
- CK-MB: >5% of total CK
- Keep in mind the possibility of false-positive results

Cause of abnormal result

Necrosis of cardiac muscle in MI causes release of CK and CK-MB into the blood.

Drugs, disorders, and other factors that may alter results

CK:

- Skeletal muscle disease (myositis, muscular dystrophy)
- Skeletal muscle injury (including intramuscular injections, surgery)
- Recent moderate to severe exercise
- Alcohol intoxication (with or without delirium tremens or convulsions)
- Hypothyroidism
- Severe hypokalemia
- Statins, particularly when used in conjunction with niacin, fibrates, or cyclosporin may cause myositis and thus elevate CK
- Renal insufficiency

CK-MB:

- Severe skeletal muscle injury (skeletal muscle also has a small amount of CK-MB) and renal insufficiency

CARDIAC TROPONINS

Description

Measurement of cardiac troponins (cTnI and cTnT) in blood sample.

Advantages/Disadvantages

Advantages:

- Very high specificity and sensitivity for cardiac muscle
- Becomes positive in 3–12h
- Prolonged time course of decay (does not return to normal for 5–10 days for cTnI and for 5–14 days for cTnT); allows late diagnosis or confirmation of MI

Normal

- cTnT: 0–0.10ng/mL
- cTnI: 0–0.15ng/mL
- Normal values may vary by laboratory

Abnormal

- cTnT: >0.10ng/mL
- cTnI: >0.15ng/mL
- Keep in mind the possibility of a false-positive result

Cause of abnormal result

Necrosis of cardiac muscle causes release of cardiac troponins into the blood.

Drugs, disorders, and other factors that may alter results

cTnT may be elevated by chronic renal insufficiency.

Imaging

CHEST RADIOGRAPHY

Advantages/Disadvantages

Advantages:

- Universally available
- Relatively inexpensive
- Fast overall evaluation of pulmonary congestion and/or cardiomegaly
- Identification of noncardiac causes of chest pain

Normal

- Clear lung fields
- Heart of normal size and shape

Abnormal

- Lung fields congested
- Cardiomegaly
- Look for radiographic findings consistent with other causes of chest pain (examine especially aortic arch for widening or other signs of dissection)

Cause of abnormal result

- Pulmonary congestion secondary to left heart failure
- Cardiomegaly – may be chronic (left ventricular hypertrophy) or acute

MYOCARDIAL PERFUSION IMAGING

Advantages/Disadvantages

Advantages:

- Noninvasive test which directly images, and can differentiate areas of ischemia and infarction
- Currently used primarily for risk stratification and/or detection of additional myocardium at risk in the post-MI period
- May be used in patients with ongoing chest pain of unclear etiology to assist in the diagnosis of cardiac abnormality

Disadvantages:

- High cost
- High level of patient cooperation required
- Requires 1–2h to arrange and interpret

Normal

- No areas (or post-MI only a single discrete area) of nonuptake without redistribution
- No abnormal uptake in lungs

Abnormal

- Multiple areas on nonuptake or delayed uptake
- Evidence of late redistribution
- Increased lung uptake
- Stress-induced left ventricular enlargement

Cause of abnormal result

- Infarcted areas cannot incorporate the radiotracer into the cells
- Ischemic areas incorporate radiotracer into cells at a slower than normal rate

Drugs, disorders, and other factors that may alter results

- False-negative result can occur in 'balanced' triple vessel disease
- Female patients may have breast attenuation of the anterior wall; the inferior wall may have diaphragmatic artifacts

RADIONUCLIDE BLOOD POOL IMAGING

Advantages/Disadvantages

Advantages:

- Noninvasive test that directly images the ventricular blood pool and which can, therefore, demonstrate ventricular function
- Currently used primarily for risk stratification in the post-MI period

Disadvantages:

- High cost
- Impractical for diagnosis of acute MI

Normal

- Normal ejection fraction
- No global or segmental dyskinesia

Abnormal

- Decreased ejection fraction
- Areas of dyskinesia/akinesia

Cause of abnormal result
- Decreased ventricular function
- Akinetic/dyskinetic segments

Drugs, disorders, and other factors that may alter results
Irregular heart rhythms may degrade images.

Other tests
ECG
Description
12-lead ECG.

Advantages/Disadvantages
Advantage: can be easily performed, universally available, and relatively inexpensive.

Disadvantages:
- Test is relatively insensitive and nonspecific in low-risk populations, i.e. the probability of false-positive and false-negative findings is high in the general population
- Classic changes may not be present
- Other ECG abnormalities (e.g. left ventricular hypertrophy, bundle branch block may mimic or obscure diagnosis of acute MI
- Findings consistent with infarct on an isolated ECG do not indicate the timing of the event; i.e. old infarcts cannot be distinguished from new infarct findings in the absence of old ECGs for comparison

Abnormal
Classic abnormalities of the ECG in MI are:
- Q wave (ST-elevation infarction – sequential changes over affected area are inverted T waves indicating ischemia, elevated ST segments indicating injury, then development of Q waves, indicating area of infarction) – develops over 12–36h
- Non-Q wave (non-ST elevation) infarction – Q waves absent; history and enzyme elevations compatible with AMI; ECG shows ST-segment depression over affected area with or without T-wave inversion
- Various arrhythmias and/or evidence of conduction abnormalities may also be present

Cause of abnormal result
- Myocardial ischemia causes abnormal 'current of injury' and changes ventricular repolarization; these effects are recorded by the ECG as ST and T-wave changes, respectively. Transmural myocardial necrosis locally abolishes electrical activity, causing Q waves
- Abnormal ECG may represent a false-positive finding in an otherwise normal patient, particularly if the patient does not have identifiable risk factors for coronary disease, and does not have clinical or other laboratory tests or findings suggestive of myocardial ischemia or infarction

Drugs, disorders, and other factors that may alter results
- Electrolyte disturbances
- Pericarditis
- Congenital heart abnormalities
- Conduction disturbances
- Noncardiac diseases, e.g. cholecystitis
- Inaccurate lead placement
- Inaccurate calibration

ECHOCARDIOGRAPHY

Description

Use of ultrasound and Doppler techniques provide two-dimensional cardiac images and assessment of blood flow velocity, valvular regurgitation, systolic and diastolic function, intracardiac pressures, cardiac chamber dimensions, and regional wall motion abnormalities.

Advantages/Disadvantages

Advanatges:

- Noninvasive evaluation of wall motion abnormalities, identification of mural thrombus and/or mitral regurgitation
- Easily performed at bedside, allowing rapid diagnosis

Disadvantages:

- More expensive than ECG, but relatively inexpensive when compared with perfusion imaging or cardiac catheterization
- Transesophageal echocardiography requires patient sedation

Normal

- No wall motion abnormalities
- Atrial and ventricular sizes normal
- No evidence of diastolic dysfunction
- Normal systolic function (ejection fraction)
- No mural thrombus identified
- No fluid in pericardial space
- No evidence of valvular regurgitation or other abnormalities
- No evidence of intracardiac shunts, e.g. atrial septal defect (ASD) or ventricular septal defect (VSD)

Abnormal

Presence of any of the above findings.

Cause of abnormal result

- Direct result of MI (e.g. wall motion abnormalities, acute enlargement of cardiac chambers, increase of intracardiac pressures)
- Complication of infarction (e.g. papillary muscle dysfunction, postinfarction VSD)

Drugs, disorders, and other factors that may alter results

- Obese patients, patients with chronic obstructive pulmonary disease and chest wall deformities may provide unsatisfactory images
- Patients with esophageal disease may not be able to undergo transesophageal echocardiography

TREATMENT

IMMEDIATE ACTION

- Time is critical
- Dose of 160–325mg oral aspirin
- Nasal oxygen 2–4L/min
- Obtain 12-lead ECG
- Place on continuous cardiac monitor
- Analgesia, morphine sulfate
- Measure heart rate and blood pressure
- Sublingual nitroglycerin unless blood pressure is <90mmHg or heart rate is <50 beats per min
- Defibrillator should be immediately available
- Thrombolytic therapy or cardiac catheterization if appropriate
- Beta-blockers if there is no contraindication
- Consult with cardiologist
- Organize emergency transfer to the emergency department

MANAGEMENT ISSUES

Goals

- Prevent attack from progressing
- Supply oxygen
- Prevent/treat arrhythmias
- Reduce burden on heart muscle
- Reduce pain and anxiety
- Prevent formation of additional thrombi
- Support blood pressure
- Prevent cardiogenic shock

Management in special circumstances

- Support blood pressure with pressors if patient is severely hypotensive (and not hypovolemic)
- Beta-adrenergic agents such as dopamine, dobutamine, and epinephrine, and alpha-adrenergic agents including phenylephrine and vasopressin, may be used in the hospital setting for hypotension. Phenylephrine is preferred for patients with reflex vasodepression; dobutamine for patients with reduced cardiac output
- Treat arrhythmias with appropriate antiarrhythmia medications
- Ventricular tachycardia or fibrillation requires immediate cardioversion
- Presentation with significant congestive heart failure (CHF) may require treatment with inotropes, diuretics, and vasodilators
- Presentation in cardiogenic shock requires urgent revascularization, and support with inotropes and vasopressors to maintain blood pressure and cardiac output
- In patients who have contraindications to thrombolytic therapy, percutaneous transluminal coronary angioplasty (PTCA) should be considered
- Thrombolytic contraindications: previous hemorrhagic stroke at any time and other strokes within 1 year, known intracranial neoplasm, active bleeding, and aortic dissection are absolute contraindications to thrombolytic therapy. These patients should be considered for PTCA
- Relative contraindications to thrombolysis include uncontrollable hypertension (>180/110mmHg), history of prior stroke or intracranial pathology, bleeding diathesis, significant trauma including head injury within 4 weeks, active peptic ulcer disease, and history of chronic hypertension. Patients with these disorders may not be suitable for thrombolysis

SPECIAL PATIENT GROUPS

- Pregnancy is a relative contraindication to thrombolysis
- Patients over 75 years may not be suitable for tissue plasminogen activator (tPA)

SUMMARY OF THERAPEUTIC OPTIONS

Choices

Patients with ST-segment elevation myocardial infarction (MI) require immediate reperfusion by thrombolytic therapy or cardiac catheterization. Guidelines for the management of patients with MI include: 1999 update: ACC/AHA guidelines for the management of patients with acute myocardial infarction. A report of the American College of Cardiology/American Heart Association Task Force on Practice Guidelines (Committee on Management of Acute Myocardial Infarction). J Am Coll Cardiol 1999;34:890–911. Also available at the National Guideline Clearinghouse.

Lifestyle changes, including cessation of smoking and weight loss, may help prevent future attacks.

Immediate management:

- Nasal oxygen, 2–4L/min, should be administered immediately
- Nitrates increase the supply of oxygen by reducing ventricular vasospasm
- Aspirin as an antiplatelet agent
- Analgesia, normally intravenous morphine
- Emergency PTCA or thrombolytics (alteplase, reteplase and streptokinase), if appropriate, with or without heparin (unfractionated heparin or low molecular weight heparin (enoxaparin or dalteparin)) and/or glycoprotein IIb/IIIa inhibitors (per local protocol)

Continuing management:

- Bed rest for 24–36h
- Liquid diet for 24h, then salt-free soft diet
- Thoughtful explanation to reduce stress
- No caffeine
- Stool softeners for constipation would be instituted in the hospital setting

Therapy instituted in a hospital:

- Beta-adrenoceptor blockers should be given to all patients who have no contraindications to beta-blockers to relieve ischemic pain and prevent tachyarrhythmias
- Calcium channel blockers, which slow heart rate, may be used in patients with preserved left ventricular ejection fraction for whom beta-blockers are contraindicated
- Angiotensin-converting enzyme (ACE) inhibitors should be given to all patients without contraindications and with left ventricular dysfunction, and/or congestive heart failure (CHF), and patients with anterior wall or large MIs after hemodynamic stability is obtained
- Continue nitrates for ischemic pain relief if necessary
- Continue aspirin as prophylaxis
- Platelet inhibitors such as ticlopidine and clopidogrel may be used if the patient has an aspirin allergy, or if aspirin is ineffective
- PTCA is an alternative to thrombolytic therapy, especially in patients with ST-elevation AMI within 12h of pain onset or after 12h of ischemic symptoms. Should be used in the case of cardiogenic shock (thrombolysis is ineffective in this group). The protocol for PTCA will vary depending on local availability
- Coronary artery bypass graft (CABG) may be used in patients unsuited for PTCA who have persistent or recurrent ischemia refractory to medical therapy, and is also suitable for patients with failed angioplasty or cardiogenic shock

Specialist in-patient management of complications:

- Digitalis derivatives and diuretics should be used to treat CHF
- Antiarrythmic medications or cardioversion may be required for the complication of arrythmias
- Permanent pacemaker implantation may be required in cases of complete heart block after MI or for symptomatic AV block at any level
- Intra-aortic balloon counterpulsation may be used as stabilizing therapy in cardiogenic shock that is not quickly reversed with pharmacologic therapy, or in acute mitral regurgitation or ventricular septal defect (VSD) complicating AMI. Also useful for hemodynamic instability secondary to recurrent intractable ventricular arrhythmias and in refractory post-MI angina as a bridge to angiography and revascularization

Clinical pearl(s)

- Treatment of acute MI should be planned in advance. A local protocol should be established and updated regularly
- Patients with ST-segment elevation MI should be rapidly referred to a center capable of tertiary care
- Avoid excessive nitrates for pain relief, especially in patients with inferior MI with probable right ventricle (RV) involvement. Use morphine liberally
- Avoid high doses of intravenous diuretics for acute CHF. Excessive diuresis frequently requires treatment for hypotension

Never

Never administer nitroglycerin or a nitrate preparation to patients who have used sildenafil within 24h without direct monitoring of arterial blood pressure.

FOLLOW UP

Plan for review

- All patients should have an assessment of left ventricular ejection fraction
- Patients with recurrent chest pain, congestive heart failure, malignant ventricular arrhythmias, depressed ejection fraction, or evidence of ischemia on functional testing should undergo cardiac catheterization
- Patients should be considered for a structured cardiac rehabilitation program
- All patients should have complete lipid evaluation and early aggressive therapy to meet NCEP III guidelines (The National Cholesterol Education Program Adult Treatment Panel II)

Information for patient or caregiver

Patients should receive instruction on their disease process; on the use and side-effects of medication; and on risk factor modification including smoking cessation and lifestyle changes.

DRUGS AND OTHER THERAPIES: DETAILS

Drugs

RETEPLASE

Although it is optimal that thrombolytic medication be given in the hospital setting, if the transport time is >90min thrombolytic therapy may need to be given prior to hospital.

Dose

tPA (given with heparin):

- Reteplase: 10U intravenously, administered over 2min, and then repeated at 30min (double bolus injection). No other medications should be administered using the same line

Efficacy

- Effective in patients with ST-elevation acute MI (>0.1mV in two or more contiguous leads) when therapy can be started within 12h of the onset of symptoms. May be considered up to 24h after symptom onset in patients with ongoing symptoms

- Bundle branch block obscuring ST-segment analysis and history suggesting acute MI may also be treated effectively
- The 'selective' agents, e.g. alteplase and reteplase, achieve best early coronary reperfusion rates (c.75% 90-min patency and 60% thrombolysis in myocardial infarction flow-grade 3)

Risks/Benefits

Risk: The risk of increased bleeding should be weighed against therapeutic benefit.

Side-effects and adverse reactions

- Cardiovascular: cardiac tamponade, electromechanical dissociation, reinfarction
- Hematalogic: internal bleeding (intracranial, retroperitoneal, surface, gastrointestinal, genitourinary)
- Skin: allergic reactions

Interactions (other drugs)

- Heparin - Vitamin K antagonists - Drugs that alter platelet function (aspirin, dipyridamole, abciximab) - Oral anticoagulants

Contraindications

- Active internal bleeding - History of cerebrovascular accident - Recent intracranial or intraspinal surgery/trauma - Intracranial neoplasm - Arteriovenous malfunction or aneurysm - Known bleeding diathesis - Severe uncontrolled hypertension

Evidence

Thrombolysis is effective in reducing mortality in patients presenting with AMI.

- A review of nine randomized controlled trials (RCTs) found that thrombolytic therapy was superior to placebo in reducing short-term mortality from MI. Benefit was greatest for patients presenting with ST-segment elevation and bundle branch block [1] *Level M*
- When thrombolytic therapy is given in the acute phase there is an increased risk of stroke in treated patients compared with placebo [1] *Level M*
- All types of MI benefit from treatment with thrombolysis, but anterior infarcts had the best mortality reduction [1] *Level M*
- In one RCT, long-term follow up showed a survival benefit with thrombolysis of up to 12 years compared with placebo [2] *Level P*
- Meta-analysis of three trials comparing streptokinase and tPA found no significant difference in the combined outcome of any stroke or death [3] *Level M*

Follow up plan

- If this therapy is instituted before hospitalization, the patient should be transferred to a hospital as soon as possible for monitoring
- ECG monitoring, vital signs, and neurologic monitoring are essential during and immediately after treatment with this medication

STREPTOKINASE

Although it is optimal that thrombolytic medication be given in the hospital setting, if the transport time is >90min thrombolytic therapy may need to be given prior to hospital.

Dose

Intravenous infusion of 1,500,000 IU diluted to a volume of 45mL and administered over 1h.

Efficacy

- Effective in patients with ST-elevation acute MI (>0.1mV in two or more contiguous leads) when therapy can be started within 12h of the onset of symptoms. May be considered up to 24h after symptom onset in patients with ongoing symptoms

- Bundle branch block obscuring ST-segment analysis and history suggesting AMI may also be treated effectively
- The 'nonselective' thrombolytic streptokinase is moderately effective (50% 90-min patency rate and 32% TIMI 3 flow) and is by far the least expensive alternative

Risks/Benefits

Risks:
- Use caution with recent surgery, obstetric delivery, trauma, subacute bacterial endocarditis, streptococcal infection, diabetic hemorrhagic retinopathy, and bleeding disorders
- Use caution with the elderly

Side-effects and adverse reactions
- Cardiovascular: hypotension, reperfusion dysrhythmias
- CNS: fever, headache
- EENT: periorbital edema
- Gastrointestinal: nausea
- Hematologic: hemorrhage, anemia
- Respiratory: bronchospasm, dyspnea, pulmonary edema
- Skin: flushing, irritation, phlebitis at injection site, urticaria

Interactions (other drugs)
- Anticoagulants (may cause bleeding complications).

Contraindications
- Active internal bleeding
- Intracranial neoplasm
- Recent cerebrovascular accident
- Recent surgery
- Severe uncontrolled hypertension

Evidence

Thrombolysis is effective in reducing mortality in patients presenting with AMI.
- A review of nine RCTs found that thrombolytic therapy was superior to placebo in reducing short-term mortality from MI. Benefit was greatest for patients presenting with ST-segment elevation and bundle branch block [1] *Level M*
- When thrombolytic therapy is given in the acute phase there is an increased risk of stroke in treated patients compared with placebo [1] *Level M*
- All types of MI benefit from treatment with thrombolysis, but anterior infarcts had the best mortality reduction [1] *Level M*
- In one RCT, long-term follow up showed a survival benefit with thrombolysis of up to 12 years compared with placebo [2] *Level P*
- Meta-analysis of three trials comparing streptokinase and tPA found no significant difference in the combined outcome of any stroke or death [3] *Level M*

Follow up plan
- If this therapy is instituted before hospitalization, the patient should be transferred to a hospital as soon as possible for monitoring
- ECG monitoring, vital signs, and neurologic monitoring are essential during and immediately after treatment with this medication

Patient and caregiver information

Patients should be informed when streptokinase has been used, in order to prevent future allergic reactions.

NITRATES

Dose

- Sublingual glyceryl trinitrate (nitroglycerin): 0.4mg every 5min, times three (three doses), until pain is relieved (sublingual tablets or spray may be used)
- Intravenous nitrates are used only in the hospital setting: start with bolus injection of 12.5–25mcg and a pump-controlled infusion of 10–20mcg/min. Increase the dosage by 5–10mcg every 5–10min, titrating to hemodynamic and clinical response. Titration end points are control of clinical symptoms or decrease in mean arterial pressure (MAP) of 10% in normotensive patients, 30% in hypertensive patients (but never a systolic pressure below 90mmHg), and increase of heart rate of 10%, or a decrease of pulmonary artery diastolic pressure of 10–30%. Infusions should be discontinued or decreased if MAP falls below 80mmHg or systolic arterial pressure below 90mmHg. Doses greater than 200mcg/min are associated with hypotension, and alternative therapy should be considered
- Slow release: isosorbide dinitrate (20–40mg 12-hourly) is used for prolonged action
- Transdermal patches are an alternative (5–15mg/24h)

Efficacy

- Nitrates are effective in relieving pain associated with myocardial ischemia
- If sublingual nitrates are ineffective, patients should be hospitalized for intravenous nitrates, or isosorbide dinitrate may be used. For acute MI pain, use morphine instead
- Modified-release preparations are effective for up to 12h

Risks/Benefits

Risks:

- Possible persistent headache
- Tolerance may occur

Benefit:

- Combination with hydralazine may improve prognosis

Side-effects and adverse reactions

- Cardiovascular: atrial fibrillation, collapse, dysrhythmias, postural hypotension, palpitations, rebound hypertension, syncope
- CNS: headache, dizziness, anxiety, dizziness
- EENT: blurred vision
- Gastrointestinal: abdominal pain, nausea, vomiting, diarrhea
- Genitourinary: dysuria, urinary frequency, impotence
- Hematologic: hemolytic anemia, methemoglobinemia
- Musculoskeletal: arthralgia
- Skin: cutaneous vasodilation, contact dermatitis

Interactions (other drugs)

■ Ergot alkaloids: opposition to coronary vasodilatory effects of nitrates ■ Ethanol: additive vasodilation could cause hypotension ■ Metronidazole: ethanol contained in intravenous nitroglycerin preparations could cause disulfiram-like reaction in some patients ■ Sildenafil: additive vasodilation may produce profound hypotension ■ A possible interaction with heparin may occur, of particular importance since heparin and nitroglycerin are frequently administered together. Several reports suggest that nitroglycerin may decrease sensitivity to heparin, necessitating larger heparin doses to achieve anticoagulation. Discontinuance of nitroglycerin during concomitant heparin infusion can potentially lead to increased bleeding risk if heparin dosing is not simultaneously adjusted

Contraindications

- Hypotension ■ Cerebral hemorrhage ■ Head trauma ■ Early MI ■ Severe anemia ■ Closed-angle glaucoma ■ Constrictive pericarditis ■ Percardial tamponade (IV)

Evidence

Nitrates are effective for symptomatic relief and may reduce short-term mortality in AMI.

- A systematic review of 10 RCTs comparing intravenous nitrates to placebo (without thrombolysis) showed that nitrates reduced mortality. The benefit was noted for the duration of the hospitalization, and there was little long-term effect on survival [4] *Level M*
- Two RCTs compared the use of nitrates with placebo in the setting of acute MI (most patients also received aspirin and/ or thrombolysis). Controlled-release mononitrate and intravenous nitrate followed by transdermal patch did not improve survival, but were useful adjunctive symptomatic treatments [5,6] *Level P*

Acceptability to patient

- Generally acceptable in the acute setting
- Long-term acceptability may be affected by headaches

Follow up plan

- Close monitoring in the hospital setting is necessary for intravenous nitrates
- Patients on long-term nitrate therapy post-MI should be monitored periodically for efficacy, side-effects, and tolerance

Patient and caregiver information

- Report any headaches or postural hypotension
- Sublingual nitrates must be taken correctly, and not swallowed
- Oral nitrates should be taken before food
- Transdermal patches should be removed for 10–12h/day

ASPIRIN

- Antiplatelet medication prevents formation of thromboxane A_2, a platelet-aggregating agent
- Other antiplatelet agents (e.g. ticlopidine or clopidogrel) may be substituted if the patient cannot tolerate or is unresponsive to aspirin

Dose

- A dose of 160–325mg should be given as soon as feasible and continued indefinitely on a daily basis as an antiplatelet agent
- The dose for long-term treatment is at least 75mg daily

Efficacy

- Aspirin has been found to be effective in reducing mortality in patients presenting with AMI
- Effective in preventing subsequent MI
- Effective in reducing the incidence of nonfatal stroke after AMI

Risks/Benefits

Risks:

- Use caution in anemia, Hodgkin's disease, gout, hepatic and renal disease, asthma, nasal polyps, nasal allergies
- Use caution with children and teenagers (Reye's syndrome)

Benefits:
- Simple daily dose
- Inexpensive

Side-effects and adverse reactions
- CNS: dizziness, headache
- EENT: hearing loss, tinnitus
- Gastrointestinal: abdominal pain, nausea, dyspepsia, hepatotoxicity, gastrointestinal bleeding
- Hematologic: bleeding disorders, thrombocytopenia
- Respiratory: hyperpnea, asthma
- Skin: angioedema, bruising, rash, urticaria

Interactions (other drugs)
- ACE inhibitors ▪ Acetazolamide ▪ Antacids ▪ Corticosteroids ▪ Diltiazem ▪ Ethanol
- Griseofulvin ▪ Methotrexate ▪ Oral anticoagulants ▪ Antigout medicines
- Warfarin (enhanced hypoprothrombinemic effect of warfarin)

Contraindications
- Gastrointestinal bleeding ▪ Bleeding disorders ▪ Bone marrow suppression
- Hypersensitivity to salicylates, nonsteroidal anti-inflammatory drugs (NSAIDs), or tartrazine

Evidence

There is evidence that aspirin is effective in reducing mortality post-AMI.
- One systematic review of RCTs showed that aspirin reduced the risk of reinfarction and death compared with placebo when given on the day of the MI, and continued for 1 month [7] *Level M*
- In a large RCT, aspirin was compared with placebo starting from the day of MI and continued for 1 month. In subsequent long-term follow up, the improvement in survival was noted for at least 4 years [8,9] *Level P*

Acceptability to patient

Generally acceptable in the short and long term.

Follow up plan
- Patients should be followed after commencement of the medication to ensure there are no gastrointestinal side-effects or asthma
- Liver function, renal function, and complete blood count should be checked when patient is on long-term therapy

Patient and caregiver information
- Dose should be taken daily
- Administer with food
- Avoid excess alcohol consumption

TICLOPIDINE

Ticlodipine and clopidogrel (thienopyridines) are antiplatelet drugs that may be used instead of, or in addition to, aspirin.

Dose

Ticlodipine: 250mg twice daily with food

Efficacy
- Effective in the prevention of vascular events and death in patients who are at risk (i.e. post-AMI)
- May have an additive effect with aspirin

Risks/Benefits
Risks:
- Use caution in peptic ulcer disease, hepatic or renal disease, trauma, and surgery
- Use caution in pregnancy
- Not recommended for use in unstable angina
- Avoid for first few days after MI or for 7 days after ischemic stroke

Benefits:
- Relatively expensive
- Reduced incidence of cerebrovascular accident as well as recurrent AMI
- Reduced gastrointestinal bleeding and upper gastrointestinal upset when compared with aspirin

Side-effects and adverse reactions
Ticlodipine has been associated with two serious reported side-effects:
- Reversible neutropenia in patients treated for more than 2 weeks
- Thrombocytopenia with thrombotic thrombocytopenic purpura. Tends to occur after 3–4 weeks of therapy but may occur earlier, and the mortality rate is quite high – 50% if untreated, 25% if treated

Also:
- Gastrointestinal: discomfort, nausea, diarrhea, gastrointestinal bleeding, ulceration, increased cholesterol levels
- Hematologic: thrombocytopenia, neutropenia, agranulocytosis
- Skin: pruritus, rash

Interactions (other drugs)
▪ Cyclosporine ▪ Phenytoin ▪ Theophylline

Contraindications
▪ Active bleeding ▪ Severe liver impairment ▪ Blood dyscrasia ▪ History of thrombotic thrombocytopenic purpura ▪ Breast-feeding ▪ Pregnancy category B

Evidence
Platelet inhibitors may be more effective than aspirin in preventing vascular events in high-risk patients.
- A systematic review of four trials comparing thienopyridines with aspirin (ticlodipine in three trials, clopidogrel in one trial) showed that thienopyridines were associated with a modest but significant reduction in the risk of a vascular event in patients at high risk for a vascular event, including patients post recent AMI. There is uncertainty about the size of the additional benefit [10] *Level M*
- Thienopyridines resulted in less gastrointestinal hemorrhage and upset than aspirin [10]
- Ticlodipine was associated with neutropenia. Ticlodipine, more than clopidogrel, was associated with rash and diarrhea [10]

Acceptability to patient
Generally acceptable.

Follow up plan

- Patients should be followed to check for the development of rash or diarrhea
- Blood testing is necessary if the patient is commenced on ticlodipine to assess for neutropenia and thrombocytopenia

Patient and caregiver information

Patients should report any adverse effects immediately (bleeding, symptoms of neutropenia).

CLOPIDOGREL

Ticlodipine and clopidogrel (thienopyridines) are antiplatelet drugs that may be used instead of, or in addition to, aspirin.

Dose

Clopidogrel: 75mg daily

Efficacy

- Effective in the prevention of vascular events and death in patients who are at risk (i.e. postacute-AMI)
- May have an additive effect with aspirin

Risks/Benefits

Risks:

- Use caution in peptic ulcer disease, hepatic or renal disease, trauma, or surgery
- Use caution in pregnancy
- Not recommended for use in unstable angina
- Avoid for first few days after MI or for 7 days after ischemic stroke

Side-effects and adverse reactions

- With clopidogrel, the incidence of reported neutropenia is very low, and thrombotic thrombocytopenic purpura is extremely rare
- Cardiovascular: hypertension, edema, chest pain
- CNS: headache, dizziness, intracranial bleeding
- Gastrointestinal: nausea, diarrhea, abdominal pain, dyspepsia, gastrointestinal bleeding, ulceration
- Hematologic: thrombotic thrombocytopenia purpura, neutropenia, purpura
- Respiratory: upper respiratory tract infection, dyspnea
- Skin: macropapular rash, urticaria, pruritus

Interactions (other drugs)

- Alosetron - Coumarins - Dipyridamole - Fluvastatin - Gingko biloba - Heparins - NSAIDs, salicylates - Other platelet inhibitors - Phenytoin - Tamoxifen - Tolbutamide - Torasemide

Contraindications

- Active bleeding - Breast-feeding - Coagulation disorders

Evidence

Platelet inhibitors may be more effective than aspirin in preventing vascular events in high-risk patients.

- A systematic review of four trials comparing thienopyridines with aspirin (ticlodipine in three trials, clopidogrel in one trial) showed that thienopyridines were associated with a modest but significant reduction in the risk of a vascular event in patients at high risk for a vascular event, including patients post recent AMI. There is uncertainty about the size of the additional benefit [10] *Level M*

- Thienopyridines resulted in less gastrointestinal hemorrhage and upset than aspirin [10]
- Ticlodipine was associated with neutropenia. Ticlodipine, more than clopidogrel, was associated with rash and diarrhea [10]

Acceptability to patient
Generally acceptable.

Follow up plan
Patients should be followed to check for the development of rash or diarrhea.

Patient and caregiver information
Patients should report any adverse effects immediately (bleeding, symptoms of neutropenia).

MORPHINE
Dose
Intravenously 2–4mg every 5–10min as needed for pain.

Efficacy
When administered subcutaneously or intravenously provides effective pain relief within 10–30min.

Risks/Benefits
Risks:
- Use with caution in the elderly and children under 18 years old
- Use with caution in hepatic and renal disease, hypothryoidism and Addison's disease, abdominal disorders, prostatic hypertrophy
- Nausea may be aggravated, and thus morphine should be given with an antiemetic

Benefits:
- Effective for pain relief
- May have an anxiolytic effect

Side-effects and adverse reactions
- Cardiovascular: bradycardia, tachycardia, palpitations, hypotension, hypertension, syncope
- CNS: drowsiness, sedation, headache, vertigo, hallucinations, dysphoria, euphoria, mood changes, dependence, anxiety, restlessness
- EENT: dry mouth, miosis, blurred vision
- Gastrointestinal: constipation, nausea, vomiting, abdominal pain, biliary spasm
- Genitourinary: urinary difficulties, decreased libido
- Respiratory: respiratory depression
- Skin: rashes, pruritus, urticaria, sweating, flushing

Interactions (other drugs)
▪ Alcohol ▪ Anticoagulants ▪ Antidepressants (tricyclic) ▪ Antihistamines ▪ Antihypertensives ▪ Antipsychotics ▪ Anxiolytics and hypnotics ▪ Cimetidine ▪ Ciprofloxacin ▪ Domperidone ▪ Esmolol ▪ Monoamine oxidase inhibitors (MAOIs) ▪ Metoclopramide ▪ Mexiletine ▪ Moclobemide ▪ Opiate antagonists ▪ Rifamycins ▪ Ritonavir

Contraindications
▪ Heart failure secondary to chronic lung disease ▪ Cardiac arrhythmias ▪ Brain tumor ▪ Acute alcoholism ▪ Delirium tremens ▪ Convulsive states ▪ Respiratory depression ▪ Hemorrhage ▪ Acute asthma attack ▪ Paralytic ileus ▪ Head injury or raised intracranial pressure ▪ Injection in pheochromocytoma

Acceptability to patient
Acceptable.

Follow up plan
Patients requiring morphine for pain relief should be transferred to hospital for further monitoring, investigation, and treatment.

ALTEPLASE
Although it is optimal that thrombolytic medication be given in the hospital setting, if the transport time is >90min, thrombolytic therapy may need to be given prior to hospital.

Dose
tPA (given with heparin):
- Alteplase: 15mg intravenous bolus, then 0.75mg/kg over 30min (maximum 50mg), then 0.5mg/kg over 60min (maximum 35mg)

Efficacy
- Effective in patients with ST-elevation acute MI (>0.1mV in two or more contiguous leads) when therapy can be started within 12h of the onset of symptoms. May be considered up to 24h after symptom onset in patients with ongoing symptoms
- Bundle branch block obscuring ST-segment analysis and history suggesting AMI may also be treated effectively
- The 'selective' agents, e.g. alteplase and reteplase, achieve best early coronary reperfusion rates (c.75% 90-min patency and 60% TIMI 3 flow)

Risks/Benefits
Risks:
- Use caution in recent major surgery
- Most common complicationt is bleeding: internal bleeding, involving intracranial and retroperitoneal sites, or the gastrointestinal, genitourinary, or respiratory tracts; and superficial bleeding, mainly at invaded or disturbed sites (e.g. venous cutdowns, arterial punctures, sites of recent surgical intervention)
- Avoid noncompressible arterial puncture
- Avoid internal jugular and subclavian venous punctures
- Minimize arterial and venous punctures
- Bleeding
- Pulmonary embolus
- Bleeding diathesis
- Cleared by the liver, if liver; function is decreased, clearance time will be affected

Benefits:
- Onset of action is rapid
- Less expensive than liver transplantation or shunt placement
- May be repeated for recurrent thrombus
- Associated with fewer hemorrhagic events

Side-effects and adverse reactions
- Cardiovascular: cardiac arrhythmias, tachycardia
- Hematologic: intracranial, retroperitoneal, surface bleeding, gastrointestinal, genitourinary bleeding, increased prothrombin time, partial prothrombin time
- Skin: rash, urticaria

Interactions (other drugs)

- Heparin (increased bleeding)
- Acetylsalicylic acid (increased bleeding)
- Dipyridamole (increased bleeding)

Contraindications

- Active bleeding
- Hemorrhagic stroke
- Severe uncontrolled hypertension
- Intracranial/intraspinal surgery
- Trauma
- Aneurysm
- Arteriovenous malformation
- Brain tumor
- Known bleeding disorder

Evidence

Thrombolysis is effective in reducing mortality in patients presenting with AMI.

- A review of nine RCTs found that thrombolytic therapy was superior to placebo in reducing short-term mortality from MI. Benefit was greatest for patients presenting with ST-segment elevation and bundle branch block [1] *Level M*
- When thrombolytic therapy is given in the acute phase there is an increased risk of stroke in treated patients compared with placebo [1] *Level M*
- All types of MI benefit from treatment with thrombolysis, but anterior infarcts had the best mortality reduction [1] *Level M*
- In one RCT, long-term follow up showed a survival benefit with thrombolysis of up to 12 years compared with placebo [2] *Level P*
- Meta-analysis of three trials comparing streptokinase and tPA found no significant difference in the combined outcome of any stroke or death [3] *Level M*

Follow up plan

- If this therapy is instituted before hospitalization, the patient should be transferred to a hospital as soon as possible for monitoring
- ECG monitoring, vital signs, and neurologic monitoring are essential during and immediately after treatment with this medication

BETA-ADRENOCEPTOR BLOCKERS

- Metoprolol, atenolol, and propranolol are commonly used beta-blockers
- Beta-blockers may be used when the patient first presents with MI, and in the long-term management post-MI for secondary prevention

Dose

- Metoprolol: three intravenous bolus injections of 5mg each may be given initially at 2min intervals as tolerated. After intravenous loading, begin oral doses of 25–50mg every 6h. Thereafter, maintenance doses of 25–100mg every 12h should be continued
- Atenolol: an intravenous dose is given in the acute stage (5mg over 5min, repeated in 10min if tolerated), followed by 50mg after 15min and 50mg at 12h. Oral dosing should be titrated up to 100mg daily
- Propranolol: 40mg four times daily for 2–3 days, then 80mg twice daily, beginning 5–21 days after infarction

Efficacy

- When used in the acute setting, may relieve pain and reduce the size of the infarct
- Effective for reducing the risk of reinfarction and mortality after an acute MI

Risks/Benefits

Risks:

- Use with caution during pregnancy and breast-feeding
- Use with caution in diabetes mellitus, liver and renal impairment, atrioventricular (AV) block, myasthenia gravis
- Do not withdraw abruptly in patients with angina

Benefits:

- Widely available
- May also treat hypertension and tachyarrhythmias

Side-effects and adverse reactions

- Cardiovascular: hypotension, bradycardia, conduction abnormalities, heart failure, peripheral vasoconstriction
- CNS: fatigue, sleep disturbances
- EENT: dry eyes
- Gastrointestinal: nausea, vomiting
- Respiratory: bronchospasm
- Skin: rashes, exacerbation of psoriasis

Interactions (other drugs)

■ Adenosine: bradycardia aggravated ■ Amoxicillin: reduced atenolol availability ■ Antacids: reduced atenolol availability ■ Calcium channel blockers: see dihydropyridine and verapamil ■ Clonidine: exacerbation of rebound hypertension on discontinuation of clonidine ■ Digoxin: concomitant slowing of AV node conduction ■ Dihydropyridines: additive hemodynamic effects; increased serum concentration of atenolol ■ Lidocaine: increased serum lidocaine possible ■ Neostigmine: bradycardia aggravated ■ NSAIDs: reduced antihypertensive effects of atenolol ■ Physostigmine: bradycardia aggravated ■ Prazosin: first-dose response to prazosin may be enhanced by beta-blockade ■ Tacrine: bradycardia aggravated ■ Theophylline: antagonistic pharmacodynamic effects ■ Verapamil: enhanced effects of both drugs

Contraindications

■ Pheochromocytoma ■ Metabolic acidosis ■ Asthma ■ Second- or third-degree AV block, sick sinus syndrome, marked bradycardia, hypotension, cardiogenic shock, peripheral arterial disease, uncontrolled heart failure, Prinzmetal's angina

Evidence

There is evidence that beta-blockers reduce mortality when used in the treatment of AMI.

- Two systematic reviews found that oral beta-blockers given early after the onset of AMI reduced the risk of death and major vascular events [11,12] *Level M*
- Long-term use of beta-blockers versus placebo showed a decrease in mortality and nonfatal reinfarction with beta-blockers. There was no difference found among different beta-blockers, but there was concern regarding the lack of efficacy of beta-blockers with intrinsic sympathomimetic activity in long-term management after MI [11] *Level M*
- One systematic review of beta-blockers versus placebo in AMI patients, found that mortality was reduced significantly over 6 months to 4 years. This evidence was obtained using propranolol, timolol, and metoprolol, and there was no difference based on the type of beta-blocker used [13] *Level M*
- Another systematic review of oral beta-blockers versus placebo that commenced within days or weeks of MI, and continued for a period of 6 weeks to 3 years, showed improved survival with beta-blockers [14] *Level M*

Acceptability to patient

Generally acceptable.

Follow up plan

- Patients should be monitored for bradycardia and hypotension
- Side-effects should be noted, and discontinuation may be necessary

Patient and caregiver information

- Patients should not discontinue the medication suddenly
- Adverse effects should be reported immediately (i.e. dyspnea, bradycardia, dizziness)

CALCIUM CHANNEL BLOCKERS

Dose

- Diltiazem: 30mg four times daily, gradually increasing to 180–360mg daily in divided doses until optimal response is obtained
- Sustained-release preparations: 60–120mg twice daily, adjust until optimal dose response is obtained
- Verapamil: 80–120mg, three times daily. The dose should be adjusted weekly, up to a maximum of 480mg daily based on response

Efficacy

- May be useful in patients with AMI with preserved left ventricular ejection fraction in whom beta-blockers are contraindicated (e.g. bronchospasm) or are ineffective in relieving ongoing ischemia or in decreasing rapid ventricular response
- Patients with non-ST-elevation infarction without pulmonary congestion or congestive heart failure (CHF) may benefit from the addition of diltiazem to standard therapy after the first 24h and continued for 1 year

Risks/Benefits

Risks: use caution in hepatic impairment and edema

Side-effects and adverse reactions

- Cardiovascular: hypotension, peripheral edema, palpitations, AV block, bradycardia, tachycardia, CHF, MI, angina
- CNS: headache, dizziness, tremor, weakness, somnolence, insomnia, paresthesias, nervousness
- Gastrointestinal: nausea, vomiting, diarrhea, constipation, hepatitis, abdominal pain, dry mouth, flatulence
- Genitourinary: sexual dysfunction, urinary disorders
- Musculoskeletal: cramps, myalgia
- Respiratory: dyspnea, cough, respiratory infection
- Skin: sweating, flushing, dermatitis, rash, pruritus, urticaria

Interactions (other drugs)

■ ACE inhibitors ■ Adrenergic neurone blockers ■ Alcohol ■ Alpha-blockers ■ Alprostadil ■ Anesthetics ■ Angiotensin II receptor antagonists ■ Antiarrhythmics ■ Antihypertensives (beta-blockers, clonidine, diazoxide, hydralazine, methyldopa, minoxidil, nitrates, nitroprusside) ■ Antipsychotics ■ Anxiolytics and hypnotics ■ Baclofen, tizanidine ■ Cimetidine ■ Corticosteroids ■ Diuretics ■ Estrogens ■ Levodopa ■ NSAIDs ■ Ritonavir ■ Theophylline

Contraindications

■ Sick sinus syndrome or second- or third-degree AV block except with a functioning pacemaker, hypotension <90mmHg systolic (diltiazem and verapamil) ■ Acute MI and pulmonary congestion (diltiazem) ■ Severe left ventricular dysfunction, cardiogenic shock, and severe CHF, unless secondary to a supraventricular tachycardia amenable to verapamil therapy and in patients with atrial flutter or atrial fibrillation and an accessory bypass tract (verapamil) ■ Do not administer intravenous verapamil concomitantly with intravenous beta-adrenergic blocking agents (within a few hours) ■ Ventricular tachycardia (verapamil) ■ Advanced aortic stenosis (nicardipine)

Evidence

There is no evidence of benefit from calcium channel blockers in patients with AMI. This class of drugs may increase mortality for some patients.

- A nonsystematic review compared short-acting nifedipine (commenced within a few days of AMI) with placebo. There was no evidence of benefit with nifedipine. The trend was towards increased mortality with this treatment [15] *Level M*
- A systematic review compared verapamil with placebo in patients post-AMI. No significant effect on mortality was noted [16] *Level P*
- Another systemic review compared calcium channel blockers (dihydropyridine, diltiazem, and verapamil) and placebo. Medications were given early or late for AMI and unstable angina, and continued in the intermediate/long term. The results showed no significant benefit or difference in RCTs comparing diltiazem or verapamil with placebo, and found decreased rates of recurrent infarction and refractory angina with active treatment. This effect was noted only for patients without evidence of heart failure. The trend was towards harm if heart failure was present [17–19] *Level P*

Acceptability to patient

Generally acceptable.

Follow up plan

Blood pressure monitoring and assessment of cardiovascular function.

Patient and caregiver information

Patients should report any side-effects immediately.

RAMIPRIL

Ramipril is one of the ACE inhibitors used.

Dose

- 2.5mg, twice daily; increased to 5mg, twice daily after 2 days
- Maintenance dose is 2.5–5mg, twice daily

Efficacy

- ACE inhibitors have been found to be effective in reducing mortality when started within 24h of AMI
- Whether they should be prescribed for all patients post-MI or only those with signs of heart failure remains controversial
- When used long-term for patients with left ventricular dysfunction following AMI, ACE inhibitors are effective in reducing the rate of death, recurrent nonfatal AMI, and hospitalization for CHF

Risks/Benefits

Risks:

- Use with caution in bilateral renal artery stenosis, renal and liver disease, diuretic therapy, CHF, hypovolemia, collagen vascular diseases
- Use with caution in the elderly
- In postrevascularization patients, ACE inhibitors may act to reduce the incidence of AMI or clinical heart failure

Side-effects and adverse reactions

- Cardiovascular: angina, hypotension, postural hypotension, palpitations
- CNS: anxiety, dizziness, headache, paresthesia
- Gastrointestinal: constipation, nausea, dry mouth, pancreatitis

- Genitourinary: sexual dysfunction
- Hematologic: agranulocytosis, neutropenia, thrombocytopenia
- Metabolic: hyperkalemia, hyponatremia, hypoglycemia
- Musculoskeletal: arthralgia, arthritis, myalgia
- Respiratory: cough, asthma, dyspnea
- Skin: alopecia, pruritus, rash

Interactions (other drugs)

■ Allopurinol ■ Alpha-adrenergic blockers ■ Aspirin ■ Cyclosporin ■ Insulin ■ Iron ■ Lithium ■ Loop diuretics ■ NSAIDs ■ Potassium/potassium-sparing diuretics

Contraindications

■ Bilateral renal artery stenosis ■ Pregnancy

Evidence

ACE inhibitors are effective in reducing morbidity and mortality in patients post-AMI.

- An overview and a systematic review compared ACE inhibitors vs placebo in post-MI patients with or without left ventricular dysfunction or heart failure. Patients who were treated were found to have a reduced mortality rate and incidence of nonfatal CHF. High-risk patients had a greater absolute benefit [20,21] *Level M*
- Three clinical trials of ACE inhibitors were conducted on post-AMI patients with CHF, patients with evidence of left ventricular failure, or both. Long-term treatment with an ACE inhibitor in such patients significantly reduced mortality and reinfarction [22–24] *Level P*

Acceptability to patient

Generally acceptable.

Follow up plan

Renal function and electrolytes must be monitored within 2 weeks of the start of treatment.

Patient and caregiver information

- Alert the primary care physician if cough or dizziness occurs
- Rise slowly from sitting to standing position to minimize postural hypotension

UNFRACTIONATED HEPARIN (UFH)

Current recommendations by the American College of Cardiology include the administration of unfractionated heparin (UFH) for the following indications:

- To prevent deep vein thrombosis (DVT) in otherwise uncomplicated MI patients
- As an adjunct to thrombolytic therapy
- As an adjunct therapy in patients undergoing percutaneous or surgical coronary revascularization
- To prevent embolic complications in patients who are at high risk, such as patients in atrial fibrillation, those with large anterior wall MI, those with known previous embolus, or patients with known left ventricular thrombus

Dose

Intravenous therapy:

- In patients undergoing thrombolytic therapy with alteplase, 60U/kg bolus followed by 12U/kg/h with a maximum bolus of 4000U and 1000U/h for patients weighing >70kg. Heparin dose should be adjusted to prolong the activated partial thromboplastin time (aPTT) to 1.5–2 times the control value

- Also recommended in patients with non-ST-elevation MI, treated with nonselective thrombolytic agents such as streptokinase, anistreplase, or urokinase, who are at high risk for embolic complications (atrial fibrillation, large anterior wall MI, previous embolic complications, or known left ventricular thrombus)

Subcutaneous therapy:
- All patients treated with nonselective thrombolytic therapy, who are not at high risk for embolic complications: 7500–12,500U twice daily
- All patients not treated with thrombolytic therapy who do not have a contraindication to heparin: 7500U twice daily (for DVT prophylaxis)

Efficacy
- In patients at high risk for systemic embolus, reports show lower in-hospital mortality (4.6%) than in untreated patients (8.8%). Stroke rates were also reduced
- In patients treated with alteplase, an 18% reduction of mortality was observed in the heparin-treated group
- Reduced risk of complications in patients undergoing angioplasty has been shown
- In patients treated with subcutaneous heparin for DVT prophylaxis, a reduction in DVT rates from 12% to 4% was observed

Risks/Benefits
Risks:
- Patients may develop white-clot syndrome (new thrombus formation)
- Use with caution in the elderly and children
- Use with caution in renal disease, subacute bacterial endocarditis, diabetes mellitus, severe hypertension, history of gastrointestinal cancer, and peptic ulcer disease

Benefits:
- Rapid onset, consistent bioavailability in intravenous form

Side-effects and adverse reactions
- Cardiovascular: shock
- CNS: fever, headache
- EENT: lacrimation, rhinitis
- Gastrointestinal: vomiting
- Genitourinary: hematuria, priapism
- Hematologic: hemorrhage, thrombocytopenia, new thrombus formation
- Metabolism: hyperlipidemia, hyperkalemia
- Musculoskeletal: osteoporosis
- Respiratory: anaphylactoid reactions, asthma
- Skin: cutaneous necrosis, alopecia, erythema, urticaria

Interactions (other drugs)
▪ ACE inhibitors ▪ Angiotensin II receptor antagonists ▪ Antiplatelet drugs (clopidogrel, dipyridamole, ticlopidine) ▪ Glyceryl trinitrate ▪ NSAIDs (aspirin, diclofenac, ketorolac)

Contraindications
▪ Hemophilia and other bleeding disorders ▪ Recent cerebral hemorrhage ▪ Thrombocytopenia ▪ Peptic ulcer ▪ Severe liver disease ▪ Severe hypertension

Evidence

There is limited evidence for the use of heparin in the treatment of AMI.

- A RCT compared heparin with placebo, both commenced within 24h of AMI. There was no difference in the rates of reinfarction; however, lower in-hospital mortality was noted in the heparin-treated patients (both with and without the addition of streptokinase) [25] *Level P*
- A systematic overview of six RCTs compared thrombolytic therapy in combination with either heparin or placebo in patients post-AMI. No significant difference was noted between reinfarction, or recurrent ischemia in heparin vs placebo groups. It was concluded that there was insufficient evidence to support or refute the use of heparin following thrombolysis [26] *Level P*

Acceptability to patient

Inpatient treatment, which requires blood testing, but is usually accepted in the acute setting.

Follow up plan

Inpatient management requires frequent blood testing for dosage adjustments.

Patient and caregiver information

Patients need to report any bleeding immediately.

ENOXAPARIN

- Enzymatically treated heparin to produce shorter-chain fragments which have similar antithrombin III effects, but reduced or absent antithrombin action, more stable anticoagulant action, and potentially lower rates of thrombocytopenia with reduced rates of heparin-induced thrombocytopenic syndrome
- Currently, dosing regimens and efficacy are under investigation, with several studies indicating improved outcomes in patients treated with low molecular weight heparin (LMWH) vs unfractionated heparin (UFH) or placebo

Dose

Enoxaparin: 1mg/kg subcutaneously twice daily.

Efficacy

- Lower rates of death, MI, and recurrent angina in enoxaparin-treated patients vs UFH-treated patients
- Lower cost per patient in enoxaparin-treated patients vs UFH patients because of lower rates of recatheterization and revascularization (average savings $1172 per patient)

Risks/Benefits

Risks:

- Use caution with bleeding disorders, gastrointestinal disease, active peptic ulceration, bacterial endocarditis, hemorrhagic stroke, recent surgery, renal impairment
- Use precaution in the elderly and children

Benefit:

- Subcutaneous injection may be given at home

Side-effects and adverse reactions

- Cardiovascular: edema
- CNS: fever, confusion
- Gastrointestinal: altered liver function tests, nausea
- Hematologic: thrombocytopenia, bleeding, anemia
- Skin: irritation, pain

Interactions (other drugs)

■ ACE inhibitors ■ Angiotensin II receptor antagonists
■ Antiplatelet drugs (clopidogrel, dipyridamole, ticlopidine) ■ Glyceryl trinitrate
■ NSAIDs (aspirin, diclofenac, ketorolac)

Contraindications

■ Active bleeding ■ Drug-related thrombocytopenia ■ Hemophilia and other bleeding disorders ■ Thrombocytopenia ■ Peptic ulcer ■ Severe hypertension ■ Recent cerebral hemorrhage ■ Severe liver disease

Evidence

LMWH combined with aspirin may reduce further ischemic cardiac events for some patients.
A blinded randomized controlled trial compared enoxaparin with heparin in the treatment of patients with non-Q wave MI or unstable angina (who were also on aspirin). Reduced rates of MI, unstable angina, death, and need for revascularization were noted in the enoxaparin group at 14 and 30 days. Enoxaparin-treated patients had a higher incidence of minor bleeding [27] *Level P*

Acceptability to patient

Does not require inpatient treatment, and may be more acceptable than UFH.

Follow up plan

Inpatient management requires frequent blood testing for dosage adjustments.

Patient and caregiver information

Patients need to report any bleeding immediately.

DALTEPARIN

- Enzymatically treated heparin to produce shorter-chain fragments which have similar antithrombin III effects, but reduced or absent antithrombin action, more stable anticoagulant action, and potentially lower rates of thrombocytopenia with reduced rates of heparin-induced thrombocytopenic syndrome
- Currently, dosing regimens and efficacy are under investigation, with several studies indicating improved outcomes in patients treated with LMWH vs UFH or placebo

Dose

Patients with unstable angina or non-Q-wave MI: 120 IU/kg body weight, not to exceed 10,000 IU, subcutaneously every 12h with concurrent oral aspirin (75–165mg once daily) therapy. Treatment should be continued until the patient is clinically stabilized. The usual duration of administration is 5–8 days. Concurrent aspirin therapy is recommended except when contraindicated.

Risks/Benefits

Risks:

- Use caution with elderly and children
- Use caution with renal or hepatic disease, subacute bacterial endocarditis, diabetes mellitus, severe hypertension, history of gastrointestinal cancer, peptic ulcer disease, bleeding disorders, thrombocytopenia, active ulceration, gastrointestinal bleeding, angiodysplastic gastrointestinal disease, recent surgery, and retinopathy

Benefit: rapid onset, consistent bioavailability in intravenous form.

Side-effects and adverse reactions
- CNS: fever, headache
- Gastrointestinal: vomiting, nausea
- Genitourinary: hematuria, priapism
- Hematologic: hemorrhage, thrombocytopenia, new thrombus formation
- Metabolism: hyperlipidemia, hyperkalemia
- Musculoskeletal: osteoporosis after prolonged treatment
- Respiratory: anaphylactoid reactions, asthma
- Skin: erythema, urticaria, skin necrosis

Interactions (other drugs)
▪ ACE inhibitors ▪ Angiotensin-II receptor antagonists ▪ Antiplatelet drugs (clopidogrel, dipyridamole, ticlopidine) ▪ Glyceryl trinitrate ▪ NSAIDs (aspirin, diclofenac, ketorolac)

Contraindications
▪ Hemophilia and other bleeding disorders ▪ Thrombocytopenia ▪ Peptic ulcer ▪ Severe hypertension ▪ Recent cerebral hemorrhage ▪ Severe liver disease

Acceptability to patient
Does not require inpatient treatment, and may be more acceptable than UFH.

Follow up plan
Inpatient management requires frequent blood testing for dosage adjustments.

Patient and caregiver information
Patients need to report any bleeding immediately

Surgical therapy

PERCUTANEOUS TRANSLUMINAL CORONARY ANGIOPLASTY

This therapy, also referred to as PTCA, may be performed in specialist centers in the setting of AMI. Stent insertion may be performed.

Efficacy
- Alternative to thrombolytic therapy, especially in patients with ST elevation, AMI within 12h of pain onset, or after 12h if ischemic symptoms persist
- 'Salvage angioplasty' for failed thrombolysis
- Should be considered as the reperfusion modality of choice in patients with cardiogenic shock
- Is effective if performed by experienced physicians in specialist centers
- Angioplasty has been shown to restore coronary flow in 95% or more of patients

Risks/Benefits
Benefits:
- Recanalization of an occluded artery
- Less risk of stroke than with thrombolysis

Evidence
There is evidence that PTCA is an effective treatment for AMI.
- A RCT compared primary angioplasty with tPA and found there was no significant difference in mortality between the groups at 30 days. However, the primary end point of death, recurrent MI, or stroke was significantly reduced in the PTCA group at 30 days. This was attenuated to a nonsignificant difference at 6 months [28] *Level P*
- A systematic review comparing primary PTCA and primary thrombolysis showed 30-day mortality of 4.4% in the PTCA group and 6.5% in the thrombolysis group [29] *Level M*

- A meta-analysis comparing thrombolytic therapy and primary angioplasty in patients with AMI showed that primary angioplasty was associated with a significant reduction in short-term mortality. The rates of reinfarction and recurrent ischemia were also reduced, as well as the combined criteria of death or reinfarction [30] *Level M*
- The frequency of strokes of any cause was significantly reduced in patients treated with angioplasty. There was no significant difference noted for the incidence of major bleeding [30] *Level M*
- It is suggested that angioplasty is superior to thrombolysis in the short term, but this effect may not be sustained. Primary angioplasty should be considered (when available in experienced centers) as the first-choice treatment option [30] *Level M*
- The benefits of primary PTCA (lower mortality and reinfarction) over thrombolysis are not conclusive. PTCA shows benefit over thrombolysis only when performed by experienced specialists. Primary PTCA may be of most benefit to patients with contraindications to thrombolysis, those with cardiogenic shock, and in elderly patients [31]

Acceptability to patient

High.

Follow up plan

6-month follow-ups after initial follow-up visits.

Patient and caregiver information

Patients should be instructed about their disease process, medications and side-effects, and risk factor modification, including smoking cessation and lifestyle changes.

CORONARY ARTERY BYPASS GRAFT

Efficacy

- May be used in patients unsuited for PTCA who have persistent or recurrent ischemia refractory to medical therapy; also, in patients with failed angioplasty or cardiogenic shock or complications of infarction
- Has been shown to reduce mortality in patients who have triple-vessel coronary disease or left-main coronary disease

Risks/Benefits

- Risks: infection, clotting, death
- Benefit: reperfusion, recanalization

Evidence

There is evidence for the use of coronary artery bypass graft (CABG) in patients post-MI.

- A systematic review compared CABG with medical treatment alone. Those treated with CABG had decreased mortality at 5, 7, and 10 years. No impact was noted on subsequent AMI [32] *Level M*
- Unfortunately, the participants in the trials were all 65 years or younger, male, and not high-risk patients. Benefits may be underestimated compared with medical treatment alone, because medical and surgical treatments were not mutually exclusive [32]

Acceptability to patient

Surgery may be less acceptable than medical therapy.

Follow up plan

Surgical follow up is required.

Patient and caregiver information

- Patients should be informed of the risks and benefits of surgery
- Patients should be aware that surgery is not curative, and that some patients will even need repeat surgery

LIFESTYLE

- Cessation of smoking
- Weight loss
- Reduction of fat consumption (especially saturated fats)
- Carefully monitored exercise program
- Treatment of hypertension
- Treatment of hyperlipidemia
- Treatment of diabetes
- Compliance with prescriptions, e.g. beta-blockers, aspirin, ACE inhibitors

RISKS/BENEFITS

Benefit: helps speed recovery and prevent future attacks.

ACCEPTABILITY TO PATIENT

- Cessation of smoking is often difficult
- Weight loss is often difficult
- Compliance is sometimes a problem with a carefully monitored exercise program
- Treatment of hypertension is usually highly acceptable
- Treatment of hyperlipidemia and diabetes is usually acceptable
- Compliance with prescription medicines is high

FOLLOW UP PLAN

- Low-risk patients should have an early noninvasive stress evaluation for assessment of prognosis and/or functional capacity
- Submaximal exercise at 4–6 days or symptom-limited thereafter
- Exercise, vasodilator stress nuclear scintigraphy, or exercise stress echocardiography may be performed when baseline abnormalities of the ECG compromise interpretation
- Dipyridamole or adenosine perfusion nuclear scintigraphy or dobutamine echocardiography may be performed in patients judged to be unable to exercise
- Ambulatory ECG (Holter) monitoring is no longer considered a necessary routine follow up measure for patients with AMI

PATIENT AND CAREGIVER INFORMATION

Patients should be instructed about their disease process; medication use and side-effects; and risk factor modification including smoking cessation, and lifestyle changes.

OUTCOMES

EFFICACY OF THERAPIES

- Thrombolysis improves short- and long-term survival
- Percutaneous transluminal coronary angioplasty (PTCA) improves survival rate, and reduces the risk of recurrent myocardial infarction (MI) and stroke
- Aspirin and thienpyridine derivatives have been shown to be effective in preventing further vascular events post-MI, including reinfarction
- There is an improvement in long-term survival with platelet inhibitors
- The use of aspirin and thienopyridines together has been shown markedly to reduce the incidence of further vascular events
- Beta-blockers reduce mortality rate and reinfarction. Survival is improved with use in the short- and long term
- Angiotensin converting enzyme (ACE) inhibitors have been shown to provide survival benefit to patients with or without associated heart failure
- Nitrates are effective in treating pain associated with MI and reducing short-term mortality, but their effect on long-term outcome is uncertain
- Provided there is no evidence of heart failure, diltiazem and verapamil may decrease reinfarction and angina
- Coronary artery bypass graft (CABG) may improve long-term outcomes
- Dietary modifications, smoking cessation, exercise programs, and cardiac rehabilitation programs are effective in reducing risk after MI

Evidence

- Intravenous nitrates may reduce symptoms and mortality in the short-term management of AMI. There is little long-term effect on survival [4] *Level M*
- Aspirin reduces the risk of reinfarction, death, and stroke in patients with AMI. Aspirin should be given immediately, and continued long term [33]
- Thienopyridines are associated with a modest but significant reduction in the risk of vascular events in patients after a recent AMI [10] *Level M*
- Patients with AMI and ST elevation or bundle branch block are effectively treated with thrombolysis, providing they present within 6h, and possibly up to 12h, after symptom onset [33]
- Long-term follow up of patients treated with thrombolytic therapy in a randomized controlled trial (RCT) showed a survival benefit of up to 12 years compared with placebo [2] *Level P*
- The use of beta-blockers confers benefit when used during, and long term after, MI. Reinfarction and mortality are reduced, and additional benefit is noted when beta-blockers are combined with thrombolysis [33]
- Calcium channel antagonists have been shown to cause harm in patients with heart failure. They do not reduce mortality for patients after AMI [33]
- Immediate management of AMI with ACE inhibitors may reduce mortality [33]
- Patients with non-Q-wave MI or unstable angina may have reduced rates of MI, unstable angina, death, and need for revascularization when enoxaparin is added to aspirin therapy [27] *Level P*
- It is suggested that angioplasty is superior to thrombolysis in the short term, but this effect may not be sustained. Primary angioplasty should be considered (when available in experienced centers) as the first-choice treatment option [30] *Level M*
- Patients treated with CABG may have decreased mortality at 5, 7, and 10 years compared with medical management, but there may be a greater risk of death in the first year. No impact is noted on the risk of subsequent AMI [33]
- Intensive dietary intervention in conjunction with multifactorial risk reduction treatment shows a decrease in progression of the extent of coronary heart disease at angiography [34] *Level P*
- Cardiac rehabilitation may result in a decrease in overall and cardiovascular mortality, and a decrease in fatal reinfarction after a mean of 3 years. There is no difference in nonfatal reinfarction [35] *Level M*

Review period

- Patients should be considered for structured cardiac rehabilitation programs beginning during admission and continued on discharge
- Patients should be followed in 4–6 weeks, sooner for patients with a complicated course, congestive heart failure, or significant comorbidities
- A symptom-limited treadmill stress test should be performed at 6 weeks for patients who have not been revascularized and for other patients to assess adequacy of anti-ischemic therapies, assess functional status prior to returning to a vigorous job, or to reassure the patient about the safety of resuming exercise
- Patients with normal lipid values during hospital admission should be reassessed at 6 weeks and lipid-lowering therapy begun as needed
- Patients with ventricular arrhythmias after the acute phase of MI, especially with a depressed ejection fraction, should be considered for an implantable defibrillator (ICD)
- Patients with coronary heart disease require lifelong follow up

PROGNOSIS

- The single most important predictor of long-term prognosis after MI is severity of left ventricular dysfunction. Other factors are:
- Age
- Significant comorbidities (diabetes, hypertension)
- Presence of high-grade ventricular arrhythmias
- Completeness of revascularization
- Evidence of continuing ischemia
- Compliance with secondary prevention strategies, including those for risk factor modification
- Reduced left ventricular ejection fraction

Clinical pearl(s)

- Aggressive lipid-lowering therapy should be started immediately
- Counseling and outcome-oriented education about the 'new medications' can help with compliance. Continued use of beta-blockers and ACE inhibitors are essential towards decreasing mortality
- Extensive counseling of the family, and encouragement of lifestyle changes, are time-consuming but critical
- Children of patients with MI should have complete cholesterol screening
- In addition to quitting smoking, patients should try to avoid second-hand smoke exposure. Encourage family members to quit

Therapeutic failure

- Patients with recurrent angina, congestive heart failure, shock, arrhythmia, or demonstrable ischemia after infarction should be considered for angiography and revascularization
- Patients with mechanical complications after MI or failed percutaneous revascularization should be considered for surgical correction

Recurrence

Mortality may occur due to reocclusion, reinfarction, or sudden cardiac death.

Deterioration

Patients with refractory symptoms may need to be considered for transplantation.

Terminal illness

For patients with terminal illness, the risk and benefit of aggressive, invasive, and expensive interventions need to be balanced against the patient's ultimate prognosis.

COMPLICATIONS

Early:

- Arrythmias are the most common acute complication associated with MI. Antiarrhythmic drugs are rarely required but, if they are, will generally be prescribed in the hospital setting. Medications that may be used include digoxin, lidocaine, procainamide, and amiodarone. Lidocaine, procainamide, or amiodarone are effective for treating sustained monomorphic ventricular tachycardia not associated with angina, pulmonary edema, or hypertension (systolic blood pressure<90mmHg). Sustained monomorphic ventricular tachycardia accompanied by these symptoms should be treated with cardioversion
- Amiodarone may be useful to treat polymorphic ventricular tachycardia
- Arrhythmias may require treatment with temporary or permanent pacing or defibrillators
- Permanent pacemaker implantation is effective in cases of complete heart block after MI or for symptomatic AV block at any level
- Pericarditis is a common early complication, and is usually effectively managed with aspirin (650mg four times daily)
- Acute congestive heart failure (CHF). Digitalis derivatives and diuretics should be used to treat CHF. Alpha-adrenergic blocking agents may also be useful
- Cardiogenic shock is managed as an inpatient with vasopressors and aortic counterpulsation
- Acute mitral regurgitation and papillary muscle rupture/dysfunction are managed surgically
- Ventricular septal defect requires early intervention with a nitroprusside infusion and intra-aortic balloon counterpulsation (i.e. inpatient treatment is required)
- Ventricular free wall rupture is almost always fatal
- Thrombosis/dissection of angioplasty site
- Systemic or pulmonary thromboembolism risk is increased in patients with an anterior infarct, severe left ventricular dysfunction, CHF, mural thrombus, atrial fibrillation, and past history of thromboembolism. The full dose of intravenous heparin followed by 3 months of warfarin therapy is indicated for these patients

Late:

- Ventricular remodeling
- Chronic CHF
- Sudden cardiac death (arrhythmia or new plaque rupture)
- Bypass graft atherosclerosis and closure
- Restenosis of PTCA site including in-stent restenosis
- Dressler's syndrome

CONSIDER CONSULT

- All patients who present with symptoms consistent with AMI should be referred immediately to the emergency department
- Patients who develop late complications should be referred to a cardiologist, if they are not already being followed up

PREVENTION

RISK FACTORS

- Smoking
- Diabetes
- Hypertension
- Thrombi
- Hyperlipidemia
- Physical inactivity
- Obesity

MODIFY RISK FACTORS

Appropriate management of diabetes, hypertension, thrombi, and hyperlipdemia should be instituted.

Lifestyle and wellness

TOBACCO

All patients should be encouraged to give up smoking.

DIET

- Patients should be encouraged to eat a healthy diet, low in fat and sodium
- Obese patients should be given advice on weight loss

PHYSICAL ACTIVITY

- Exercise regularly three to four times a week for 30–60min under a physician's guidance as required
- Consider cardiac rehabilitation

FAMILY HISTORY

Patients with a family history of heart disease should be especially careful to follow a healthy lifestyle.

SCREENING

- Routine screening of asymptomatic individuals for significant coronary artery disease by exercise stress testing is not recommended (low yield and high rate of false-positives)
- Exercise stress testing is, however, recommended for screening purposes in males over 40 with one or more risk factors
- Additionally, screen for/identify major recognized risk factors and treat appropriately: high blood pressure; tobacco use; dyslipidemias (particularly high total and LDL cholesterol, and low HDL cholesterol); diabetes; obesity; and family history of premature coronary artery disease

PREVENT RECURRENCE

Ensure adherence to lifestyle measures.

Reassess coexisting disease

Reassess management of diabetes, hypertension, and hyperlipdemia.

INTERACTION ALERT

Following a myocardial infarction, patients are often started and discharged on several new medications – review previous medications for potential interactions. Also review with patient the potential interactions with over-the-counter medications and health food and herbal therapies.

ASSOCIATIONS

American Heart Association
National Center
7272 Greenville Avenue
Dallas, TX 75231
Tel: (800) 242-8721
http://www.americanheart.org

National Heart, Lung, and Blood Institute
PO Box 30105
Bethesda, MD 20824-0105
Tel: (301) 592-8573
Fax: (301) 592-8563
http://www.nhlbi.nih.gov

American College of Cardiology
Heart House
9111 Old Georgetown
Bethesda, MD 20814-1699
Tel: (800) 253-4636
Fax: (301) 897-9745
http://www.acc.org

KEY REFERENCES

- American College of Cardiology/American Heart Association Guidelines for the Management of Patients with Acute Myocardial Infarction: 1999 Update; A Report of the ACC/AHA Task Force on Practice Guidelines, available at www.acc.org
- American Heart Association Guidelines 2000 for Cardiopulmonary Resuscitation and Emergency Cardiac Care. Circulation 2000;102(suppl 1):I1–I384
- Braunwald E, ed. Heart disease: a text book of cardiovascular medicine, 5th edn. Philadelphia: WB Saunders, 1997

Evidence references

1 Fibrinolytic Therapy Trialists' (FTT) Collaborative Group. Indications for fibrinolytic therapy in suspected acute myocardial infarction: collaborative overview of early mortality and major morbidity results of all randomized trials of more than 1000 patients. Lancet 1994;343:311–22. Reviewed in: Clinical Evidence 2001;5:8–23
2 French, JK, Hyde, TA, Patel, H, et al. Survival 12 years after randomization to streptokinase: the influence of thrombolysis in myocardial infarction flow at three to four weeks. J Am Coll Cardiol 1999;34:62–9. Reviewed in: Clinical Evidence 2001;5:8–23
3 Collins R, Peto R, Baigent BM, Sleight DM. Aspirin, heparin and fibrinolytic therapy in suspected acute myocardial infarction. N Engl J Med 1997;336:847–60. Reviewed in: Clinical Evidence 2001;5:8–23
4 Yusuf S, Collins R, MacMahon S, et al. Effect of intravenous nitrates on mortality in acute myocardial infarction: an overview of the randomised trials. Lancet 1988;i:1088–1092. Reviewed in: Clinical Evidence 2001;5:8–23
5 Fourth International Study of Infarct Survival (ISIS-4) Collaborative Group. ISIS-4: a randomised factorial trial assessing early oral captopril, oral mononitrate, and intravenous magnesium sulfate in 58,050 patients with suspected acute myocardial infarction. Lancet 1995;345:669–685. Reviewed in: Clinical Evidence 2001;5:8–23
6 GISSI-3 effects of lisinopril and transdermal glyceryl trinitrate singly and together on 6-week mortality and ventricular function after acute myocardial infarction. Lancet 1994;343:1115–22. Reviewed in: Clinical Evidence 2001;5:8–23
7 Antiplatelet Trialists' Collaboration. Collaborative overview of randomized trials of antiplatelet therapy I: prevention of death, myocardial infarction, and stroke by prolonged antiplatelet therapy in various categories of people. BMJ 1994;308:81–106. Reviewed in: Clinical Evidence 2001;5:8–23

8 Second International Study of Infarct Survival (ISIS-2) Collaborative group. Randomised trial of intravenous streptokinase, oral aspirin, both, or neither among 17,187 cases of suspected acute myocardial infarction. Lancet 1988;ii:349–360. Reviewed in: Clinical Evidence 2001;5:8–23
9 Baigent BM, Collins, R. ISIS-2: four year mortality of 17,187 patients after fibrinolytic and antiplatelet therapy in suspected acute myocardial infarction study. Circulation 1993;(suppl 1):1–291. Reviewed in: Clinical Evidence 2001;5:8–23
10 Hankey GJ, Sudlow CLM, Dunbabin DW. Thienopyridine derivatives (ticlodipine, clopidogrel) versus aspirin for preventing stroke and other serious vascular events in high vascular risk patients (Cochrane Review). In: The Cochrane Library, 3, 2001. Oxford: Update Software
11 Yusuf S, Peto R, Lewis J, et al. Beta blockade during and after myocardial infarction: an overview of the randomized trials. Prog Cardiovasc Dis 1985;27:355–71. Reviewed in: Clinical Evidence 2001;5:8–23
12 Sleight P for the ISIS Study Group. Beta blockade early in acute myocardial infarction. Am J Cardiol 1987;60:6A–12A. Reviewed in: Clinical Evidence 2001;5:8–23
13 Freemantle N, Cleland J, Young P, et al. Beta blockade after myocardial infarction: systematic review and meta regression analysis. BMJ 1999;318:1730–37. Reviewed in: Clinical Evidence 2001;5:8–23
14 Teo KK, Yusuf S, Furberg CD. Effects of prophylactic antiarrhythmic drug therapy in acute myocardial infarction. JAMA 1993;270:1589–95. Reviewed in: Clinical Evidence 2001;5:95–126
15 Opie LH, Yusuf S, Kubler W. Current status of safety and efficacy of calcium channel blockers in cardiovascular diseases: a critical analysis based on 100 studies. Prog Cardiovasc Dis 2000;43:171–96. Reviewed in: Clinical Evidence 2001;5:8–23
16 Pepine Cj, Faich G, Makuch R. Verapamil use in patients with cardiovascular disease: an overview of randomized trials. Clin Cardiol 1998;21:633–41. Reviewed in: Clinical Evidence 2001;5:8–23
17 Gibson R, Boden WE, Therouux P, et al. Diltiazem and reinfarction in patients with non-Q wave myocardial infarction. N Engl J Med 1986;315:423–9. Reviewed in: Clinical Evidence 2001;5:95–126
18 Multicentre Diltiazem Postinfarction Trial Research Group. The effect of diltiazem on mortality and reinfarction after myocardial infarction. N Engl J Med 1988;319:385–92. Reviewed in: Clinical Evidence 2001;5:95–126
19 Danish Study Group on Verapamil in Myocardial Infarction. Effect of verapamil on mortality and major events after acute myocardial infarction: the Danish verapamil infarction trial II (DAVIT II). Am J Cardiol 1990;66:779–85. Reviewed in: Clinical Evidence 2001;5:95–126
20 ACE Inhibitor Myocardial Infarction Collaborative Group. Indications for ACE inhibitors in the early treatment of acute myocardial infarction: systemic overview of individual data from 100,000 patients in randomized trials. Circulation 1998;97:2202–12. Reviewed in: Clinical Evidence 2001;5:8–23
21 Domanski MJ, Exner DV, Borkowt CB, et al. Effect of angiotensin converting enzyme inhibition on sudden cardiac death in patients following acute myocardial infarction. A meta-analysis of randomized clinical trials. J Am Coll Cardiol 1999;33:598–604. Reviewed in: Clinical Evidence 2001;5:8–23
22 Pfeffer MA, Braunwald E, Moye CA, et al. Effect of captopril on mortality and morbidity in patients with left ventricular dysfunction after myocardial infarction. N Engl J Med 1992;327:669–77. Reviewed in: Clinical Evidence 2001;5:8–23
23 Acute Infarction Ramipril Efficacy (AIRE) Study Investigators. Effect of ramipril on mortality and morbidity of survivors of acute myocardial infarction with clinical evidence of heart failure. Lancet 1993;342:821–8. Reviewed in: Clinical Evidence 2001;5:8–23
24 Trandolapril Cardiac Evaluation (TRACE) Study Group. A clinical trial of the ACE inhibitor trandolapril in patients with left ventricular dysfunction after MI. N Engl J Med 1995;333:1670–76. Reviewed in: Clinical Evidence 2001;5:8–23
25 Randomised controlled trial of subcutaneous calcium-heparin in acute myocardial infarction: the SCATI (Studio sulla Calciparina nell-Angina e nella Thrombosi ventricolare nell'Infarto) Group. Lancet. 1989;ii:182–86. Medline
26 Mahaffey KW, Granger CB, Collins R, et al. Overview of randomized trials of intravenous heparin in patients with acute myocardial infarction treated with thrombolytic therapy. Am J Cardiol 1996;77:551–6. Medline
27 Cohen M, Demers C, Gurfinkel EP, et al. A comparison of low-molecular-weight heparin with unfractionated heparin for unstable coronary artery disease. Efficacy and Safety of Subcutaneous Enoxaparin in Non-Q-Wave Coronary Events Study Group. N Engl J Med 1997;337:447–52. Medline
28 The GUSTO IIb Angioplasty Substudy Investigators. A clinical trial comparing primary coronary angioplasty with tissue plasminogen activator for acute myocardial infarction. N Engl J Med 1997;336:1621–8. Reviewed in: Clinical Evidence 2001;5:8–23
29 Weaver WD, Simes RJ, Betriu A, et al. Comparison of primary coronary angioplasty and intravenous thrombolytic therapy for acute myocardial infarction: a quantitative review. JAMA 1997;278:2093–8. Reviewed in: Clinical Evidence 2001;5:8–23

30 Cucherat M, Bonnefoy E, Tremeau, G. Primary angioplasty versus intravenous thrombolysis for acute myocardial infarction (Cochrane Review). In: The Cochrane Library, 3, 2001. Oxford: Update Software
31 Van de Werf F, Topol EJ, Lee KL, et al. Variations in patient management and outcomes for acute myocardial infarction in the United States and other countries: results from the GUSTO trial. JAMA 1995;273:1586–91. Reviewed in: Clinical Evidence 2001;5:8–23
32 Yusuf S, Zucker D, Peduzzi P, et al. Effect of coronary artery bypass graft surgery on survival: overview of 10 year results form randomized trials by the coronary artery bypass graft surgery trialists collaboration. Lancet 1994;344:563–70. Reviewed in: Clinical Evidence 2001;5:8–23
33 Mehta, S. Acute myocardial infarction: cardiovascular disorders. In: Clinical Evidence 2001;5:8–233. London: BMJ Publishing Group.
34 Waters D. Lessons from coronary atherosclerosis 'regression' trials. Cardiol Clin 1996;14:31–50. Reviewed in: Clinical Evidence 2001;5:95–126
35 O'Connor GT, Buring JE, Yusuf S, et al. An overview of randomized trials of rehabilitation with exercise after myocardial infarction. Circulation 1989;80:234–44. Reviewed in: Clinical Evidence 2001;5:95–126

FAQS

Question 1

Why is time so critical in the diagnosis of acute myocardial infarction?

ANSWER 1

Irreversable myocardial damage is ongoing until reperfusion is accomplished. Many studies have established systolic ventricular function as the most important prognostic factor for patients with coronary artery disease. Myocardial salvage is, therefore, critical. The most salvage occurs if reperfusion can be accomplished within 1h, with little benefit seen after 4–6h.

Question 2

Why is it that a patient can have a normal stress test one day and then an acute MI the next day?

ANSWER 2

Coronary artery disease has two distinct presentations. Stable angina pectoris results from severe coronary stenosis. Acute coronary syndromes (including acute MI) typically involve less severe, lipid-rich plaques which suddenly rupture resulting in thrombosis. Stress testing can only detect severe stenoses, but does not screen for vulnerable plaques.

Question 3

What is the best role of the primary care physician in the management of acute MI?

ANSWER 3

The patient and his or her family need reassurance and counseling about the impact on the patient's life. Many studies have shown that aggressive and attentive post-MI risk factor modification can significantly (i.e. a 45% decreased risk of death at 5 years) alter patient outcome. These measures add at least as much or possibly more to the ultimate care of the patient than anything done in the initial hospital phase by specialists.

Question 4

How can post-MI complications be prevented?

ANSWER 4

Many cannot; however, careful twice-daily examinations and patient checks can often pick up the early signs of complications. New murmurs, rubs, rales, and edema can be quickly evaluated. Evaluation of left ventricular systolic function, monitoring for nonsustained ventricular tachycardia, and a very low threshold for cardiac catheterization allow intervention for prevention of sudden death or reocclusion.

Question 5

How important are minor troponin leaks or ECG changes?

ANSWER 5

The ECG during ischemic pain is prognostic for outcome. Contrary to popular belief, ST elevation has one of the best prognostic outcomes. ST depression is actually a more ominous finding. Similarly, even minor troponin elevations confer a 3–4-fold increase in short-term mortality. Thus, any troponin leak or even subtle ECG change should be aggressively pursued.

CONTRIBUTORS

Kathleen M O'Hanlon, MD
John McB Hodgson, MD, FACC, FSCAI
Gail A Van Norman, MD

ORTHOSTATIC HYPOTENSION

SUMMARY INFORMATION

DESCRIPTION

- Sudden drop in blood pressure that is provoked by standing. Condition may be asymptomatic, or it may induce dizziness, light-headedness, diaphoresis, vision changes, head and neck pain, and syncope
- Most prevalent among the elderly. Causes include prescription medications and over-the-counter drugs, hypovolemia, vasodilation, prolonged bed rest, and disorders of the autonomic nervous system
- Treatment should seek to remove underlying causes. When this is not possible, as is the case with neurogenic disease, patients may require a combination of medication, nonpharmacologic aids, and lifestyle changes

URGENT ACTION

Severe orthostatic hypotension from hypovolemia may require intravenous fluid resuscitation.

ICD9 CODE
458.0 Hypotension, orthostatic (chronic).

SYNONYMS
Postural hypotension.

CARDINAL FEATURES
- Fall in systolic blood pressure of at least 20mmHg or diastolic blood pressure of at least 10mmHg within 3min of rising to a standing position
- May cause cerebral hypoperfusion, resulting in dizziness, blurred vision, light-headedness, headache, neckache, palpitations, weakness, fatigue, diaphoresis, cognitive impairment, nausea, and/or syncope

CAUSES
Common causes
- Medications: phenothiazines, monoamine oxidase inhibitors, tricyclic antidepressants, diuretics, levodopa, bromocriptine, beta-blockers, calcium channel blockers, nitrates, sildenafil, and some chemotherapeutic drugs
- Hypovolemia (including that caused by dehydration, overdiuresis, diarrhea, hemorrhage, burns, fever, and hot environment)
- Decreased baroreceptor sensitivity – most common in the elderly
- Common general neuropathies affecting the peripheral autonomic nervous system, including diabetes mellitus, alcohol abuse, and amyloidosis
- Prolonged bed rest
- Salt-free diet
- Anemia

Rare causes
- Disorders involving blood vessels, including severe varicose veins, vasospastic disorders, and atherosclerosis
- Primary adrenal insufficiency (Addison's disease)
- Generalized neurologic disorders that affect the autonomic nervous system, including Parkinson's disease, multiple strokes, brainstem lesions, multiple system atrophy (MSA), e.g. Shy–Drager syndrome, and multiple sclerosis
- Specific autonomic nervous system disorders, including Riley–Day syndrome (familial dysautonomia), and pure autonomic failure (PAF) – previously called Bradbury–Eggleston syndrome, and postural orthostatic tachycardia syndrome (POTS)
- Uncommon disorders affecting primarily autonomic nervous system, including, Guillain–Barré syndrome, dopamine–beta hydroxylase deficiency, AIDS, porphyria, and paraneoplastic syndromes
- Damage to the spinal cord, including that associated with syringomyelia and tabes dorsalis

Serious causes
All symptomatic orthostatic hypotension must be taken seriously as patients may develop syncope. Medication- and volume-induced hypotension are easier to treat than autonomic nervous system disorders.

Contributory or predisposing factors
- Normal aging process: aging is associated with reduced cerebral blood flow, possible impairment of the baroreflex, and reduced renal salt and water conservation
- Hypertension: age-related elevation in systolic blood pressure may impair the baroreflex. Moreover, drugs used to treat hypertension may cause orthostatic hypotension as a side-effect

EPIDEMIOLOGY

Incidence and prevalence

PREVALENCE

Among elderly individuals, prevalence is estimated at 130–300 per 1000.

Demographics

AGE

Most common among people aged 65 years and older.

GENDER

Younger patients tend more often to be women.

GENETICS

May be caused by the following inherited disorders: dopamine–beta-hydroxylase deficiency, Riley–Day syndrome, and familial amyloidosis.

DIFFERENTIAL DIAGNOSIS

Vasovagal syncope

FEATURES

- Fainting caused by temporary decline in blood circulation in the brain
- Occurs at irregular intervals, rather than as a result of postural change
- May be provoked by emotional stress, pain, or shock

Cardiac syncope

FEATURES

- Resulting from a sudden decrease in cardiac output, most often due to an arrhythmia or mechanical cause
- Not specifically associated with postural changes

SIGNS & SYMPTOMS

Signs

- Decline in systolic blood pressure of at least 20mmHg or diastolic blood pressure of at least 10mmHg within 3min of standing
- Failure of a compensatory rise in heart rate suggests an autonomic dysregulation in contrast to hypovolemia

Symptoms

On standing suddenly, patients may experience any of the following symptoms:

- Light-headedness
- Dizziness
- Blurred vision
- Head or neck pain
- Syncope
- Diminished hearing
- Diaphoresis

ASSOCIATED DISORDERS

- Supine hypertension (particularly in orthostatic hypotension associated with autonomic failure)
- Postprandial hypotension
- Signs of diffuse autonomic dysfunction, including impotence, constipation, and urinary retention

INVESTIGATION OF THE PATIENT

Direct questions to patient

Q **What medications do you take, including over-the-counter drugs?** Side-effects of medications are common causes of orthostatic hypotension. Of particular concern are drugs that cause hypovolemia or vasodilation, or that impair the baroreflex. Drugs that have been implicated in orthostatic hypotension include diuretics, phenothiazines, monoamine oxidase inhibitors, tricyclic antidepressants, levodopa, bromocriptine, vasodilators, beta-blockers, calcium channel blockers, nitrates, sildenafil, and some chemotherapeutic agents. Barbiturates and alcohol may also contribute to the condition

Q **Have you experienced any of the following: prolonged bed rest, extensive bleeding, or circumstances that would cause dehydration?** All of these conditions are reversible causes of orthostatic hypotension

Q **Are you on a salt-free diet?** Inadequate salt intake may cause this condition

Q **Is the problem exacerbated by exercise or straining?** Typical of the condition

Q **Was the onset of problems gradual or sudden?** Gradual onset, particularly in middle-aged patients, provides increased cause to suspect failure of autonomic reflexes

- **Q** **Do you have problems with bowel or bladder control, impotence, loss of peripheral sensation, constipation, and have you noticed a decline in sweating?** Affirmative answer may suggest autonomic failure
- **Q** **Do your symptoms interfere with your daily activities?** After treatable causes have been removed, therapy should be geared toward improving functionality rather than altering blood pressure. Patients with mild symptoms may not require treatment, and treatment is not recommended for asymptomatic patients
- **Q** **Does the condition become worse after meals?** Postprandial hypotension may also be present; lifestyle changes may help with this problem

Contributory or predisposing factors

- **Q** **What medications do you take, including over-the-counter drugs?** Side-effects of medications are common causes of orthostatic hypotension. Of particular concern are drugs that cause hypovolemia or vasodilation, or that impair the baroreflex. Drugs that have been implicated in orthostatic hypotension include diuretics, phenothiazines, monoamine oxidase inhibitors, tricyclic antidepressants, levodopa, bromocriptine, vasodilators, beta-blockers, calcium channel blockers, nitrates, sildenafil, and some chemotherapeutic agents. Barbiturates and alcohol may also contribute to the condition
- **Q** **Have you experienced any of the following: prolonged bed rest, extensive bleeding, or circumstances that would cause dehydration?** All of these conditions are reversible causes of orthostatic hypotension
- **Q** **Are you on a salt-free diet?** Inadequate salt intake may cause this condition
- **Q** **Do you have any other medical disorders?** Related conditions may include: cardiac impairment (pump failure, unrecognized myocardial infarction, arrhythmias, myocarditis, constrictive pericarditis, and aortic stenosis); adrenal insufficiency, including Addison's disease, diabetes insipidus; alcoholism; blood vessel disorders, including severe varicose veins, atherosclerosis, and vasospastic disorders; primary autonomic system failure; secondary autonomic system failure; disorders of the brain and brainstem, including tumor, multiple strokes, and multiple sclerosis; disorders of the spinal cord, including transverse myelitis, syringomyelia, tumor, and tabes dorsalis; and disorders involving the peripheral nervous system, including diabetes mellitus, Guillain–Barré syndrome, alcoholic polyneuropathy, AIDS, amyloidosis, and porphyria

Family history

- **Q** **Do any relatives have the following conditions: dopamine-beta-hydroxylase (DBH) deficiency, Riley–Day syndrome, porphyria, or amyloidosis?** All these disorders may cause orthostatic hypotension. DBH deficiency and Riley–Day syndrome are genetic syndromes, and a familial form of amyloidosis exists.

Examination

- Review patient's medications
- Assess coexisting disorders
- Check for signs of blood volume depletion
- Determine supine and standing blood pressure and pulse after 2–3min in each position. Pulse changes may be indicative of etiology. Normally, pulse rate increases by roughly 10–30 beats/min on standing. A higher increase may indicate non-neurogenic causes of the condition, particularly hypovolemia. Additionally, it may signal postural orthostatic tachycardia syndrome. Lack of any increase is indicative of autonomic neuropathy
- A cardiac examination can determine whether the rhythm is regular and whether there are any murmurs suggesting valvular disorders
- A careful neurologic examination, including a mental status examination, cranial nerve assessment, motor examination, and sensory evaluation must be performed to look for signs of CNS disorder

- If other findings from the examination are inclusive, autonomic function tests should be performed. These include the Valsalva maneuver and assessment of the heart rate variation that occurs with deep breathing (sinus arrhythmia). Tilt-table testing may be advisable for patients who undergo syncope of uncertain cause

Summary of investigative tests

- If autonomic failure is suspected, Valsalva maneuver may be indicated (typically performed in a specialized testing laboratory)
- Sinus arrhythmia testing can also reveal autonomic function (typically performed in a specialized testing laboratory)
- Plasma norepinephrine levels, measured when patient is supine and standing, may indicate pure autonomic failure (typically performed in a specialized testing laboratory)
- Tilt-table testing may be indicated for recurrent syncope of uncertain cause (typically performed in a cardiac testing facility)

DIAGNOSTIC DECISION

Decline in systolic blood pressure of at least 20mmHg or diastolic pressure of at least 10mmHg within 3min of standing.

Guidelines

- Consensus Committee of the American Autonomic Society and the American Academy of Neurology. Consensus statement on the definition of orthostatic hypotension, pure autonomic failure, and multiple system atrophy. Neurology 1996;46(5):1470 [1]
- The American Academy of Family Physicians has produced the following: Engstrom JW, Aminoff MJ. Evaluation and treatment of orthostatic hypotension. Am Fam Physician 1997;56:1378–84 [2]

CLINICAL PEARL(S)

- Orthostatic hypotension secondary to impaired baroreflexes is very common in the elderly patient
- Reassess all medications in patients with orthostatic hypotension, as drugs that decrease extracellular volume or impair sympathetic nervous system transmission may be the cause
- Consider secondary medical conditions that may result in orthostasis, such as diabetes mellitus

THE TESTS

Body fluids

PLASMA NOREPINEPHRINE LEVELS

Description

Blood drawn when patient has been in a restful supine position for 30min and after the patient has stood for 5min. Is performed only occasionally, because diagnosis can normally be made without it.

Advantages/Disadvantages

Advantage: can signal peripheral autonomic failure.

Normal

Basal plasma norepinephrine level 0.9–1.8nmol/L.

Abnormal

Low supine levels, or a <2–3-fold rise in levels after 5min of standing.

Cause of abnormal result

Pure autonomic failure.

Drugs, disorders, and other factors that may alter results

Any stimulation of the patient will increase adrenergic hormones.

Tests of function

VALSALVA RESPONSE

Advantages/Disadvantages

- Advantage: can be performed noninvasively; indicates integrity of the baroreceptor reflex
- Disadvantage: requires appropriate testing facility and is impractical in most settings. Diagnosis can typically be made without test

Normal

- Maneuver involves patient's exhalation against a constant expiratory pressure of about 40mmHg for 15s while continual blood pressure and heart rates are recorded
- Two important phases of the normal response include the initial tachycardia in phase II due to decreased venous return and cardiac output, and the postexhalation brachycardia of phase IV which is mediated by an intact baroreceptor that reacts to the supranormal blood pressure. The Valsalva ratio is the maximum tachycardia in phase II divided by the minimum bradycardia in phase IV

Abnormal

The phase II tachycardia and phase IV hypertension signify an intact autonomic baroreceptor response. Normal ratio is >1.45 in young patients.

Cause of abnormal result

Any disorder in the baroreceptor neural arc.

Drugs, disorders, and other factors that may alter results

Normal ratios vary with age and position. Congestive heart failure, asthma, or emphysema may interfere with results.

SINUS ARRHYTHMIA TEST

Description

Test to evaluate the parasympathetic effect on cardiac rate by having patient breathe deeply (forced vital capacity 1.5L or more) for 1min while monitoring heart rate. Results are contrasted with those of normal age-matched control subjects.

Advantages/Disadvantages

- Advantage: noninvasive test used in patients with orthostatic hypotension and suspected autonomic dysfunction
- Disadvantage: requires appropriate testing facility and is impractical in most settings. Diagnosis can typically be made without test

Normal

Deep breathing typically causes a faster heart rate during inspiration and a slower rate with expiration. If autonomic function is normal, this difference in heart rate is >9 beats/min in the elderly and >15 beats/min in younger patients.

Abnormal

Sinus arrhythmia <9 beats/min in patients over 60 and <15 beats/min in younger patients.

Cause of abnormal result

Abnormality of vagal efferent function.

Drugs, disorders, and other factors that may alter results
Atropine abolishes normal respiratory variation in heart rate.

Special tests

TILT-TABLE TESTING

Description
Test to assess neurocardiogenic syncope by allowing venous pooling when head is tilted up.

Advantages/Disadvantages
- Advantage: used when patient experiences syncope of uncertain cause. Can confirm outpatient diagnosis
- Disadvantage: typically performed in a cardiac testing facility

Normal
Reduction of systolic blood pressure of <20mmHg or diastolic blood pressure of <10mmHg within 3min of resting in a tilt-table in the head-up position, at an angle of at least 60°.

Abnormal
Reduction of systolic blood pressure by at least 20mmHg or diastolic blood pressure by at least 10mmHg within 3min of resting in a tilt-table in the head-up position, at an angle of at least 60°. Lack of increase in heart rate to compensate indicates excessive vagal tone or defective baroreceptor.

Cause of abnormal result
Vasovagal (neurocardiogenic syncope).

Drugs, disorders, and other factors that may alter results
Any drugs or other factors that typically cause orthostatic hypotension.

TREATMENT

PATIENT AND CAREGIVER ISSUES

Patient or caregiver request

- Increased salt intake (10–20g/day) is often helpful; however, many people believe that salt should be avoided
- Some patients mistakenly fear that the drug fludrocortisone is an anabolic steroid

Health-seeking behavior

Have you developed strategies that are helpful in coping with this condition? Examples may be flexing calf muscles and rising extremely slowly to a standing position. Prescription-strength support stockings may also be helpful.

MANAGEMENT ISSUES

Goals

- Identify and alleviate any treatable underlying causes
- Help patient to enhance functionality in daily life, possibly utilizing a combination of medications and nonpharmacologic measures

Management in special circumstances

- Bedridden patients should sit up in bed for short periods of time each day.

COEXISTING DISEASE

- Supine hypertension is common among people with orthostatic hypotension related to autonomic failure. This necessitates caution when administering drugs that may increase blood pressure. Elevating the head of the bed when supine can help to alleviate this problem
- Coexisting coronary disease provides increased cause for treatment, because asymptomatic myocardial ischemia may occur on standing

COEXISTING MEDICATION

Orthostatic hypotension may signal a need to change medications or reduce the dosage of medications for pre-existing conditions. Some of the medications that may cause orthostatic hypotension as a side-effect include: diuretics, phenothiazines, monoamine oxidase inhibitors, tricyclic antidepressants, levodopa, bromocriptine, vasodilators, beta-blockers, calcium channel blockers, nitrates, barbiturates, sildenafil, and some chemotherapeutic agents.

PATIENT SATISFACTION/LIFESTYLE PRIORITIES

Therapy should seek to support patients' lifestyle priorities.

SUMMARY OF THERAPEUTIC OPTIONS

Choices

- First-choice treatment is the removal of any non-neurologic causes of condition, including medication side-effects
- Second-choice treatment is the use of nonpharmacologic aids and lifestyle changes. These include rising slowly, wearing compression stockings, sleeping in a head-up tilt position, avoiding straining, drinking adequate fluids, increasing salt intake, and carrying a collapsible chair
- Third-choice treatment is a combination of nonpharmacologic measures with one or more drugs. Drugs used for this condition include fludrocortisone, midodrine, erythropoietin, and caffeine
- Nonsteroidal anti-inflammatory drugs (NSAIDs) are useful as supplemental therapy with fludrocortisone

Clinical pearl(s)

- Reassess all medications if a patient has orthostatic hypotension
- Rule out secondary causes such as diabetes mellitus
- Nonpharmacologic aids may be quite effective in controlling symptoms of orthostatic hypotension

Never

Never initiate drug therapy without assessing the risk of an exaggerated hypertensive response due to the supine hypertension that often coexists with orthostatic hypotension.

FOLLOW UP

Careful follow up is required in patients who receive drugs to control this condition, by following symptoms and blood pressure readings. Repeating physiologic tests after treatment may be useful if hypotension is due to autonomic dysfunction.

Information for patient or caregiver

Patients can take numerous steps to minimize the impact of this disorder. These include:

- Changes in patterns of movement: rising slowly, flexing calf muscles when standing, standing with one foot placed before the other, avoiding straining, and avoiding strenuous exercise
- Dietary changes: drinking adequate fluids, adding salt to diet (10–20g/day), avoiding alcohol, and eating multiple small meals instead of three large ones

Further measures are to raise the head of the bed, carry a collapsible chair, wear compression stockings, and avoid hot environments, including taking hot showers and baths.

DRUGS AND OTHER THERAPIES: DETAILS

Drugs

FLUDROCORTISONE

This is an off-label indication.

Dose

- Initially, 0.1mg orally once or twice daily
- Dosage may be increased every 1–2 weeks

Efficacy

Potent mineralocorticoid.

Risks/Benefits

Risks:

- Use extreme caution in patients with cardiac disease, congestive heart failure, hypertension, recent myocardial infarction, renal disease, ulcerative colitis, peptic ulcer, or esophagitis
- Use caution in children and the elderly, and in patients with psychosis, seizure disorders, or myasthenia gravis
- Use caution in trauma, severe illness, or surgery
- Do not withdraw medication abruptly

Benefit:

- Increases renal sodium reabsorption and heightens the sensitivity of arterioles to norepinephrine

Side-effects and adverse reactions

- Cardiovascular: hypertension, edema, congestive heart failure, ECG changes
- CNS: dizziness, headache
- Gastrointestinal: nausea, vomiting, anorexia

- Metabolic: fluid imbalance, hypokalemia, metabolic alkalosis, hypernatremia
- Musculoskeletal: cramps, weakness
- Skin: bruising, sweating, hives, rash

Interactions (other drugs)

- Amphotericin B
- Androgens
- Barbiturates
- Cardiac glycosides
- Diuretics (loop and thiazide)
- Dofeltilide
- Nondepolarizing neuromuscular blockers
- NSAIDs
- Phenytoin
- Rifampin

Contraindications

- Systemic fungal infections
- Avoid during pregnancy and breast-feeding

Acceptability to patient

Weight gain, headache, and peripheral edema may reduce compliance.

Follow up plan

Evaluation needed to monitor for heart failure, hypokalemia, and supine hypertension.

Patient and caregiver information

Effectiveness requires increased salt intake and weight gain caused by the expansion of intravascular fluid volume.

MIDODRINE

Dose

- Initially 2.5mg/day
- Increase to a maximum of 30mg/day in two or three divided doses

Efficacy

Drug is a vasopressor that improves vascular tone and elevates blood pressure.

Risks/Benefits

Risks:

- Excessive increase in supine blood pressure
- Use caution in patients with urinary retention problems, diabetes, and renal and hepatic impairment
- Use caution in patients with increased intraocular pressure and glaucoma

Side-effects and adverse reactions

- Cardiovascular: supine and sitting hypertension
- CNS: dizziness, drowsiness, headache, irritability, paresthesia, restlessness
- Gastrointestinal: nausea, vomiting
- Genitourinary: dysuria, urinary retention, and urinary frequency
- Metabolism: increase in body weight
- Skin: pruritus, piloerection

Interactions (other drugs)

- Alpha-adrenergic agonists
- Alpha-adrenergic antagonists
- Cardiac glycosides

Contraindications

- Severe organic heart disease
- Congestive heart failure
- Hypertension
- Acute renal disease
- Acute nephritis
- Pheochromocytoma
- Thyrotoxicosis

Evidence

A blinded randomized controlled trial compared midodrine with placebo in patients with neurogenic orthostatic hypotension. The treatment group had a greater improvement in symptoms and standing systolic blood pressure than the placebo group [3] *Level P*

Acceptability to patient

Drug is a vasopressor that improves vascular tone and elevates blood pressure.

Follow up plan

Supine and standing blood pressure should be regularly monitored weekly at least during several initial weeks.

Patient and caregiver information

Patients should report symptoms that may signal supine hypertension.

ERYTHROPOIETIN

- Epoetin alfa (human recombinant erythropoietin)
- This is an off-label indication

Dose

25–75U/kg, administered subcutaneously three times weekly.

Efficacy

Stimulates red blood cell production in patients who have orthostatic hypotension, anemia, and low serum erythropoietin levels. Take with iron supplementation.

Risks/Benefits

Risks:

- May cause hypertension
- Use caution in patients with severe anemia and seizure disorder

Side-effects and adverse reactions

- Cardiovascular: hypertension, tachycardia, edema
- CNS: headache, seizures, fatigue
- Gastrointestinal: diarrhea, nausea, vomiting
- Metabolism: iron deficiency, hyperkalemia
- Musculoskeletal: arthralgia, myalgia
- Respiratory: shortness of breath
- Skin: stinging at injection site

Interactions (other drugs)

- No known drug interactions.

Contraindications

- Uncontrolled hypertension
- Hypersensitivity to mammalian-derived products or to human albumin

Evidence

Patients with orthostatic hypotension were treated with erythropoietin for 6–10 weeks in a small prospective trial. Erythropoietin increased the standing systolic and diastolic blood pressure. The average supine blood pressure was not increased, although three of the eight patients developed supine hypertension. Symptoms of orthostatic dizziness improved in six patients. Long-term effects are not known [4] *This trial does not meet the criteria for level P*

Acceptability to patient

Patients should not drive during the first 90 days of treatment.

Follow up plan

- Monitor for hypertension
- Monitor for rise in hematocrit

Patient and caregiver information

Should be prepared to report signs of hypertension and signals of possibly impending seizures.

CAFFEINE

Dose

250mg (two cups) with meals.

Efficacy

Reduces postprandial hypotension.

Risks/Benefits

Risks:

- Use caution in patients with nervousness, insomnia, and depression
- Use caution in patients with dysrythmias, ulcers, and diabetes mellitus

Benefit:

- Reduces postprandial hypotension

Side-effects and adverse reactions

- Cardiovascular: dysrhythmias, palpitations, tachycardia
- CNS: insomnia, hyperactivity, dizziness
- Gastrointestinal: anorexia, diarrhea, gastric irritation, nausea, vomiting
- Genitourinary: diuresis
- Metabolism: hyperglycemia
- Skin: hyperesthesia

Interactions (other drugs)

- Beta-adrenergic agents ▪ Cimetidine ▪ Clozapine ▪ Contraceptives ▪ Disulfiram ▪ Fluoroquinolones ▪ Fluconazole ▪ Mexiletine ▪ Phenylpropanolamine ▪ Phenytoin ▪ Pipemidic acid ▪ Terbinafine ▪ Theophylline

Contraindications

- Cardiac arrhythmias and palpitations

Acceptability to patient

Good.

Follow up plan

Check with physician about results.

Patient and caregiver information

Patients should be encouraged to try caffeine but to be prepared to discontinue it if adverse effects occur, as may sometimes happen in patients with neurally mediated hypotension.

NSAIDS

NSAID: indomethacin. Non-FDA-approved use.

Dose
25–50mg 2–4 times daily, not to exceed 200mg/day.

Efficacy
Useful as supplemental therapy with fludrocortisone by possibly reducing levels of the vasodilator prostaglandin.

Risks/Benefits
Risks:
- Use caution in patients with hepatic and cardiac failure, epilepsy, psychiatric disorders, parkinsonism, and bleeding disorders
- Use caution in patients who are pregnant and breast-feeding

Benefit:
- Potentiates fludrocortisone therapy

Side-effects and adverse reactions
- Cardiovascular: cardiac abnormalities, congestive heart failure
- CNS: headache, dizziness, tinnitus, somnolence
- Gastrointestinal: anorexia, nausea, vomiting, abdominal pain, diarrhea, constipation, dyspepsia, peptic ulceration, gastritis, gastrointestinal bleeding
- Genitourinary: renal dysfunction, hyperuricemia
- Hematologic: blood cell disorders
- Hypersensitivity: rashes, bronchospasm, angioedema

Interactions (other drugs)
■ Aminoglycosides ■ Anticoagulants ■ Antidiabetics ■ Antihypertensives ■ Baclofen ■ Corticosteroids ■ Cidofovir ■ Cyclosporine, tacrolimus ■ Digoxin ■ Diuretics ■ Ethanol ■ Gentamicin ■ Haloperidol ■ Lithium ■ Methotrexate ■ Phenylpropanolamine ■ Probenecid ■ Triamterene ■ Vancomycin ■ Warfarin

Contraindications
■ Severe renal, hepatic, or cardiac disease ■ Hypertension ■ Peptic ulceration, gastrointestinal bleeding, ulcerative colitis ■ Hypersensitivity to NSAIDs ■ Coagulation defects ■ Untreated infection ■ Thrombocytopenia ■ Cidofovir

Follow up plan
Check with physician about results.

Other therapies
COMPRESSION STOCKINGS
Efficacy
Prevent venous pooling.

Risks/Benefits
Benefit: prevents venous pooling in the legs and compress the abdomen; particularly effective if the stockings are waist-high.

Acceptability to patient
Regular users grow comfortable with them. Can be time-consuming to put on initially. May be hot and uncomfortable, particularly if they are waist-high.

Patient and caregiver information

Patient should be told to avoid wearing stockings during sleep.

LIFESTYLE

A variety of lifestyle changes may be helpful. These include:

- Raising the head of the bed
- Rising slowly when standing up
- Flexing calves when standing
- Standing with one foot in front of the other
- Avoiding straining, strenuous exercise, and alcohol
- Avoiding hot environments, including hot showers and baths
- Increasing fluid intake and salt intake
- Eating several small meals instead of three large ones

RISKS/BENEFITS

Benefits:

- Contraction of leg muscles helps pump blood back to the heart
- Elevating the bed helps the body retain fluid at night
- Increased salt intake also helps with fluid retention
- Reducing the size of meals can avert postprandial hypotension

ACCEPTABILITY TO PATIENT

Patients may need to be persistent to continue with some of these measures.

PATIENT AND CAREGIVER INFORMATION

Patients should understand why lifestyle changes may be beneficial.

EFFICACY OF THERAPIES

Outcome depends on the cause of the condition.

Evidence

- PDxMD is unable to cite evidence that meets our criteria for evidence for most therapies used in orthostatic hypotension
- Midodrine was shown in one randomized controlled trial to improve symptoms and increase standing systolic blood pressure in patients with neurogenic orthostatic hypotension [3] *Level P*

PROGNOSIS

- Dependent on underlying cause
- If cause is neurologic, condition may be chronic

Clinical pearl(s)

- Orthostatic hypotension can result from medication use or a number of medical or neurologic disorders
- Medications and nonpharmacologic aids may need to be used in combination to minimize the symptoms
- The goal of therapy is to decrease the frequency and severity of the symptoms, and to prevent syncope

COMPLICATIONS

- Injuries from accidental falls
- Ischemic organ injury caused by hypoperfusion

CONSIDER CONSULT

Patients should be referred if they have signs of more pervasive neurologic disorders or if, after reversing potential causes such as dehydration, patients remain symptomatic despite lifestyle modification.

PREVENTION

Orthostatic hypotension is not specifically preventable.

PREVENT RECURRENCE

- For causes other than neurogenic, avoid the conditions that caused the initial condition (e.g. dehydration, salt-free diet)
- Neurogenic disease tends to be chronic. Symptoms can be lessened but not entirely prevented

ASSOCIATIONS

National Organization for Rare Disorders
P.O. Box 8923
New Fairfield, CT 06812-8923
Tel: (800) 999-6673
http://www.rarediseases.org

KEY REFERENCES

- Engstrom JW, Aminoff MJ. Evaluation and treatment of orthostatic hypotension. Am Fam Physician 1997;56:1378–84
- Mathias CJ. Orthostatic hypotension: causes, mechanisms, and influencing factors. Neurology 1995;45:(4 Suppl 5):S6–11
- The Consensus Committee of the American Autonomic Society and the American Academy of Neurology. Consensus statement on the definition of orthostatic hypotension, pure autonomic failure, and multiple system atrophy. Neurology 1996;46(5):1470
- Neurally Mediated Hypotension Working Group, Johns Hopkins Hospital. General information brochure on neurally mediated hypotension and its treatment. Available online: http://www.med.jhu.edu (Note: this is a good reference for patients, and possibly useful for doctors)
- Onrot J, Goldberg MR, Hollister AS, et al. Management of chronic orthostatic hypotension. Am J Med 1986;80(3):454–64

Evidence references and guidelines

1 Consensus Committee of the American Autonomic Society and the American Academy of Neurology. Consensus statement on the definition of orthostatic hypotension, pure autonomic failure, and multiple system atrophy. Neurology 1996;46(5):1470.

2 Engstrom JW, Aminoff MJ. Evaluation and treatment of orthostatic hypotension. Am Fam Physician 1997;56:1378–84

3 Low PA, Gilden JL, Freeman R, et al. Efficacy of midodrine vs placebo in neurogenic orthostatic hypotension. A randomized, double-blind multicenter study. Midodrine Study Group. JAMA 1997;277:1046–51. Medline

4 Hoeldtke, RD, Streeten DH. Treatment of orthostatic hypotension with erythropoietin. N Engl J Med 1993;329:611–5. Medline

FAQS

Question 1

When should I refer to a specialist?

ANSWER 1

Refer to a specialist if the patient has persistent symptoms despite initial nonpharmacologic aids (e.g. increased fluids, increased salt) and initial medications (fludrocortisone), or if a neurologic etiology is suspected.

Question 2

What is the most common cause of orthostatic hypotension?

ANSWER 2

Hypovolemia.

Question 3

What initial laboratory work should be done in a patient presenting with orthostatic hypotension?

ANSWER 3

A complete blood count and chemistry panel are very helpful to look for anemia, electrolyte derangements, and as an index of volume status.

CONTRIBUTORS

Kathleen M O'Hanlon, MD
John McB Hodgson, MD, FACC, FSCAI
Benjamin M Scirica, MD

PERICARDITIS

SUMMARY INFORMATION

DESCRIPTION

- Inflammatory or infective disease of the pericardial sac, which may be acute or chronic
- The acute form typically presents with chest pain relieved by leaning forward, a pathognomonic friction rub, and widespread ST-segment elevation on ECG
- The chronic form is insidious, painless, characterized by dyspnea and fatigue, and accompanied by signs of right and/or left heart failure

URGENT ACTION

Sudden development of cardiac tamponade (classic triad of raised jugular venous pressure, pulsus paradoxus, and hypotension) is a surgical emergency.

KEY! DON'T MISS!

Do not mistake the signs and symptoms of developing cardiac tamponade (hypotension, pulsus paradoxus, and raised jugular venous pressure) for right heart failure.

BACKGROUND

ICD9 CODE
- 420 Acute pericarditis
- 420.9 Other and unspecified acute pericarditis

SYNONYMS
Myopericarditis.

CARDINAL FEATURES
Acute pericarditis:
- Central chest pain radiating to the neck and shoulders, particularly to the left
- Pericardial friction rub (pathognomonic), best heard with patient leaning forward in expiration
- Characteristic ECG changes of widespread concave-upward ST-segment elevation not corresponding to a coronary artery territory

Chronic pericarditis:
- Chronic inflammation of the pericardium, which is often asymptomatic until a large pericardial effusion or the onset of pericardial constriction causes hemodynamic compromise

CAUSES
Common causes
- Viral: coxsackievirus and echovirus
- Early after myocardial infarction: up to 20% of patients with transmural acute myocardial infarction develop clinical signs of pericarditis at 2–4 days postinfarct, often associated with low-grade fever. This is usually self-limiting and clinically not significant
- Late postmyocardial infarction pericarditis (Dressler's syndrome): now disputed as a separate entity and regarded as a severe, prolonged form of early postmyocardial infarction pericarditis
- Uremia: up to 20% of uremic patients develop signs of pericarditis, particularly in the first 3 months of dialysis; one-fifth will go on to develop cardiac tamponade
- Metastatic disease: most commonly breast, lung, leukemia, Hodgkin's lymphoma
- Post-traumatic: e.g. after blunt chest injury or cardiac surgery
- Postsurgical: e.g. after cardiac surgery
- Postradiation: 5% of patients develop pericarditis, particularly after radiotherapy for breast cancer and Hodgkin's lymphoma
- Chronic water and salt retention states, such as heart failure, hepatic cirrhosis
- Tuberculosis: present in 1–2% of patients with tuberculosis and may not be associated with signs of pulmonary tuberculosis
- HIV: multiple pathogeneses, including tuberculosis, fungal infection, viral infection, and Kaposi's sarcoma
- Idiopathic: many cases of viral pericarditis in which serologic confirmation of the causative organism has not been obtained will fall into this group

Rare causes
- Drugs (hydralazine, procainamide, methysergide, isoniazid, anticoagulants)
- Connective tissue disease: rheumatoid arthritis (17% of patients within 3 years of diagnosis); systemic lupus erythematosus (SLE; 50% of patients at some stage in the disease); ankylosing spondylitis, Reiter's disease, panarteritis nodosa
- Familial Mediterranean fever (familial recurrent polyserositis)
- Bacterial pericarditis due to *Staphylococcus* or *Haemophilus influenzae*, particularly in children with septic arthritis
- Fungal pericarditis, endemic histoplasmosis, and coccidioidomycosis
- Myxedema
- Primary pericardial tumors (extremely rare)

Serious causes
- Purulent pericarditis after pericardiocentesis, surgery, penetrating trauma, and immunosuppression
- Hemorrhagic pericarditis after aortic dissection

Contributory or predisposing factors
Previous acute pericarditis is a predisposing factor to chronic pericarditis.

EPIDEMIOLOGY
Incidence and prevalence
- True incidence in nonselected population is unknown
- Approximately 6% of patients have signs of pericarditis at autopsy
- Hospital diagnosis for pericarditis accounts for approximately 1/1000 admissions

Demographics
AGE

More common in adults.

GENDER

More common in males.

RACE

Tuberculous pericarditis is more common in African-Americans with HIV infection.

GEOGRAPHY
- Histoplasmosis pericarditis is endemic in Mississippi and Ohio river valleys and in Western Appalachian Mountains
- Coccidioidomycosis pericarditis is endemic in the southwest US and Argentina

DIAGNOSIS

DIFFERENTIAL DIAGNOSIS

Acute myocardial infarction

Acute myocardial infarction is the most important differential diagnosis for acute pericarditis.

FEATURES

- Acute crushing central chest pain radiating to jaw and/or arms
- Often associated with systemic symptoms of sweating, nausea, and breathlessness
- ECG changes of convex upwards ST-segment elevation

Dissection of thoracic aorta

- Aortic dissection is a rare but important differential diagnosis for acute pericarditis
- In its acute form, dissection of the thoracic aorta is a catastrophic event associated with cardiovascular collapse
- More protracted forms with slow leakage of blood retrograde into the pericardial sac may present with symptoms of pericarditis
- Patients with atypical history for either myocardial infarction or pericarditis should have diagnostic imaging to exclude the diagnosis

FEATURES

- Severe chest pain radiating between shoulder blades
- Cardiovascular collapse
- ECG may or may not show myocardial ischemia, depending on whether the origin of the coronary arteries is involved in the dissection
- Chest X-ray shows mediastinal widening in 90% of cases

Pleurisy

All causes of pleuritic chest pain are a potential differential diagnosis to acute pericarditis that presents with predominantly pleuritic chest pain. Careful history to exclude pulmonary causes is mandatory.

FEATURES

- No pericardial rub
- Productive or nonproductive cough
- Shortness of breath
- Tachypnea
- Physical signs of lung disease on auscultation

Musculoskeletal chest pain

Precipitating event in history. Pain can be reproduced by direct pressure over affected muscle group.

Left and right ventricular failure

Owing to its varying pathophysiology (constrictive, constrictive-effusive, effusive) and its insidious onset, chronic pericarditis may mimic almost any cause of left- and right-sided cardiac failure. Although rare, it should be considered in patients with known predisposing factors.

FEATURES

- Pump failure (ischemic heart disease, cardiomyopathy)
- Left ventricular outflow obstruction (aortic stenosis, subvalvular aortic stenosis)
- Left atrial outflow obstruction (mitral valve stenosis)

- Right heart outflow obstruction (pulmonary hypertension due to chronic lung disease, recurrent pulmonary emboli, pulmonary valve disease)
- Right atrial outflow obstruction (tricuspid valve disease, atrial myxoma)
- Right atrial inflow obstruction (superior vena cava obstruction)

SIGNS & SYMPTOMS

Signs

Acute pericarditis:

- Pathognomonic: pericardial friction rub that is best heard with patient leaning forward in expiration

Chronic pericarditis:

- Signs of pulmonary venous congestion (dyspnea and pleural effusion)
- Signs mimicking right heart failure (raised jugular venous pressure, hepatomegaly, and peripheral edema)
- Tachycardia
- Kussmaul's sign (marked swelling of the neck veins during inspiration)
- Pulsus paradoxus
- Atrial fibrillation
- Friedreich's sign (sharp diastolic collapsing jugular venous pressure), absent apex beat, and soft heart sounds (due to effusion)

Purulent pericarditis:

- Severely ill
- High, swinging fever

Cardiac tamponade:

- Hypotension
- Pulsus paradoxus
- Tachycardia
- Raised jugular venous pressure
- Signs of right heart failure

Symptoms

Acute pericarditis:

- Systemic symptoms of viral infection
- Central chest pain radiating to either side of the neck into the trapezius muscles, often aggravated by deep inspiration

Chronic pericarditis:

- The hallmark of chronic pericarditis is the onset of dyspnea; other symptoms depend on the degree of reduction of cardiac output and pulmonary and systemic venous pressure
- Dyspnea
- Orthopnea
- Dizziness
- Progressive reduction in exercise tolerance
- Fatigue
- Weakness
- Ankle swelling

Purulent pericarditis:

- Severely ill
- High, swinging fever

Cardiac tamponade:
- Extreme fatigue
- Sweating
- Shortness of breath

KEY! DON'T MISS!
Do not mistake the signs and symptoms of developing cardiac tamponade (hypotension, pulsus paradoxus, and raised jugular venous pressure) for right heart failure.

CONSIDER CONSULT
- All patients with hypotension (may be developing cardiac tamponade)
- All patients in whom differential diagnosis cannot clearly be excluded (particularly if acute myocardial infarction cannot be ruled out)
- All patients with recurrent pericarditis (require investigation for underlying causes)
- All patients who are on anticoagulant medication for known underlying disease (mechanical heart valves, after thromboembolism): such patients are at a higher risk for acute hemorrhagic pericarditis with cardiac tamponade
- All patients who are clinically unwell or known to be immunocompromised (the main risk is missing a clinically silent, tuberculin-negative, tuberculous pericarditis)
- All patients with known malignancies: 50% will not have a pericarditis due to the malignancy, and establishing exact diagnosis is mandatory before commencing treatment
- All children with acute pericarditis (the most common causes all require specialist investigation and treatment)
- Even presumed viral and idiopathic pericarditis has a 1:7 risk of developing cardiac tamponade, and referral should be considered when patient presents with signs of hemodynamic compromise or with moderate to large pericardial effusion. Patients managed in the community must be monitored closely for signs of developing cardiac tamponade

INVESTIGATION OF THE PATIENT
Direct questions to patient
Acute pericarditis:
- **Q** **Do you have any chest pain?** Cardinal symptom of acute pericarditis
- **Q** **Does the chest pain go anywhere?** Radiation to either side of the neck into the trapezius muscles is a typical sign of pericardial pain; unlike ischemic pain, pericardial pain rarely radiates down the left arm
- **Q** **Does the chest pain get any better when you lean forward?** Pericardial pain is typically relieved by leaning forward and aggravated by leaning backward
- **Q** **Does the pain get any worse when you breathe in?** Pleuritic-type chest pain is common in pericardial disease
- **Q** **Do you get any palpitations?** Cardiac arrhythmias are normally a sign of underlying cardiac disease
- **Q** **Do you get short of breath?** Dyspnea is partly due to pleuritic chest pain
- **Q** **Did you travel recently to Ohio, Mississippi, the US southwest, or Argentina?** Consider rarer forms of histoplasmosis pericarditis and coccidioidomycosis pericarditis specific to endemic areas

Constrictive pericarditis:
- **Q** **Do your ankles swell up?** Signs of systemic venous congestion are usually present and appear before signs of pulmonary venous congestion
- **Q** **Do you get short of breath? Can you lie flat?** Signs of pulmonary venous congestions appear when left heart filling pressures start to rise; this is particularly relevant in suspected chronic pericarditis with cardiac tamponade
- **Q** **Have you been feeling very tired and listless recently?** This may indicate onset of persistently reduced cardiac output in cardiac tamponade

Contributory or predisposing factors

- **Q Have you had flu-like symptoms recently?** Viral pericarditis is often preceded by flu-like illness
- **Q Have you hurt your chest recently?** Exclude post-traumatic pericarditis, particularly after road traffic accidents with chest impact on steering wheel
- **Q Have you had a heart attack?** Exclude postmyocardial infarction pericarditis
- **Q Have you felt unwell generally? Lost weight? Lost your appetite?** Nonspecific signs of underlying systemic illness
- **Q Have you had a cough recently? Did you bring up phlegm? Was it bloodstained?** Nonspecific signs of possible underlying cancer or tuberculosis
- **Q Have you noticed any lumps in your breast?** Exclude undiagnosed breast cancer
- **Q Do you get any joint pains? Have you had a rash?** Common manifestation of connective tissue diseases
- **Q Do you practise safe sex? Do you inject drugs?** Look for risk factors for HIV infection
- **Q Have you had symptoms like this before?** Constrictive pericarditis usually follows an episode of acute pericarditis, although it may not have been diagnosed at the time
- **Q Have you had tuberculosis?** Tuberculosis can cause constrictive pericarditis

Family history

- **Q Does anyone in the family have tuberculosis?** Identify high-risk patient groups who may require tuberculin testing.

Examination

- **Is the patient generally well?** Patients with chronic tamponade and bacterial pericarditis are usually unwell
- **Listen for pericardial friction rub:** scratchy sound best heard on the left sternal border with patient leaning forward after expiration (this is pathognomonic for acute pericarditis but will be absent in chronic or constrictive pericarditis)
- **Check blood pressure:** hypotension below 100mmHg systolic is suggestive of tamponade or severe constrictive pericarditis
- **Check for enlarged lymph nodes:** indicates metastatic disease
- **Look for signs of systemic venous congestion:** indicates hemodynamically significant pericardial effusions
- **Look for signs of pulmonary venous congestion:** indicates pericardial constriction, due either to constrictive pericarditis or large effusion
- **Check for pulsus paradoxus:** this is an exaggeration of the normal fall in systolic blood pressure during inspiration; values of >15mmHg are abnormal and may indicate tamponade

Summary of investigative tests

- Full blood count: nonspecific screening test useful for monitoring the course of acute pericarditis and the activity of underlying disease
- Serum blood urea nitrogen and/or creatinine: nonspecific screening test indicated to exclude uremia
- Creatinine kinase MB fraction: indicated to exclude acute myocardial infarction in acute pericarditis
- Cardiac troponins: indicated to exclude myocardial infarction in acute pericarditis
- ECG: indicated in all cases of suspected pericarditis
- Chest X-ray: in chronic pericarditis, there may be a large globular shadow with sharp outlines. It may give clues to underlying pathology (tuberculous calcification, neoplasms)
- Viral serology: indicated in initial stages of pericarditis in which the differential diagnosis is not yet clear
- Antinuclear antibodies and rheumatoid factor: indicated in patients who have pointers in the history toward underlying collagen vascular disease

- Echocardiography: 'gold standard' for the diagnosis of pericardial effusion and investigation of choice in the differential diagnosis of chronic pericarditis. Mandatory prior to pericardiocentesis
- Computed tomography and magnetic resonance imaging and MRI scans (normally ordered by cardiologist) are alternatives to echocardiography if results are inconclusive or suggest structural abnormalities of the pericardium (metastases, constrictive pericarditis)
- Gallium-67 or indium-111 leukocyte nuclear scans (normally ordered by cardiologist) are useful to confirm purulent pericardial effusions before surgery
- Pericardiocentesis (normally performed by specialist) is useful in diagnosing underlying causes, particularly for tuberculous and purulent pericarditis. It can be combined with pericardial biopsy
- Cardiac catheterization (normally ordered by specialist), although invasive, provides objective confirmation of cardiac tamponade and the degree of its hemodynamic significance. It also confirms the presence of coexisting hemodynamically important factors (cardiomyopathies, coronary heart disease) that will not be relieved by decompression of the pericardial sac
- Pericardioscopy is still a new technique and may prove useful to determine macroscopic alterations of the pericardium

DIAGNOSTIC DECISION

- The diagnosis of acute pericarditis rests on the combination of the typical history, the detection of a pericardial friction rub, and typical changes on ECG. Patients should be admitted to hospital or referred urgently for investigation to a cardiologist depending on their clinical condition. If symptoms abate within 1–3 weeks and serious underlying illness has been ruled out, it is safe to assume a viral or idiopathic etiology
- Patients with acute pericarditis who have pointers in the history toward underlying causes and patients with recurrence require a more aggressive diagnostic approach
- The diagnosis of chronic pericarditis (constrictive and effusive) is clinically very difficult, and requires investigation to prove the diagnosis. It should be suspected in patients with known causes or predisposing factors for pericarditis who develop dyspnea and signs of cardiac failure, regardless of whether the history of an index episode can be elicited. Echocardiography is the investigation of choice; depending on the result, more invasive diagnostic tests, including cardiac catheterization and open pericardial biopsy, may be indicated
- Purulent pericarditis, if undiagnosed, is rapidly fatal and its poor prognosis is largely due to failure to consider the diagnosis. It should be suspected in immunocompromised and debilitated patients who develop signs of sepsis with no clinically identifiable focus
- Cardiac tamponade is a complication of all forms of pericarditis at any stage of the disease. The diagnosis can be suspected in the presence of the triad of hypotension, raised jugular venous pressure, and pulsus paradoxus. In practice, it is difficult to distinguish the syndrome from cardiogenic shock, however, and echocardiography is required to confirm the presence of fluid

Guidelines

- Information on pericarditis is available from the American Academy of Family Physicians: Marinella M. Electrocardiographic manifestations and differential diagnosis of acute pericarditis. Am Fam Physician 1998;57:699–704

CLINICAL PEARL(S)

- Cardiac tamponade requires immediate echocardiography and pericardiocentesis
- Echocardiography is a key test for all patients with suspected pericarditis

THE TESTS

Body fluids

CREATINE KINASE MB FRACTION

Description

Venous blood sample.

Advantages/Disadvantages

Advantages:

- Routine test
- Easy to collect

Normal

5ng/mL.

Abnormal

- Value above the normal reference range but usually only a small elevation above normal and much less than in a patient with a large ST-segment elevation myocardial infarction
- A raised level may be seen in both acute pericarditis with myocardial involvement and myocardial infarction
- Keep in mind the possibility of a false-positive result

Cause of abnormal result

- Pericarditis with myocardial involvement
- Acute myocardial infarction

FULL BLOOD COUNT

Description

Venous sample.

Advantages/Disadvantages

Advantages:

- Routine test
- Inexpensive
- Useful for monitoring

Disadvantage: Nondiagnostic screening test.

Normal

- Red cell count: 4.3–5.5x10^{12}/L
- White cell count: 3.5–11x10^9/L
- Platelet count: 150–400x10^9/L

Abnormal

- Values outside the normal reference range
- Keep in mind the possibility of a falsely abnormal result

Cause of abnormal result

- All causes and predisposing factors to pericarditis
- Abnormal results can occur with any infectious or inflammatory disease process

SERUM BLOOD UREA NITROGEN AND CREATININE

Description

Venous sample.

Advantages/Disadvantages

Advantages:

- Routine test
- Inexpensive
- Reliably excludes uremia as underlying cause

Normal

- Blood urea nitrogen: 8–18mg/dL (3–6.5mcmol/L)
- Serum creatinine: 0.6–1.2mg/dL (120–400mcmol/L)

Abnormal

Values outside normal reference range.

Cause of abnormal result

- Dehydration
- Uremia

CARDIAC TROPONINS

Description

Venous sample taken 6–72h after onset of symptoms.

Advantages/Disadvantages

Advantage: emerging standard in diagnosis of myocardial ischemia and infarction.

Normal

Value below reference range of laboratory.

Abnormal

- Value above the normal reference range but usually only a small elevation above normal and much less than in a patient with a large ST-segment elevation myocardial infarction
- May be positive in pericarditis with myocardial involvement

Cause of abnormal result

- Myocardial damage
- Keep in mind the possibility of a false-negative result, particularly if the sample was not taken within the timespan in which troponin levels rise

VIRAL SEROLOGY

Description

Venous sample; two specimens 6 weeks apart.

Advantages/Disadvantages

Advantage: Simple specimen collection.

Disadvantages:

- Requires at least two specimens
- Only provides retrospective diagnosis

Normal

Absence of pathogenic viral titers.

Abnormal

Significant rise in viral titers between samples proves infection in interim.

Cause of abnormal result

Infection with organism tested in interim.

ANTINUCLEAR ANTIBODIES AND RHEUMATOID FACTOR

Description

Venous sample. Positive results should be followed up with more specific autoantibody testing.

Advantages/Disadvantages

Advantages:

- Simple specimen collection
- Most helpful result is a negative one because it virtually excludes active autoimmune disease

Disadvantage: A positive result does not mean a patient has autoimmune disease or rheumatoid arthritis.

Normal

Values below the reference range for laboratory and test.

Abnormal

- Positive antinuclear antibody (ANA) and rheumatoid factor (RF) titers
- Keep in mind the possibility of a false-positive result (the underlying diseases are rare)

Cause of abnormal result

Positive ANA and RF titers are relatively nonspecific and can be found in many rheumatologic diseases, as well as in chronic infection and chronic pulmonary, hepatic, and renal disease. The interpretation of a positive ANA depends also on the specific pattern seen, with a peripheral, or 'rim', pattern more indicative of the presence of antibodies against double-stranded DNA.

Causes of abnormal results include the following:

- Active autoimmune disease
- Chronic infection
- Chronic hepatic, renal, and pulmonary diseases
- The administration of certain drugs: procainamide, hydralazine, quinidine

Imaging

ECHOCARDIOGRAPHY

Advantages/Disadvantages

Advantages:

- Gold standard technique to demonstrate pericardial effusion
- May be normal in acute pericarditis with only fibrinous exudate
- Noninvasive, relatively inexpensive

Normal

Absence of fluid excludes pericardial effusion.

Abnormal

- The presence of echolucent area adjacent to cardiac structures
- If tamponade is present, right atrial collapse until late into systole, right ventricular filling, and septal wall motion toward the left ventricle during inspiration, dilated inferior vena cava
- Keep in mind the possibility of a falsely abnormal result

Cause of abnormal result

- Pericardial effusion
- Impeded atrial and left ventricular filling due to pericardial fluid or constriction; augmentation of right heart filling with inspiration

CHEST X-RAY

Advantages/Disadvantages

Advantages:

- Noninvasive, relatively inexpensive, low radiation exposure
- May provide clues to underlying causes

Disadvantages:

- Of little use in viral and idiopathic pericarditis
- Does not demonstrate hemodynamic impact of pericardial effusion or constrictive pericarditis
- A large heart shadow does not prove pericardial effusion, and a small heart shadow does not exclude it

Abnormal

- May show pericardial calcification, pleural effusion, metastatic deposits, pulmonary congestion, enlarged heart
- No individual finding is diagnostic, and any abnormality must be interpreted in the light of the clinical picture (i.e. the presence of pericardial calcification does not prove constrictive pericarditis, nor does its absence exclude it)

Other tests

ECG

Advantages/Disadvantages

Advantages:

- Noninvasive
- Relatively inexpensive

Disadvantages:

- If normal, may require serial use to demonstrate the typical abnormalities
- Abnormal findings can mimic other cardiac abnormalities: conduction delays, myocardial ischemia, myocardial infarction

Abnormal

ECG is abnormal in about 90% of cases of acute pericarditis. Changes typically occur in four phases:

- Phase 1: diffuse, concave, upward ST elevation in all leads except aVR and V1, which have reciprocal ST-segment depression
- Phase 2: ST-segment changes revert to normal and T waves flatten, giving at times a normal ECG
- Phase 3: deep symmetric inversion of T waves throughout
- Phase 4: normal ECG

Other ECG signs include:

- Depression of PR interval (all leads except aVR and V1), if present, is typical of pericarditis
- Arrhythmias are a sign of underlying cardiac disease
- Electric alternans (variation of height of QRS complex) is typically seen in pericardial effusion

TREATMENT

CONSIDER CONSULT

- All patients should be admitted for assessment and treatment if they are acutely unwell, if they are relatively well and the diagnosis is in doubt, if they present with moderate to severe pericardial effusion, or if they present with hemodynamic compromise

IMMEDIATE ACTION

Clinical suspicion of cardiac tamponade is an indication for urgent referral.

MANAGEMENT ISSUES

Goals

- Diagnose and manage underlying causes
- Provide symptomatic relief for pain and fever
- Diagnose and treat cardiac tamponade promptly

Management in special circumstances

COEXISTING DISEASE

- Postmyocardial infarction and postsurgery pericarditis often necessitate corticosteroids for pain management and to aid resolution
- Pericarditis in uremia should be treated with a vigorous course of dialysis, which is usually sufficient to promote resolution of the pericardial effusion
- Pericardial effusion in severe hypothyroidism does not necessarily imply pericarditis, particularly if the lung fields show congestion. The effusion resolves if underlying cardiac failure and hypothyroidism are treated
- Pericardial effusion in the presence of any form of malignancy will require referral in order to establish the cause (infective due to immunosuppression, direct involvement due to metastatic disease, differentiation from superior vena cava obstruction) before commencing treatment
- Despite advances in chemotherapy, tuberculous pericarditis has a mortality rate of up to 50%, and patients should be hospitalized for treatment. In addition to the normal drug regimen for tuberculosis, this may include surgical drainage. Suggested treatment is with isoniazid 300mg/day with pyridoxine 50mg/day for 9 months, and another drug, either rifampin 600mg/day or ethambutol 50mg/kg/day. There is at present insufficient evidence to support the routine use of corticosteroids for pericarditis of confirmed tuberculous origin
- Pericarditis in immunocompromised or debilitated patients should always raise the suspicion of tuberculous pericarditis, even if tuberculin test is negative. Referral for investigation is indicated in all cases

COEXISTING MEDICATION

- Anticoagulants are relatively contraindicated in acute and chronic pericarditis due to the risk of hemorrhage into the pericardial sac. If anticoagulation is required (mechanical heart valves, previous pulmonary embolus), referral to a cardiologist for risk/benefit in the specific circumstance is recommended
- The exception is postmyocardial infarction pericarditis, where anticoagulation may be desired for infarct management

SPECIAL PATIENT GROUPS

- In pregnant women, asymptomatic pericardial effusion is a well described entity, and the presence of a pericardial effusion does not imply pericarditis
- Pericarditis in children is extremely rare, is often bacterial in origin, has a higher mortality rate than in adults, and more often requires surgical intervention for drainage of pus
- Patients with known cancer and echocardiographically proven pericardial effusion should not be assumed to have malignant pericarditis: some 50% of patients have other causes. These patients benefit from referral for full evaluation

SUMMARY OF THERAPEUTIC OPTIONS

Choices

- Acute viral, idiopathic, and postmyocardial infarction forms of pericarditis are benign, self-limiting diseases; in the absence of contraindications, aspirin, indomethacin, or nonsteroidal anti-inflammatory drugs (NSAIDs) are the first-choice treatments to control symptoms of pain and fever
- If aspirin, indomethacin, or NSAIDs are insufficient to control symptoms, then a short course of corticosteroids may provide symptomatic relief
- There is increasing evidence that colchicine is effective in preventing recurrent pericarditis
- Pericardiocentesis is required for relief of cardiac tamponade. This may be carried out through needle or catheter aspiration under echocardiographic control or surgically as a pericardiotomy (performed by a specialist)
- Purulent pericarditis is managed surgically with pericardiocentesis, with or without indwelling catheter for lavage (performed by a specialist)
- Open pericardiotomy with pericardiectomy is reserved for all but the most refractory cases of recurrent pericarditis with hemodynamically compromising pericardial effusions and intractable low cardiac output states of constrictive pericarditis (performed by a specialist)

Clinical pearl(s)

- For viral/idiopathic pericarditis with evidence of tamponade or some hemodynamic compromise, a single diagnostic pericardiocentesis is needed
- Patients with malignant effusions usually require a more definitive surgical drainage after the initial tap

Never

- Never attempt blind pericardiocentesis to drain a presumed cardiac tamponade in the community unless the patient is moribund and unlikely to reach the nearest emergency room alive (and even then, remember that the condition is very difficult to distinguish clinically from cardiogenic shock). The procedure carries high morbidity and mortality rates due to lacerations of lung and cardiac structures
- Blind pericardiocentesis should be reserved for use in the resuscitation room within the framework of resuscitation protocols or carried out by a trained interventional cardiologist using fluoroscopy-guided pericardiocentesis

FOLLOW UP

Plan for review

Acute pericarditis, in 80% of cases, is a benign, self-limiting disease. Patients should be asked to report back if symptoms have not settled on treatment after 48h and be instructed to report back immediately if symptoms of breathlessness and increasing fatigue develop.

Information for patient or caregiver

- Patients should be informed that progressive dyspnea may indicate progression of pericarditis and development of tamponade
- Risk of recurrence of pericarditis after an acute episode is 15–32%

DRUGS AND OTHER THERAPIES: DETAILS

Drugs

ASPIRIN (OTC)

Dose

Up to 650mg every 4h, not exceeding 4g/day.

Efficacy

Effectively controls pain and reduces the pericardial inflammation of acute pericarditis.

Risks/Benefits

Risks:

- Use caution in anemia, Hodgkin's disease, gout, hepatic and renal disease, asthma, nasal polyps, nasal allergies
- Use caution with children and teenagers (Reye's syndrome)

Benefits:

- Inexpensive, readily available, and generally well tolerated
- Simple dosing regimen allows for better patient compliance

Side-effects and adverse reactions

- Gastrointestinal: abdominal pain, nausea, dyspepsia, hepatotoxicity, gastrointestinal bleeding
- EENT: hearing loss and tinnitus
- Hematologic: bleeding disorders, thrombocytopenia
- Respiratory: hyperpnea, asthma
- Skin: angioedema, bruising, rash, urticaria
- CNS: dizziness, headache

Interactions (other drugs)

- Angiotensin-converting enzyme (ACE)
- Acetazolamide
- Antacids
- Corticosteroids
- Diltiazem
- Ethanol
- Griseofulvin
- Methotrexate
- Oral anticoagulants
- Antigout medicines
- Warfarin

Contraindications

- Gastrointestinal bleeding
- Active peptic ulcer disease
- Bleeding disorders
- Bone marrow suppression
- Hypersensitivity to salicylates, NSAIDs, or tartrazine

Evidence

- There is evidence for and/or general agreement that aspirin is effective in the treatment of pericarditis following acute myocardial infarction [1] *Level C*
- Results of a retrospective and prospective trial were reported in one paper. The small randomized controlled trial (RCT) compared aspirin and indomethacin in the treatment of postmyocardial infarction pericarditis. Aspirin and indomethacin were found to be equally effective, and relief from discomfort was noted at 48h [2] *Level P*

Acceptability to patient

Good.

Follow up plan

Ask patient to report back to surgery if symptoms do not settle within 48h.

Patient and caregiver information

- Avoid alcohol
- Take tablets with food

NONSTEROIDAL ANTI-INFLAMMATORY DRUGS (OTC)

Dose

- Depends on preparation. Use anti-inflammatory dose
- Ibuprofen: usual dose 1200–2400mg/day in divided doses (maximum dose 3200mg/day)

Efficacy

Effective in controlling nonspecific symptoms of pain and fever, and reduces the pericardial inflammation in acute pericarditis.

Risks/Benefits

Risks

- Caution in the elderly
- Use caution in renal, cardiac, and hepatic impairment
- Use caution in patients with a history of peptic ulcer disease
- Use caution in bleeding disorders
- There is substantial individual variation in clinical response to NSAIDs

Benefit: has a range of actions: anti-inflamatory, anti-pyretic, analgesic.

Side-effects and adverse reactions

- Gastrointestinal: anorexia, nausea, vomiting, diarrhea, dyspepsia, peptic ulceration and perforation, gastritis, gastrointestinal bleeding
- CNS: headache, dizziness, tinnitus, decreased hearing
- Cardiovascular: hypertension, peripheral edema, congestive heart failure
- Genitourinary: nephrotoxicity
- Hematologic: blood cell disorders
- Hypersensitivity: rashes, urticaria, bronchospasm, angioedema

Interactions (other drugs)

■ Aminoglycosides ■ Anticoagulants (heparin, warfarin, phenindione) ■ Antihypertensives ■ Antiplatelet agents (clopidogrel, ticlopidine) ■ Aspirin ■ Baclofen ■ Calcium channel blockers ■ Corticosteroids ■ Cyclosporine, tacrolimus ■ Digoxin ■ Diuretics ■ Lithium ■ Methotrexate ■ Phenylpropanolamine

Contraindications

■ Active peptic ulceration ■ Hypersensitivity to NSAIDs or aspirin ■ Coagulation defects ■ Severe renal or hepatic disease

Acceptability to patient

Usually well tolerated.

Follow up plan

Patient should report to the physician if no improvement of symptoms after 48h.

Patient and caregiver information

Take the pills with food.

INDOMETHACIN

Dose

25–75mg, four times a day.

Efficacy

Effective symptomatic relief in most cases within 2–3 days.

Risks/Benefits

Risks:

- Use caution in hepatic, renal, and cardiac failure, epilepsy, psychiatric disorders, parkinsonism, and bleeding disorders
- Use caution in pregnancy and breast-feeding

Benefit: safe, effective, relatively inexpensive.

Side-effects and adverse reactions

- Gastrointestinal: anorexia, nausea, vomiting, abdominal pain, diarrhea, constipation, dyspepsia, peptic ulceration, gastritis, gastrointestinal bleeding
- CNS: headache, dizziness, tinnitus, somnolence
- Genitourinary: renal dysfunction, hyperuricemia
- Cardiovascular: cardiac abnormalities, congestive heart failure
- Hypersensitivity: rashes, bronchospasm, angioedema
- Hematologic: blood cell disorders

Interactions (other drugs)

■ Aminoglycosides ■ Anticoagulants ■ Antidiabetics ■ Antihypertensives ■ Baclofen ■ Corticosteroids ■ Cidofovir ■ Cyclosporine, tacrolimus ■ Digoxin ■ Diuretics ■ Ethanol ■ Gentamicin ■ Haloperidol ■ Lithium ■ Methotrexate ■ NSAIDs ■ Phenylpropanolamine ■ Probenecid ■ Triamterene ■ Vancomycin ■ Warfarin

Contraindications

■ Severe renal, hepatic, or cardiac disease ■ Active peptic ulceration, gastrointestinal bleeding, ulcerative colitis ■ Hypersensitivity to NSAIDs or aspirin ■ Coagulation disorders ■ Cidofovir

Evidence

- Indomethacin is recommended in the management of postmyocardial infarction pericarditis, although its efficacy is less well established by efficacy/opinion [1] *Level C*
- Results of a retrospective and prospective trial were reported in one paper. The small RCT compared aspirin and indomethacin in the treatment of postmyocardial infarction pericarditis. Aspirin and indomethacin were found to be equally effective, and relief from discomfort was noted at 48h [2] *Level P*

Acceptability to patient

Usually well accepted and tolerated.

Follow up plan

Initial follow-up within 3–4 days to determine clinical response.

Patient and caregiver information

- Patient should be cautioned about the development of edema (may indicate decreased renal function from indomethacin or clinical deterioration of pericarditis) and be instructed to stop the medication and contact the physician immediately to determine whether the symptoms are drug-related or related to progression of pericarditis
- Patient should be informed to stop medication if dyspnea, rash, dark stools, or tinnitus develop and to follow up immediately with the physician to determine whether symptoms are drug-related

CORTICOSTEROIDS

Prednisone and prednisolone.

Dose

- For severe acute pericarditis not responding to anti-inflammatory medication, begin 60mg/day in divided doses for 2–3 days, followed by a rapid taper
- For recurrent pericarditis, 40–60mg/day in divided doses for 1–3 weeks, then gradually taper to 15mg/day. Very slow taper thereafter

Efficacy

- Indicated in patients with severe symptoms of acute uncomplicated pericarditis not controlled by aspirin or NSAIDs alone
- Most patients with acute or recurrent pericarditis respond quickly to corticosteroids when anti-inflammatory medication has failed
- In recurrent pericarditis, symptoms recur in many patients when corticosteroids are tapered below 15mg/day
- Some patients with recurrent pericarditis may require dosage of 2–5mg/day for several months
- In rare cases, therapy has been required for more than 1 year to prevent recurrences

Risks/Benefits

Risks:

- Slow acting
- False-negative skin allergy tests.
- Overwhelming septicemia if patient has an infection
- Loss of control of blood glucose in those with diabetes
- Use caution in elderly due to risk of diabetes and osteoporosis
- Use caution in patients with psychosis, seizure disorders, or myasthenia gravis
- Use caution in congestive heart failure, renal disease, hypertension, ulcerative colitis, peptic ulcer, or esophagitis
- Use caution in patients with a history of tuberculosis; in those with active tuberculosis use only in fulminant or disseminated cases in conjunction with an anti-tuberculous drug regimen
- Prolonged use causes adrenal suppresion
- May mask the signs of an acute abdomen or intussusception

Benefit: relatively inexpensive.

Side-effects and adverse reactions

- Side-effects are minimized by short duration of therapy
- Gastrointestinal: dyspepsia, peptic ulceration, esophagitis, oral candidiasis
- Cardiovascular: hypertension, thromboembolism
- Endocrine: adrenal suppression, impaired glucose tolerance, growth suppression in children
- Musculoskeletal: proximal myopathy, osteoporosis
- CNS: insomnia, euphoria, depression, psychosis, seizures
- Skin: delayed healing, acne, striae, fragile skin
- EENT: cataract, glaucoma, blurred vision

Interactions (other drugs)

■ Aminoglutethimide: increased clearance of prednisone ■ Antidiabetics: hypoglycemic effect inhibited ■ Antihypertensives: may antagonize hypotensive effect ■ Barbiturates: increased clearance of prednisone ■ Cardiac glycosides: increased toxicity if hypokalemia occurs ■ Cholestyramine, colestipol: may reduce absorption of corticosteroids ■ Clarithromycin, erythromycin, troleandomycin: may enhance steroid effect ■ Cyclosporine: levels of both drugs may be increased; may cause seizures ■ Diuretics: may antagonize diuretic effect ■ Isoniazid: reduced plasma levels of isoniazid ■ Ketoconazole ■ NSAIDs: increased risks of bleeding ■ Oral contraceptives: enhanced effect of corticosteroids ■ Rifampin: may inhibit hepatic clearance of prednisone ■ Salicylates: increased clearance of salicylates ■ Warfarin: altered clotting time

Contraindications

■ Systemic infection ■ Avoid live virus vaccines in those receiving immunosuppressive doses ■ Cushing's syndrome ■ Recent myocardial infarction

Evidence

Corticosteroids may be an effective treatment for pericarditis, but further studies are required.

- A systematic review examined the effectiveness of steroid treatment in the management of tuberculous pericarditis. The study concluded that, while steroids may have a potentially large impact on survival, the RCTs in the meta-analysis were too small to test this. Further RCTs are required [3] *Level M*
- Corticosteroids are recommended in the management of postmyocardial infarction pericarditis, although their efficacy is less well established by efficacy/opinion [1] *Level C*

Acceptability to patient

- May be less tolerable to patients who are aware of concerns about chronic steroid use
- Patients may not tolerate cosmetic effects of chronic steroid therapy

Follow up plan

Ask patient to return at weekly intervals to determine efficacy and decide best time for withdrawal.

Patient and caregiver information

Reassure patient that widespread fear of corticosteroids is not justified for short courses of corticosteroids.

COLCHICINE

Indicated for the treatment of mild, acute, and recurrent pericarditis.

Dose

- For acute cases, 1mg, followed by 0.5mg every 2–3h to a maximum of 10mg. Then maintenance of 0.5mg twice a day
- 1mg/day for 1 year for recurrent pericarditis

Efficacy

- Recurrence rates are significantly reduced
- Colchicine appears both effective and safe in treatment of recurrent pericarditis and acute pericarditis

Risks/Benefits

Risks:

- Use caution in elderly and children
- Use caution in alcoholism, gastrointestinal disease, bone marrow suppression, and dental disease
- Use caution in cardiac, hepatic, and renal impairment

Benefits:

- May be used in patients who cannot tolerate NSAIDs
- Relatively inexpensive and well tolerated
- Gastrointestinal side-effects, although usually mild, are relatively common

Side-effects and adverse reactions

- Gastrointestinal: nausea, vomiting, anorexia, abdominal pain, diarrhea, adynamic ileus
- Genitourinary: nephrotoxicity
- Hematologic: blood cell disorders
- CNS: peripheral neuropathy, neuritis
- Musculoskeletal: myopathy
- Skin: injection site reaction, tissue necrosis, urticaria, angioedema, rashes, alopecia, purpura
- Metabolic: hypothyroidism

Interactions (other drugs)

- Cyclosporine - Ethanol - Macrolide antibiotics - NSAIDs - Tacrolimus - Vitamin B12

Contraindications

- Pregnancy and breast-feeding - Severe cardiac, renal, hepatic, or gastrointesinal disorders
- Concurrent hepatic and renal disease - Blood dyscrasias - Intramuscular injections

Evidence

Cohort studies have shown that colchicine may be useful in the treatment of recurrent pericarditis. RCTs are required to evaluate the effectiveness of colchicine [4] *Level P*

Acceptability to patient

- Patients may be reluctant to take 'plant poison' long-term. They can be reassured that, in the recommended dose, colchicine does not cause toxicity and was well tolerated by patients in the trials
- Colchicine may be more acceptable to patients who have fears about corticosteroid therapy

Follow up plan

Check full blood count, platelets, and reticulocytes before commencing therapy and at 3-monthly intervals thereafter.

Patient and caregiver information

- Patients must be advised to report symptoms of skin bruising
- Female patients of childbearing potential must be advised that colchicine is a known teratogen and that appropriate contraception must be used

OUTCOMES

EFFICACY OF THERAPIES

- Aspirin, indomethacin,* or nonsteroidal anti-inflammatory drugs control symptoms of pain and fever, usually within 48h in patients with acute viral, idiopathic, and postmyocardial infarction forms of pericarditis
- Indomethacin provides effective symptomatic relief in most cases within 2–3 days
- Most patients with acute or recurrent pericarditis respond quickly to corticosteroids when anti-inflammatory medication has failed; however, in recurrent pericarditis, symptoms recur in many patients when corticosteroids are tapered below 15mg/day, and some patients with recurrent pericarditis may require dosage of 2–5mg/day for several months
- Colchicine appears both effective and safe in treatment of recurrent pericarditis and acute pericarditis; recurrence rates are significantly reduced

Evidence

- Use of corticosteroids for severe acute and recurrent pericarditis that does not respond to anti-inflammatory medication is supported in the general literature and by abundant clinical experience
- Use of NSAIDs is supported by the general literature and by long-standing clinical experience
- There is limited evidence that aspirin and indomethacin are effective in the management of postmyocardial infarction pericarditis [2] *Level P*
- Steroids may have a potentially large impact on survival in patients with tuberculous pericarditis; however, further randomized controlled trials (RCTs) are required to provide evidence [3] *Level M*
- There is limited evidence that colchicine may be useful in the treatment of recurrent pericarditis. Further RCTs are required to provide definitive evidence [4] *Level P*

Review period

Acute pericarditis should respond to treatment within 48h. Patients should be asked to report after that time if there has been little or no symptomatic improvement.

PROGNOSIS

Idiopathic and viral pericarditis:

- 60% recover in 1 week
- 18% recover in 3 weeks
- 3% take more than 3 weeks to recover
- 16% have recurrence within 1 year
- 3% have recurrence beyond 1 year

The prognosis of pericarditis associated with other disorders is dependent on the underlying disorder.

Clinical pearl(s)

- High-dose aspirin or NSAIDs are usually effective for viral/idiopathic pericarditis
- Such patients can usually be monitored clinically, although consider a follow up echocardiogram to determine whether the effusion was reduced in size
- Although patients may become asymptomatic within a few weeks, it may take 3–6 months before the effusion has completely resolved

PREVENTION

RISK FACTORS

- Patients on dialysis are at higher risk of developing pericarditis within the first 3 months of starting dialysis
- Patients with a history of pericarditis are prone to recurrence and should be advised to report recurrence of symptoms or onset of dyspnea
- Patients with a history of open heart surgery are at risk of developing constrictive pericarditis. Consider the diagnosis if they develop dyspnea that is not explained by congestive cardiac failure alone

MODIFY RISK FACTORS

SCREENING

Screening is not required.

PREVENT RECURRENCE

- For acute viral and idiopathic pericarditis, there is no intervention that prevents recurrence
- In recurrent pericarditis, colchicine has been shown to be effective in reducing recurrences in small series of patients studied

RESOURCES

ASSOCIATIONS

American Heart Association
National Center
7272 Greenville Avenue
Dallas, TX 75231
Tel: (800) AHA-USA-1, (800) 242-8721
www.americanheart.org

American College of Cardiology
Heart House
9111 Old Georgetown
Bethesda, MD 20814-1699
Tel: (800) 253-4636
Fax: (301) 897-9745
www.acc.org

KEY REFERENCES

- Rosen P, ed. Emergency medicine: concepts and clinical practice, 4th edn. St Louis (MO): Mosby, 1998
- Roberts JR, Hedges JR, eds. Clinical procedures in emergency medicine, 3rd edn. Philadelphia (PA): WB Saunders, 1998
- Braunwald E, Zipes DP, Libby P, eds. Heart disease: a book of cardiovascular medicine, 5th edn. Philadelphia (PA): WB Saunders, 1997
- Mayosi BM, Volmink JA, Commerford PJ. Interventions for treating tuberculous pericarditis (Cochrane Review). In: The Cochrane Library, 1, 2002. Oxford: Update Software
- Marcolongo R, Russo R, Laveder F, et al. Immunosuppressive therapy prevents recurrent pericarditis. J Am Coll Cardiol 1995;26:1276–9
- Roodpeyma S, Sadeghian N. Acute pericarditis in childhood: a 10-year experience. Pediatr Cardiol 2000;21,363–7
- Marinella MA. Electrocardiographic manifestations and differential diagnosis of acute pericarditis. Am Fam Physician 1998;57:699–704
- American College of Cardiology/American Heart Association. ACC/AHA guidelines for the clinical application of echocardiography: a report of the American College of Cardiology/American Heart Association Task Force on Practice Guidelines (Committee on Clinical Application of Echocardiography). Circulation 1997;95:1686–744
- Mayosi BM, Volmink JA, Patrick J. Pericardial disease: an evidence based approach to diagnosis and treatment. In: Yusuf S, Cairns JA, Camm AJ, et al., eds. Evidence based cardiology. London: BMJ Publishing Group, 1998
- Sagristà-Sauleda J, Angel J, Permanyer-Miralda G, Soler-Soler J. Long-term follow-up of idiopathic chronic pericardial effusion. N Engl J Med 1999;341:2054–9
- Ling LH, Oh JK, Breen JF, et al. Calcific constrictive pericarditis: is it still with us? Ann Intern Med 2000;132:444–50
- Ling LH, Oh JK, Schaff HV, et al. Constrictive pericarditis in the modern era: evolving clinical spectrum and impact on outcome after pericardiectomy. Circulation 1999;100:1380–6
- Chen Y, Brennessel D, Walters J, et al. Human immunodeficiency virus-associated pericardial effusion: report of 40 cases and review of the literature. Am Heart J 1999;137:516–21
- Sagristà-Sauleda J, Merce J, Permanyer-Miralda G, Soler-Soler J. Clinical clues to the causes of large pericardial effusions. Am J Med 2000;109:95–101
- Roodpeyma S, Sadeghian N. Acute pericarditis in childhood: a 10-year experience. Pediatr Cardiol 2000;21:363–7
- Shabetai R. Acute pericarditis. Cardiol Clin 1990;8:639–44
- Fowler NO, Manitas GT. Infectious pericarditis. Prog Cardiovasc Dis 1973;16:323–36
- Fowler NO. Recurrent pericarditis. Cardiol Clin 1990;8:621–6
- Adler Y, Finkelstein Y, Guindo J, et al. Colchicine treatment for recurrent pericarditis: a decade of experience. Circulation 1998;97:2183–5
- Oakley CM. Myocarditis, pericarditis and other pericardial diseases. Heart 2000;84:449–54
- Brockington GM, Zebede J, Pandian NG. Constrictive pericarditis. Cardiol Clin 1990;8:645–61

Evidence references

1 1999 update: ACC/AHA guidelines for the management of patients with acute myocardial infarction. A report of the American College of Cardiology/American Heart Association Task Force on Practice Guidelines (Committee on Management of Acute Myocardial Infarction). J Am Coll Cardiol 1999;34:890–911

2 Berman J, Haffajee CI, Alpert JS. Therapy of symptomatic pericarditis after myocardial infarction: retrospective and prospective studies of aspirin, indomethacin, prednisone, and spontaneous resolution. Am Heart J 1981;101:750–3. Medline

3 Mayosi BM, Volmink JA, Commerford PJ. Interventions for treating tuberculous pericarditis (Cochrane Review). In: The Cochrane Library, 3, 2001. Oxford: Update Software

4 Mayosi BM, Volmink JA, Commerford PJ. Pericardial disease: an evidence based approach to diagnosis and treatment. In: Yusuf S, Cairns JA, Camm AJ, et al., eds. Evidence based cardiology. London: BMJ Publishing Group, 1998

FAQS

Question 1

Should all patients with suspected pericarditis be hospitalized?

ANSWER 1

Probably not. Most patients will present with pericardial chest pain and fatigue. In the absence of severe symptoms or moderate to large pericardial effusion, or findings of hemodynamic compromise, patients may not need inpatient management.

Question 2

What should my next line of therapy be if anti-inflammatory medications fail to resolve symptoms?

ANSWER 2

At this time, evidence supporting the use of colchicine is limited to a relatively small number of patients. However, in mild cases, a trial of colchicine in preference to corticosteroids is probably warranted because colchicine is well tolerated and has fewer side-effects.

CONTRIBUTORS

Eric F Pollak, MD, MPH
Christopher P Cannon, MD
Gail A Van Norman, MD

PERIPHERAL VASCULAR DISEASE

SUMMARY INFORMATION

DESCRIPTION

- Chronic, peripheral manifestation of atherosclerosis, usually affecting the lower limbs
- Associated with the history or presence of intermittent claudication
- Strongly linked in lower limbs to an ankle:brachial index of 0.95 or less (or a toe systolic pressure index of less than 0.60 in diabetics)
- Affected patients are at increased risk of stroke or myocardial infarction

URGENT ACTION

- Critical limb ischemia, characterized by the 'five Ps' (pain, pallor, pulselessness, paresthesias, and paralysis), is a surgical emergency
- Patients should also be hospitalized if they present with gangrenous lesions or infected ischemic ulcers

KEY! DON'T MISS!

- Critical limb ischemia, characterized by the 'five Ps' (pain, pallor, pulselessness, paresthesias, and paralysis), is a surgical emergency
- Patients should also be hospitalized if they present with gangrenous lesions or infected ischemic ulcers

ICD9 CODE

443.9 Peripheral vascular disease, unspecified

SYNONYMS

PVD, peripheral arterial disease (PAD), peripheral arterial occlusive disease (PAOD), occlusive arterial disease, chronic occlusive arterial disease, obliterative arteriosclerosis, arteriosclerosis obliterans, atherosclerotic occlusive disease.

CARDINAL FEATURES

- History or presence of intermittent claudication, provoked by exercise and relieved by rest
- History consistent with atherosclerosis
- Pulses decreased or absent distal to the occlusion
- Bruits audible over the affected artery
- Ankle:brachial index of 0.95 or less (or toe systolic pressure index of less than 0.60 in diabetics)
- Most often occurs in elderly patients and smokers
- In severe disease, ischemic appearance of affected region (hair loss; thickened brittle nails; shiny and smooth skin; changed skin color, especially in the digits; muscular atrophy; presence of ulcers or gangrene)
- Pain not relieved by sitting and leaning forward

CAUSES

Common causes

Atherosclerosis

Contributory or predisposing factors

As for atherosclerosis:

- Diabetes mellitus or glucose intolerance: diabetics have the greatest risk of developing peripheral vascular disease, the relative risk being 3–4
- Smoking: smokers are 2.5–3 times more likely to develop peripheral vascular disease than nonsmokers
- Hyperhomocysteinemia: individuals with this disorder have a relative risk of 1.7–2.6 of developing peripheral vascular disease
- Hypertension: hypertensives have a relative risk of 1.5–2.5 of developing peripheral vascular disease
- Hyperlipidemia: for every 10mg/dL increase in total cholesterol there is a relative risk increase of 1.1
- Age: intermittent claudication affects 1–2% of men under 50 years of age, but affects 5% of men over this age. A similar trend is seen in women
- Male gender: the prevalence of intermittent claudication is twice as great in men as women
- Obesity: a recognized risk factor for atherosclerosis
- Familial history: peripheral vascular disease is more likely in those with a family history of this disorder or other manifestations of atherosclerosis
- Sedentary lifestyle: a recognized risk factor for atherosclerosis; exercise is very effective in reducing symptoms of peripheral vascular disease

EPIDEMIOLOGY

Incidence and prevalence

INCIDENCE

Annual incidence of symptomatic disease: 2.6 per 1000 men; 1.2 per 1000 women (increased in individuals >75 years old).

PREVALENCE

- Prevalence in individuals 45–70 years old: 1–5% in men; 1–2% in women
- Increases with age; in those aged 55–74 years, 50 per 1000 have intermittent claudication and a further 100 per 1000 have asymptomatic peripheral vascular disease

Demographics

AGE

Risk increases with age: most often occurs in patients of 60–80 years of age.

GENDER

Male patients generally affected twice as often as women. (In the Framingham Heart Study, the incidence was 2-fold greater in men than in women regardless of age.)

GENETICS

Incidence tends to be higher in those with a familial history of peripheral vascular disease, myocardial infarction, coronary heart disease, or stroke.

SOCIOECONOMIC STATUS

- Less education
- Lower income
- Unemployment

DIFFERENTIAL DIAGNOSIS

Osteoarthritis

FEATURES

- Pain may be present at rest
- Pain associated with exercise starts immediately on joint-loading and is made worse by movement
- Pain not reliably produced by a constant amount of exercise, and not completely relieved by rest
- Pain intensity varies from day to day
- Does not affect ankle:brachial index or toe systolic pressure index
- Pulses normal peripherally

Venous insufficiency

FEATURES

- Swelling and discomfort in the calf brought on by standing, which is often exacerbated by exercise
- Prominent superficial veins
- Stasis dermatitis
- Ulcers typically proximal to or in the region of the ankle
- Ulcers associated with only mild pain that is relieved (not exacerbated) by elevation
- Does not affect ankle:brachial index or toe systolic pressure index
- Pulses normal peripherally

Nocturnal leg cramps

FEATURES

- Only occurs at night
- Does not affect ankle:brachial index or toe systolic pressure index

Spinal stenosis

FEATURES

- Pain relieved not just by rest, but by sitting or squatting, and leaning forward to straighten the lumbar spine
- Lower extremity numbness and weakness induced by standing or increasing lumbar lordosis, not by exercise alone
- History of chronic back pain or surgery on the lumbar spine
- Does not affect ankle:brachial index or toe systolic pressure index
- Pulses normal peripherally
- The disorder most commonly confused with peripheral vascular disease

Raynaud's phenomenon

FEATURES

- Symptoms not related to exercise and rest
- Induced by cold, emotional stress, working with vibrating machinery, or smoking
- Intermittent, short-term attacks of triphasic color changes: pallor to cyanosis to rubor
- Only the digits are normally affected
- Gangrene is absent or is minimal and limited to the skin
- More prevalent in women than in men

Neuropathy

FEATURES

- Does not affect ankle:brachial index or toe systolic pressure index
- Ulcers found in sites of repeated trauma, especially the metatarsal heads

- Associated with a continuous burning sensation that is unaffected by exercise or by elevating or lowering the affected limb
- History of diabetes mellitus or alcoholism is common

Arterial embolism

FEATURES

- Associated with atrial fibrillation, valvular disease, or recent myocardial infarction
- Sudden, severe, 'shocking' pain not associated with exercise
- Sharply demarcated, chalk-white pallor in affected region
- Numbness and paralysis

Arterial thrombosis

FEATURES

- Acute onset
- Pain unaffected by exercise
- History of atherosclerosis
- Usually of subacute severity

Trauma

FEATURES

- History often clear-cut
- Acute pain not affected by exercise

Thromboangiitis obliterans

FEATURES

- Usually associated with young male smokers
- Painful, tender, reddened, or dark nodules over an artery whose pulse is either decreased or absent

SIGNS & SYMPTOMS

Signs

Mild disease:

- Limping gait
- Pulses decreased or absent distal to the occlusion (but note that the dorsalis pedis artery is congenitally absent in up to 10% of the population)
- Bruits audible over the affected artery (disappears with complete occlusion)
- Ankle:brachial index of 0.95 or less (or toe systolic pressure index of less than 0.60 in diabetics), even in the absence of symptoms
- Pallor in the extremities on raising the limb, and reactive hyperemia when lowered

Severe disease (in addition to the above):

- Ischemic appearance over affected region (hair loss; thickened, brittle nails; shiny and smooth skin; changed skin color, especially in the digits – white, blue, or red; muscular atrophy)
- Ischemic ulcers (resulting from even minor trauma) usually distal to the ankle and taking 6 weeks or longer to heal
- Gangrenous lesions
- Peripheral edema (due to keeping the limb lowered)
- Hyporeflexia (due to ischemic neuritis)

Symptoms

In mild disease:

- Intermittent claudication (muscular cramp, ache, numbness, tightness, tingling, or weakness provoked by exercise and relieved by rest (5min or less))

- Claudication reliably occurs in the same region (usually in the calf, but also in the thigh, hip, or buttock, or rarely in the arm) by a constant amount of exercise
- Occurs distal to the site of vascular stenosis or occlusion. May affect one or both limbs. Not relieved by sitting and leaning forward
- Persistently cold feet (or hands) at night

In severe disease (in addition to the above):

- Rest pain that worsens when the affected limb is raised and is relieved when it is lowered
- Common at night from leg elevation in bed; the patient may be able to sleep only with the affected limb lowered
- Typically felt in the toes or forefoot
- Not relieved by sitting and leaning forward
- Ischemic appearance over affected region (hair loss; thickened, brittle nails; shiny and smooth skin; changed skin color, especially in the digits; muscular atrophy)
- Nonhealing sores (resulting from even minor trauma) or gangrenous lesions
- Peripheral edema (due to keeping the limb lowered)
- Sexual dysfunction in men (Leriche syndrome) in severe aortoiliac occlusion
- Numbness and/or paralysis, indicating limb-threatening ischemia

ASSOCIATED DISORDERS

- Mostly associated with general atherosclerosis
- Myocardial infarction
- Coronary heart disease
- Stroke
- Renal artery stenosis
- Sexual dysfunction in men (Leriche syndrome) in severe aortoiliac occlusion
- Cardiac arrhythmias, including atrial fibrillation
- Hypercoagulable states

KEY! DON'T MISS!

- Critical limb ischemia, characterized by the 'five Ps' (pain, pallor, pulselessness, paresthesias, and paralysis), is a surgical emergency
- Patients should also be hospitalized if they present with gangrenous lesions or infected ischemic ulcers

CONSIDER CONSULT

- Refer to a vascular medicine specialist (usually a vascular surgeon or intervention cardiologist or radiologist) if signs and symptoms become prominent and patient's lifestyle is impacted significantly, or for immediate hospitalization for critical limb ischemia

INVESTIGATION OF THE PATIENT

Direct questions to patient

The Edinburgh Claudication Questionnaire is thought to be the most robust questionnaire to determine the presence of intermittent claudication (Wilt TJ. J Gen Intern Med 1992;7:87–101), although the World Health Organization/Rose Questionnaire appears to be the most widely used (Rose GA. The diagnosis of ischemic heart pain and intermittent claudication in field surveys. Bull WHO 1962; 27: 645–58). Otherwise, the following questions can aid the physician in diagnosing peripheral vascular disease:

Q **Have you ever had discomfort, numbness, or weakness in the affected area that was regularly brought on by exercise and relieved by rest?** Intermittent claudication is the classic symptom of this disorder

Q **Where is the pain felt?** The location of the pain reflects the site of occlusion

- **Is the affected limb numb? Can you move it?** Numbness and paralysis indicates limb-threatening ischemia and constitute a surgical emergency
- **Have you ever had a heart attack or stroke?** History of atherosclerosis helps to confirm the diagnosis
- **Is the affected limb persistently cold, especially at night?** Coldness reflects poor perfusion
- **Does the affected limb hurt at night, particularly in the extremities?** Night pain reflects poor perfusion
- **Are you in constant pain?** Constant pain reflects severe arterial occlusion
- **Was the pain brought on suddenly?** Peripheral vascular disease is a gradual, chronic disorder
- **Is any pain you feel aggravated by raising the affected limb and relieved by lowering it?** Poor perfusion is made worse by elevating the limb
- **Do you have painful ulcers or sores that do not seem to heal?** This is indicative of ischemia
- **(In a man) Do you have difficulties getting sexually aroused?** Sexual dysfunction in men may indicate severe aortoiliac occlusion

Contributory or predisposing factors

As for atherosclerosis:

- **Do you have diabetes mellitus or glucose intolerance?** Diabetes mellitus is the greatest risk factor for this condition
- **Do you have a history of smoking?** Current or past smoking is a strong risk factor for this disorder
- **Are there signs of hyperhomocysteinemia?** Hyperhomocysteinemia is a risk factor for atherosclerosis
- **Is blood pressure normal?** Hypertension is a risk factor for atherosclerosis
- **Are there signs of hyperlipidemia?** Hyperlipidemia is a risk factor for atherosclerosis
- **Are you 50 years of age?** The disorder is more common with increasing age
- **Are you overweight?** Obesity is a risk factor for atherosclerosis
- **Do you have a sedentary lifestyle?** This is also a risk factor for atherosclerosis

Family history

- **Is there a family history of this disorder, diabetes mellitus, coronary heart disease, myocardial infarction, or stroke?** Family history of atherosclerosis is associated with this disorder.

Examination

- Note any changes in skin color over the affected area, indicative of ischemia. A sharply defined chalk-white area, especially of sudden onset, differentiates this disorder from arterial embolism, which is a surgical emergency
- Check whether the patient can feel light brushing over the affected area, and check voluntary movement. Numbness and paralysis suggest severe arterial occlusion, which is a surgical emergency
- Check pulses and look for bruits around the affected area. Weak or absent pulses help to confirm the diagnosis and locate the occlusion. Bruits can be heard over an occluded artery. (Note that the dorsalis pedis artery is absent in up to 10% of the population)
- Use a Doppler examination to listen for pulses that are not palpable
- Check the appearance of the limb for other signs of ischemia
- Check whether the affected area feels cool. Coolness indicates poor perfusion
- Test for poor perfusion in the affected region by raising the limb and flexing the muscles. In the ischemic patient, this produces pallor, which changes to rubor when the limb is lowered again
- Measure brachial and ankle (or toe, in diabetics) blood pressure. Hypertension is a risk factor for atherosclerosis. An ankle:brachial index of 0.95 or less (or a toe systolic pressure index of less than 0.60) is strongly diagnostic of peripheral vascular disorder

Summary of investigative tests

- Fasting total cholesterol: if hyperlipidemia suspected but not confirmed
- Lipid profile: including low-density lipoprotein (LDL) and high-density lipoprotein (HDL) and triglycerides. Note the LDL level can be calculated by the laboratory if the triglycerides are <400mg/dL
- Fasting glucose: if diabetes mellitus or glucose intolerance suspected but not confirmed and fasting glucose borderline, hemoglobin A1c is useful
- Consider serum homocysteine levels: if hyperhomocysteinemia suspected but not confirmed
- Ankle:brachial index is used to assess patency of the lower limb arteries, allowing detection of decreased blood flow in the artery from the blood pressure ratio of the ankle and upper arm
- Toe systolic pressure index results reflect presence and severity of peripheral vascular disease in diabetics, who are not suitable for ankle:brachial index testing
- Treadmill test can detect peripheral vascular disease in those with normal ankle:brachial or toe systolic pressure index values at rest
- Segmental pressure recordings help to confirm a diagnosis of peripheral vascular disease. Useful for studying noncompressible vessels of diabetic patients
- ECG can reveal cardiac irregularities that may be coexistent with peripheral arterial disease. Evidence of prior myocardial infarction or ongoing ischemia indicates the presence of coronary atherosclerotic disease – a predisposing factor for peripheral vascular disease

DIAGNOSTIC DECISION

- Presence or history of intermittent claudication is strongly indicative of peripheral vascular disease. An ankle:brachial index of less than 0.95 or a toe systolic pressure index of less than 0.60 confirms the diagnosis.
- Guidelines for the diagnosis of peripheral vascular disease are published by the American Heart Association: Weitz JI, Byrne J, Clagett GP, et al. Diagnosis and treatment of chronic arterial insufficiency of the lower extremities: a critical review. Circulation 1996;94:3026–49 [1]

CLINICAL PEARL(S)

- The majority of patients with peripheral vascular disease will have either diabetes or be cigarette smokers
- The diagnosis can almost always be made with the clinical history (e.g. claudication – see above) and physical examination (e.g. decreased pulses)

THE TESTS

Body fluids

FASTING TOTAL CHOLESTEROL

Description

Fasting serum cholesterol.

Advantages/Disadvantages

- Blood can be taken immediately and in the primary care practice. Inexpensive
- Not directly diagnostic of peripheral vascular disease. Hyperlipidemia is a predisposing factor for atherosclerosis and helps to confirm this underlying condition
- Results are not immediately available

Normal

Traditional definition is less than 240mg/dL. However, if total cholesterol >200mg/dL, a full lipid profile should be checked. Normal is LDL less than or equal to 100mg/dL.

Abnormal

- Greater than 240mg/dL
- Treatment is indicated for patients with LDL >100mg/dL and known vascular disease
- Keep in mind the possibility of a false-positive result

Cause of abnormal result

Hyperlipidemia.

Drugs, disorders, and other factors that may alter results

- The patient should not have received food for 12h beforehand
- Both low- and high-density lipoprotein levels are depressed for several weeks following a myocardial infarction or unstable angina, beginning 24h after the onset of the acute event
- Lipid-lowering drugs will obviously affect the results
- Hormone therapy will affect the results

LIPID PROFILE

Description

This includes total cholesterol, but also includes LDL, HDL, and triglycerides. Note that the LDL level can be calculated by the laboratory if the triglycerides are <400mg/dL.

Advantages/Disadvantages

- The advantage is that LDL is the true marker of increased risk, as is low HDL. In addition, the target for treatment recommended by the National Cholesterol Education Program (NCEP) Guidelines is based solely on LDL levels
- The only disadvantage is that it is more costly than total cholesterol. However, given the potency of these markers for prognosis, and their importance in directing lipid-lowering therapy, the increased cost is very much worth it and is strongly recommended

Normal

For patients with documented peripheral vascular disease, this is evidence of atherosclerosis, and a normal LDL would be <100mg/dL. The normal range for HDL is >35mg/dL.

Abnormal

For patients with documented peripheral vascular disease, this is evidence of atherosclerosis, and an abnormal LDL would be >100mg/dL. An abnormal HDL is <35mg/dL, although in the treatment guidelines treatment is largely based on LDL not HDL level.

Cause of abnormal result

Hyperlipidemia is the cause of elevated LDL or decreased HDL. Note that if the sample was taken soon after the patient had eaten, this will alter triglycerides more than LDL or HDL, and thus is not as critical in patients (compared with outpatients without coronary risk factors, where having a fasting blood sample – to make an initial diagnosis of hyperlipidemia – would be more important).

Drugs, disorder, and other factors that may alter results

If patients are on lipid-lowering agents, this will affect blood levels.

FASTING GLUCOSE

Description

Fasting serum glucose level.

Advantages/Disadvantages

Simple test that provides useful information on how to proceed with diagnosis and treatment. If present, either diabetes mellitus or glucose intolerance must be managed aggressively to reduce the risk of developing progression of atherosclerotic disease. Affected individuals may develop calcified, noncompressible arteries, which are not well suited to evaluation with ankle:brachial index testing.

Normal
Fasting (overnight): <140mg/dL

Abnormal
- Diabetes mellitus: fasting (overnight): >140mg/dL
- Glucose intolerance: fasting (overnight): >140mg/dL
- Keep in mind the possibility of a false-positive result

Cause of abnormal result
Diabetes mellitus or glucose intolerance.

Drugs, disorders, and other factors that may alter results
Stress, coexisting illness, use of steroids, poor diet, or lack of exercise can all give false-positive results.

SERUM HOMOCYSTEINE LEVELS
Advantages/Disadvantages
- Blood can be taken immediately in the primary care practice
- Inexpensive
- Not directly diagnostic of peripheral vascular disease
- Hyperhomocysteinemia is a predisposing factor for atherosclerosis and helps to confirm this underlying condition
- Results are not immediately available

Normal
4.5–12.4mcmol/L.

Abnormal
- Greater than 12.4mcmol/L
- Keep in mind the possibility of a false-positive result

Cause of abnormal result
Hyperhomocysteinemia.

Drugs, disorders, and other factors that may alter results
Folate supplementation may reduce systemic homocysteine levels.

Special tests
ANKLE:BRACHIAL INDEX
Description
Resting blood pressure recordings at the ankle and upper arm using Doppler-velocity stethoscopy techniques. In the event of symptoms of peripheral vascular disease in the arm, bilateral brachial measurements can be taken and compared.

Advantages/Disadvantages
- May be performed by the primary care physician
- Results reflect presence and severity of peripheral vascular disease
- Provides baseline values for follow up measures
- No cost
- Tester may require training

Normal
Ankle:arm blood pressure ratio of at least 0.95.

Abnormal

Ankle:brachial blood pressure ratio:

- 0.95 – normal
- 0.5–0.8 – typically associated with exertional symptoms
- <0.5 – often associated with symptoms at rest, ulceration, gangrene

(An absolute ankle systolic blood pressure of less than 50mmHg confirms marginal perfusion to the foot.)

Cause of abnormal result

Arterial stenoses (e.g. caused by atherosclerotic disease) diminish blood flow and pressure to distal portions of affected vessel. By comparing the ankle blood pressure to that in the brachial artery, relative burden of disease in lower vs upper extremity can be estimated.

Drugs, disorders, and other factors that may alter results

In diabetes mellitus, peripheral arteries may become calcified and noncompliant; often more pronounced in the distal vasculature of the lower extremities than elsewhere. Thus measurement of ankle vs brachial blood pressure may appear 'elevated', since affected vessels are not easily compressed with a sphygmomanometer. Consider alternative methods for measuring pressure and flow in lower extremity, e.g. toe systolic pressure index or pulse-volume recording technique.

TOE SYSTOLIC PRESSURE INDEX

Description

Resting blood pressure recordings at the toe and upper arm using a strain gauge sensor or a photoplethysmograph.

Advantages/Disadvantages

- May be performed by the primary care physician at consultation
- Results reflect presence and severity of peripheral vascular disease in diabetics, who are not suitable for ankle:brachial index testing
- Provides baseline values for follow up measures
- Minimal cost
- Tester may need training

Normal

Toe systolic pressure index of more than 0.60.

Abnormal

- Toe systolic pressure index of less than 0.60
- (An absolute ankle blood pressure of less than 30mmHg indicates that the healing potential of any ulcers present is very low)

Cause of abnormal result

Low blood pressure in the toe indicates that there is obstruction (i.e. arterial disease) at some point in the lower extremity proximal to the toe.

TREADMILL TEST

Description

Supine ankle blood pressure recordings before and after 5min exercise on a treadmill set to a speed of 2 miles per h and a gradient of 12°.

Advantages/Disadvantages

- Allows reproduction and clinical examination of intermittent claudication, if present
- Can detect peripheral vascular disease in those with normal ankle:brachial or toe systolic pressure index values at rest
- Allows simultaneous evaluation of coronary heart disease
- Cannot usually be performed by the primary care physician
- The patient may have to travel to the testing center

Normal

- No intermittent claudication on exercise
- Supine ankle blood pressure remains steady or increases during exercise

Abnormal

- Intermittent claudication on exercise
- Supine ankle blood pressure falls by more than 20% of the baseline value during exercise and does not return to baseline for more than 3min

Cause of abnormal result

Treadmill test reproduces, in a measurable way, exercise-induced reduction in blood flow and pressure across a significant peripheral arterial stenosis with consequent symptoms and signs.

SEGMENTAL PRESSURE RECORDINGS

Description

Recordings taken at multiple levels on the affected limb using continuous-wave Doppler, typically in conjunction with digital pulse-volume recording, or Doppler flow velocity waveform analysis techniques.

Advantages/Disadvantages

- Helps to localize the site of occlusion
- Helps to confirm a diagnosis of peripheral vascular disease
- Useful for studying noncompressible vessels of diabetic patients
- Requires training or referral
- Patient may have to travel to a testing center

Normal

- Segmental blood pressures do not vary along the length of an extremity
- Pulse-volume recordings have characteristic sharp systolic upstroke, rapid rise to peak, followed by gradual decline to baseline with dicrotic notch
- Doppler velocity waveform demonstrates triphasic velocity signal

Abnormal

- Segmental blood pressures diminish at an identifiable point along the extremity (vascular territory) under examination
- Pulse-volume assessment reveals more rounded shape, attenuation of speed of rise to peak, more gradual descent, and absence of dicrotic notch
- Doppler velocity waveform is damped, with degree of loss of component signal phases reflecting severity of arterial occlusion

Cause of abnormal result

- Arterial occlusion reduces flow at the site of the lesion. Blood pressure measured distal to the lesion is lower than that measured proximal to the lesion

- Loss of vascular compliance affects properties of fluid mechanics and flow through the affected arterial segments. Pulse-volume recording and Doppler velocity waveform analysis may identify changes in flow mechanics that indicate underlying atherosclerotic disease and vascular noncompliance

Other tests

ECG

Advantages/Disadvantages

Routine test for cardiac health.

Cause of abnormal result

- Cardiac irregularities that may be coexisting with peripheral arterial disease
- Evidence of prior myocardial infarction or ongoing ischemia indicates the presence of coronary atherosclerotic disease – a predisposing factor for peripheral vascular disease
- Left ventricular hypertrophy may be associated with hypertension – a predisposing factor for peripheral vascular disease
- Arrhythmias may be detected by ECG. Atrial fibrillation may be associated with the presence of peripheral vascular disease
- Antiarrhythmic drugs may cause abnormalities on ECG
- Electrolyte or metabolic disturbances may result in an abnormal ECG
- Pericardial disease may invoke changes seen on ECG

TREATMENT

CONSIDER CONSULT

- Critical limb ischemia, characterized by the 'five Ps' (pain, pallor, pulselessness, paresthesias, and paralysis), is a surgical emergency

IMMEDIATE ACTION

- Critical limb ischemia, characterized by the 'five Ps' (pain, pallor, pulselessness, paresthesias, and paralysis), is a surgical emergency
- Aspirin is effective in chronic management – but not sufficient for acute emergencies

PATIENT AND CAREGIVER ISSUES

Patient or caregiver request

- **Will the limb have to be amputated?** Only 4% of patients with intermittent claudication require amputation over a 5-year period
- **Will I die from this disease without medical attention?** The annual mortality rate is 5%, usually due to coronary or cerebrovascular complications
- **Has peripheral vascular disease been in the news recently?**

Health-seeking behavior

- **Waited too long?** The disease has a gradual onset and the patient may wait until the pain is severe before seeing a primary care physician
- **Self-medications?** The patient may have tried to treat the pain with over-the-counter medications. *Ginkgo biloba* is one reported alternative therapy
- **Visited ER?** Patient not indicated for surgery or intravascular intervention may be given aspirin and told to visit the primary care physician

MANAGEMENT ISSUES

Goals

- Eradicate symptoms due to ischemia and prevent progression to complete vascular occlusion
- Prevent cardiovascular complications arising from general atherosclerosis, including myocardial infarction and stroke

Management in special circumstances

Diabetic patients with peripheral vascular disease are at particular risk of morbidity and mortality from all complications of atherosclerosis. Disease management should be aggressive in these patients.

COEXISTING DISEASE

Treatment for coronary heart disease, atherosclerosis, myocardial infarction, hypertension, or diabetes mellitus is beneficial and should be maintained.

COEXISTING MEDICATION

Aspirin should be used with caution with angiotensin-converting enzyme (ACE) inhibitors: may reduce the effect of the ACE inhibitor, but evidence on this issue is conflicting.

Large doses of aspirin may:

- Increase the effect of sulfonylurea hypoglycemic drugs
- Affect the insulin requirements of diabetics, owing to a hypoglycemic action

Pentoxifylline (oxpentifylline) may increase the action of:

- Antihypertensive drugs
- Insulin

SPECIAL PATIENT GROUPS

- Aspirin should be avoided by women in the third trimester of pregnancy
- Clopidogrel, pentoxifylline, or cilostazol should be used during pregnancy only if clearly needed
- Nursing mothers taking clopidogrel, pentoxifylline, or cilostazol should discontinue the drug or nursing, depending on individual need
- Smoking decreases cilostazol exposure by about 20%

PATIENT SATISFACTION/LIFESTYLE PRIORITIES

- Gastrointestinal side-effects are common with aspirin, clopidogrel, and pentoxifylline
- Headache may affect up to a third of patients taking cilostazol
- The risks of percutaneous endovascular therapy or revascularization may discourage patients from undergoing such treatment
- Amputation is not welcomed by most patients and may severely affect mobility

SUMMARY OF THERAPEUTIC OPTIONS

Choices

- Antiplatelet therapy should be initiated and aspirin is the best-documented and most cost-effective treatment
- Clopidogrel, like aspirin, is an antiplatelet agent that is effective in preventing stroke, myocardial infarction, or death in patients with peripheral vascular disease. Clopidogrel is more expensive than aspirin, but may be particularly useful in patients who cannot tolerate aspirin (in a large trial clopidogrel was superior to aspirin in long-term secondary prevention in patients with peripheral arterial disease)
- Cilostazol reduces intermittent claudication symptoms and can be coprescribed with an antiplatelet drug
- Pentoxifylline is approved by the FDA for relief of intermittent claudication, but reviews of the clinical evidence have questioned its efficacy. May be effective in selected patients
- Exercise therapy is an extremely effective means to reduce symptoms of intermittent claudication and increase mobility
- Advise patient on lifestyle changes that would help, especially smoking cessation
- *Ginkgo biloba* may reduce capillary fragility, inhibit platelet aggregation, inhibit lipid peroxidation of cell membranes – resulting in increased blood fluidity and improved circulation
- Optimize the management of conditions that predispose to development of peripheral vascular disease – especially diabetes mellitus, hyperlipidemia, and hypertension
- The NCEP (National Cholesterol Education Program) advises use of lipid-lowering therapy for low-density lipoprotein (LDL) levels >100mg/dL in patients with evidence of peripheral arterial disease
- The patient must be counseled on foot care to prevent ischemic ulceration. Ischemic ulcers must be treated promptly
- The patient's bed can be adjusted to reduce night pain and so aid sleep
- Referral for invasive treatment should be considered in cases of severe or disabling symptoms, and ischemia at rest. This may also be necessary for patients whose occupations require that they be symptom-free. Based on technical considerations, percutaneous endovascular therapy or surgical revascularization may be recommended. Amputation is reserved for management of limb ischemia that is not amenable to revascularization

Guidelines

Guidelines for treatment of peripheral vascular disease are published by the American Heart Association:

- Weitz JI, Byrne J, Clagett GP, et al. Diagnosis and treatment of chronic arterial insufficiency of the lower extremities: a critical review. Circulation 1996;94:3026–49 [1]

Guidelines for the use of antithrombotic drugs were developed at the Sixth American College of Chest Physicians Consensus Conference on Antithrombotic Therapy:

- Jackson MR, Clagett GP. Antithrombotic therapy in peripheral arterial occlusive disease. Chest 2001;119(1 Suppl):283S–299S; a summary is available online at the National Guideline Clearinghouse [2]

Further guidelines on the management of peripheral arterial disease have been published:

- Anonymous. Management of peripheral arterial disease (PAD). TransAtlantic Inter-Society Consensus (TASC). Eur J Vasc Endovasc Surg 2000;19(Suppl A):Si–Sxxviii, S1–250 [3]

Clinical pearl(s)

- The ankle:brachial index is a very powerful tool for prognosis. One series of 1000 patients with peripheral arterial disease showed 90% of them had some degree of coronary artery disease
- Medical management of peripheral vascular disease is limited but, in general, aspirin (or clopidogrel), exercise, cholesterol lowering, and smoking cessation can make the biggest difference. Without invasive treatment or surgery, however, the amount of improved exercise capacity is generally very small
- Use caution when prescribing vasodilators to treat severe peripheral vascular disease. These drugs have not proved effective in treating this condition, and may even make the condition worse by diverting blood away from the affected area

FOLLOW UP

Plan for review

Patients should be evaluated on a regular basis to monitor the progress of the disease, the success of any treatment, and to provide support for recommended lifestyle changes. Postoperative recovery must be followed especially closely. Supervised exercise sessions, if available, should be used.

Information for patient or caregiver

The disease is a chronic one and can only be managed, not cured. Treatment is lifelong and requires commitment from the patient. The patient must be educated about signs and symptoms that require immediate medical assessment.

DRUGS AND OTHER THERAPIES: DETAILS

Drugs

ASPIRIN

Salicylate derivative.

Dose

160–325mg per day.

Efficacy

The efficacy is excellent:

- Delays the progression of established peripheral vascular disease and decreases the need for surgery
- Reduces risk of nonfatal stroke and myocardial infarction by one-third and all deaths from vascular causes by one-sixth

Risks/Benefits

- Well-documented efficacy
- Inexpensive
- May cause severe side-effects, especially in elderly patients
- Simple dosing regimen allows for better patient compliance
- Use caution in anemia, Hodgkin's disease
- Use caution with gout, hepatic and renal disease

- Use caution with asthma, nasal polyps, nasal allergies
- Use caution with children and teenagers (Reye's syndrome)

Side-effects and adverse reactions

- Gastrointestinal: abdominal pain, nausea, dyspepsia, hepatotoxicity, gastrointestinal bleeding
- EENT: hearing loss and tinnitus
- Hematologic: bleeding disorders, thrombocytopenia
- Respiratory: hyperpnea, asthma
- Skin: angioedema, bruising, rash, urticaria
- CNS: dizziness, headache

Interactions (other drugs)

■ ACE inhibitors ■ Acetazolamide ■ Antacids ■ Corticosteroids ■ Diltiazem ■ Ethanol ■ Griseofulvin ■ Methotrexate ■ Oral anticoagulants ■ Other nonsteroidal anti-inflammatory drugs (NSAIDs) ■ Antigout medicines ■ Warfarin

Contraindications

■ Active gastrointestinal bleeding ■ Bleeding disorders ■ Bone marrow suppression ■ Hypersensitivity to salicylates, NSAIDs, or tartrazine

Evidence

- A review of 145 randomized trials of prolonged antiplatelet therapy (principally with 'medium-dose' aspirin) found that in high-risk patients (including those with peripheral vascular disease) long-term therapy gives worthwhile protection against myocardial infarction, stroke, and death, and that no other therapy appeared significantly more effective at preventing myocardial infarction, stroke, or death [4] *Level M*
- A double-blind randomized trial of 240 patients with occlusive lower-limb arterial disease carried out over 2 years found that treatment with aspirin plus dipyridamole and with aspirin alone both slowed disease progression compared with placebo [5] *Level P*
- A review and statement from the American College of Chest Physicians on antithrombotic therapy in peripheral arterial occlusive disease notes that aspirin alone or in combination with dipyridamole may modify the natural history of intermittent claudication; it also recommends treatment with lifelong aspirin therapy [2] *Level C*
- A statement from the American Heart Association confirms the role of aspirin in patients with peripheral vascular disease [1] *Level C*

Acceptability to patient

Good, but compliance may be difficult, as for all preventive therapies.

Follow up plan

As clinically warranted, assess for signs of aspirin intolerance, particularly with respect to bleeding complications.

Patient and caregiver information

Chronic, lifelong therapy.

CLOPIDOGREL

Dose

75mg per day.

Efficacy

- Very good
- Evidence from one large trial suggests clopidogrel may be more effective than aspirin in reducing incidence of myocardial infarction, stroke, or vascular death in patients with peripheral vascular disease

Risks/Benefits

- More expensive than aspirin
- Efficacy less well documented than for aspirin
- Limited evidence suggests may be more effective than aspirin and have less severe side-effects
- Use caution in peptic ulcer disease
- Use caution in hepatic or renal disease
- Use caution in trauma or surgery
- Use caution in pregnancy
- Not recommended for use in unstable angina
- Avoid for first few days after myocardial infarction or for 7 days after ischemic stroke

Side-effects and adverse reactions

- Gastrointestinal: nausea, diarrhea, abdominal pain, dyspepsia, gastrointestinal bleeding, and ulceration
- Hematologic: thrombotic thrombocytopenic purpura, neutropenia, purpura
- Cardiovascular: hypertension, edema, chest pain
- CNS: headache, dizziness, intracranial bleeding
- Skin: macropapular rash, urticaria, pruritus
- Respiratory: upper respiratory tract infection, dyspnea

Interactions (other drugs)

- Alosetron
- Coumarins
- Dipyridamole
- Fluvastatin
- Gingko biloba
- Heparins
- NSAIDs, salicylates
- Other platelet inhibitors
- Phenytoin
- Tamoxifen
- Tolbutamide
- Torsemide

Contraindications

- Active bleeding
- Breast-feeding
- Coagulation disorders

Evidence

- One large randomized controlled trial (RCT) of more than 19,000 patients suggests that clopidogrel may be more effective than aspirin in reducing the incidence of myocardial infarction, stroke, or vascular death in patients with peripheral vascular disease. The incidence of side-effects was also lower. [6] *Level P*
- A review and statement from the American College of Chest Physicians on antithrombotic therapy in peripheral arterial occlusive disease confirms the role of clopidogrel in the management of patients with peripheral vascular disease [2] *Level C*

Acceptability to patient

Good, but compliance may be difficult, as for all preventive therapies.

Follow up plan

Consider checking complete blood count at 1 month after institution of therapy to ensure that thrombocytopenia has not developed.

Patient and caregiver information

The treatment is preventive and should be lifelong.

CILOSTAZOL

Quinolinone derivative.

Dose

100mg twice daily.

Efficacy

Good for the symptom of intermittent claudication. Can substantially increase walking distance.

Risks/Benefits

- No known effect on atherosclerotic morbidity or mortality
- May be coadministered with aspirin
- Reduces intermittent claudication
- Use caution in hypotension or history of cardiac disease including angina, uncontrolled hypertension, recent myocardial infarction, etc
- Use caution in renal or hepatic impairment
- Use caution in breast-feeding and pregnancy
- Use caution in tasks that require alertness
- Do not administer with food

Side-effects and adverse reactions

- Gastrointestinal: nausea, diarrhea, loose stools, dyspepsia, abdominal pain, flatulence
- Cardiovascular: edema, palpitations, sinus tachycardia, PVCs, or ventricular tachycardia
- Respiratory: cough, rhinitis, pharyngitis
- Skin: rash, pruritus, urticaria
- CNS: vertigo, dizziness, headache
- Musculoskeletal: myalgia, back pain

Interactions (other drugs)

■ Antiretroviral protease inhibitors ■ Azole antifungals ■ Cannabinoids ■ Cimetidine ■ Diltiazem ■ Erythromycin, clarithromycin ■ Fluoxetine, fluvoxamine, sertraline ■ Grapefruit juice ■ Nefazadone ■ Norfloxacin ■ Omeprazole ■ Other platelet inhibitors, anticoagulants, or thrombolytic agents ■ Verapamil ■ Warfarin ■ Zafirlukast

Contraindications

■ Congestive heart failure ■ Should not be used in women trying to conceive

Evidence

A consensus statement on the use of antithrombotic drugs from the American College of Chest Physicians recommends a trial of cilostazol therapy for patients experiencing disabling claudication, particularly when lifestyle modification alone is ineffective and revascularization cannot be offered or is declined by the patient [2] *Level C*

Acceptability to patient

High, but it must be stressed that the benefit is not immediate.

Patient and caregiver information

- Treatment for up to 12 weeks may be needed before any benefit is noticed
- Grapefruit juice should be avoided because it interferes with the metabolism of cilostazol. The treatment is lifelong

PENTOXIFYLLINE

Dose

400mg three times a day with meals, for at least 8 weeks.

Efficacy

Overall, modest efficacy, but may increase walking distance in severely affected patients who are not responsive to exercise therapy.

Risks/Benefits

- No known effect on atherosclerotic morbidity or mortality
- Not as effective as cilostazol in reducing intermittent claudication
- Use caution in pregnancy or breast-feeding
- Use caution in hepatic or renal impairment
- Use caution in chronic occlusive areterial disease of the limbs
- Use caution in children and the elderly
- Use caution in peptic ulcer disease
- Use caution in recent surgery
- Incidence of side-effects decreases with the controlled-release formulation

Side-effects and adverse reactions

- Gastrointestinal: nausea, vomiting, dyspepsia, constipation, dry mouth, cholecystitis, anorexia, bloating
- Cardiovascular: hypotension, dyspnea, angina, chest pain, tachycardia, arrhythmias
- Hematologic: blood cell disorders
- CNS: headache, dizziness, tremor, agitation, sleep disturbances
- EENT: conjunctivitis, visual disturbances, scotomata, earache, sore throat, epistaxis
- Respiratory: laryngitis, nasal congestion, flu-like symptoms
- Skin: rash, urticaria, brittle fingernails, pruritus

Interactions (other drugs)

- Antihypertensives
- Cimetidine
- Fluoroquinolones
- Ketorolac
- NSAIDs
- Platelet inhibitors
- Theophylline
- Warfarin

Contraindications

- Intracranial or retinal bleeding
- Acute myocardial infarction
- Intolerance to pentoxifylline or methylxanthine derivatives

Evidence

- A medical statement from the American Heart Association notes that the actual improvement in walking distance attributable to pentoxifylline is often unpredictable, may not be clinically important compared with the effects of placebo, and does not justify the added expense for most patients [1] *Level C*
- A review of RCTs of pentoxifylline in the treatment of intermittent claudication concluded that the limited amount and quality of reported data precluded an overall, reliable estimate of it efficacy [7] *Level M*

Acceptability to patient

- Average
- Gastrointestinal side-effects are common
- Any benefit that does occur may not be seen immediately

Follow up plan

Treatment must be reassessed regularly.

Patient and caregiver information

Treatment for up to 8 weeks may be needed before any benefit is noticed. The treatment is lifelong.

Surgical therapy

PERCUTANEOUS ENDOVASCULAR THERAPY

Synonym: percutaneous transluminal angioplasty or stenting.

Efficacy

Initial procedural success rate is 90%. Subsequent restenosis results in patency rates of 80% at 1 year, 70% at 3 years, and 60% at 5 years. Overall outcome is more favorable when the procedure is performed for amelioration of symptoms of claudication, in vessels that are not totally occluded, and for treatment of proximal, short (less than 10cm), localized lesions.

Risks/Benefits

Procedural complication rate is lower than that for surgical revascularization, costs less, and requires shorter recovery period. Depending on technical considerations, surgical revascularization may have greater immediate and long-lasting success rates. The use of endoluminal stents may prove to have a more durable effect than angioplasty alone.

Evidence

- The efficacy and safety of these therapies have been investigated in a number of case-series studies, which are summarized in a medical statement from the American Heart Association, which notes that it is appropriate only when arterial disease is localized to a vessel segment less than 10cm in length and when there is a skilled vascular interventionalist available to perform the procedure [1] *Level C*
- A literature review concluded that the results, which are limited, suggest that angioplasty may have had a short-term benefit but that this benefit may not have been sustained [8] *Level M*
- A prospective, randomized comparison of percutaneous angioplasty and surgery in 263 men with occlusive disease of the iliac, superficial femoral, or popliteal arteries found that both were effective at increasing the ankle:brachial index but that surgery had a higher rate of complications [9] *This trial does not meet the criteria for level P*

Acceptability to patient

High. These options present less risk than surgical revascularization, are less invasive, and require only 1–2 days of hospitalization.

Follow up plan

Recovery must be monitored closely for vascular complications.

Patient and caregiver information

Patients must be encouraged to exercise as soon as possible following surgery, and maintain compliance with treatment and lifestyle.

SURGICAL REVASCULARIZATION

Efficacy

High. Success rate depends on the site and extent of disease and on the operative procedure selected. Aortoiliac revascularization may have 10-year patency rates of 85%. Femoropopliteal bypass grafting is estimated to confer a 5-year patency rate of 80–85%. Infrapopliteal bypass procedures have patency rates of 60% in the long term.

Risks/Benefits

Higher success rate than percutaneous endovascular therapy, but the risk of vascular complications is also greater. As many as 5% may experience myocardial infarction, and the mortality rate is 2–3%. Only recommended in refractory cases of severe ischemia when all less invasive treatments have been tried.

Evidence

- The indications, efficacy, and safety of surgical revascularization are discussed a medical statement from the American Heart Association [1] *Level C*
- A prospective, randomized comparison of percutaneous angioplasty and surgery in 263 men with occlusive disease of the iliac, superficial femoral, or popliteal arteries found that both were effective at increasing the ankle:brachial index but that surgery had a higher rate of complications [9] *This trial does not meet the criteria for level P*

Acceptability to patient

Intermediate. These treatments have higher risk than percutaneous endovascular therapy, and require longer convalescence.

Follow up plan

Recovery must be monitored closely for vascular complications.

Patient and caregiver information

Patients must be encouraged to exercise as soon as possible following surgery, and to maintain compliance with treatment and lifestyle changes.

AMPUTATION

Efficacy

High.

Risks/Benefits

Removes the lesion, but is an extreme measure. No advantage over revascularization in terms of cost or operative risk. Only indicated in severe circumstances when the limb cannot be salvaged by any other means.

Evidence

The indications, efficacy, and safety of amputation for peripheral vascular disease are discussed a medical statement from the American Heart Association [1] *Level C*

Acceptability to patient

Very low. Severely affects mobility and self-image. Convalescence is prolonged.

Follow up plan

Recovery must be monitored closely for vascular complications.

Patient and caregiver information

Patients must be encouraged to exercise as soon as possible following surgery, and to maintain compliance with treatment and lifestyle changes.

Complementary therapy

GINKGO BILOBA

Efficacy

Ginkgo may reduce capillary fragility, inhibit platelet aggregation, inhibit lipid peroxidation of cell membranes – resulting in increased blood fluidity and improved circulation.

Risks/Benefits
Risks:
- Should be discontinued prior to any surgery
- Avoid in patients with known risk of intracranial hemorrhage
- Some individuals are hypersensitive to *Ginkgo biloba*

Interactions
- Aspirin
- Warfarin
- Papaverine
- Monoamine oxidase inhibitors

Evidence
A RCT compared 6 months of *Ginkgo biloba* extract with placebo in the management of peripheral vascular disease. The treatment group had significantly improved pain at 24 weeks, and claudication distance was significantly improved when compared with placebo. No difference was noted in A/B ratio or Doppler ankle response to exercise, or in post-exercise recovery time [10] *Level P*

Acceptability to patient
Well tolerated.

Follow up plan
Usual care.

Patient and caregiver information
Dose recommended is 120mg once or twice daily of extract standardized to 24% flavone glycosides.

Other therapies

METICULOUS FOOT CARE

Efficacy
Good.

Risks/Benefits
Requires cooperation from the patient. Reduces the risk of ulceration.

Acceptability to patient
Compliance may be difficult.

Follow up plan
Regular contact with the patient may be necessary to maintain compliance.

Patient and caregiver information
The feet should be washed daily and treated with moisturizing cream to prevent excessive drying. Only well-fitting, protective shoes that allow the feet to breathe should be worn.

ULCER TREATMENT

Efficacy
High in preventing progression of ulcers.

Risks/Benefits
Prevents ischemic ulceration from progressing to the extent that it becomes limb-threatening.

Acceptability to patient
High.

Follow up plan
Any ulcers should be monitored closely for any signs of improvement or deterioration.

Patient and caregiver information
Any ulcers should be reported to the physician promptly.

BED ADJUSTMENT
Efficacy
May provide some relief of pain during the night.

Risks/Benefits
In cases of severe disease, may improve arterial circulation and relieve night pain. A simple measure.

Acceptability to patient
High.

Patient and caregiver information
The head of the bed can be raised by 4–6 inches and a canopy placed over the feet.

LIFESTYLE

- Smoking cessation, if relevant, is critical
- Restrictive leg garments (such as elastic support hose, self-support stockings, elastic socks, or garters) should not be worn
- Regular exercise may markedly increase pain-free walking distances and improve muscular efficiency and general mobility (American Heart Association Medical Statement)

RISKS/BENEFITS
Slows progression of underlying atherosclerosis and reduces risk of all atherosclerotic events, including myocardial infarction. Loose clothing encourages blood flow.

ACCEPTABILITY TO PATIENT
Recommendations including smoking cessation, weight loss, adherence to a prescribed (and restricted) diet, and maintenance of a regular exercise program are limited by compliance issues.

FOLLOW UP PLAN
Regular contact with the patient may encourage compliance with lifestyle changes.

PATIENT AND CAREGIVER INFORMATION
Lifestyle modification may have a dramatic impact on the progression of atherosclerotic disease.

OUTCOMES

EFFICACY OF THERAPIES

- Antiplatelet therapies such as aspirin and clopidogrel are effective at preventing complications and slowing progression and should generally be initiated
- Cilostazol and pentoxifylline may be effective at reducing intermittent claudication, especially in selected patients
- Invasive treatment is often effective in cases of severe or disabling symptoms, and in patients who have ischemia at rest.
- Amputation is reserved for the management of limb ischemia that is not amenable to revascularization or other treatments

Evidence

- Antiplatelet therapy with aspirin has been shown to protect against peripheral vascular disease in high-risk patients [4] *Level M*
- Aspirin has also been shown to slow disease progression [5] Level P
- Clopidogrel may be more effective than aspirin in reducing the incidence of myocardial infarction, stroke, and vascular death in patients with peripheral vascular disease, and the incidence of side-effects is lower with clopidogrel [6] *Level P*
- Angioplasty is beneficial, although the benefit may not be sustained [8] *Level M*
- *Ginkgo biloba* extract may decrease ischemia in patients with peripheral vascular disease [11] *Level P*
- PDxMD are unable to cite evidence for surgical revascularization and amputation that meets our criteria

Review period

The need for follow-up must be tailored to the individual patient. Regular review of reported symptoms, activity tolerance, physical examination, and laboratory studies should be used to steer therapeutic and diagnostic strategies.

PROGNOSIS

- After 5 years, 73% have no change in the severity of intermittent claudication symptoms, 16% deteriorate, 7% require surgery, and 4% have a major amputation
- Mortality rates from all causes are three times higher for patients with peripheral vascular disease compared with disease-free controls. Relative risks for cardiovascular mortality and coronary death are 5.9 and 6.6, respectively, in patients with peripheral vascular disease. 75% of such patients will die from a vascular event
- Prognosis is worse for persistent smokers: in those who have undergone surgery, survival at 5 years is 36%, compared with 66% in nonsmokers. Moreover, amputation rate is 28% in smokers and 11% in nonsmokers. Diabetes has a similar impact on prognosis in conjunction with peripheral arterial disease

Clinical pearl(s)

- Patients with with peripheral vascular disease are at risk of progression of disease, but of more importance, are at increased risk of coronary events
- One recent large study found that among smokers with with peripheral vascular disease, patients who continue to smoke have a worse prognosis than those who quit, thus emphasizing the importance of talking to your patient about quitting smoking

Deterioration

If the clinical condition deteriorates despite medical therapy, lifestyle modification, and regular exercise, referral to a cardiologist should be requested for consideration of percutaneous endovascular treatments, surgical revascularization, or amputation.

COMPLICATIONS

Ischemia can lead to necrosis and gangrene that may ultimately necessitate amputation.

PREVENTION

RISK FACTORS

- **Diabetes mellitus or glucose intolerance:** diabetics have the greatest risk of developing peripheral vascular disease, the relative risk being 3–4
- **Smoking**: smokers are 2.5–3 times more likely to develop peripheral vascular disease than nonsmokers
- **Hyperhomocysteinemia**: individuals with this disorder have a relative risk of 1.7–2.6 of developing peripheral vascular disease
- **Hypertension:** hypertensives have a relative risk of 1.5–2.5 of developing peripheral vascular disease
- **Hyperlipidemia:** for every 10mg/dL increase in total cholesterol there is a relative risk increase of 1.1 in cardiovascular mortality
- **Age**: intermittent claudication affects 1–2% of men under 50 years of age, but affects 5% of men over this age. A similar trend is seen in women
- **Male gender:** the prevalence of intermittent claudication is twice as great in men as women
- **Obesity:** a recognized risk factor for atherosclerosis
- **Familial history:** peripheral vascular disease is more likely in those with a family history of this disorder or other manifestations of atherosclerosis
- **Sedentary lifestyle:** a recognized risk factor for atherosclerosis; exercise is very effective in reducing symptoms of peripheral vascular disease

MODIFY RISK FACTORS

- Patients with diabetes mellitus or glucose intolerance should be managed aggressively and educated about the risks of their condition
- Those with hypertension should be managed with drugs and lifestyle changes appropriate to their condition
- Patients with identified hyperhomocysteinemia should be prescribed oral pyridoxine (25–500mg per day)
- Hyperlipidemia should be managed with diet and usually also with lipid-lowering agents
- National Cholesterol Education Program

Lifestyle and wellness

TOBACCO

All patients should be encouraged not to smoke.

DIET

Obese patients should be encouraged to attain a healthy weight, and all patients should eat a nutritious diet that is low in saturated fat.

PHYSICAL ACTIVITY

Patients should be encouraged to exercise regularly.

FAMILY HISTORY

Patients who have a family history of this disorder or other manifestations of atherosclerosis should be questioned about symptoms at consultations.

SCREENING

CHOLESTEROL SCREENING

- High serum cholesterol levels are a risk factor for all manifestations of atherosclerosis and may play a role in a general screening program. This should not be a screening measure for peripheral vascular disease alone
- Dyslipidemia is well known to be a risk factor for development of atherosclerosis. Lipid screening plays a critical role in the primary prevention of vascular disease, but should not be considered a 'diagnostic' modality for identifying the presence of peripheral vascular disease

ANKLE:BRACHIAL INDEX

Ankle:brachial index or toe systolic pressure index should be determined in any patient with clinical evidence (by history or physical examination) of with peripheral vascular disease.

PREVENT RECURRENCE

Some patients achieve remission of symptoms, but the condition is not cured and treatment is lifelong.

RESOURCES

ASSOCIATIONS

American College of Cardiology
Heart House
9111 Old Georgetown Road
Bethesda, MD 20814–1699
Tel: (800) 253-4636/(301) 897-5400
Fax: (301) 897-9745
http://www.acc.org

American Heart Association
National Center
7272 Greenville Avenue
Dallas, Texas 75231, USA.
Tel: (800) AHA-USA1
http://www.americanheart.org

KEY REFERENCES

- de Vries SO, Visser K, de Vries JA, et al. Intermittent claudication: cost-effectiveness of revascularization versus exercise therapy. Radiology 2002;222:25–36
- Donnelly R, Yeung JM. Management of intermittent claudication: the importance of secondary prevention. Eur J Vasc Endovasc Surg 2002;23:100–7

Evidence references and guidelines

1 Weitz JI, Byrne J, Clagett GP, et al. Diagnosis and treatment of chronic arterial insufficiency of the lower extremities: a critical review. Circulation 1996;94:3026–49

2 Jackson MR, Clagett GP. Antithrombotic therapy in peripheral arterial occlusive disease. Chest 2001;119(1 Suppl):283S–299S; a summary is available online at the National Guideline Clearinghouse

3 Anonymous. Management of peripheral arterial disease (PAD). TransAtlantic Inter-Society Consensus (TASC). Eur J Vasc Endovasc Surg 2000;19(Suppl A):Si–Sxxviii, S1–S250

4 Antiplatelet Trialists' Collaboration. Collaborative overview of randomised trials of antiplatelet therapy. Prevention of death, myocardial infarction, and stroke by prolonged antiplatelet therapy in various categories of patients. BMJ 1994;308:81–106

5 Hess H, Mietaschk A, Deichsel G. Drug-induced inhibition of platelet function delays progression of peripheral occlusive arterial disease. A prospective double-blind arteriographically controlled trial. Lancet 1985;i:415–19

6 CAPRIE Steering Committee. A randomised, blinded, trial of clopidogrel versus aspirin in patients at risk of ischaemic events (CAPRIE). Lancet 1996;348:1329–39

7 Radack K, Wyderski RJ. Conservative management of intermittent claudication. Ann Intern Med 1990;113:135–46

8 Fowkes FGR, Gillespie IN. Angioplasty (versus non surgical management) for intermittent claudication (Cochrane Review). In: The Cochrane Library, 4, 2001. Oxford: Update Software

9 Wilson SE, Wolf GL, Cross AP. Percutaneous transluminal angioplasty versus operation for peripheral arteriosclerosis. Report of a prospective randomized trial in a selected group of patients. J Vasc Surg 1989;9:1–9

10 Thomson GJ, Vohra RK, Carr MH, Walker MG. A clinical trial of *Ginkgo biloba* extract in patients with intermittent claudication. Int Angiol 1990;9:75–8. Medline

11 Mouren X, Caillard P, Schwartz F. Study of the antiischemic action of EGb 761 in the treatment of peripheral arterial occlusive disease by TcPo2 determination. Angiology 1994;45:413–17

FAQS

Question 1

When should a patient with intermittent claudication be referred to a vascular surgeon?

ANSWER 1

As long as there is no evidence of foot ischemia or nonhealing ulcers, this is a decision based on the patient's degree of comfort with lifestyle limitations. If the patient is happy with limitations, this can be managed medically. For the more active patient, or where work needs are impacted, earlier intervention is warranted.

Question 2

If a patient with peripheral vascular disease is going to have vascular surgery, how should their coronary risk be investigated?

ANSWER 2

In general, if they have previous coronary disease, are over 70, and diabetic, or have other high-risk considerations, they should have a pharmacologic stress test prior to surgery (for example, a dobutamine echocardiogram) because they would be unable to walk well enough to do a standard treadmill test.

Question 3

If my coronary patient is taking a beta-blocker, should this be stopped if intermittent claudication develops?

ANSWER 3

Although beta-blockers can theoretically worsen intermittent claudication, they should be continued if there is coronary artery disease present because of their importance here. In general, beta-blockers have little effect one way or the other on the clinical course of intermittent claudication.

Question 4

Should patients with peripheral arterial disease receive aspirin or clopidogrel?

ANSWER 4

Data for aspirin in secondary prevention of cardiac events are strong, although the number of patients with peripheral arterial disease who have been studied is limited. In one large study, clopidogrel was significantly better than aspirin with about a 20% relative risk reduction in vascular death, myocardial infarction, or stroke. Although clopidogrel is more expensive than aspirin, strong consideration of use of this agent should be taken for patients with peripheral arterial disease.

CONTRIBUTORS

Randolph L Pearson, MD
Jane L Murray, MD
Christopher P Cannon, MD
Doug Drachman, MD

RAYNAUD'S PHENOMENON

SUMMARY INFORMATION

DESCRIPTION

- Raynaud's phenomenon is a vasospastic disorder characterized by episodic ischemia of the digits of the hands and feet that is precipitated by cold exposure or emotional distress
- Manifested clinically by a sequential triphasic discoloration of the fingers and toes comprising digital blanching and cyanosis following cold exposure and rubor of the digits on subsequent rewarming
- The phases of pallor and cyanosis are often accompanied by sensations of cold, numbness, or paresthesias of the digit, while a throbbing, painful sensation is often experienced during the subsequent hyperemic phase
- Classified as either the primary form (Raynaud's disease, idiopathic Raynaud's phenomenon, primary Raynaud's phenomenon) when no underlying cause can be found or the secondary form (secondary Raynaud's phenomenon, Raynaud's phenomenon), which is always associated with an underlying disease or some aspect of the patient's lifestyle
- Primary Raynaud's phenomenon is more common than secondary Raynaud's phenomenon, is generally milder in severity, occurs more frequently in women than in men (4:1), and is more common in the young (<40 years of age) than in the old
- Between 5 and 15% of patients thought to have primary Raynaud's phenomenon will subsequently develop a secondary cause (frequently a connective tissue disorder)

URGENT ACTION

Although rare, critical ischemia of the digits may complicate Raynaud's phenomenon – this complication should prompt immediate referral and aggressive treatment.

BACKGROUND

ICD9 CODE

- 443.0 Raynaud's syndrome, Raynaud's disease, Raynaud's phenomenon (secondary)
- 785.4 If gangrene is present

SYNONYMS

- Primary Raynaud's phenomenon
- Raynaud's disease
- Idiopathic Raynaud's phenomenon
- Secondary Raynaud's phenomenon

CARDINAL FEATURES

- Classic clinical manifestation of the disease is the sequential development of blanching, cyanosis, and rubor of the fingers and/or toes following exposure to cold temperatures and subsequent rewarming
- In rare cases, may involve the tongue, nose, ears, or nipples

CAUSES

Common causes

When no underlying cause can be found, phenomenon is classified as primary Raynaud's phenomenon (Raynaud's disease). Secondary Raynaud's phenomenon is associated with a number of disorders, particularly a variety of connective tissue diseases, including:

- Scleroderma, mixed connective tissue disease, polymyositis and dermatomyositis. Raynaud's phenomenon is seen in approx. 85–95% of patients with scleroderma and mixed connective tissue disease
- CREST (calcinosis cutis, Raynaud's phenomenon, esophageal involvement, sclerodactyly, and (esonophilia) telangiectasia) syndrome
- Systemic lupus erythematosus (SLE) – Raynaud's phenomenon is present in approx. one-third of patients with SLE
- Rheumatoid arthritis
- Sjögren's syndrome
- A variety of neurogenic disorders, including intervertebral disk disease, syringomyelia, carpal tunnel syndrome, thoracic outlet syndrome
- Vaso-occlusive diseases, including arteriosclerosis obliterans, peripheral emboli. Atherosclerosis of the extremities is frequently associated with Raynaud's phenomenon in men over age 50
- Hematologic disorders, including cryoglobulinemia, cold agglutinins, dysproteinemias
- A number of drugs, including ergot preparations, methysergide, beta-adrenergic antagonists, oral contraceptives, bleomycin, vinblastine, cisplatin
- A severe form of Raynaud's phenomenon is seen in up to one-third of patients receiving bleomycin and vincristine in combination and this persists even with discontinuance of the drugs
- Estrogen replacement therapy without progestogen
- Trauma to the digits including electric shock and frostbite
- Workers operating vibrating machinery on a regular basis can develop a type of Raynaud's phenomenon called vibration-induced white finger
- Typists, pianists, and others whose fingers are exposed to repeated physical stress are susceptible to the disease

Rare causes

- Poliomyelitis
- Thromboangiitis obliterans. This should be considered in young men who smoke cigarettes

Serious causes

- Primary pulmonary hypertension
- Occult carcinoma, particularly spinal cord tumors
- Thromboangiitis obliterans. Raynaud's phenomenon usually occurs in only one or two digits when associated with this disorder, and may result in critical limb-threatening ischemia and infarction
- Peripheral emboli

Contributory or predisposing factors

- Connective tissue diseases
- Smoking: the nicotine in cigarettes causes skin temperature to drop, which may precipitate an attack
- Stress and emotional upsets may trigger an attack
- Workers operating vibrating machinery on a regular basis can develop a type of Raynaud's phenomenon called vibration-induced white finger
- Typists, pianists, and others whose fingers are exposed to repeated physical stress are susceptible to the disease
- A number of drugs, including ergot preparations, methysergide, beta-adrenergic antagonists, oral contraceptives, bleomycin, vinblastine, cisplatin

EPIDEMIOLOGY

Incidence and prevalence

PREVALENCE

- Raynaud's phenomenon (either primary or secondary) is estimated to affect between 5 and 20% of the population, with women accounting for over 75% of reported cases
- It is estimated that up to 20–25% of young women have some form of Raynaud's phenomenon
- Between 5 and 15% of patients thought to have primary Raynaud's will develop a secondary cause

Demographics

AGE

- Women: onset occurs typically between the ages of 15 and 40
- Men: onset typically occurs later in life

GENDER

Women are affected with primary Raynaud's phenomenon more often than men (4:1).

GEOGRAPHY

- Appears to be more common in people living in cold climates
- Patients who live in milder climates have more attacks during periods of cold weather

SOCIOECONOMIC STATUS

- Workers operating vibrating machinery on a regular basis can develop a type of Raynaud's phenomenon called vibration-induced white finger
- Typists, pianists, and others whose fingers are exposed to repeated physical stress are susceptible to the disease

DIFFERENTIAL DIAGNOSIS

It is important to differentiate Raynaud's disease from Raynaud's phenomenon and the numerous disorders associated with Raynaud's phenomenon. The history and examination will differentiate the diagnosis of Raynaud's disease from rheumatoid arthritis, systemic sclerosis (including CREST syndrome), systemic lupus erythematosus, and mixed connective tissue disease, which are common causes of Raynaud's phenomenon.

Thromboangiitis obliterans

Also called Buerger's or Winiwarter–Buerger disease.

FEATURES

- Generally a disease of men
- Associated with cigarette smoking
- Peripheral pulses are often diminished or absent
- Raynaud's phenomenon usually occurs in only one or two digits when in association with thromboangiitis obliterans

Thoracic outlet syndromes

Thoracic outlet syndromes are a group of poorly categorized syndromes characterized by a variety of pain and paresthesias in the neck, shoulder, arms, and hand.

FEATURES

- Raynaud's phenomenon may occur in patients with thoracic outlet syndromes
- Involvement is usually unilateral and symptoms referable to brachial plexus compression are evident

Carpal tunnel syndrome

Carpal tunnel syndrome is caused by compression of the median nerve at the wrist.

FEATURES

- Often seen in individuals with a history of repetitive use of their hands or following injuries of the wrist
- Pain, which may be burning and tingling, in the distribution of the median nerve

Acrocyanosis

An uncommon symmetric condition involving the skin of the hands and feet, and occasionally the forearms and legs.

FEATURES

- Associated with arteriolar vasoconstriction combined with dilation of the subpapillary venous plexus of the skin
- Exacerbated in cold weather but does not disappear completely during warm weather
- Occurs in both males and females, most commonly in teenagers and those in their 20s
- Characterized by coldness, sweating, slight edema, and cyanotic discoloration of the involved areas

Cryoglobulinemia

A disorder in which serum proteins aggregate in the cooler distal circulation.

FEATURES

- May be idiopathic or associated with multiple myeloma and other hyperglobulinemic states
- Diagnosis based on a positive serum test for cryoglobulins

SIGNS & SYMPTOMS

Signs

- Well-demarcated, triphasic digit discoloration induced by cold exposure: sequential development of blanching, cyanosis, and rubor of the fingers and/or toes following exposure to cold temperatures and subsequent rewarming
- Fingers are involved more frequently than toes, although thumbs are rarely affected
- The tips of the ears and nose can be affected but this is uncommon
- Sensations of cold, numbness or paresthesias of the digits often accompany the phases of pallor and cyanosis
- A throbbing, painful sensation sometimes accompanies the hyperemic phase
- Sclerodactyly develops in 10% of patients
- Primary Raynaud's phenomenon usually affects both hands and both feet
- Secondary Raynaud's phenomenon usually affects both hands or both feet
- Primary Raynaud's phenomenon is usually associated with a normal nailfold capillary pattern, a negative antinuclear antibody test, normal erythrocyte sedimentation rate (ESR), the absence of pitting scars or ulcerations on the skin of the digits
- Secondary Raynaud's phenomenon is usually associated with an abnormal nailfold capillary pattern, a positive antinuclear antibody test, abnormal ESR and the presence of pitting scars or ulcerations on the skin of the digits. Rarely, gangrene in the digits is seen
- Secondary Raynaud's phenomenon may be associated with clinical manifestations of the underlying disease process, e.g. scleroderma

Symptoms

- Well-demarcated, triphasic digit discoloration induced by cold exposure: sequential development of blanching, cyanosis, and rubor of the fingers and/or toes following exposure to cold temperatures and subsequent rewarming
- Sensations of cold, numbness, or paresthesias of the digits often accompany the phases of pallor and cyanosis
- A throbbing, painful sensation sometimes accompanies the hyperemic phase
- Gastroesophageal reflux and diminished peristaltic clearance which are often associated with connective tissue disorders are sometimes observed

ASSOCIATED DISORDERS

Secondary Raynaud's phenomenon is associated with a number of disorders, particularly a variety of connective tissue diseases, including:

- Scleroderma, mixed connective tissue disease, polymyositis, and dermatomyositis – Raynaud's phenomenon is seen in approx. 85–95% of patients with scleroderma and mixed connective tissue disease
- CREST (calcinosis cutis, Raynaud's phenomenon, esophageal involvement, sclerodactyly, and (esonophilia) telangiectasia) syndrome
- Systemic lupus erythematosus (SLE) – Raynaud's phenomenon is present in approx. one-third of patients with SLE
- Rheumatoid arthritis
- Sjögren's syndrome
- Sclerodactyly, which develops in 10% of patients
- A variety of neurogenic disorders, including intervertebral disk disease, syringomyelia, carpal tunnel syndrome, thoracic outlet syndrome
- Vaso-occlusive diseases, including arteriosclerosis obliterans, peripheral emboli, atherosclerosis of the extremities (which is a frequent cause of Raynaud's phenomenon in men over age 50 years)
- Hematologic disorders including cryoglobulinemia, cold agglutinins, dysproteinemias
- Migraine or variant angina (Raynaud's phenomenon occurs frequently in patients with these disorders)

CONSIDER CONSULT

- Rheumatology consult is indicated in the case of secondary collagen-vascular disease diagnosis
- Immediate vascular surgery consult is indicated if ulcers, gangrene, or threatened autoamputation is evident

INVESTIGATION OF THE PATIENT

Direct questions to patient

- Q **Do you regularly operate machinery or tools that produce vibration?** Workers operating vibrating machinery on a regular basis can develop a type of Raynaud's phenomenon called vibration-induced white finger
- Q **Do you spend a lot of time typing, playing the piano, sewing, or doing any other activities that involve repeated physical stress to the fingers?** People whose fingers are exposed to repeated physical stress are susceptible to the disease
- Q **Do you smoke?** Nicotine in cigarettes causes the skin temperature to drop, which can lead to an attack
- Q **Are you currently taking any prescription medications?** A number of drugs can induce Raynaud's phenomenon
- Q **Are you under a lot of stress at home or at work?** Stress and emotional upsets may trigger an attack

Contributory or predisposing factors

- Q **Is there a history of connective tissue diseases?** Raynaud's syndrome may be secondary to other disorders
- Q **What prescription medicines is the patient taking?** A number of drugs, including ergot preparations, methysergide, beta-adrenergic antagonists, oral contraceptives, bleomycin, vinblastine, and cisplatin may induce Raynaud's phenomenon

Examination

- Inspect hands for signs of ulceration on digits
- May place hands in ice water to precipitate an attack for diagnostic purposes

Summary of investigative tests

- Initial evaluation should include routine laboratory tests, including complete blood count, electrolytes, creatinine, and blood urea nitrogen, urinalysis, ESR, and antinuclear antibody test. These tests will confirm or rule out a potential secondary cause, e.g. connective tissue or other autoimmune disorders commonly associated with Raynaud's phenomenon. This initial evaluation also assesses renal function, which can be impaired in patients with connective tissue disease
- If initial testing suggests a secondary cause, more specific serologic testing may be performed, including anticentromere antibodies, anti-Scl-70 antibodies, cryoglobulins, and protein electrophoresis. A more specific diagnosis of the underlying cause of secondary Raynaud's can then be made
- Nailfold capillaroscopy can also help to distinguish between primary and secondary Raynaud's phenomenon

DIAGNOSTIC DECISION

- A history of well-demarcated digit discoloration associated with cold exposure is the diagnostic criterion for primary or secondary Raynaud's phenomenon. The triphasic discoloration can sometimes be induced in the office by placing the hand in an icebath
- Differentiation of primary from secondary Raynaud's phenomenon is important for determining treatment and prognosis

- Diagnostic criteria for primary Raynaud's phenomenon include: normal nailfold capillary pattern, negative antinuclear antibody test, normal ESR, no evidence of pitting scars, ulceration, or gangrene of the skin on the fingers or toes
- Diagnostic criteria for secondary Raynaud's phenomenon include: abnormal nailfold capillary pattern, positive antinuclear antibody test, abnormal ESR, presence of pitting scars, ulceration, or (in severe cases) gangrene in the skin of the fingers or toes

CLINICAL PEARL(S)

- Although the triphasic color change (white-blue-red) is classic, most patients will not report all three colors. Pallor, followed by cyanosis, is a common history
- Idiopathic Raynaud's is especially common among young women
- Patients with connective tissue disease will almost always have other symptoms besides Raynaud's

THE TESTS

Body fluids

COMPLETE BLOOD COUNT

Description

Venous blood sample.

Advantages/Disadvantages

Advantages:

- Inexpensive, routine, readily available test
- Easy to interpret
- Provides baseline information

Disadvantage: not diagnostic.

Normal

- Hemoglobin: males, 3.6–17.7g/dL (8.4–11.0mmol/L); females, 12.0–15.0g/dL (7.4–9.3mmol/L)
- Hematocrit: 39–49% (males); 33–43% (females)
- Mean corpuscular volume: 76–100mcm^3 (76–100fL)
- White cell count: 3200–9800/mm^3 (3.2–9.8x10^9/L)
- Platelet count: 130–400x10^3/mm^3 (1.3–4.0x10^9/L)

Abnormal

Values outside the normal ranges.

ELECTROLYTES, CREATININE, AND BLOOD UREA NITROGEN

Description

Venous blood sample.

Advantages/Disadvantages

Advantages:

- Inexpensive, routine, readily available test
- Easy to interpret
- Provides baseline information

Disadvantage: not diagnostic.

Normal

- Sodium: 135–147mEq/L (135–147mmol/L)
- Potassium: 3.5–5.0mEq/L (3.5–5.0mmol/L)
- Calcium: 8.8–10.3mg/dL (2.2–2.6mmol/L)
- Urea: 8–18mg/dL (1.3–3.0mmol/L)
- Creatinine: 0.6–1.2mg/dL (53.0–106.1mcmol/L)

Abnormal

Values outside the normal range.

URINALYSIS

Description

Urine sample.

Advantages/Disadvantages

Advantages:

- Inexpensive, routine, readily available test that can be performed in the office
- Easy to interpret
- Provides baseline information

Disadvantage: not diagnostic.

Normal

- Color: light straw-colored
- Appearance: clear
- pH: 4.5–8.0
- Specific gravity: 1.005–1.030
- No protein, ketones, glucose, or blood

Microscopic examination:

- Up to five red blood cells per high-power field
- Up to five white blood cells per high-power field
- No bacteria
- Up to four hyaline casts per low-power field

Abnormal

Features outside the normal parameters.

ANTINUCLEAR ANTIBODY TEST

Description

Serum.

Advantages/Disadvantages

Advantage: may help distinguish between primary and secondary Raynaud's phenomenon.

Normal

No antibodies will be detected in the sample.

Abnormal

- Antibodies will be present in the sample
- Keep in mind the possibility of a false-positive result

Cause of abnormal result
Increased probability that patient has a connective tissue or other autoimmune disorder, particularly SLE.

ERYTHROCYTE SEDIMENTATION RATE
Description
Whole blood.

Advantages/Disadvantages
Advantages:
- May help distinguish primary from secondary Raynaud's phenomenon
- A normal ESR is associated with primary Raynaud's phenomenon
- An elevated ESR may be associated with secondary Raynaud's phenomenon; however, this test is nonspecific and can be elevated for many other reasons such as infections and neoplasms

Disadvantage: test will not provide information regarding the specific disorder associated with secondary Raynaud's.

Normal
- Males: <10mm/h
- Females: <15mm/h

Abnormal
- Values are elevated above normal (any inflammation will elevate the ESR)
- Keep in mind the possibility of a falsely abnormal result

Cause of abnormal result
Inflammation, infections, neoplasms.

ANTICENTROMERE ANTIBODY
Description
Serum.

Advantages/Disadvantages
Advantage: rule out or confirm scleroderma or related disease, e.g. CREST syndrome.

Normal
Anticentromere antibody is absent in sample.

Abnormal
- Anticentromere antibody is detected in sample
- Keep in mind the possibility of a false-positive result

Cause of abnormal result
Increased probability that patient has scleroderma or related connective tissue disease.

ANTI-SCL-70 ANTIBODY
Description
Serum.

Advantages/Disadvantages
Advantage: specific test to confirm or rule out a diagnosis of scleroderma.

Normal

Anti-Scl-70 antibodies are absent from sample.

Abnormal
- Anti-Scl-70 antibodies are detected in sample
- Keep in mind the possibility of a false-positive result

Cause of abnormal result
Patient has scleroderma.

CRYOGLOBULINS
Description
Serum.

Advantages/Disadvantages
Advantage: confirm or rule out possibility of cryoglobulinemia.

Normal
Less than 0.12mg/dL.

Abnormal
- Levels are elevated above normal values
- Keep in mind the possibility of a false-positive result

Cause of abnormal result
Cryoglobulins in the blood support a diagnosis of cryoglobulinemia.

PROTEIN ELECTROPHORESIS
Description
Serum.

Advantages/Disadvantages
Advantage: confirms or rules out possible secondary causes for Raynaud's phenomenon, e.g. cryoglobulinemia.

Normal
- Albumin: 3.3–4.7g/dL (33–47g/L)
- $Alpha_1$: 0.1–0.4g/dL (1–4g/L)
- $Alpha_2$: 0.3–0.9g/dL (3–9g/L)
- $Beta_2$: 0.7–1.5g/dL (7–15g/L)
- Gamma: 0.5–1.4g/dL (5–14g/L)

Abnormal
- Elevated levels of any globulins
- Keep in mind the possibility of a false-positive result

Cause of abnormal result
- Hypergammaglobulinemia often associated with scleroderma
- Multiple myeloma and other hyperglobulinemic states associated with cryoglobulinemia

Imaging

NAILFOLD CAPILLAROSCOPY

Advantages/Disadvantages

Advantages:

- Test may differentiate between primary and secondary Raynaud's phenomenon
- A normal result points towards a diagnosis of primary Raynaud's phenomenon
- An abnormal result suggests a diagnosis of secondary Raynaud's phenomenon associated with a connective tissue disorder

Normal

Capillaries supplying patient's nailfolds appear normal.

Abnormal

Capillaries supplying nailfolds are enlarged or deformed.

Cause of abnormal result

Probable connective tissue disorder.

TREATMENT

CONSIDER CONSULT

- If nonpharmacologic and drug measures fail, referral to a microvascular surgeon is warranted

PATIENT AND CAREGIVER ISSUES

Health-seeking behavior

Has patient implemented nonpharmacologic measures to ameliorate an attack of Raynaud's? For example, keeping warm in cold weather by dressing appropriately, reducing stress at home or work.

MANAGEMENT ISSUES

Goals

- To reduce the number and severity of attacks
- To prevent tissue damage in the fingers and toes

SUMMARY OF THERAPEUTIC OPTIONS

Choices

Patients with either primary or secondary Raynaud's will benefit from a number of general lifestyle, nonpharmacologic measures:

- Avoidance of cold exposure and stress reduction
- The use of warm dress to keep the whole body warm including thermal underwear, hat, mittens
- Knowledge of techniques to help terminate an attack, including placing the hands under warm water or in a warm place, rotating the arms in a whirling or windmill pattern
- Avoidance of smoking and sympathomimetic drugs including decongestants, amphetamines, diet pills, herbs containing ephedra

Pharmacologic therapy may ultimately be necessary, particularly for patients with secondary Raynaud's phenomenon, which is the more severe form of the disease:

- Calcium channel blockers are the most effective treatment for Raynaud's phenomenon. Nifedipine is the calcium channel blocker that is most often recommended. If side-effects occur, other calcium channel blockers can be used, including diltiazem, felodipine, amlodipine, nicardipine, and nisoldipine. Verapamil has not been shown to be effective in Raynaud's phenomenon
- The sympatholytic drugs prazosin and phenoxybenzamine have shown some effectiveness in treating Raynaud's phenomenon
- Direct vasodilators including nitroglycerin have been used topically in the treatment of Raynaud's phenomenon
- Intravenous epoprostenol (prostacyclin) (PG12) has been reported to be beneficial in the short term in the treatment of severe Raynaud's phenomenon. Alprostadil (PGE1) failed to show a significant clinical benefit
- Localized digital sympathectomy should be limited to patients who have failed medical treatment and who have some benefit from temporary chemical sympathectomy but continue to experience ischemia or threat of losing digit

Clinical pearl(s)

- Almost all patients with limited or diffuse scleroderma will have a positive test for antinuclear antibody
- An abnormal nailfold capillary examination strongly points to the presence of a connective disease
- Be sure the whole body is warmed including a scarf, facemask, and hat

FOLLOW UP

Plan for review

- Almost all patients with limited or diffuse scleroderma will have a positive test for antinuclear antibody
- An abnormal nailfold capillary examination strongly points to the presence of a connective disease
- Be sure the whole body is warmed including a scarf, facemask, and hat

Information for patient or caregiver

The patient should be instructed about exposure to cold, methods for staying warm, and the importance of smoking cessation.

DRUGS AND OTHER THERAPIES: DETAILS

Drugs

NIFEDIPINE

This is an off-label indication.

Dose

- Nifedipine is most often prescribed at a dose of 10–20mg by mouth 30min before going outside, or may be given in three divided doses up to 60mg/day
- For symptoms that have a long duration, nifedipine XL 30–90mg by mouth once daily is effective

Efficacy

Reduces both frequency and severity of attacks.

Risks/Benefits

Risks:

- Nifedipine should be used during pregnancy only if the potential benefit justifies the potential risk to the fetus
- Use caution in congestive heart failure, hypotension, aortic stenosis, hepatic and renal disease, and recent beta-blocker withdrawal
- Use caution in the elderly

Side-effects and adverse reactions

- Cardiovascular: bradycardia, peripheral edema, palpitations
- CNS: dizziness, headache, paresthesias
- Gastrointestinal: constipation, nausea, dry mouth, dyspepsia
- Genitourinary: nocturia, polyuria, sexual dysfunction
- Respiratory: cough, dyspnea
- Skin: alopecia, pruritus, rash

Interactions (other drugs)

■ Anticoagulants ■ Barbiturates ■ Beta-blockers ■ Cimetidine, ranitidine ■ Carbamazepine ■ Cardiac glycosides ■ Diltiazem ■ Doxasozin ■ Fentanyl ■ Grapefruit juice ■ Histamine H_2 antagonists ■ Insulin ■ Lansoprazole ■ Magnesium ■ Phenytoin ■ Quinidine ■ Theophylline ■ Vincristine

Contraindications

■ Severe coronary artery disease ■ Recent myocardial infarction ■ Hypertensive emergencies ■ Pregnancy category C ■ Safety and efficacy in pediatric patients have not been established

Acceptability to patient

High.

DILTIAZEM

This is an off-label indication.

Dose

30mg by mouth four times initially, gradually increased up to a maximum dose of 120mg by mouth four times daily until optimum response is obtained.

Efficacy

Reduces frequency and severity of attacks.

Risks/Benefits

Risks:

- Use caution in congestive heart failure, hypotension, aortic stenosis, hepatic and renal disease
- Use caution in the elderly and children

Side-effects and adverse reactions

- Cardiovascular: peripheral edema, palpitations, arrhythmia, atrioventricular block, congestive heart failure
- CNS: dizziness, headache, paresthesia
- Gastrointestinal: constipation, nausea, dry mouth, dyspepsia
- Skin: alopecia, pruritus, rash

Interactions (other drugs)

▪ Adrenergic blockers (alpha- and beta-blockers) ▪ Antidysrhythmics (amiodarone, cardiac glycosides) ▪ Anticonvulsants (carbemazepine, phenobarbital, phenytoin) ▪ Aspirin ▪ Azole antifungals ▪ Cyclosporine, tacrolimus ▪ Erythromycin, troleandomycin ▪ Fentanyl ▪ H_2 receptor antagonists ▪ Lithium ▪ Neuromuscular blockers ▪ Nitroprusside ▪ Rifampin ▪ Tricyclic antidepressants

Contraindications

▪ Recent myocardial infarction, severe bradycardia, ventricular tachycardia, atrial fibrillation, hypotension, sick sinus syndrome, second- or third-degree atrioventricular block ▪ Pregnancy and breast-feeding

Acceptability to patient

High.

FELODIPINE

This is an off-label indication.

Dose

2.5mg by mouth once daily, up to 10mg once daily.

Efficacy

Reduces frequency and severity of attacks.

Risks/Benefits

Risks:

- May cause significant hypotension and, rarely, syncope
- Patients over 65 years of age or patients with impaired liver function may have elevated plasma concentrations of felodipine and may respond to lower doses of felodipine; therefore a starting dose of 2.5mg once daily is recommended
- May cause peripheral edema

Side-effects and adverse reactions

- Cardiovascular: peripheral edema, palpitation
- CNS: asthenia, headache, dizziness, paresthesia
- Gastrointestinal: nausea, vomiting, constipation
- Respiratory: sneezing, rhinorrhea, infection
- Skin: rash, flushing

Interactions (other drugs)

- Beta-blockers
- Cimetidine
- Anticonvulsants

Contraindications

- Hypersensitivity to felodipine
- Pregnancy category C
- Breast-feeding
- Safety and effectiveness in pediatric patients have not been established

Acceptability to patient

High.

Patient and caregiver information

- Administer as whole tablet; not to be crushed or chewed
- Grapefruit juice should be avoided

AMLODIPINE

This is an off-label indication.

Dose

5mg by mouth once daily initially, may increase up to 10mg by mouth once daily.

Efficacy

Reduces frequency and severity of attacks.

Risks/Benefits

Risks:

- Use caution in congestive heart failure, aortic stenosis, hypotension, hepatic insufficiency
- Use caution in the elderly

Side-effects and adverse reactions

- Cardiovascular: bradycardia, arrhythmias (including ventricular tachycardia and atrial fibrillation), hypotension, palpitations, chest pain, peripheral edema, syncope, tachycardia, postural dizziness
- CNS: anxiety, asthenia, depression, fatigue, headache, insomnia, malaise, tremor
- Gastrointestinal: constipation, dyspepsia, diarrhea, flatulence, pancreatitis, vomiting, gingival hyperplasia
- Genitourinary: nocturia, polyuria
- Musculoskeletal: arthralgia, arthrosis, muscle cramps, myalgia
- Skin: angiodema, erythema multiforme, pruritus, rash, erythematous rash, maculopapular rash

Interactions (other drugs)

■ Barbiturates ■ Diltiazem ■ Erythromycin ■ Fentanyl ■ H_2 receptor antagonists ■ Proton pump inhibitors ■ Quinidine ■ Rifampin ■ Vincristine ■ Grapefruit juice

Contraindications

■ Sensitivity to amlodipine ■ Cardiogenic shock ■ Unstable angina ■ Significant aortic stenosis ■ Pregnancy and breast-feeding

Acceptability to patient

High.

Patient and caregiver information

Advise patient to notify physician of:

- Irregular heartbeat
- Shortness of breath
- Swelling of feet or hands
- Pronounced dizziness or hypotension

NICARDIPINE

This is an off-label indication.

Dose

20mg by mouth three times a day up to 40mg by mouth three times a day.

Efficacy

Reduces frequency and severity of attacks.

Risks/Benefits

Risks:

- Effective antianginal and antihypertensive medications
- Use caution in congestive heart failure, hypotension, aortic stenosis, hepatic and renal disease
- Use caution in the elderly

Side-effects and adverse reactions

- Cardiovascular: angina, bradycardia, peripheral edema, palpitations
- CNS: depression, dizziness, headache, paresthesia
- Gastrointestinal: constipation, nausea, dry mouth, dyspepsia, vomiting
- Genitourinary: nocturia, polyuria, sexual dysfunction
- Respiratory: cough, dyspnea
- Skin: alopecia, pruritus, rash

Interactions (other drugs)

■ Beta-blockers ■ Calcium ■ Cyclosporine, tacrolimus ■ H_2 antagonists ■ Fentanyl ■ Neuromuscular blocking agents

Contraindications

■ Cardiogenic shock ■ Advanced aortic stenosis ■ Unstable or acute attacks of angina ■ Pregnancy and breast-feeding. Avoid within 1 month of myocardial infarction

Acceptability to patient

High.

NISOLDIPINE

This is an off-label indication.

Dose

20mg once daily by mouth, may increase by 10mg/week to a maximum of 60mg/day.

Efficacy

Reduces frequency and severity of attacks.

Risks/Benefits

Risks:

- Increased angina and/or myocardial infarction in patients with coronary artery disease
- Blood pressure should be carefully monitored
- Use caution in patients with severe hepatic dysfunction

Side-effects and adverse reactions

- Cardiovascular: peripheral edema, vasodilation, palpitation, chest pain
- CNS: dizziness, headache
- EENT: laryngitis, sinusitis
- Gastrointestinal: nausea

Interactions (other drugs)

- Cimetidine
- Quinidine

Contraindications

- Known hypersensitivity to dihydropyridine calcium channel blockers
- Pregnancy category C
- Breast-feeding

Patient and caregiver information

Do not take with high-fat meals or grapefruit juice.

PRAZOSIN

This is an off-label indication.

Dose

1mg by mouth twice a day, up to 4mg by mouth twice a day. Initial dose should be taken at bedtime to minimize risk of hypotension.

Efficacy

Modestly effective in reducing episodes in secondary Raynaud's.

Risks/Benefits

Risks:

- May cause syncope with sudden loss of consciousness
- May cause drowsiness – avoid driving or operating machinery

Side-effects and adverse reactions

- Cardiovascular: palpitations
- CNS: dizziness, headache, drowsiness, lack of energy, weakness
- Gastrointestinal: nausea

Interactions (other drugs)

- Cardiac glycosides
- Hypoglycemics
- Tranquilizers and sedatives
- Antigout drugs
- Antiarrhythmics
- Analgesics, antipyretics, and anti-inflammatories

Contraindications

- Known sensitivity to quinazolines, prazosin, or any of the inert ingredients
- Pregnancy category C
- Breast-feeding
- Safety and effectiveness in children have not been established

Patient and caregiver information

- Alert patient to the possibility of syncopal and orthostatic symptoms, particularly following the first dose
- Take initial dose at bedtime

PHENOXYBENZAMINE

This is an off-label indication.

Dose

10mg by mouth twice a day initially; usual dosage range 20–40mg two or three times daily.

Risks/Benefits

Risk: first-dose effect resulting in profound hypoytension may occur with first dose – recommend taking first dose at bedtime and not prior to any activity where dizziness would be a significant hazard.

Side-effects and adverse reactions

- Cardiovascular: syncope, orthostatic hypotension
- CNS: dizziness, headache, drowsiness
- Genitourinary: urinary incontinence

Interactions (other drugs)

- Angiotensin-converting enzyme (ACE) inhibitors
- Indomethacin
- Beta-blockers
- Verapamil

Contraindications

- Avoid in pregnancy.

Patient and caregiver information

- Patient should avoid alcohol
- Dizziness may result from sudden changes in posture
- Cough, cold, or allergy medications containing sympathomimetics should be avoided

NITROGLYCERIN

This is an off-label indication.

Dose

Topical application of 1–2 inches every 8h, up to 4–5 inches every 4h.

Efficacy

Reduces severity and frequency of attacks in both primary and secondary Raynaud's.

Risks/Benefits

Risks:

- Risk of persistent headache
- Tolerance may occur

Side-effects and adverse reactions

- Cardiovascular: atrial fibrillation, collapse, dysrhythmias, postural hypotension, palpitations, rebound hypertension, syncope
- CNS: headache, dizziness, anxiety, dizziness
- EENT: blurred vision
- Gastrointestinal: abdominal pain, nausea, vomiting, diarrhea
- Genitourinary: dysuria, urinary frequency, impotence
- Hematologic: hemolytic anemia, methemoglobinemia
- Musculoskeletal: arthralgia
- Skin: cutaneous vasodilation, contact dermatitis

Interactions (other drugs)

■ Ergot alkaloids: opposition to coronary vasodilatory effects of nitrates ■ Ethanol: additive vasodilation could cause hypotension ■ Metronidazole: ethanol contained in intravenous nitroglycerin preparations could cause disulfiram-like reaction in some patients ■ Sildenafil: additive vasodilation may produce profound hypotension ■ A possible interaction with heparin may occur: this is of particular importance because heparin and nitroglycerin are frequently administered together. Several reports suggest that nitroglycerin may decrease sensitivity to heparin, necessitating larger heparin doses to achieve anticoagulation. Discontinuance of nitroglycerin during concomitant heparin infusion can potentially lead to increased bleeding risk if heparin dosing is not simultaneously adjusted

Contraindications

■ Hypotension ■ Cerebral hemorrhage ■ Head trauma ■ Early myocardial infarction ■ Severe anemia ■ Closed-angle glaucoma ■ Constrictive pericarditis ■ Percardial tamponade (intravenous)

Acceptability to patient

Headache may limit use.

Patient and caregiver information

- Alcohol should be avoided
- Patient should notify physician if persistent headache occurs
- A thin layer of ointment should be spread on skin using an applicator or dose-measuring papers; patient should not use fingers, rub, or massage

EPOPROSTENOL (PROSTACYCLIN)

This is an off-label indication.

Dose

- Chronic infusion should be initiated at 2ng/kg/min and increased in increments of 2ng/kg/min every 15min or longer until dose-limiting pharmacologic effects are elicited, or until a tolerance limit to the drug is established and further increases in the infusion rate are not clinically warranted
- Increments in dose should be considered if symptoms of pulmonary hypertension persist or recur after improving. The infusion should be increased by 1–2ng/kg/min increments at intervals sufficient to allow assessment of clinical response; these intervals should be at least 15min

Efficacy

- Short-term palliation of severe Raynaud's phenomenon
- Reduces frequency and severity of attacks
- Prevents or speeds healing of ulceration

Risks/Benefits

Risks:

- Must be reconstituted only as directed using sterile diluent for preparation and must not be reconstituted or mixed with any other parenteral medications or solutions prior to or during administration
- Abrupt withdrawal (including interruptions in drug delivery) or sudden large reductions in dosage may result in symptoms associated with rebound pulmonary hypertension

Side-effects and adverse reactions

- Cardiovascular: flushing, hypotension, chest pain, bradycardia
- CNS: headache, anxiety, dizziness
- Gastrointestinal: nausea, vomiting, abdominal pain
- Musculoskeletal: pain
- Respiratory: dyspnea

Interactions (other drugs)

- Diuretics ■ Antihypertensive agent ■ Other vasodilators

Contraindications

- Known hypersensitivity to the drug or to structurally related compound
- Congestive heart failure ■ Pulmonary hypertension ■ Pregnancy category B
- Breast-feeding ■ Safety and effectiveness in pediatric patients have not been established

Surgical therapy

LOCALIZED DIGITAL SYMPATHECTOMY

Should be limited to patients who have failed medical treatment and who have some benefit from temporary chemical sympathectomy but continue to experience ischemia or threat of losing digit.

Efficacy

- Moderate improvement in cold intolerance
- Sustained effect over 2.5 years
- May allow narcotic analgesics to be discontinued, but unlikely to result in a vasodilator medication change
- Digital ulcers often heal postoperatively

Risks/Benefits

Risk: few complications following digital sympathectomy.

Acceptability to patient

Most patients feel their quality of life is improved and would have surgery again.

LIFESTYLE

Patients should be advised to:

- Avoid cold exposure
- Reduce stress
- Use warm clothes to keep the whole body warm in cold conditions, including thermal underwear, hat, mittens
- Learn techniques to help terminate an attack (e.g. placing the hands under warm water or in a warm place, rotating the arms in a whirling or windmill pattern)
- Avoid smoking and sympathomimetic drugs, including decongestants, amphetamines, diet pills, herbs containing ephedra
- Avoid drugs and medications known to cause the phenomenon

RISKS/BENEFITS

Benefit: patients with either primary or secondary Raynaud's will benefit from general lifestyle measures.

ACCEPTABILITY TO PATIENT

High, except in the case of avoidance of smoking for addicted smokers.

OUTCOMES

EFFICACY OF THERAPIES
Most therapies are moderately effective in reducing frequency and severity of attacks. Complete relief is unlikely, especially in secondary Raynaud's.

Review period
Dependent on symptom relief and associated diseases.

PROGNOSIS
Between 40 and 60% of patients with primary Raynaud's phenomenon respond to management techniques.

Clinical pearl(s)
- Before pharmacologic therapy is considered, patients should be advised to be diligent in maintaining extremity warmth, including covering the head in cold weather
- The calcium channel blockers, especially those of the dihydropyridine class, are the agents of choice in managing Raynaud's phenomenon
- Patients should be counseled that no medications are likely to be effective in patients who do not cease smoking

Therapeutic failure
Vascular inflow should be assessed in severe cases. If significant obstruction is found, surgical correction is indicated.

Recurrence
This is a chronic disease. Digital ulcers rarely recur after surgical therapy.

Deterioration
Digital sympathectomy can be used in the case of severe secondary Raynaud's phenomenon.

COMPLICATIONS
Digital ulceration, gangrene, amputation, narcotic dependence.

CONSIDER CONSULT
- Referral is indicated in refractory cases with developing narcotic dependence or digital ulcers. May also need referral for management of the secondary associated disease

PREVENTION

RISK FACTORS

Risk factors for attacks in susceptible patients include:

- Exposure to cold temperatures
- Smoking
- Sympathomimetic drugs including decongestants, amphetamines, diet pills, herbs containing ephedra

MODIFY RISK FACTORS

Patients should be warned to:

- Avoid exposure to cold temperatures
- Dress appropriately if cold exposure cannot be avoided
- Avoid smoking and sympathomimetic drugs including decongestants, amphetamines, diet pills, herbs containing ephedra

Lifestyle and wellness

TOBACCO

Patients should be strongly encouraged to give up smoking.

ENVIRONMENT

Exposure to cold may precipitate attacks in susceptible people.

FAMILY HISTORY

A family history of predisposing factors or associated disorders may indicate an increased risk of developing Raynaud's phenomenon.

DRUG HISTORY

Sympathomimetic drugs (e.g. decongestants, amphetamines, diet pills, herbs containing ephedra) may precipitate attacks in susceptible people.

PREVENT RECURRENCE

Avoid situations which the patient knows can precipitate an attack, e.g. cold or stressful situations.

ASSOCIATIONS

Arthritis Foundation
1330 West Peachtree Street
Atlanta, GA 30309
Tel: (404) 872-7100
Toll-free: (800) 283-7800
www.arthritis.org

United Scleroderma Foundation, Inc
PO Box 350
Watsonville, CA 95077-0350
Tel: (408) 728-2202

American Lupus Society
23751 Madison Street
Torrance, CA 90505
Tel: (213) 373-1335

KEY REFERENCES

- National Institute of Arthritis and Musculoskeletal and Skin Diseases (http://www.nih.gov/niams). Questions and answers about Raynaud's disease (http://www.nih.gov/niams/healthinfo/ar125fs.htm)
- Tierey LM, McPhee SJ, Papadakis MA. Current medical diagnosis and treatment, 38th edn. New York: McGraw-Hill, 1998
- Wigley FM. Treatment of Raynaud's phenomenon. located at: http://www.medscape.com/
- Raynaud's phenomena. Harvard Health Letter 1992;17(3)
- Block JA, Sequeira W. Raynaud's phenomenon. Lancet 2001;357:2042–8
- Thompson AE, Shea B, Welch V, et al. Calcium-channel blockers for Raynaud's phenomenon in systemic sclerosis. Arth Rheum 2001;44:1841–7
- Pope J, Fenlon D, Thompson A, et al. Iloprost and cisaprost for Raynaud's phenomenon in progressive systemic sclerosis (Cochrane Review). In: The Cochrane Library, 1, 2002. Oxford: Update Software
- Tomaino MM, Goitz RJ, Medsger TA. Surgery for ischemic pain and Raynaud's phenomenon in scleroderma: description of treatment protocol and evaluation of results. Microsurgery 2001;21:75–9

FAQS

Question 1

How frequently does Raynaud's phenomenon progress to a full-blown connective tissue disease?

ANSWER 1

Patients presenting with mild symptoms, normal erythrocyte sedimentation rate (ESR) and normal serology have a 6.3% risk over 10 years of developing a secondary disease.

Question 2

What diagnostic work-up should be done for a new patient who appears otherwise healthy?

ANSWER 2

ESR, antinuclear antibodies (ANA), nailbed capillaroscopy. If the ANA and capillaroscopy are abnormal, the patient is highly likely to have preclinical scleroderma.

Question 3

What is the role of antithrombotic agents?

ANSWER 3
Anticoagulation should not be routinely used, and there is almost no role in primary syndrome. Sporadic reports of benefit with thrombolysis or low-molecular-weight heparin have been seen in severe cases of ischemia; however, treatment should be individualized.

Question 4
My patients are quite unhappy with the symptoms and have found a number of reports of 'cures'. What nontraditional therapy is worth looking into?

ANSWER 4
Plasmapheresis, estrogens, acupuncture, biofeedback, and antioxidants have all been anecdotally reported to help. Probucol has also been shown to be of benefit.

Question 5
What about endothelial function?

ANSWER 5
Endothelial function and, in secondary cases, the endothelial structure is deranged in Raynaud's. Short-term infusion of L-arginine has improved acute symptoms, but has not provided lasting results. Calcitonin gene-related protein has also been beneficial in the short term. Cold-sensitive $alpha_2$ adrenergic receptor blocking agents are under development. Currently, there are no viable substitutes for traditional therapy.

CONTRIBUTORS
Fred F Ferri, MD, FACP
John McB Hodgson, MD, FACC, FSCAI
Richard Brasington Jr, MD, FACP
James Orford, MD

RHEUMATIC FEVER

SUMMARY INFORMATION

DESCRIPTION

- Delayed sequela of upper respiratory infection with group A streptococcus, occurring 2–3 weeks after infection
- Characterized by nonsuppurative inflammatory lesions involving primarily the heart, joints, subcutaneous tissues, and central nervous system
- Classic form is acute, febrile, and self-limiting
- Damage to heart valves can occur, be chronic and progressive, and lead to heart failure and death many years after the initial episode

URGENT ACTION

Congestive heart failure, a rare complication, requires immediate treatment.

KEY! DON'T MISS!

Do not fail to miss signs or symptoms suggestive of congestive heart failure, which can complicate carditis. Immediate attention and referral is indicated.

BACKGROUND

ICD9 CODE
390 Rheumatic fever.

SYNONYMS
- Acute rheumatic fever
- Rheumatic carditis

CARDINAL FEATURES
- Acute episodes occur about 2–3 weeks after group A streptococcal pharyngitis
- Clinical presentation is highly variable, possibly including carditis, Sydenham's chorea, migratory polyarthritis, erythema marginatum, and subcutaneous nodules
- Initial treatment involves eradication of residual group A streptococci, reduction of inflammation, and treatment of congestive heart failure if present
- Prophylaxis against additional group A streptococcal infections necessary for at least 5 years (length of treatment reflects degree of cardiac involvement)

CAUSES
Common causes
- In all instances, occurs as a delayed sequela of group A streptococcal pharyngitis, including pharyngitis associated with scarlet fever
- Never results from group A streptococcal skin infections

Contributory or predisposing factors
- Repeated upper respiratory infections
- Family history of rheumatic fever
- Crowded living or working conditions, such as military bases

EPIDEMIOLOGY
Incidence and prevalence
INCIDENCE
- The incidence of rheumatic fever is very low in the West (e.g. in Scotland, 6/million per year; in the US <2/100,000). In developing countries it may exceed 100/100,000
- Overall incidence is 0.18 per 1000 in ages 5–17; more rare in adults
- Peak incidence in Europe and US is in the spring
- An estimated 3% of military recruits with untreated streptococcal pharyngitis develop rheumatic fever, compared with 0.4% of untreated children

PREVALENCE
- 6.8 per 1000
- Affects approximately 1 in 1,800,000 Americans

Demographics
AGE
- In children, peak incidence between ages 5–15
- Adults more likely to have recurrent than primary disease
- In adults, peak incidence of primary adult disease is end of the second to the beginning of the third decade of life

Adults:
- More likely than children to have accompanying severe arthritis
- Less likely than children to have accompanying chorea

GENDER
Females more often affected.

RACE
Higher incidence among the following groups:
- African-Americans
- Puerto Ricans
- Hispanic-Americans
- Native Americans
- Native Hawaiians

GENETICS
Familial pattern of occurrence often seen; one or more genes may confer susceptibility.

GEOGRAPHY
- Rare in developed countries
- Rampant in Middle East, Indian subcontinent, and parts of Africa and South America

SOCIOECONOMIC STATUS
- Outbreaks have occurred at military bases
- Historically linked to inner-city poor; however, this population has become less at risk due to improved access to medical care
- Outbreaks in the 1980s affected middle-class populations in urban and rural areas

DIFFERENTIAL DIAGNOSIS

Bacterial endocarditis

The main features of bacterial endocarditis are as follows:

FEATURES

- Valvular endocardium most often involved
- Abrupt onset with high fever and systemic toxicity
- New or altered heart murmur in some cases
- Endocarditis affecting native valves, most often seen in patients above age 50, frequently with a predisposing cardiac lesion
- Bacterial endocarditis can complicate pre-existing rheumatic heart disease

Viral myocarditis

FEATURES

- Usually follows viral illness by 2 weeks
- May present with fatigue, palpitations, dyspnea with exertion, chest pain (35% of cases), fever (20% of cases)
- Fulminant congestive heart failure in some instances

Systemic lupus

The main features of systemic lupus are as follows:

FEATURES

- Most cases are in women of childbearing age
- Nearly any organ system may be affected
- Common manifestations are fever, fatigue, rash (often facial 'butterfly' rash), inflammatory arthritis, anemia, cardiopulmonary symptoms (pleuritis, pericarditis, myocarditis, endocarditis), nephritis, peritonitis, and organic brain syndromes
- Presence of antinuclear antibodies a cardinal feature

Serum sickness

FEATURES

- Serum sickness occurs 6–21 days after injection of foreign protein or serum
- Usual symptoms are fever, arthralgia, lymphadenopathy, and skin eruption
- Possible chest pain and dyspnea
- Systemic disease usually preceded by pain, pruritus, and swelling at injection site

Rheumatoid arthritis

The main features of rheumatoid arthritis are as follows:

FEATURES

- Characterized by persistent inflammatory synovitis, usually affecting peripheral joints
- Most cases seen in women in fourth and fifth decades
- Early morning stiffness, arthritis involving at least three joints, subcutaneous nodules, occasional rash, thick synovium

Infectious arthritis

The main features of infectious arthritis are as follows:

FEATURES

- Presents as a monoarticular process involving large joints
- Swelling, pain, warmth, and restricted movement
- Predisposing factors include immunosuppression, alcoholism, intravenous drug use, and former joint damage

SIGNS & SYMPTOMS

Signs

MAJOR MANIFESTATIONS

Carditis (65% of patients):

- When present, usually appears early in the course of disease
- New murmur of mitral or aortic insufficiency
- Mitral regurgitation typically of moderate to high intensity throughout systole
- Aortic insufficiency (less common), signaled by basal diastolic murmur
- Pancarditis and pericardial friction rub, with pericardial and myocardial involvement, may accompany valvulitis
- Cardiomegaly
- Congestive heart failure
- Transient mitral diastolic murmur

Migratory polyarthritis (75% of patients):

- Most often affects large joints of extremities
- Extremely painful, with redness, heat, swelling, and limitation of motion
- Typically disappears in less than 4 weeks

Sydenham's chorea, St. Vitus' dance (5–10% of patients):

- Rapid, uncontrolled motions of face and upper extremities
- Sometimes cease during sleep
- Onset may be delayed for months, presenting after other signs have resolved
- Attacks can last 2–4 months
- Rare in adult females; almost nonexistent in adult males

Subcutaneous nodules (10% of patients):

- Firm, painless nodules typically on wrists, elbows, knees, and Achilles tendons, from a few millimeters to about 2cm in size
- Resemblance to the nodules associated with systemic lupus erythematosus
- Nodules nearly always occur in conjunction with carditis
- Usually persist 1–2 weeks

Erythema marginatum (less than 5% of patients):

- Nonpruritic, nonpainful eruption
- Raised or flat erythematous patches, commonly on trunk and proximal parts of extremities
- Evanescent in nature; patterns can change before the observer's eyes
- Center of each patch returns to normalcy in advance of the margins
- Generally associated with subcutaneous nodules; nearly always seen in conjunction with carditis
- Lesions may for last minutes to hours; entire process may occur over weeks to months

MINOR MANIFESTATIONS

- Arthralgia
- Fever: 101–104°F (38.3–40.0°C)
- Elevated acute-phase reactants (C-reactive protein and erythrocyte sedimentation rate [ESR])
- Prolonged PR interval on electrocardiogram
- Leukocytosis (indicative of previous rheumatic fever)

Symptoms

NONSPECIFIC SYMPTOMS

- Fever
- Aching joints
- Abdominal pain, sometimes severe
- Possible nosebleeds
- Weakness
- Fatigue

SPECIFIC SYMPTOMS

- Arthritis that affects numerous joints but emerges in one joint at a time
- Abnormal heartbeat
- Chest pain
- Possible shortness of breath
- Red patches on skin, possibly with normal skin in the center of each patch
- Small, painless lumps beneath skin
- Rapid, involuntary movements in muscles of extremities and/or face (rare in adults)

KEY! DON'T MISS!

Do not fail to miss signs or symptoms suggestive of congestive heart failure, which can complicate carditis. Immediate attention and referral is indicated.

CONSIDER CONSULT

- Pre-existing heart disease
- Pregnancy
- Severe carditis, associated with signs or symptoms of congestive heart failure

INVESTIGATION OF THE PATIENT

Direct questions to patient

- Q **Did you have a sore throat in recent weeks?** About 70% of adults with acute rheumatic fever can recall pharyngitis. In others, infection may have been subclinical
- Q **Do you have chest pain, unusual weakness, irregular heartbeats, or shortness of breath?** May signal cardiac involvement
- Q **Do you have aching joints?** Arthralgia is designated as a minor manifestation of rheumatic fever in the diagnostic Jones criteria
- Q **If polyarthritis is present, did it emerge in different joints simultaneously or at different times?** Arthritis associated with rheumatic fever is considered migratory because it emerges in one joint at a time. (However, it may persist temporarily in one joint after emerging in another)
- Q **How painful is your arthritis?** Arthritis associated with rheumatic fever is extremely painful, although it responds dramatically to salicylates

Contributory or predisposing factors

- Q **Do you get sore throats often?** Affirmative answer may signal increased vulnerability to rheumatic fever
- Q **Have you had a previous acute attack of rheumatic fever?** Patients who have once had rheumatic fever are vulnerable to recurrent disease
- Q **Do you live or work in crowded conditions?** Risk increased at military bases and other crowded environments

Family history

Q Have any family members had rheumatic fever? Susceptibility to rheumatic fever is thought to have a genetic component, although specific genes causing susceptibility have not been identified. Those with currently affected family members may have been infected with group A streptococci by their relatives

Examination

- **Are cardiac irregularities evident with auscultation?** Mitral insufficiency is the most likely cardiac manifestation. Mitral regurgitation is most evident at apex; occurs throughout systole; intensity is moderate to high. Aortic insufficiency manifests with a basal diastolic murmur, usually high-pitched and blowing. Pulmonic, tricuspid valves rarely involved
- **Does patient have signs of rheumatic arthritis?** Check knees, ankles, elbows, and wrists for swelling, erythema, heat, severe pain, and restricted motion
- **Does patient have chorea?** (Usually occurs after, rather than in association with, acute disease.) Observe for involuntary motions and lack of muscle coordination. Ask patient to squeeze your fingers. A squeezing and relaxing motion known as 'milkmaid's grip' suggests Sydenham's chorea
- **Does skin display erythema marginatum?** Check for nonpruritic rash that forms red patches with normal skin at the center
- **Are subcutaneous nodules present?** Check elbows, knees, and wrists; the occipital scalp; and spinous processes. Nodules are firm and freely movable; overlying skin is not discolored or inflamed
- **Does patient have fever?** Check temperature. Like arthralgia, fever can support the diagnosis when only a single major manifestation is present

Summary of investigative tests

- Throat culture: useful in all cases for evidence of a preceding group A streptococcal infection
- Rapid antigen test: commonly used to screen for group A streptococcal infection, but throat culture is more definitive
- Serologic antibody tests: used when throat culture and rapid antigen tests are negative. Antistreptolysin O (ASO) titer most commonly used, but anti-DNase B and antihyaluronidase titers may also be obtained
- Acute-phase reactants: ESR and C-reactive protein. Test results may assist diagnosis by fulfilling a minor manifestation of the Jones criteria
- Chest X-ray: indicates cardiomegaly and congestive heart failure, if present
- Echocardiography: may confirm evidence of cardiac involvement
- Electrocardiography: may indicate pericarditis, or prolonged PR interval, which is identified by the revised Jones criteria as a minor manifestation of rheumatic fever

DIAGNOSTIC DECISION

Rheumatic fever should be considered highly probable in patients with evidence of a preceding group A streptococcal infection of the upper respiratory tract in conjunction with either two major manifestations, or one major and two minor manifestations. Lack of evidence of a preceding group A streptococcal infection makes the diagnosis doubtful in nearly all instances. Guidelines not intended to substitute for clinical judgment.

MAJOR MANIFESTATIONS

- Carditis
- Polyarthritis
- Chorea
- Erythema marginatum
- Subcutaneous nodules

MINOR MANIFESTATIONS

- Arthralgia
- Fever
- Laboratory findings of elevated acute-phase reactants, ESR, C-reactive protein
- Electrocardiographic findings of prolonged PR interval

SUPPORTIVE EVIDENCE OF ANTECEDENT GROUP A STREPTOCOCCAL INFECTION

- Positive throat culture or rapid streptococcal antigen test
- Elevated or rising streptococcal antibody titer

EXCEPTIONS TO THE ABOVE CRITERIA

- Chorea may be the sole manifestation of rheumatic fever
- Indolent carditis may be the sole manifestation in patients who seek medical treatment months after the onset of rheumatic fever
- In individuals with a history of rheumatic fever or rheumatic heart disease, pre-emptive diagnosis of a rheumatic recurrence may be based on a single major or several minor manifestations, provided supporting evidence of a recent group A streptococcal infection exists

Guidelines

- Guidelines for the diagnosis of rheumatic fever. Jones criteria, 1992 update. Special writing group of the committee on Rheumatic Fever, Endocarditis, and Kawasaki Disease of the Council on Cardiovascular Disease in the Young of the American Heart Association. JAMA 1992;268:2069–73 [1]

CLINICAL PEARL(S)

- Avoid use of echocardiography to 'overdiagnose' valvular regurgitation in the absence of clinical manifestations
- Myocarditis or pericarditis in the absence or valvular involvement is not likely to be rheumatic fever
- Failure of the arthritis to respond dramatically to anti-inflammatory agents should indicate a re-evaluation of the diagnosis

THE TESTS

Body fluids

THROAT CULTURE

Description

Swab of pharynx, particularly areas of inflammation or exudates.

Advantages/Disadvantages

Advantages:

- More sensitive than rapid antigen tests
- Relatively noninvasive and inexpensive

Disadvantages:

- Results are often negative by the time patient seeks treatment
- Positive result does not differentiate between recent infection and chronic pharyngeal carriage, which is more likely to occur in children than adults

Normal

No growth of group A streptococcus.

Abnormal

- Growth of group A streptococcus
- Keep in mind the possibility of a false-positive result

Cause of abnormal result

Suggests prior infection with group A streptococcus.

Drugs, disorders, and other factors that may alter results

Time elapsed since initial infection. Rheumatic fever typically latent for 10 days or more following pharyngitis. Accordingly, positive throat cultures seen in only about 25% of patients with acute rheumatic fever.

RAPID ANTIGEN TESTING

Description

Throat culture taken from inflamed, purulent, or ulcerated areas.

Advantages/Disadvantages

Advantages:

- Faster results than is possible with throat culture
- Relatively noninvasive and inexpensive

Disadvantages: results considered less definitive than those of throat culture, particularly if negative.

Normal

Negative results for group A streptococcus.

Abnormal

- Positive results for group A streptococcus
- Keep in mind the possibility of a false-positive result

Cause of abnormal result

Suggests that patient had streptococcal pharyngitis prior to the onset of acute disease.

Drugs, disorders, and other factors that may alter results

Test must be performed precisely according to instructions on the package insert, otherwise its sensitivity and specificity will be reduced.

STREPTOCOCCAL ANTIBODY TESTS

Description

- Venous blood sample
- Most frequently used test is antistreptolysin O (ASO)
- Anti-DNase B used less commonly

Advantages/Disadvantages

Advantages:

- Relatively inexpensive and noninvasive
- Elevated or rising titers indicated by any of these tests fulfill the Jones criteria for evidence of a recent group A streptococcal infection

Disadvantages:

- Mild discomfort associated with blood draw
- About 20% of patients evaluated within the first 2 months of acute onset of rheumatic fever have low or borderline ASO titers. However, when three different antibody tests are used, about 95% of patients show an elevated titer in at least one test

Normal
- For all tests, lack of a significant antibody increase. Significant increase is defined as a rise in titer of two or more dilution increments between acute-phase and convalescent-phase specimens
- ASO titer <240 Todd units in adults is not considered elevated
- Anti-DNase B titer <120 Todd units in adults is not considered elevated
- Antihyaluronidase titer <1:256 is not considered elevated

Abnormal
- Elevated or rising titers
- A significant increase is defined as a rise in titer of two or more dilution increments between acute-phase and convalescent-phase specimens
- ASO titer ≥240 Todd units in adults is considered elevated
- Anti-DNase B titer ≥120 Todd units in adults is considered elevated
- Antihyaluronidase titer >1:256 is considered elevated
- Keep in mind the possibility of a false-positive result

Cause of abnormal result
Recent infection with group A streptococcus.

Drugs, disorders, and other factors that may alter results
Time elapsed since infection. A patient who waits months or years before seeking medical attention is less likely to show an elevated titer.

ERYTHROCYTE SEDIMENTATION RATE
Description
Venous blood sample.

Advantages/Disadvantages
Advantages:
- Relatively noninvasive and inexpensive
- If elevated, fulfils a minor manifestation for the Jones criteria

Disadvantages:
- Results not in themselves of significant diagnostic value
- Can be elevated by many different causes of systemic inflammation

Normal
- Males: 0–15mm/h
- Females: 0–20mm/h

Abnormal
- Values above normal
- Keep in mind the possibility of a false-positive result

Drugs, disorders, and other factors that may alter results
- Pregnancy
- Advanced age
- Increase in globulin proteins
- Extensive tissue necrosis
- Anemia
- Heparinized blood

C-REACTIVE PROTEIN

Description

Venous blood sample.

Advantages/Disadvantages

Advantages:

- Relatively inexpensive and noninvasive
- Positive result fulfils a minor diagnostic criteria for rheumatic fever

Disadvantage:

- Can be elevated by many different causes of inflammation

Normal

Negative.

Abnormal

- Positive
- Keep in mind the possibility of a false-positive result

Cause of abnormal result

In patients with other indications of acute rheumatic fever, abnormal result increases cause to suspect this diagnosis.

Drugs, disorders, and other factors that may alter results

Elevation likely to occur in response to a variety of acute insults, including surgery.

Imaging

CHEST X-RAY

Description

Advantages/Disadvantages

Advantages:

- Noninvasive, relatively inexpensive
- Reveals cardiomegaly and congestive heart failure

Disadvantages:

- Low-level radiation exposure (about 6nrem). However, the risk of harmful effects is low
- Findings not specific to rheumatic fever

Abnormal

- Cardiomegaly
- Congestive heart failure, Kerly B lines
- Increased pulmonary vascularity, possible pleural effusion
- Keep in mind the possibility of a false-positive result

Cause of abnormal result

Myocardial dysfunction secondary to carditis; valvular malfunction such as mitral regurgitation.

Drugs, disorders, and other factors that may alter results

Patients with coronary artery disease, viral myocarditis, or any other cause of cardiomyopathy can exhibit similar results.

ECHOCARDIOGRAM

Description

- Ultrasound waves are used to produce a visual image of intracardiac structures, allowing for evaluation of cardiac function and valvular integrity
- Transthoracic echocardiogram is accomplished via a transducer that is passed over specific areas of the thorax
- Transesophageal echocardiogram is accomplished via a transducer introduced into the patient's esophagus; this procedure may require sedation and intravenous access

Advantages/Disadvantages

Advantages:

- Relatively noninvasive
- Can detect valvular dysfunction and pericardial effusions, and can evaluate myocardial performance

Disadvantages:

- Moderately expensive
- Results are not specific to rheumatic heart disease: any disorder that causes valvular abnormalities, pericardial effusion, or myocardial dysfunction can produce similar results

Abnormal

- Valvular regurgitation most likely abnormal finding with rheumatic fever
- Valvular thickening and/or restriction of leaflet mobility
- Focal valvular nodes reported in acute stage of rheumatic fever
- Pericardial effusion
- Global or segmental myocardial dysfunction

Cause of abnormal result

- Inflammation associated with carditis can cause pericardial effusion
- Myocardial involvement can lead to cardiac dysfunction
- Inflammation of cardiac valves can lead to structural or functional abnormalities

Drugs, disorders, and other factors that may alter results

Any disorder involving cardiac valvular abnormalities (including congenital heart disease), myocardial inflammation (including viral infections), and myocardial dysfunction (such as coronary artery disease) can produce similar results.

Other tests

ELECTROCARDIOGRAM

Advantages/Disadvantages

Advantages:

- Noninvasive, relatively inexpensive
- May demonstrate ST or T-wave changes suggestive of myocarditis or pericarditis, or prolonged PR interval, a minor diagnostic manifestation of rheumatic fever

Disadvantage: insensitive, nonspecific test.

Normal

- Normal PR interval: 0.12–0.20
- Isoelectric ST segments, normal T-wave repolarization

Abnormal

- PR interval in excess of normal range
- Diffusely elevated ST-segment changes, or T-wave inversions
- Keep in mind the possibility of a false-positive result

Cause of abnormal result

Carditis can result in diffuse inflammation with generalized ST-segment and T-wave changes, and prolonged AV block.

Drugs, disorders, and other factors that may alter results

- Hyperthyroidism
- Any cause of pericarditis, or myocarditis
- Pre-existing conduction system disease
- Any drug associated with increased PR interval: beta and calcium channel blockers, procainamide, digitalis, quinidine, amiodarone, etc

TREATMENT

CONSIDER CONSULT

- Referral is indicated in all cases in which signs and/or symptoms of congestive heart failure intervene

IMMEDIATE ACTION

Congestive heart failure requires immediate treatment.

PATIENT AND CAREGIVER ISSUES

Patient or caregiver request

Didn't rheumatic fever disappear from the US a long time ago? Rheumatic fever was extremely rare in the 1970s, but outbreaks occurred in the 1980s. Changing patterns of disease may reflect changes in the virulence of strains of the bacteria that cause this disease (group A streptococci).

Health-seeking behavior

Have you taken any medications to reduce the symptom of swollen, painful joints? Aspirin may be sufficiently effective against rheumatic polyarthritis to remove this manifestation, making it harder for the physician to determine whether the diagnostic Jones criteria are fulfilled.

MANAGEMENT ISSUES

Goals

- Reduce constitutional symptoms
- Monitor cardiac function and refer as necessary
- Provide long-term prophylaxis

Management in special circumstances

COEXISTING DISEASE

Cardiology referral should be considered for patients with pre-existing heart disease.

COEXISTING MEDICATION

Reassess any coexisting medication with regard to its compatibility with long-term antibiotic prophylaxis.

SPECIAL PATIENT GROUPS

Cardiology referral is necessary in pregnancy.

PATIENT SATISFACTION/LIFESTYLE PRIORITIES

- The need for long-term prophylaxis may be dismaying to some patients. Patients should understand the reasons for this treatment
- Patients with cardiac impairment may need extensive support and education

SUMMARY OF THERAPEUTIC OPTIONS

Choices

- Penicillin: 10-day course of therapy is recommended for all patients with acute rheumatic fever even though throat culture is likely to be negative. Following this treatment, patient should begin long-term prophylaxis with penicillin
- Erythromycin: possible alternative for patients allergic to penicillin; used both for initial 10-day therapy and subsequent long-term prophylaxis
- Sulfadiazine: possible alternative to penicillin for long-term prophylaxis
- Aspirin: used in patients with mild or no carditis to relieve joint pain
- Corticosteroids: used in patients with significant carditis
- Bed rest: recommended for all patients during acute phase

Guidelines

Dajani A, Taubert K, Ferrieri P, et al. Treatment of acute streptococcal pharyngitis and prevention of rheumatic fever. A statement for health professionals. Committee on Rheumatic Fever, Fndocarditis, and Kawasaki Disease of the Council on Cardiovascular Disease in the Young, the American Heart Association. Pediatrics 1995;96:758–64

Clinical pearl(s)

- Duration of therapy is based on symptoms of inflammation and does not influence the development of future heart damage
- Early treatment may sufficiently suppress the clinical manifestations so that a diagnosis cannot be made

Never

Never fail to educate patients with valvular damage about the need for endocarditis prophylaxis prior to dental and other procedures that could infect heart valves. Antibiotic regimens for preventing recurrence of acute rheumatic fever are not sufficient for preventing bacterial endocarditis. If penicillin is used for long-term prophylaxis, then another antibiotic should be used for endocarditis prophylaxis because alpha-hemolytic streptococci in the upper respiratory tract may have become resistant to oral penicillin.

FOLLOW UP

- If possible, patient should be hospitalized for close observation during acute phase of illness
- After acute phase has resolved, follow up should occur as needed to assist patient's compliance with long-term prophylaxis. Patients with residual rheumatic heart disease should be followed by a cardiologist

Information for patient or caregiver

After having a diagnosis of rheumatic fever, both episodic antibiotic prophylaxis to prevent valve infection after procedures (e.g. dental work) AND long-term general prophylaxis to prevent recurrent rheumatic fever are needed. Any exposure to persons with strep throat, or personal occurrence of strep throat, should be reported to your doctor.

DRUGS AND OTHER THERAPIES: DETAILS

Drugs

PENICILLIN

Dose

For initial treatment during acute disease, either:

- Benzathine penicillin G, one intravenous injection of 1,200,000U for patients above 60lb, OR
- Penicillin V (oral), 500mg two to three times/day for 10 days

For long-term prophylaxis, either intramuscular or oral administration.

Intramuscular administration:

- For most circumstances, injection of 1,200,000U of intramuscular benzathine penicillin G every 4 weeks
- In high-risk individuals, injection of 1,200,000U intramuscular benzathine penicillin G every 3 weeks

Oral administration:

- Penicillin V: 250mg twice daily (oral administration usually limited to patients at lower risk of rheumatic fever recurrence)

Duration of long-term prophylaxis:

- Rheumatic fever without carditis: 5 years or until age 21, whichever is later
- Rheumatic fever with carditis but no residual heart disease (no valvular disease): 10 years or well into adulthood, whichever is longer
- Rheumatic fever with carditis and persistent valvular disease: at least for 10 years since most recent episode and at least until age 40; sometimes lifelong prophylaxis

Efficacy

Active against group A streptococci.

Risks/Benefits

Risks:

- Use caution in patients allergic to cephalosporins
- Use caution in severe renal failure

Benefits:

- Narrow spectrum of activity
- Proven efficacy
- Inexpensive

Side-effects and adverse reactions

- Gastrointestinal: diarrhea, nausea, vomiting
- Respiratory: anaphylaxis
- Skin: erythema multiforme, rash, urticaria
- Hematologic: bone marrow suppression, coagulation disorders
- Renal: interstitial nephritis
- CNS: anxiety, coma, seizures
- Hypersensitivity reactions

Interactions (other drugs)

- Chloramphenicol ■ Glucocorticoids ■ Macrolide and tetracycline antibiotics
- Methotrexate ■ Oral contraceptives ■ Phenindione ■ Probenecid ■ Warfarin

Contraindications

- Penicillin hypersensitivity

Evidence

- Penicillin is the treatment of choice in the prevention of rheumatic fever in patients with group A beta-hemolytic streptococcal pharyngitis [2] *Level C*
- Penicillin is also the agent of choice for secondary prophylaxis in patients who have had an attack of rheumatic fever [2] *Level C*

Acceptability to patient

Long-term prophylaxis with intramuscular injections is painful and inconvenient. Pain of injection may be reduced by warming medication to room temperature. Oral agents may be preferred, but these are more appropriate for patients at a lower risk for recurrence of rheumatic fever.

Follow up plan

Will be individual to each patient, depending on age, history of recurrences, and presence of cardiac involvement.

Patient and caregiver information

Patients with rheumatic valvular heart disease should understand that long-term prophylaxis does not substitute for short-term antibiotic prophylaxis prior to certain surgical and dental procedures (endocarditis prophylaxis).

ERYTHROMYCIN

Dose

For initial treatment of acute rheumatic fever (recommended for patients allergic to penicillin):
- Erythromycin estolate: 20–40mg/kg two to four times/day (max 1g/day) for 10 days, OR Erythromycin ethylsuccinate: 40mg/kg two to four times/day (max 1g/day) for 10 days

For long-term prophylaxis:
- 250mg twice daily

Duration of long-term prophylaxis:
- Rheumatic fever without carditis: 5 years or until age 21, whichever is later
- Rheumatic fever with carditis but no residual heart disease (no valvular disease): 10 years or well into adulthood, whichever is longer
- Rheumatic fever with carditis and persistent valvular disease: at least for 10 years since most recent episode and at least until age 40; sometimes lifelong prophylaxis

Efficacy

Active against group A streptococci.

Risks/Benefits

Risks:
- Use caution in hepatic and renal impairment, porphyria
- Avoid concomitant administration with terfenadine, astemizole, and cisapride
- Use caution with repeated or prolonged therapy

Benefit: acceptable alternative to penicillin for allergic patients.

Side-effects and adverse reactions
- Gastrointestinal: anorexia, nausea, diarrhea, abdominal pain, vomiting, heartburn, hepatitis
- Cardiovascular: dysrhythmias (uncommon)
- Skin: rashes, pruritus, vaginal candidiasis
- EENT: deafness, tinnitus

Interactions (other drugs)

■ Alfentanil ■ Antiarrhythmic drugs (digoxin, disopyramide) ■ Antihistamines (terfenadine, astemizole) ■ Anticonvulsants (carbamazepine, valproic acid) ■ Antiviral agents ■ Benzodiazepines ■ Bromocriptine ■ Buspirone ■ Cisapride ■ Clozapine ■ Colchicine ■ Cyclosporine, tacrolimus ■ Ergotamine ■ Ethanol ■ Felodipine ■ Itraconazole ■ Methylprednisolone ■ Penicillin ■ Quinidine ■ Sildenafil ■ Statins ■ Theophylline ■ Warfarin ■ Zopiclone

Contraindications

■ Liver disease ■ Various infections (vaccinia, varicella, mycobacterial, fungal, viral)

Evidence

- Erythromycin is a suitable alternative for penicillin-allergic patients in primary prevention of rheumatic fever in patients infected with group A beta-hemolytic streptococcus [2] *Level C*
- Erythromycin may be used for secondary prophylaxis of rheumatic fever in patients allergic to penicillin [2] *Level C*

Acceptability to patient

Patients may appreciate oral administration. Nevertheless, long-term compliance is necessary.

Follow up plan

- No official guidelines exist for follow up
- Eradication failures after antimicrobial treatment can occur in up to 28% of patients in some studies

Patient and caregiver information

Patients with rheumatic valvular heart disease should understand that long-term prophylaxis does not substitute for short-term antibiotic prophylaxis prior to certain surgical and dental procedures.

SULFADIAZINE

Dose

For long-term prophylaxis only (cannot be used for initial 10-day regimen of group A streptococcal eradication): 1g once daily for patients weighing more than 27kg.

Duration of long-term prophylaxis:

- Rheumatic fever without carditis: 5 years or until age 21, whichever is later
- Rheumatic fever with carditis but no residual heart disease (no valvular disease): 10 years or well into adulthood, whichever is longer
- Rheumatic fever with carditis and persistent valvular disease: at least for 10 years since most recent episode and at least until age 40; sometimes lifelong prophylaxis

Efficacy

Prevents new infection, although does not eradicate existing group A streptococci.

Risks/Benefits

Risks:

- Impaired renal or hepatic function
- Bronchial asthma or severe allergy

Benefit: prevents new infection, although does not eradicate group A streptococci.

Side-effects and adverse reactions

- CNS: headache, convulsions, depression, hallucinations, tinnitus, insomnia, vertigo
- Gastrointestinal: nausea, abdominal pain, anorexia, diarrhea
- Metabolism: anemia, agranulocytosis, thrombocytopenia, leukopenia
- Skin: arthralgia, allergic myocarditis, erythema multiforme, urticaria, pruritus, serum sickness, anaphylactoid reactions

Interactions (other drugs)

- Cyclosporine ▪ Clozapine ▪ Coumarins ▪ Estrogens ▪ Methotrexate ▪ Phenytoin ▪ Potassium aminobenzoate ▪ Prilocaine ▪ Pyrimethamine ▪ Sulfonylureas ▪ Thiopental

Contraindications

- Hypersensitivity to sulfonamides
- Infants <2 months
- During pregnancy and lactation

Evidence

Sulfadiazine may be used for secondary prophylaxis of rheumatic fever in patients allergic to penicillin [2] *Level C*

Acceptability to patient

Patients may value oral administration, although some may fail to comply with long-term administration.

Follow up plan

- No specific guidelines
- Reculture after completion of antibiotics

Patient and caregiver information

Patients with rheumatic valvular heart disease should understand that long-term prophylaxis does not substitute for short-term antibiotic prophylaxis prior to certain surgical and dental procedures.

ASPIRIN (OTC)

Dose

100mg/kg per day, divided into four or five doses, typically for about 1 month or until sufficient evidence of inflammatory inactivity.

Efficacy

Typically relieves joint pain within 24h.

Risks/Benefits

Risks:

- Use caution in anemia, Hodgkin's disease, gout, hepatic and renal disease, asthma, nasal polyps, nasal allergies
- Use caution with children and teenagers (Reye's syndrome)

Benefits: simple dosing regimen allows for better patient compliance.

Side-effects and adverse reactions

- Gastrointestinal: abdominal pain, nausea, dyspepsia, hepatotoxicity, gastrointestinal bleeding
- EENT: hearing loss and tinnitus
- Hematologic: bleeding disorders, thrombocytopenia
- Respiratory: hyperpnea, asthma
- Skin: angioedema, bruising, rash, urticaria
- CNS: dizziness, headache

Interactions (other drugs)

- Angiotensin-converting enzyme (ACE) inhibitors
- Antigout medicines
- Acetazolamide
- Antacids
- Corticosteroids
- Diltiazem
- Ethanol
- Griseofulvin
- Methotrexate
- Oral anticoagulants
- Warfarin

Contraindications

- Gastrointestinal bleeding
- Bleeding disorders
- Bone marrow suppression
- Hypersensitivity to salicylates, nonsteroidal anti-inflammatory drugs (NSAIDs), or tartrazine

Evidence

A meta-analysis (dominated by one large negative trial) was performed to determine whether salicylates or corticosteroids are more likely to prevent valvular damage in patients with established rheumatic carditis. No significant advantage was noted with corticosteroid treatment in preventing a pathologic murmur at 1 year [3] *Level M*

Acceptability to patient

Highly acceptable.

Follow up plan

Patient's progress should be closely monitored during acute phase of disease, which corresponds to the period of aspirin administration.

Patient and caregiver information

Patient should understand the reason for aspirin therapy.

CORTICOSTEROIDS

Dose

- See instructions for individual product
- Usual corticosteroid is prednisone, in dosage of 1–2mg/kg per day
- Should be continued until adequate evidence shows inflammatory inactivity; sometimes this may take 2–3 months
- Following prolonged therapy, dosage should be tapered before drug is discontinued

Efficacy

Reduces symptoms of inflammation; considered preferable to aspirin for patients with significant cardiac involvement.

Risks/Benefits

Risks:

- Slow acting
- False-negative skin allergy tests. Overwhelming septicemia if patient has an infection
- Loss of control of blood glucose in those with diabetes
- Use caution in elderly due to risk of diabetes and osteoporosis
- Use caution in patients with psychosis, seizure disorders, myasthenia gravis, congestive heart failure, hypertension, ulcerative colitis, peptic ulcer, or esophagitis

Benefit: reduces symptoms of inflammation.

Side-effects and adverse reactions

- Side-effects are minimized by short duration of therapy
- Gastrointestinal: dyspepsia, peptic ulceration, esophagitis, oral candidiasis, nausea, diarrhea
- Cardiovascular: hypertension, thromboembolism
- CNS: insomnia, euphoria, depression, psychosis
- Endocrine: adrenal suppression, impaired glucose tolerance, growth suppression in children, Cushing's syndrome
- Musculoskeletal: proximal myopathy, osteoporosis
- Skin: delayed healing, acne, striae
- EENT: cataract, glaucoma, blurred vision

Interactions (other drugs)

- Adrenergic neurone blockers, alpha-blockers, beta-blockers, $beta_2$ agonists
- Aminoglutethimide
- Anticonvulsants (carbamazepine, phenytoin, barbiturates)
- Antidiabetics
- Antidysrhythmics (calcium channel blockers, cardiac glycosides)
- Antifungals (amphotericin, ketoconazole)
- Antihypertensives (ACE inhibitors, diuretics: [loop and thiazide], acetazolamide, angiotensin II receptor antagonists, clonidine, diazoxide, hydralazine, methyldopa, minoxidil)
- Cyclosporine
- Erythromycin
- Methotrexate
- NSAIDs
- Nitrates
- Nitroprusside
- Oral contraceptives
- Rifampin
- Ritonavir
- Somatropin
- Vaccines

Contraindications

- Systemic infection
- Avoid live virus vaccines in those receiving immunosuppressive doses

Evidence

A meta-analysis was performed to determine whether salicylates or corticosteroids are more likely to prevent valvular damage in patients with established rheumatic carditis. No significant advantage was noted with corticosteroid treatment in preventing a pathologic murmur at 1 year; however, the meta-analysis was dominated by one large negative trial [3] *Level M*

Acceptability to patient

Some patients may fear adverse effects.

Follow up plan

Close follow up should be provided in the acute phase of disease, which corresponds to the time of corticosteroid administration.

Patient and caregiver information

Patients should understand the benefits of corticosteroids.

Other therapies

BED REST

Efficacy

Reduces joint pain; recommended until fever abates.

Acceptability to patient

Generally acceptable.

Follow up plan

Patient should be closely followed during acute phase of disease, which is when bed rest is advocated.

Patient and caregiver information

Patient should understand the reason for bed rest.

OUTCOMES

EFFICACY OF THERAPIES

Acute episodes usually resolve in 10–12 weeks, but some patients may have rheumatic activity for longer than 6 months.

Evidence

PDxMD are unable to cite evidence meeting our criteria for evidence.

While definitive evidence for the management of rheumatic fever is not available, practical application of bed rest and aspirin for symptom relief as well as prevention of recurrence with antibiotic therapy has resulted in dramatic declines in adult rheumatic heart disease. Perhaps the best justification for this approach is the very low rate of rheumatic heart disease in countries where such a program has been followed compared with the much higher rates in countries where it has not.

Review period

During acute phase, intense observation in a hospital setting is desirable.

PROGNOSIS

- Acute episodes usually resolve in 10–12 weeks, but some patients may have rheumatic activity for longer than 6 months
- Death from myocarditis in acute phase is extremely rare
- Likelihood of residual rheumatic heart disease correlates with severity of carditis during the acute attack
- Prognosis is most serious for those with pre-existing heart disease and those who experienced more than one attack of acute rheumatic fever during a 10-year period

Clinical pearl(s)

- Patients should be counseled on the possible late development of valvular cardiac disease (most commonly mitral stenosis)
- Occasionally, acute valvular regurgitation is so severe that surgery is necessary to correct heart failure

Therapeutic failure

- Failure of therapy to improve cardiac function necessitates referral to a cardiologist and possible hospitalization
- Failure of arthritis to respond to salicylates within 24h may signal that the patient does not in fact have rheumatic arthritis; referral may be needed to obtain correct diagnosis

Recurrence

Hospitalization and cardiac referral: patients with more than one attack at higher risk of cardiac involvement.

Deterioration

Hospitalization and urgent cardiac referral.

COMPLICATIONS

- Congestive heart failure
- Chronic valvular disease (most likely mitral stenosis)
- Subsequent attacks of acute rheumatic fever

CONSIDER CONSULT

Cardiac referral necessary for:

- Any patients who experience two or more acute episodes of rheumatic fever within a 10-year interval
- Patients whose heart function declines after initial presentation

PREVENTION

RISK FACTORS

Untreated sore throat: if a sore throat is caused by group A streptococci, it has the potential to result in rheumatic fever unless the person receives appropriate antibiotic treatment.

MODIFY RISK FACTORS

Untreated sore throat: by examining a sore throat and sometimes culturing the bacteria that grow in it, a doctor can determine whether preventive treatment for rheumatic fever is necessary.

SCREENING

No screening test exists for rheumatic fever.

PREVENT RECURRENCE

Any patient with a history of acute rheumatic fever is at heightened risk of recurrence. Long-term antibiotic prophylaxis is required as follows:

- Rheumatic fever without carditis: 5 years or until age 21, whichever is later
- Rheumatic fever with carditis but no residual heart disease (no valvular disease): 10 years or well into adulthood, whichever is longer
- Rheumatic fever with carditis and persistent valvular disease: for at least 10 years since most recent episode and at least until age 40; sometimes lifelong prophylaxis

Reassess coexisting disease

INTERACTION ALERT

Ensure that patient's existing drugs do not have undesired interactions with the antibiotic used for long-term prophylaxis.

RESOURCES

ASSOCIATIONS

American Heart Association
National Center
7272 Greenville Ave
Dallas, TX 75231
Tel: (800) AHA-USA1
http://www.americanheart.org

KEY REFERENCES

- Bisno AL. Nonsuppurative poststreptococcal sequelae: rheumatic fever and glomerulonephritis. In: Mandell's principles and practice of infectious diseases, 5th edn. Edinburgh: Churchill Livingstone, 2000
- Bisno AL. Rheumatic fever. In: Goldman C, ed. Textbook of medicine, 21st edn. Philadelphia, PA: WB Saunders, 2000
- Centers for Disease Control, Vital and Health Statistics, Series 10, No. 200, Table 58 Number of selected reported chronic conditions per 1000 persons, by sex and age: United States, 1996-Con. and Table 59 Number of selected reported chronic conditions per 1000 persons, by race and age: United States, 1996-Con
- Dajani AS. Rheumatic fever. In: Braunwald E, ed. Heart disease: a textbook of cardiovascular medicine, 5th edn. Philadelphia, PA: WB Saunders, 1997
- Dajani A, Taubert K, Ferrieri P, et al. Treatment of acute streptococcal pharyngitis and prevention of rheumatic fever: a statement for health professionals. Pediatrics 1995;96:758–64
- Diehl AM, Hamilton TR, Keeling IC. Long acting repository penicillin in prophylaxis of recurrent rheumatic fever. JAMA 1954;155:1466–70
- Foggo BA. Sore throat, antibiotics and rheumatic fever. Fam Pract 1985;2:101–7
- Guidelines for the diagnosis of rheumatic fever, Jones criteria, 1992 update. Special writing group of the Committee on Rheumatic Fever, Endocarditis, and Kawasaki Disease of the Council on Cardiovascular Disease in the Young of the American Heart Association. JAMA 1992;268(15):2069
- Janicki RS, Garnham JC, Worland MC, et al. Comparison of erythromycin ethyl succinate, stearate, and estolate treatments of group A streptococcal infection of the upper respiratory tract. Clin Pediatr 1975;14(12):1098–107
- Mirkinson L. The diagnosis of rheumatic fever. Pediatr Rev 1998;19:310–1
- Onion DK. Primary care, pearls and references, 3rd edn. Malden, MA: Blackwell Science, 1999
- Schrock CG. Clarithromycin versus penicillin in the treatment of streptococcal pharyngitis. Fam Pract 1992;35(6):622–6
- Toth PP. Cardiology: rheumatic fever and rheumatic carditis. In: University of Iowa family practice handbook, 3rd edn. http://www.vh.org/
- Vason RS. Echocardiographic evaluation of patients with acute rheumatic fever and rheumatic carditis. Circulation 1996;1:94(1):73–82
- Wood HF, Feinstein AR, Taranta A, et al. Rheumatic fever in children and adolescents. A long term epidemiological study of subsequent prophylaxis, streptococcal infections and clinical sequelae. III. Comparative effectiveness of three prophylaxis regimens in preventing streptococcal infections and rheumatic recurrences. Ann Intern Med 1964;6(Suppl 5):31–46
- Wenger NK, Miller FM, Brim A. A study of the oral flora of children receiving sulfadiazine prophylaxis against rheumatic fever. Am Heart J 1966;72(3):420–2

Evidence references and guidelines

1 Guidelines for the diagnosis of rheumatic fever, Jones criteria, 1992 update. Special writing of the Committee on Rheumatic Fever, Endocarditis, and Kawasaki Disease of the Council on Cardiovascular Disease in the Young of the American Heart Association. JAMA 1992;268(15):2069

2 Dajani A, Taubert K, Ferrieri P, et al. Treatment of acute streptococcal pharyngitis and prevention of rheumatic fever. A statement for health professionals. Committee on Rheumatic Fever, Endocarditis, and Kawasaki Disease of the Council on Cardiovascular Disease in the Young, the American Heart Association. Pediatrics 1995;96:758–64

3 Albert DA, Harel L, Karrison T. The treatment of rheumatic carditis: a review and meta-analysis. Medicine (Baltimore) 1995;74:1–12

FAQS

Question 1

Should I refer all patients who have rheumatic fever to a cardiologist?

ANSWER 1

Not unless they have signs of congestive heart failure or evidence on echocardiography of more than mild valve regurgitation.

Question 2

How likely is someone with rheumatic fever to develop subsequent valve disease requiring treatment (valve replacement or valvuloplasty)?

ANSWER 2

Several longitudinal studies place the percentage of acute cases progressing to symptomatic valve disease at between 17 and 39% over 5–15 years. Mitral regurgitation is the most common late problem.

Question 3

Does the chronic prophylaxis for recurrence obviate the need for procedure-specific endocarditis prophylaxis?

ANSWER 3

No, the doses for rheumatic fever recurrence prophylaxis are inadequate for endocarditis prophylaxis.

CONTRIBUTORS

Gordon H Baustian, MD
John McB Hodgson, MD, FACC, FSCAI
Gail A Van Norman, MD

SUPERIOR VENA CAVA SYNDROME

SUMMARY INFORMATION

DESCRIPTION

- Superior vena cava syndrome (SVCS) is an uncommon condition caused by obstruction of the venous return from the upper body to the heart
- The clinically distinctive features of swelling of the face, arms, and upper torso lead to the diagnosis
- Leading cause is lung cancer (70% of cases)
- Treatment is directed at underlying cause of the venous obstruction. SVCS is usually investigated and treated on an urgent basis

URGENT ACTION

- Patients with SVCS who experience laryngeal edema with stridor, hoarseness, or hypoxemia require immediate endotracheal intubation or, if not feasible, tracheostomy
- In the emergency situations of airway restriction or cerebral edema (suggested by a change in mental status, seizures, or syncope), endovascular techniques including thrombolysis, stent placement, and angioplasty can lead to rapid resolution of symptoms
- If this technology is not available, prompt initiation of radiation therapy and administration of corticosteroids and diuretics is recommended

KEY! DON'T MISS!

Unilateral upper extremity swelling may be due to selective compression of the ipsilateral subclavian vein.

BACKGROUND

ICD9 CODE
453.2 Vena cava thrombosis

SYNONYMS
Superior vena cava obstruction.

CARDINAL FEATURES
- Dyspnea and sensation of fullness in the cervical region and head are the major symptoms
- Clinically distinctive features that lead to diagnosis of superior vena cava syndrome (SVCS) are facial, upper torso, and arm swelling but absence of edema in lower extremities
- Distention of veins of head, neck, arms, or upper thorax
- Periorbital swelling and a roaring in the ears
- Many signs and symptoms are exacerbated by orthostatic changes induced by lying or bending over
- Treatment is directed at underlying cause of venous obstruction
- SVCS is investigated and treated on an urgent basis

CAUSES
Common causes
- Lung cancer (80% of malignant cases), especially bronchogenic carcinoma
- Metastatic carcinoma within the mediastinum, including breast, thyroid, and melanoma (10% of malignant cases)
- Lymphoma (10% of malignant cases)
- Thrombus around central venous catheters (commonest nonmalignant cause; reported with increasing frequency)

Rare causes
- Thrombus around pacemaker wires
- Thymoma
- Mediastinal granulomatous disease
- Aortic aneurysm (in the preantibiotic era, an infective syphilitic aneurysm was the most common etiology of SVCS)
- Substernal goiter
- Atrial myxoma
- Idiopathic mediastinal fibrosis
- Fungal or bacterial infection
- Teratoma
- Repair of congenital vascular transposition
- Trauma

Serious causes
- Lung and metastatic cancers
- Lymphoma and thymoma
- Mediastinal granulomatous disease
- Aortic aneurysm
- Substernal goiter
- Atrial myxoma
- Idiopathic mediastinal fibrosis
- Fungal or bacterial infection
- Teratoma
- Repair of congenital vascular transposition
- Trauma

Contributory or predisposing factors
Predisposing factors to lung cancer, as most cases of SVCS are a result of lung cancer.

EPIDEMIOLOGY
Incidence and prevalence
Demographics of SVCS parallel those of lung cancer.

INCIDENCE
15,000 new cases in the US per year.

PREVALENCE
3–5% of lung cancer patients.

DIFFERENTIAL DIAGNOSIS

The following conditions can present with similar clinical features but can be ruled out by the absence of lower extremity edema.

Congestive heart failure

Congestive heart failure is congestion of the pulmonary and systemic circulation due to ischemic heart disease, cardiomyopathy, and myocarditis. It is the most common diagnosis leading to admission in the elderly.

FEATURES

- Dyspnea on exertion progressing to being present at rest
- Orthopnea and paroxysmal nocturnal dyspnea
- Nocturnal angina secondary to increased venous return
- Fatigue and lethargy

Angioneurotic edema

Vasoactive chemicals are released, leading to swelling of the cutaneous tissues. Mast cell activation and degranulation occurs. Immunologic and nonimmunologic mechanisms implicated.

FEATURES

- Nonpruritic, burning swelling of the skin
- Involves eyelids, tongue, lips, and extremities
- Larynx can be involved leading to respiratory distress
- Resolves slowly

Cirrhosis

Cirrhosis is the histologic definition of fibrosis and regeneration nodules in the liver.

FEATURES

- Classified as micronodular, macronodular, and mixed
- All forms can be seen in a patient as disease progresses
- Clinical features include jaundice, tender hepatomegaly or small nodular liver, ascites, and hemorrhoids
- Alcoholism is the common cause
- Complications include hepatic encephalopathy, portal hypertension, and variceal bleeding

Constrictive pericarditis

Fibrotic constriction of the pericardium.

FEATURES

- Clinical features include jugular venous distension, Kussmaul's sign, pericardial knock, and clear lungs
- Ascites, tender hepatomegaly, and pedal edema can occur
- Causes include infectious agents, collagen diseases, and ischemic heart disease

SIGNS & SYMPTOMS

Signs

- Plethora of the face (facial swelling)
- Periorbital edema
- Enlargement of the neck, most frequently noted because shirts become tight around the collar
- Blue or purple discoloration of the skin

- Distension of the veins of the neck, arms, and upper torso
- Collateral venous channels of the arms and torso
- Swelling of the arms and upper torso
- Tachypnea, cough, or hemoptysis caused by underlying disease
- Hoarseness or stridor (signs of laryngeal edema)
- Syncope, seizures, or coma (signs of cerebral edema)

Symptoms

- Dyspnea or orthopnea
- Roaring in the ears and distorted vision
- Dysphagea or odynophagia
- Chest pain
- Headache, light-headedness, dizziness, and drowsiness
- Fatigue and anorexia

KEY! DON'T MISS!

Unilateral upper extremity swelling may be due to selective compression of the ipsilateral subclavian vein.

CONSIDER CONSULT

- Refer to a radiologist or interventional cardiologist for imaging of the SVCS (chest X-ray and computed tomography [CT] scan) and endovascular interventions
- Refer to an oncologist if malignant diagnosis is confirmed
- Refer to a respiratory physician for bronchoscopy if indicated
- Refer to a surgeon or interventional electrophysiologist if superior vena cava bypass is indicated or for removal of a central venous pacemaker lead

INVESTIGATION OF THE PATIENT

Direct questions to patient

- Q **Have you suffered from a cough, breathlessness, or weight loss?** All these symptoms are related to lung cancer, which is the commonest cause
- Q **Have you suffered from a hoarse voice or roaring in your ears?** These symptoms are associated with SVCS
- Q **Have you had problems swallowing?** Dysphagia and odynophagia are associated with SVCS
- Q **Have you had any swelling of the face?** Facial swelling is common in SVCS

Contributory or predisposing factors

- Q **Do you smoke cigarettes?** This is associated with lung cancer
- Q **Have you suffered from any lung or heart conditions?** Lung and heart disease can lead to SVCS
- Q **Have you been fitted with a pacemaker or central venous line?** These can cause thrombus formation leading to SVCS

Examination

- **Is the patient dyspneic and tachypneic?** Both signs are indicative of lung disease leading to SVCS
- **Is there swelling of the face, arms, or upper torso, and distension of the veins?** These signs are diagnostic of SVCS
- **Is there evidence of laryngeal edema, including hoarseness of the voice and stridor?** These signs can be present in SVCS
- **Are there signs of cerebral edema, including seizures and syncope?** SVCS can lead to cerebral edema

Summary of investigative tests

The goals of the investigative tests are:

- Identification of the underlying etiology of SVCS
- Determination of extent of superior vena cava compression

Investigations include:

- Chest X-ray: widened mediastinum and lung lesion
- CT scan of larynx and chest
- Bronchoscopy of lesion leading to SVCS (normally performed by a specialist)
- Fine-needle biopsy of the obstruction leading to SVCS
- Invasive contrast venography

DIAGNOSTIC DECISION

Most patients can be diagnosed with SVCS on the basis of physical examination alone. The severity of the illness is a function of the rapidity of superior vena cava obstruction and the development of contralateral vessels. If SVCS leads to gradual compression, then contralateral circulation develops, leading to subtle signs of the disease.

CLINICAL PEARL(S)

Once a diagnosis is established with noninvasive imaging, venography should be performed by an specialist capable of intervention at the same setting.

THE TESTS

Imaging

CHEST X-RAY

Description

- Useful as chest X-ray is abnormal in 80% of SVCS cases
- Diagnoses lung lesions and pleural effusions

Advantages/Disadvantages

Advantages:

- Routine noninvasive procedure
- Noninvasive
- Can be diagnostic of SVCS
- Can be diagnostic for lesions in the lung – a major cause of SVCS
- Cost-effective

Disadvantages:

- Radiation exposure for patient
- Cannot diagnose actual cause of lesion

Abnormal

- Abnormal in 80% of patients
- Widened mediastinum
- Lesion in right lung field
- Pleural effusion is the most common abnormality associated with SVCS

Cause of abnormal result

- SVCS
- Lung cancer

CT SCAN OF THE LARYNX AND CHEST

Description

- Two-dimensional computer-assisted imaging of the larynx and chest
- Useful to delineate soft tissue lesions

Advantages/Disadvantages

Advantages:

- Identifies location and extent of lesion in chest or larynx, including in the vocal cords and lungs
- Useful to guide attempts at biopsy using bronchscopy and fine-needle biopsy
- Noninvasive

Disadvantages:

- Expensive
- Radiation exposure
- Unpleasant experience for patient – claustrophobia can be a problem

Abnormal

- Mass lesions in the lung and other soft tissues
- Widened mediastinum

Cause of abnormal result

- Lung cancer
- SVCS

CONTRAST VENOGRAPHY

Description

- Venous imaging with injection of radio-opaque contrast material
- Phlebogram to study the superior vena cava: it is helpful to determine the degree of obstruction and anatomy of the veins

Advantages/Disadvantages

Advantages:

- Identifies precisely the site of vascular obstruction
- Aids in surgical planning and management
- Guides therapeutic decision-making

Disadvantages:

- Expensive and specialized procedure
- Invasive
- Anaphylactic risk
- Risk of inducing renal failure, particularly in patients with existing renal disease, dehydration, diabetes
- Requires specialized interpretation
- Unpleasant experience for patient

Abnormal

Obstruction of venous flow in the superior vena cava.

Cause of abnormal result

- SVCS
- Lung or other soft tissue mass

TREATMENT

CONSIDER CONSULT

- Refer if evidence of cerebral edema or airway obstruction as these are considered medical emergencies. All other patients are treated on an urgent basis

IMMEDIATE ACTION

- Endotracheal intubation or tracheostomy if there is evidence of airway compromise
- Emergent consideration of endovascular intervention in life-threatening situations

PATIENT AND CAREGIVER ISSUES

Forensic and legal issues

In making decisions about intervening in superior vena cava syndrome (SVCS) it is important for the patient (or family/power of attorney if patient is unable to make decisions) to consider balance between probable dramatic short-term improvement in patient's condition and the usually poor longterm prognosis.

Impact on career, dependants, family, friends

The patient and family often need to deal with two different issues that may be hard to understand and assimilate: first, immediate relief for the problem for which care is sought (the SVCS), and, second, usually a malignancy with poor prognosis.

Patient or caregiver request

- Information should be given on SVCS, including its causes
- Patient should be informed of serious nature of this disease

Health-seeking behavior

Patient will normally present as the SVCS develops.

MANAGEMENT ISSUES

Goals

- To treat SVCS to relieve symptoms
- To treat underlying disorder

Management in special circumstances

- Patients with a poor prognosis need to balance the risk of invasive procedures with short-term improvement in the face of a terminal illness
- In many patients, palliation (particularly pain control) and improving the quality of life are principal concerns

PATIENT SATISFACTION/LIFESTYLE PRIORITIES

- Patients should have rapid relief of the SVCS
- The cause should be treated but cure may not be possible
- Palliation should be optimal

SUMMARY OF THERAPEUTIC OPTIONS

Choices

Treatment should be guided by:

- Severity of symptoms
- Etiology of obstruction
- Prognosis of patient
- Patient preference
- Treatment goals

- Medical management includes elevation of the head of the bed, steroids (dexamethasone), diruretics (furosemide), urokinase
- Radiation therapy is used as the main treatment for SVCS due to malignancy and most patients will be treated with this modality. Severe SCVS is usually treated with emergency radiation therapy
- Chemotherapy is sometimes preferable if the causal tumor is chemosensitive – particularly small cell cancer of the lung and lymphoma
- Thrombolysis is required if a thrombus is the causal agent or if endovascular therapy is performed
- Surgical bypass of the superior vena cava is rarely indicated
- Endovascular therapy: endovascular removal of pacemaker leads or central lines, or endovascular balloon or stent-assisted angioplasty may be indicated. This is a new approach that has been increasingly used. It is indicated especially for mildly symptomatic patients who do not have yet a histopathologic diagnosis. The long-term results of this modality are not yet known

Clinical pearl(s)

- Most treatments are palliative, given the high mortality rate associated with the usual underlying disease
- Most patients will be treated with radiation and will achieve significant relief of symptoms

Never

- Never delay treatment of a severe case of SCVS even if a histologic diagnosis has not been made
- Never remove a central venous catheter causing SCVS without consultation with the radiologist, cardiologist, or surgeon

FOLLOW UP

The cause of the SVCS determines the follow up.

Plan for review

Regular review of the patient to check for:

- Complications
- Recurrence
- Treatment of the underlying cause

Information for patient or caregiver

It is most important for the patient and family to understand the palliative nature of the initial intervention and of follow up care for the underlying disorder.

DRUGS AND OTHER THERAPIES: DETAILS

Drugs

DEXAMETHASONE

Symptomatic management of cerebral and laryngeal edema.

Dose

- Dosage must be individualized
- Adult dose: 8–40mg intravenously immediately, then 4–6mg intravenous/oral every 4h

Efficacy

- Reduces swelling due to tumors
- Can be very useful if tumor is a lymphoma, in which case patient can even achieve a remission

Risks/Benefits

Risks:

- Overwhelming septicemia if patient has an infection
- Loss of control of blood glucose in those with diabetes
- Use caution in renal disease, esophagitis, peptic ulcer, and ulcerative colitis
- Use caution in cerebral malaria, latent tuberculosis, and AIDS

Benefits:

- Rapid reduction of symptoms due to edema
- Its use does not preclude local therapy with radiation/endovascular procedures

Side-effects and adverse reactions

- Side-effects are minimized by short duration of therapy
- Cardiovascular: hypertension, thromboembolism
- CNS: insomnia, euphoria, depression, psychosis, headache
- Endocrine: adrenal suppression, impaired glucose tolerance, growth suppression in children
- EENT: cataract, glaucoma, blurred vision
- Gastrointestinal: dyspepsia, peptic ulceration, oesophagitis, oral candidiasis
- Musculoskeletal: proximal myopathy, osteoporosis
- Skin: delayed healing, acne, striae

Interactions (other drugs)

- Aldesleukin ■ Aminoglutethimide ■ Antibiotics ■ Anticholinesterases ■ Anticoagulants ■ Antidiabetics ■ Antifungals ■ Barbiturates ■ Bismuth subsalicylate ■ Colestyramine ■ Colestipol ■ Diltiazem ■ Ephedrine ■ Estrogens ■ Formoterol ■ Imitanib mesylate ■ Insulin ■ Mifepristone ■ Nondepolarizing muscle relaxants ■ Oral contraceptives ■ Phenytoin ■ Rifabutin ■ Rifampin ■ Rifapentine ■ Salicylates ■ Troleandomycin ■ Verpamil ■ Xanthine derivatives

Contraindications

- Lack of a definite diagnosis ■ Systemic infection
- Avoid live virus vaccines in those receiving immunosuppressive doses

Acceptability to patient

Most patients accept treatment with corticosteroids readily. If there are symptoms indicating patient compromise, radiation should be added.

Follow up plan

Patients with SCVS undergoing treatment with corticosteroids must be carefully followed and educated. If new symptoms appear, radiation therapy must be initiated.

Patient and caregiver information

Must be aware that this treatment is temporary, and if new symptoms develop radiation must be started.

FUROSEMIDE

- Symptomatic management of SVCS
- Reduces venous return to the heart by reducing the preload
- Relieves increased pressure in the superior vena cava

Dose

Adult dose: 20–80mg orally immediately, 40–120mg as required 6h after initial dose.

Efficacy

Reduces edema, but direct effect on the disease is very limited and this therapy alone is not enough to treat SVCS.

Risks/Benefits

Risks:

- Excessive diuresis may cause dehydration and blood volume reduction with circulatory collapse and possibly vascular thrombosis and embolism, particularly in elderly patients
- Use caution with diabetes mellitus
- Use caution with renal and liver disease
- Use caution with systemic lupus erythematosus
- Use caution with pregnancy and nursing mothers
- Use caution with hypertension and gout
- Use caution with porphyria

Benefit: temporary symptomatic relief.

Side-effects and adverse reactions

- Cardiovascular: chest pain, circulatory collapse, orthostatic hypotension
- CNS: dizziness, headache, paresthesia, fever
- EENT: visual disturbances, ototoxicity, tinnitus, hearing impairment, thirst
- Gastrointestinal: ischemic hepatitis, vomiting, pancreatitis, nausea, diarrhea, anorexia
- Genitourinary: glycosuria, hyperuricemia, bladder spasm, polyuria
- Hematologic: blood disorders
- Metabolic: hyperglycemia, hyponatremia, hypokalemia, hypomagnesemia, hypovolemia, hypochloremia, hypercholesterolemia, hypertriglyceridemia
- Skin: erythema multiforme, exfoliative dermatitis, urticaria

Interactions (other drugs)

▪ Angiotensin-converting enzyme (ACE) inhibitors ▪ Alpha-adrenergic antagonists ▪ Amphotericin ▪ Antibiotics (aminoglycosides, polymixins, vancomycin, cephalosporins) ▪ Antidiabetics ▪ Antidysrhythmics (amiodarone, cardiac glycosides, disopyramide, flecainide, mexelitine, quinidine, sotalol) ▪ Beta$_2$ adrenergic agonists ▪ Carbenoxolone ▪ Cholestyramine, colestipol ▪ Cisplatin ▪ Clofibrate ▪ Corticosteroids ▪ Diuretics (thiazides, metolazone, acetazolamide) ▪ Lidocaine ▪ Lithium ▪ Nonsteroidal anti-inflammatory drugs (NSAIDs) ▪ Phenobarbital ▪ Phenytoin ▪ Pimozide ▪ Reboxetine ▪ Seratonin-selective reuptake inhibitors (SSRIs) ▪ Terbutaline ▪ Tubocurarine

Contraindications

▪ Renal failure with anuria ▪ Hepatic coma

Acceptability to patient

Due to lack of evidence and increased risk of thrombosis, most patients will accept diuretic therapy only for initial relief of symptoms.

Follow up plan

Patients with SCVS treated with diuretics should be carefully evaluated and followed to avoid dehydration.

Patient and caregiver information

- Should be aware of signs and symptoms of dehydration
- Should be instructed to contact their physician if symptoms worsen

UROKINASE

- Indicated for known thrombus formation leading to SVCS
- Lyses the thrombus leading to rapid dissolution
- Major indication for nonmalignant SCVS

Dose

Adult dose: 4400 IU/kg intravenously over 10min as a loading dose followed by 4400 IU/kg/h at a rate of 15mL/h for 12h.

Efficacy

- Powerful antifibrinolytic leading to thrombus degradation in 60% if cases
- Degrades fibrin clots, fibrinogen, and other plasma proteins
- Effective in nonmalignant SVCS caused by thrombus, especially those associated with a catheter
- 73% of patients undergoing endovascular surgery plus thrombolysis had a response

Risks/Benefits

Risks:

- Use caution with recent surgery, obstetric delivery, and trauma
- Use caution with subacute bacterial endocarditis and streptococcal infection
- Use caution with diabetic hemorrhagic retinopathy and bleeding disorders
- Use caution with elderly
- Use caution with hypertension

Benefit: rapid reduction of symptoms due to thrombus.

Side-effects and adverse reactions

- Cardiovascular: hypotension, hypertension, myocardial infarction, reperfusion dysrhythmias
- Gastrointestinal: nausea
- Hematologic: hemorrhage, surface bleeding
- Metabolism: acidosis
- Respiratory: bronchospasm, dyspnea
- Skin: rash

Interactions (other drugs)

■ Anticoagulants ■ Antiplatelet agents

Contraindications

■ Active bleeding ■ Intraspinal surgery ■ Intracranial tumor ■ Ulcerative colitis ■ Enteritis ■ Coagulation defects ■ Rheumatic valvular heart disease ■ Cerebral embolism ■ Thrombosis or hemorrhage within 2 months ■ Intra-arterial diagnostic procedure ■ Surgery or trauma within 10 days ■ Severe hypertension

Acceptability to patient

In rare nonmalignant cases, this therapy can be curative, or at least provide significant benefit. If patient does not have major contraindications, it should be readily accepted.

Follow up plan

After thrombolysis, all invasive procedures must be avoided. Patients must take extra care to avoid accidents.

Patient and caregiver information

Must be aware that if new symptoms develop, radiation must be initiated.

Surgical therapy

- Rarely patients with SVCS require surgery
- Surgical venous bypass of the superior vena cava can relieve venous obstruction. Bypass is performed from a patent vein above the obstruction to the right atrium with autologous vein or synthetic conduits
- Surgical intervention may be required for the safe removal of a central venous catheter
- Palliation surgery is sometimes offered when chemotherapy and radiotherapy fail

SURGICAL BYPASS

Efficacy

5-year patency rate is 80% for surgical bypass patients with benign conditions.

Risks/Benefits

Risks:

- High morbidity: patients who have a malignant cause of SVCS are poor candidates for surgical resection and are rarely cured
- Significant recovery period
- Indications for procedure are unclear and more research is needed to identify who can benefit from this approach

Acceptability to patient

This is an experimental therapy and most patients will agree to it only as a last resort.

Radiation therapy

RADIATION THERAPY

- Radiation therapy is considered first-line treatment in patients with SVCS
- Useful for SVCS caused by malignancy

Efficacy

- 90% of patients experience a partial or complete response with a 3-week regimen of 8Gy given once a week for a total dose of 24Gy
- Radiation can lead to palliation in 70% of lung cancers and 95% of lymphomas

Risks/Benefits

Risks:

- Esophagitis and skin irritation
- Weight loss
- Initial worsening of symptoms from radiation-induced edema

Benefits:

- Rapid dissolution of symptoms
- Tumor reduction

Acceptability to patient

This is the major modality, and even with some small risk it will be accepted by most patients given the prompt clinical response usually seen.

Follow up plan

Patients undergoing radiation therapy should be followed for complications by a specialized team. Attention should be paid to the skin, leukocyte count, and adequate protection of healthy tissues.

Patient and caregiver information

Should be aware of risk of burns, dysphagia, and other complications of radiation.

Chemotherapy

CHEMOTHERAPY

- Effective for sensitive tumors including lymphoma or small-cell lung cancer
- Most patients will be treated with radiation, but chemosensitive tumors can be treated with chemotherapy only

Efficacy

Response rates are up to 80%.

Risks/Benefits

Risks:

- Myelosuppression
- Alopecia
- Nausea and vomiting
- Stomatitis
- Opportunistic infection

Benefit: rapid symptom resolution if causal agent is chemosensitive.

Follow up plan

Patients should be followed by a specialized team. Special attention should be given to monitoring for fever, which can be a sign of febrile neutropenia and is a potentially life-threatening situation.

Patient and caregiver information

- Patients should be educated about signs of complications of chemotherapy; particular attention should be given to monitoring for fever
- Nausea and vomiting can be prevented
- If the symptoms of SVCS worsen or do not respond to chemotherapy, patients should receive radiation

Endoscopic therapy

Thrombolysis, stent placement, and angioplasty can result in prompt resolution of signs and symptoms of SVCS: breathing may improve within hours of successful stent placement; edema resolves in 1–7 days.

Other therapies

THROMBOLYSIS

Thrombolysis is considered when thrombus is present in the superior vena cava, either as a primary event, such as occlusion of the SVCS as a result of central line placement, or thrombus formation in a partially occluded superior vena cava.

Efficacy

Central line-induced thrombosis treated with thrombolytic therapy alone has a success rate of up to 60%.

Risks/Benefits

Risks:

- Bleeding
- Intracranial hemorrhage
- Rethrombosis

Acceptability to patient
It should be offered to patients with nonmalignant SVCS. The acceptability in these cases will be high as it spares patients from radiation therapy. Most cases will be resolved.

Follow up plan
Patients should be followed by a specialized team. Maintenance of vein patency is the major aim.

Patient and caregiver information
Risk of bleeding is high and avoidance of accidents must be a rule.

ENDOVASCULAR THERAPY
Stent placement.

Efficacy
Small studies have reported a response in up to 90% of patients.

Risks/Benefits
Risks:
- Recurrence of symptoms in up to 40% of patients
- Stent migration
- Stent occlusion
- Pulmonary edema

Benefit: immediate response if successful.

Acceptability to patient
This is a new therapeutic approach with high success rates and it spares patients from surgery.

Follow up plan
Patients should be followed by a specialized team. Maintenance of vein patency is the major aim. Collapse of the stent can occur. There is no consensus about need for anticoagulation.

Patient and caregiver information
Should be informed that this treatment is still experimental.

ELEVATION OF THE HEAD OF THE BED
Efficacy
Low: this is a palliative measure with the aim of immediate relief only.

Risks/Benefits
Benefit: there is no risk, and patient can achieve relief of symptoms.

Acceptability to patient
High. No risk or cost is involved.

OUTCOMES

EFFICACY OF THERAPIES

- Life expectancy in patients with malignant superior vena cava syndrome (SVCS) is <1 year
- Most cases are palliative
- Palliation goals are to improve quality of life, particularly with pain control

Review period

Patients should be followed by an experienced team that will assist him or her during course of the disease, including any complications arising from SVCS.

PROGNOSIS

- Immediate mortality rate resulting from superior vena cava obstruction is 1–2%
- 90% of patients will die from the underlying disease within 2 years

Clinical pearl(s)

- Most treatments are palliative given the severe nature of the causative disease
- Despite a poor long-term prognosis, endovascular treatment should not necessarily be withheld as symptom relief is often dramatic and improves quality of life

Recurrence

If SVCS recurs, other modalities of therapy should be offered, if the underlying condition permits.

Deterioration

Palliative care should include the participation of the radiologist, interventional cardiologist, and surgeon.

Terminal illness

- Palliative care should include the participation of the radiologist, interventional cardiologist, and surgeon
- Pain control and comfort measures are paramount considerations in these patients

PREVENTION

RISK FACTORS

Tobacco smoking: lung cancer is the major cause of superior vena cava syndrome (SVCS).

MODIFY RISK FACTORS

Lifestyle and wellness

TOBACCO

Stop smoking.

RESOURCES

ASSOCIATIONS

Society for Cardiac Angiography and Interventions
9111 Old Georgetown Rd
Bethesda, MD 20814
Phone: (800) 992-7224 or (301) 897-5400
Fax: (301) 581-3408
e-mail: info@scai.org
http://www.scai.org

Society of Cardiovascular & Interventional Radiology
10201 Lee Highway
Suite 500
Fairfax, VA 22030
Phone: (800) 488-7284 or (703) 691-1805
Fax: (703) 691-1855
e-mail: info@scvir
http://www.scvir.org

KEY REFERENCES

- Schindler N, Vogelzang RL. Endovascular and minimally invasive vascular surgery. Surgical Clin North Am 1999;79:683–94
- Chen JC, Bongard F, Klein SR. A contemporary perspective of superior vena cava syndrome. Am J Surg 1990;160:207–11
- Abner A. Approach to the patient who presents with superior vena cava obstruction. Chest 1993;103(Suppl 4):394S–7S
- Doty D. Bypass of superior vena cava with spiral vein graft. Ann Thorac Surg 1976;22:490–3
- Yim CD, Sane SS, Bjarnason H. Superior vena cava stenting. Radiol Clin North Am 2000;38:409–24
- Valji K. Vascular and interventional radiology. Philadelphia: WB Saunders, 1999
- Hochrein J, Bashore TM, O'Laughlin MP, Harrison JK. Percutaneous stenting of superior vena cava syndrome: a case report and review of the literature. Am J Med 1998;104:78–84

FAQS

Question 1

How can I ensure that I do not miss this diagnosis, given that many of its symptoms are vague?

ANSWER 1

Patients with known thoracic pathology must have all symptoms investigated with a high index of suspicion.

Question 2

How can superior vena cava syndrome (SVCS) be differentiated from constrictive pericarditis, another rare condition?

ANSWER 2

In pericardial disease, symptoms and signs in the lower extremities predominate. Cerebral pressure is much less elevated and therefore CNS symptoms are rare. A history of pericarditis, prior cardiac surgery, or heart failure out of proportion to chest X-ray and lung findings should alert you to the possibility of constriction.

Question 3
Why do unilateral symptoms occur?

ANSWER 3
Occasionally, the compression can be high enough to impede blood flow selectively from one subclavian. Alternatively, collateral flow may be better developed on one side, especially the right. Anomalous venous anatomy can also lead to unusual patterns of obstruction.

Question 4
How should patients with pacer leads be treated?

ANSWER 4
If imaging suggests pacer-lead fibrosis as the cause of SVCS, consultation with the electrophysiologist is indicated. It may be possible to remove the leads using laser techniques. Alternatively, surgical bypass may be necessary. This form of SVCS has a much better prognosis as the cause is benign.

CONTRIBUTORS
Russell C Jones, MD, MPH
John McB Hodgson, MD, FACC, FSCAI
Otavio A Clark, MD

THROMBOPHLEBITIS

SUMMARY INFORMATION

DESCRIPTION

- The presence of thrombus with an accompanying inflammatory response in a superficial or deep vein
- Predisposing factors: stasis of blood, vascular damage, hypercoagulability
- Increased risk for venous thrombosis: immobilization, trauma or surgery, cancer, pregnancy or estrogen use, hypercoagulable states
- 10% of patients with idiopathic deep venous thrombosis go on to develop cancer

URGENT ACTION

Urgent diagnosis and treatment of proximal deep vein thrombosis (DVT) is indicated, because approx. 50% of untreated individuals may develop pulmonary embolism.

KEY! DON'T MISS!

- Signs and symptoms suggestive of proximal DVT (deep femoral vein, superficial femoral vein or saphenous vein) are an indication for urgent work-up and therapy, because 50% of proximal DVTs are associated with subsequent pulmonary embolism
- Development of a cyanotic hue to the limb, or pallor, may indicate that massive thrombosis has occurred, with associated arterial insufficiency, which can lead to 'venous gangrene' and subsequent death
- Signs and symptoms of pulmonary embolism are indications for institution of treatment even before establishment of diagnosis of DVT
- Patients with superficial venous thrombosis and positive blood cultures should be evaluated for possible endocarditis or suppurative thrombophlebitis (infected blood clot)

BACKGROUND

ICD9 CODE

- 451 Phlebitis and thrombophlebitis
- 451.0 Phlebitis and thrombophlebitis of superficial vessels of lower extremities
- 451.1 Phlebitis and thrombophlebitis of deep vessels of lower extremities
- 451.11 Phlebitis of the femoral vein
- 451.19 Phlebitis and thrombophlebitis of deep vessels of lower extremities, other
- 451.8 Of lower extremities, unspecified
- 451.81 Iliac vein
- 451.82 Of superficial veins of upper extremities
- 451.83 Of deep veins of upper extremities
- 451.84 Of upper extremities, unspecified
- 451.89 Other
- 451.9 Unspecified site

SYNONYMS

- Deep venous thrombosis/thrombophlebitis
- Superficial venous thrombosis/thrombophlebitis
- Phlebitis
- Phlebothrombosis
- Deep vein thrombosis
- 'Economy class syndrome'
- DVT

CARDINAL FEATURES

- Single or multiple blood clots in the deep or superficial veins of the extremities or pelvis
- Thrombosis is usually accompanied by inflammation of the vessel wall
- Clinical features: unilateral swelling, warmth, and erythema of the affected extremity, sometimes associated with tenderness and a palpable cord
- Embolization of clot can complicate deep venous thrombosis of the lower extremity, leading to life-threatening pulmonary embolism

CAUSES

Common causes

- Immobilization, trauma, or surgery (particularly orthopedic surgeries involving the hip or knee, intra-abdominal and intrathoracic surgeries)
- Pregnancy
- Estrogen therapy or oral contraceptive use
- Cancer, particularly cancer of the pancreas, lungs, genitourinary tract, stomach, and breast
- Hypercoagulable states: resistance to activated protein C (factor V Leiden), antithrombin III deficiency, protein C and protein S deficiencies, antiphospholipid syndrome, systemic lupus erythematosus (SLE), myeloproliferative diseases, dysfibrinogenemia, disseminated intravascular coagulation, hyperhomocysteinemia
- Indwelling venous catheters and infusions (superficial thrombophlebitis); associated with *Staphylococcus* or Enterobacteriaceae
- Varicose veins (superficial thrombophlebitis)

Rare causes

- Venulitis: thromboangiitis obliterans, Behçet's disease, homocysteinuria, Mondor's disease
- Infectious: syphilis and psittacosis

Serious causes

Immobilization, trauma or surgery:

- Can occur in more than 50% of patients having orthopedic surgery of the hip and knee, and in 10–40% of patients having intra-abdominal or intrathoracic surgery
- 10–20% of patients with idiopathic deep vein thrombosis (DVT) develop clinically apparent cancer
- Immobilization probably explains the high incidence of DVT following myocardial infarction, episodes of congestive heart failure, and prolonged air travel (also known as 'economy class syndrome')

Hypercoagulable states:

- Of patients with venographically proven spontaneous DVT, 25–50% have a measurable thrombophilic state
- Elevated factor VIII:C (above 150% of normal): 25% of unselected DVT patients
- Factor V Leiden (resistance to activated protein C): 21% of unselected DVT patients
- Factor XI elevations above the 90th percentile: 19% of unselected DVT patients
- Lupus anticoagulant (in non-SLE patients): 14% of unselected DVT patients
- Hyperhomocysteinemia: 10% of unselected DVT patients
- Prothrombin gene 20210A allele: 2.8% of unselected DVT patients
- Antithrombin III deficiency: 2.8% of unselected DVT patients
- Protein S and C deficiency: 1.3% and 2.5% of unselected DVT patients, respectively
- Dysfibrinogenemia
- Factor XII deficiency

Pregnancy:

- 49-fold increase in incidence of phlebitis

Contributory or predisposing factors

- Estrogen or oral contraceptive therapy
- Recent surgery or trauma
- Thrombocytosis, polycythemia vera
- 20% of cases of superficial thrombophlebitis are associated with occult DVT

EPIDEMIOLOGY

Incidence and prevalence

INCIDENCE

- Affects 1–2% of hospitalized patients in the US annually
- Source of emboli that causes approx. 200,000 deaths per year in the US
- Annual incidence of catheter-related thrombophlebitis in the US: 0.88/1000

PREVALENCE

- Approx. 2 million cases of DVT/year in the US
- 1.6 cases/1000 annually

Demographics

AGE

- Septic thrombophlebitis more common in childhood
- DVT more common overall after age 40 years
- Thrombophlebitis associated with protein C or S deficiency is more common before age 30 years
- Thrombophlebitis associated with antithrombin III deficiency first occurs usually between ages 20 and 30 years

- Mondor's disease (development of thrombosis in a superficial draining vein of the breast, often after breast augmentation surgery): women aged 21–55 years
- Thromboangiitis obliterans: onset age 20–50 years

GENDER

- Female:male incidence of DVT 1.2:1
- Female:male equal in cases of suppurative superficial thrombophlebitis
- Female:male incidence 2:1 in Mondor's disease
- Thromboangiitis obliterans is rare in females

RACE

- Genetic resistance to factor V Leiden, the most common genetic risk factor for venous thrombosis, is more common in European populations (5% prevalence) but rarely occurs in native Asian or African populations
- Thromboangiitis obliterans is more common in Japan, India, and southeast Asian populations

GENETICS

Genetically mediated diseases associated with hypercoagulable states are as follows.

Inherited:

- Factor V resistance (Leiden): most common genetic risk factor for venous thrombosis. Present in 20–60% of patients with spontaneous venous thrombosis
- Antithrombin III deficiency: autosomal dominant, prevalence of 0.2–0.4% of persons with this defect, 50% will experience venous thrombosis
- Protein C deficiency: autosomal dominant with variable penetrance, prevalence 0.2–0.5%. Of persons with this deficiency, 75% will experience a venous thrombosis (50% by age 50 years)
- Protein S deficiency: similar inheritance, prevalence, and incidence to those of protein C deficiency
- Disorders of defective fibrinolysis (plasminogen, plasminogen activator, or plasminogen activator inhibitor): rare
- Dysfibrinogenemia: autosomal dominant
- Factor XII deficiency: autosomal recessive
- Antiphospholipid syndrome: acquired defect with genetic predisposition

Acquired:

- Lupus anticoagulant (in non-SLE patients)
- Cancer
- Estrogen
- Renal disease
- Congestive heart failure

DIAGNOSIS

DIFFERENTIAL DIAGNOSIS

Cellulitis

Cellulitis is an acute infection of the deep subcutaneous tissues.

FEATURES

- Superficially spreading, warm, erythematous lesion
- Local tenderness and adenopathy
- 85% of cases occur in the legs and feet
- May be associated with bullae
- Fever and lymphadenopathy

Venous stasis

Venous stasis results from incompetent venous valves that cause pooling of the blood in the lower extremities.

FEATURES

- Unilateral, but is often bilateral and is chronic in nature, unlike deep vein thrombosis
- Skin changes such as hyperpigmentation and lichenification with loss of hair
- Not usually painful and is improved with elevation

Edema

Edema is due to fluid overload from congestive heart failure, liver failure, or renal insufficiency.

FEATURES

- Usually bilateral but may sometimes be worse in one leg
- Skin changes such as hyperpigmentation and lichenification with loss of hair
- Not usually painful and is improved with elevation
- Improves with diuretics and compression stockings

Ruptured Baker's cyst (pseudothrombophlebitis syndrome)

Pseudothrombophlebitis syndrome, or ruptured Baker's cyst, is caused by rupture of the membranous sac that encloses a Baker's cyst.

FEATURES

- Pain in the popliteal space
- Knee swelling
- Leg edema
- Prominence of the popliteal fossa
- Decreased range of motion and locking of the knee
- Foucher's sign: the cyst becomes hard with knee extension and soft with flexion
- Neuropathic lancinating pain radiating from the knee down the back of the leg
- Associated with DVT

Lymphedema

Lymphedema is chronic edema of the extremities due to accumulation of interstitial fluid. This may be unilateral or bilateral and is caused by obstruction or disorders of the lymphatic system.

FEATURES

- Edema
- Can be extremely painful and progressive
- Often results from pelvic or inguinal lymph node resections

- Elevation of leg produces relief in early stages but not in advanced stages
- Stemmer's sign (squaring of toes) may be seen
- Loss of ankle contour giving 'tree trunk' legs
- Humped appearance of dorsal surface of foot
- Thickened, hard, or leathery skin (lichenification)

Superficial venous thrombosis

Superficial venous thrombosis is the most common type of venous thrombosis, and seldom causes serious complications.

FEATURES

- Localized pain in the area of thrombus (in DVT, pain – if present – is less localized)
- Reddened, warm, and tender cord extending along a superficial vein

Lymphangiitis

Lymphangiitis is inflammation of a lymph vessel or vessels.

FEATURES

- May be associated with bacterial cellulitis
- May be associated with a site of skin trauma
- Erythema, edema, tenderness of the limb, with erythematous streaks extending proximally to regional lymph nodes
- Fever
- Lymphadenitis
- Associated with group A streptococci, chronic lymphedema, and chronic superficial fungal infections (such as tinea pedis)
- More common in the Midwest (associated with *Sporothrix schenckii* and *Francisella tularensis* infections)

Achilles tendinitis

Tendinitis of the Achilles tendon.

FEATURES

- Pain and/or tenderness in the back of the leg near the heel
- Pain at its worst with the first steps of out bed in the morning
- Pain is often worse after long periods of sitting
- Pain usually improves with activity

Hematoma

Hematoma is a blood clot or localized collection of blood in an organ, space or tissue, caused by leakage from a blood vessel.

FEATURES

- Often associated with direct trauma
- Pain and tenderness at the site of the hematoma
- Discoloration of the tissues
- Palpable mass or swelling at the site of tenderness

Muscle or soft tissue injury

Muscle or soft tissue injury may result from a variety of causes, including physical assault.

FEATURES
- History of trauma
- Similar features to hematoma
- May or may not be associated with discoloration of tissues

Varicose veins
Varicose veins are distended and permanently distorted veins, usually found in the subcutaneous tissues of the leg.

FEATURES
- Dull ache, burning, or cramping in the leg
- Discomfort worse with standing, warm temperatures, menses
- Tortuous dilation of superficial veins
- Edema of the leg
- Can be associated with superficial ulceration
- Darkened pigmentation of the skin (dermatitis pigmentation)

Arterial insufficiency, peripheral arterial disease
Peripheral arterial disease is brought about by atherosclerosis, leading to insufficient blood supply to limb and working muscles.

FEATURES
- Decreased pulses in the affected extremity
- Pallor of the affected limb
- Claudication of the affected limb; increasing activity causes pain, which resolves slowly at rest
- Edema

Postphlebitic syndrome (post-thrombotic syndrome)
The postphlebitic syndrome occurs following a blood clot in the vein to the leg (DVT).

FEATURES
- Chronic swelling of the limb
- Dull, aching pain in the leg, which is worse after periods of standing
- Glossy appearance to the skin
- In severe cases, skin ulceration due to chronic venous stasis

SIGNS & SYMPTOMS
Signs
Superficial venous thrombosis:
- Reddened, warm, tender cord extending along a superficial vein
- Erythema and edema of the surrounding area may be present

Deep venous thrombosis (upper extremity deep venous thrombosis is uncommon compared with lower extremity DVT; findings are similar to those found in the legs):
- Posterior calf tenderness
- Edema and erythema
- Warmth, increased tissue turgor, or modest swelling
- Rarely, a cord may be palpable
- Homan's sign (increased resistance or pain during dorsiflexion of the foot) is unreliable
- Superficial veins of the affected limb may appear dilated
- Cyanosis may occur in the affected limb from the presence of deoxygenated hemoglobin in the stagnant veins (phlegmasia cerulea dolens)
- Pallor in the affected limb can result when marked edema causes interstitial pressure to exceed capillary perfusion pressure (phlegmasia alba dolens)

Symptoms

- Both superficial and deep venous thrombosis are associated with pain in the affected limb
- Fever may or may not be present
- Redness and swelling of the affected limb may or may not be present

ASSOCIATED DISORDERS

- Hypercoagulable states
- Immobility
- Pulmonary embolus

KEY! DON'T MISS!

- Signs and symptoms suggestive of proximal DVT (deep femoral vein, superficial femoral vein or saphenous vein) is an indication for urgent work-up and therapy, because 50% of proximal DVTs are associated with subsequent pulmonary embolism
- Development of a cyanotic hue to the limb, or pallor, may indicate that massive thrombosis has occurred, with associated arterial insufficiency, which can lead to 'venous gangrene' and subsequent death
- Signs and symptoms of pulmonary embolism are indications for institution of treatment even before establishment of diagnosis of DVT
- Patients with superficial venous thrombosis and positive blood cultures should be evaluated for possible endocarditis or suppurative thrombophlebitis (infected blood clot)

CONSIDER CONSULT

- When moderate to high suspicion of DVT exists, tests such as duplex ultrasound and venous plethysmography are nondiagnostic and more sophisticated diagnostic testing is needed
- Referral is warranted when the diagnosis of idiopathic DVT is made in a patient under the age of 50 years, and there is suspicion of hypercoagulable state (requiring a coagulation specialist)

INVESTIGATION OF THE PATIENT

Direct questions to patient

Q **Do you have any recent history of injury to your leg (or arm), including scratches, punctures, blunt trauma, or possible muscle strain?** Suggestive of predisposing factors to DVT, superficial thrombosis, and other causes of limb pain and swelling, such as cellulitis and lymphangiitis

Q **Do you have a history of knee pain, arthritis in the knee, or injury to the knee?** Suggestive of predisposing factors to DVT and possible presence of Baker's cyst

Q **Have you had a fever, generalized muscle aches, or generalized rash?** Suggestive of infectious causes of extremity pain or lymphangiitis

Q **Have you recently had major surgery, such as hip or knee surgery, or abdominal or chest surgery?** Predisposing factors for DVT

Q **Have you ever had a previous blood clot in your veins?** Suggestive of either a predisposition to venous thrombophlebitis or of postphlebitic syndrome

Q **Are you, or have you recently been, pregnant?** Predisposing factor

Q **Have you recently been exposed to any unusual animals?** Tick bites, animal carcass exposure can indicate exposure to rare causes of infectious phlebitis (e.g. tularemia)

Q **Do you have pain in the leg that radiates down the calf?** Suggestive of Baker's cyst rupture

Q **Have you experienced chest pain, especially with deep breaths, or shortness of breath?** Suggestive of possible pulmonary embolism

Contributory or predisposing factors

Q **Have you recently been forced to sit for long periods of time or to stay immobile, such as a long car or airplane ride, or recent inability to move around due to surgery, trauma, or heart condition?** Predisposing factors for DVT

Q **Have you recently taken medication such as estrogens or oral contraceptives?** Predisposing factor for DVT

Q **Have you recently had any intravenous catheters placed (for intravenous fluids, antibiotics, procedural sedation, chemotherapy)?** Predisposing factor for superficial thrombophlebitis

Family history

Q **Has anyone in your family ever had blood clots in their veins or arteries?** Suggestive of familial condition predisposing to thrombophlebitis

Q **If so, at what age did it occur?** Suggestive of specific inherited disorder if it occurred under age 50 years, vs immobility or other disease factors in older age groups

Examination

Examine for swelling, erythema, and/or tenderness of the limb:

- **Is tenderness well localized, or associated with a palpable cord?** This is suggestive of superficial phlebitis
- **Does the limb have significant cyanosis or pallor?** Indicative of secondary arterial insufficiency
- **Is there swelling in the popliteal fossa and does it soften with flexion of the knee?** Suggestive of Baker's cyst
- **Does the pain increase with dorsiflexion of the foot of the affected leg?** Homan's sign; unreliable indicator of possible DVT
- **Is the patient tachypneic, pale, tachycardic, or in respiratory distress?** Suggestive of pulmonary embolism

Summary of investigative tests

Diagnosis of venous thrombosis:

- **Duplex ultrasonography:** for diagnosis of thrombus involving the iliac, femoral, or popliteal veins. Performed by radiologist or ultrasonographer, and usually available in primary care setting
- **Venography:** when the diagnosis of thrombosis cannot be established or ruled out by duplex ultrasonography. Performed by a radiologist, and usually available in the primary care setting
- **Plethysmography:** acceptable accuracy in diagnosing thrombotic obstruction of major proximal veins of the extremities. Cannot detect DVT of the calf. Can be done by a trained technician. Usually available in the primary care setting
- **Magnetic resonance imaging (MRI):** useful in patients with suspected thrombosis of the superior and inferior vena cava or pelvic veins. Interpreted by a specialist, and may not be available in all primary care settings
- **Serum blood test for D-dimers:** can be helpful in cases where clinical suspicion is high but other test results are inconsistent. Available in the primary care setting
- **Serial testing** (when clinically indicated) should be performed to exclude DVT when using duplex ultrasonography or plethysmography since these tests are generally sensitive for proximal DVT and become positive with distal DVT when the thrombosis has propagated to the proximal veins

Diagnosis of complications:

- **Pulmonary nuclear scan (V/Q):** when pulmonary embolism is suspected. Performed by a nuclear medicine specialist, and may not be available in all primary care settings
- **Pulmonary arteriogram:** for suspected pulmonary embolism when nuclear scan is unavailable or nondiagnostic. Usually performed by a specialist
- **Arterial blood gases:** only in cases of suspected pulmonary embolism

Diagnosis of underlying causes:

- **Complete blood count (CBC) with differential:** may show anemia suggestive of underlying disorder
- **Pregnancy testing:** may uncover underlying predisposition; certain therapies for DVT are contraindicated in pregnancy

- **Serum coagulation studies:** in any patient with major thrombosis occurring before age 50, a familial history of venous thrombosis, an unusual site of spontaneous thrombosis, or massive thrombosis
- **Bacterial cultures:** of blood, indwelling venous catheters
- **Venereal Disease Research Laboratory (VDRL):** in cases of suspected syphilis

DIAGNOSTIC DECISION

Diagnosis of thrombophlebitis is not an easy matter. Objective tests aimed at establishing the presence of venous thrombosis, discovering underlying causes that may require further or prolonged treatment, and diagnosis of the presence of complications, such as pulmonary embolism or arterial insufficiency, should be carried out.

Establishing the diagnosis of superficial thrombophlebitis:

- Diagnosis is usually obvious from history and classic findings on physical examination
- Further imaging techniques are seldom indicated

Establishing the diagnosis of deep venous thrombophlebitis:
Clinical pretest probability of DVT of lower extremity can be estimated using Wells' criteria (Wells PS, Anderson DR, Bormanis J, et al. Value of assessment of pretest probability of deep vein thrombosis in clinical management. Lancet 1997;350:1795–98).

Score 1 point each for the presence of any of the following:

- Active cancer
- Paralysis, paresis, or recent plaster immobilization of lower extremity
- Recently bedridden for >3 days or major surgery within 4 weeks
- Localized tenderness along the distribution of the deep venous system
- Entire leg swollen
- Calf swollen by more than 3cm when compared with unaffected leg (measured 10cm below tibial tuberosity)
- Pitting edema (greater in the symptomatic leg)
- Collateral, nonvaricose, superficial veins

Subtract 2 points from the total if an alternative diagnosis is as likely or greater than that of DVT. If both legs are symptomatic, score on the more severe side.

The final score should be interpreted as follows:

- High risk: 3 points or more
- Moderate risk: 1–2 points
- Low risk: 0 or less

Comments regarding Wells' criteria:

- When Wells' criteria indicate moderate or high probability of DVT, noninvasive imaging techniques provide sufficient diagnostic accuracy in most cases to evaluate lower-extremity thrombosis
- Imaging ultrasound has slightly lower accuracy in evaluation of venous structures of the upper extremity, where MRI imaging may be useful. MRI has yet to be evaluated in large clinical series for diagnosis of lower-extremity venous thrombosis; however, preliminary studies suggest sensitivity and specificity in the 85–95% range
- Contrast venography may be needed wherever noninvasive imaging techniques fail

Diagnosis of predisposing conditions requiring treatment:
(Hypercoagulable states)

- Patients should be tested for hypercoagulable states in consultation with a hematologist

- Patients who should be tested include those with first idiopathic DVT who are under age 50 years, have a family history of venous thromboembolism in one or more first-degree relatives, have an unusual site of spontaneous thrombosis, or have massive thrombosis
- Laboratory test for hypercoagulable states should be done at least 2 weeks after discontinuation of anticoagulation

(Cancer)
- Although some patients presenting with idiopathic DVT have occult malignancy, extensive work-up of asymptomatic patients beyond appropriate cancer screening has not been shown to be beneficial

Diagnosis of major complications:
- Pulmonary embolism
- Arterial insufficiency

CLINICAL PEARL(S)
- Risk for DVT following surgery can be assessed by type of procedure, with hip or knee operations the highest risk, prolonged general surgery and long bone fractures intermediate, and short procedures low risk
- The complication of pulmonary embolism is often missed. A high index of suspicion is needed for all at-risk patients who complain of dyspnea or develop unexplained hypoxia
- Patients presenting with upper extremity DVT should be carefully screened for indwelling catheters, pacemakers, and mediastinal carcinoma

THE TESTS
Body fluids
COMPLETE BLOOD CELL COUNT (CBC) WITH DIFFERENTIAL BLOOD COUNT

Description

Venous blood sample.

Advantages/Disadvantages

Advantages:
- Relatively noninvasive and inexpensive
- Useful if infectious or septic cause of thrombosis is suspected
- May reveal thrombocytosis
- Needed before institution of anticoagulation

Disadvantages:
- Nonspecific and nonsensitive test
- Mild patient discomfort associated with test

Normal
- Hematocrit: males 42%–52%, females 37%–48%
- White bloodcell count (WBC): 4.5–10.5x109/L
- Neutrophils: 60%
- Lymphocytes: 40%
- Platelets: 130–400x10^6/L

Abnormal

Values outside the normal ranges.

Cause of abnormal result

- Elevations and depressions in platelet, WBC count, and differential counts can occur due to multiple factors including infection, inflammation, hematologic malignancy, and primary hematopoietic disorders
- WBC may be elevated in cases of superficial venous thrombosis, due to septic or infectious causes
- Keep in mind he possibility of a false-positive or false-negative result

Drugs, disorders, and other factors that may alter results

Steroids and sympathomimetic drugs can cause elevations of WBC and differential counts.

SERUM PREGNANCY TEST

Description

Venous blood sample.

Advantages/Disadvantages

Advantage: relatively inexpensive and noninvasive.

Disadvantages:

- Mild patient discomfort associated with test
- False-negative tests can occur in very early pregnancy

Normal

- Nonpregnant: human chorionic gonadotropin (hGC) <5mU/mL
- First week of pregnancy: hGC 5–50mU/mL
- Second week of pregnancy: hGC 50–550mU/mL
- 2–3 weeks: hGC up to 5000mU/mL
- 3–4 weeks: hGCup to 10,000mU/mL
- 4–5 weeks: hGC >10,000mU/mL

Abnormal

In the nonpregnant patient, hGC levels are below 5mU/mL.

Cause of abnormal result

- Pregnancy
- Hydatidiform mole
- Choriocarcinoma
- Germ cell tumors of testicle
- Occasionally, neoplasms of the cervix, gastrointestinal tract, ovary, lung, and breast

COAGULATION STUDIES

Description

Venous blood sample for functional coagulation studies (e.g. prothrombin time (PT), partial thromboplastin time (PTT), and specific factor levels).

Advantages/Disadvantages

Advantages:

- Relatively noninvasive
- In patients at risk of having hypercoagulable states predisposing to DVT, may identify risk and help direct therapy
- Specific and sensitive

Disadvantage: hypercoagulable laboratory tests are relatively expensive and should be ordered only in consultation with a coagulation specialist, who can direct economical testing.

Abnormal
Results considered abnormal vary among local laboratories and require interpretation by a coagulation specialist.

Cause of abnormal result
- Coagulation abnormalities, either congenital or acquired (lupus anticoagulant causes prolongation of PTT)
- Anticoagulant therapy
- Recent hemorrhage or transfusion
- Requires interpretation by a coagulation specialist

Drugs, disorders, and other factors that may alter results
- Dietary insufficiency of vitamin K
- Herbal supplements, which may contain cascara or warfarin-related compounds, can inhibit platelet activity, may be weakly estrogenic, or have other pharmacologic properties that can alter test results
- Prescription anticoagulants

D-DIMERS
Description
Venous blood sample.

Advantages/Disadvantages
Advantages:
- Relatively noninvasive
- Relatively inexpensive

Disadvantages:
- Insensitive and nonspecific
- 2–5% of the time a negative test does not rule out DVT
- Useful only in a patient with a moderate risk of DVT and normal duplex ultrasound result

Normal
Negative.

Abnormal
Positive for D-dimers.

Cause of abnormal result
Any fibrinolytic state:
- Recent severe hemorrhage
- Disseminated intravascular coagulation
- Thrombolytic therapy
- DVT

Drugs, disorders, and other factors that may alter results
Recent thrombolytic therapy.

BLOOD OR TISSUE BACTERIAL CULTURES

Description

Specimens:

- Venous blood samples
- Swabs of suspected infection site
- Culture of extracted venous catheter material

Advantages/Disadvantages

Advantages:

- Relatively noninvasive and inexpensive
- Most useful in superficial thrombosis, when septic cause is suspected
- Both sensitive and specific for common bacterial sources of infection, such as *Staphylococcus*, group A streptococci
- Can be used to determine antibiotic sensitivity profiles of infectious agents for appropriately directed drug therapy

Disadvantage: may be insensitive for detecting fungal infections, mycobacteria, and others.

Normal

No bacterial growth.

Abnormal

Bacterial growth suggestive of infection, and not contamination.

Cause of abnormal result

Septic cause of thrombosis.

Drugs, disorders, and other factors that may alter results

Concurrent antibiotic therapy may inhibit growth of culture. Advise laboratory of concomitant antibiotic therapy.

VDRL

Description

Venous blood sample. Syphilis is a rare cause of migratory thrombosis.

Advantages/Disadvantages

Advantage: relatively inexpensive and noninvasive.

Normal

Negative test.

Abnormal

Positive test.

Cause of abnormal result

- Syphilis
- Other treponemal disease: yaws, pinta, bejel
- False-positives can occur in patients with SLE, lupus anticoagulant, infectious mononucleosis, HIV, atypical pneumonia, malaria, leprosy, typhus, relapsing fever

Imaging

DUPLEX ULTRASONOGRAPHY

Description

Combined B-mode and color Doppler ultrasound. With patient reclining, ultrasound Doppler transducer is applied on the surface of the limb to image deep venous structures while light compression is applied at intervals along the veins.

Advantages/Disadvantages

Advantages:

- First choice test for diagnosis of either upper or lower extremity venous thrombosis
- Noninvasive, safe, portable, and available in most places
- Relatively inexpensive
- 91–94% sensitive in detecting deep venous thrombosis of lower extremities (common and superficial femoral veins), with no false positives
- May help diagnose other pathology, such as Baker's cyst, hematoma or abscess, lymphadenopathy, superficial thrombophlebitis

Disadvantages:

- Less accurate in detecting venous thrombosis of the upper extremities but still the first choice test. A negative result with high suspicion should lead to further tests (magnetic resonance imaging or possibly venography) or repeat ultrasound in a week
- Operator dependent
- Less sensitive to detect thrombosis of veins of the calf
- Can remain abnormal for 6 months or more following an acute episode of thrombosis
- Less sensitive in massively obese or edematous patients
- Cannot be used if casts or immobilization devices are in use on the extremity

Normal

No findings suggestive of venous obstruction or thrombosis and normal compressibility of the veins.

Abnormal

- Visible thrombi or obstruction
- Abnormal compressibility of the veins
- Loss of flow phasicity in response to Valsalva
- Absence of color Doppler flow signal from the vein lumen

Cause of abnormal result

- Thrombus or other obstruction of the venous system
- Thrombophlebitis within the previous 6 months

PLETHYSMOGRAPHY

Description

Evaluates rate of venous return from the lower extremity. Relies on the principle that a volume of blood in the leg affects its ability to conduct an applied electric current.

A small current is passed between a set of electrodes, while another set of electrodes measures changes in voltage. A cuff is inflated around the thigh to obstruct venous outflow but not arterial inflow. Electrical impedance is measured in the leg as blood accumulates in the leg (impedance falls), until venous pressure equals cuff pressure (impedance plateaus), and after release of the cuff with venous outflow (impedance rises sharply). If venous obstruction is present in the legs, the venous outflow is lower than normal, and the rise in impedance after cuff release is significantly slower.

Advantages/Disadvantages

Advantages:

- Noninvasive, low risk
- Relatively inexpensive
- Portable
- Sensitive to the presence of proximal deep venous thrombosis (multiple studies indicate sensitivity 91–98%, specificity 93–98%)
- Available most places

Disadvantages:

- Insensitive to the presence of nonobstructing thrombi, such as calf thrombi
- Test accuracy is operator dependent
- False-positive results can occur with other causes of slow venous outflow, such as elevated central venous pressure
- Not useful for upper extremity DVT
- Casts or immobilization devices on the limb preclude use
- Normal return to baseline impedance with release of thigh cuff

Abnormal

Slow rate of return to baseline impedance.

Cause of abnormal result

- Obstruction to venous outflow of the lower extremity
- Decreased arterial inflow to the lower extremity

Drugs, disorders, and other factors that may alter results

Nonthrombotic causes of decreased venous outflow can cause false-positive results, such as:

- Increased abdominal pressure due to obesity or ascites
- Increased central venous pressure due to vena caval obstruction, cor pulmonale, pericardial tamponade, congestive heart failure
- Decreased arterial inflow to lower extremity due to peripheral arterial disease or cardiogenic shock
- Nonthrombotic venous outflow obstruction, such as pregnancy, abdominal or pelvic masses, abnormal leg muscle tension

CONTRAST VENOGRAPHY

Description

Invasive study, requiring injection of contrast into deep venous system with concomitant radiographic imaging.

Advantages/Disadvantages

Advantages:

- Diagnostic 'gold standard', considered 100% sensitive and specific
- Useful in cases where less invasive studies, such as plethysmography or ultrasound, are inconclusive
- Available in most healthcare settings
- Less operator dependent than ultrasound and plethysmography

Disadvantages:

- Requires expert interpretation
- Carries risk of intravenous contrast injection
- Requires venous access, with moderate discomfort to the patient
- Relatively expensive

- Relatively contraindicated in patients with acute and chronic renal failure, or creatinine >2.0, and in patients with known contrast allergy

Normal
Normal venous flow pattern, without intraluminal defects.

Abnormal
- Intraluminal defects in venous filling in two or more views
- Abrupt 'cutoff' of venous filling

Cause of abnormal result
- Intraluminal venous obstruction due to thrombus or other obstruction
- Previous deep venous thrombosis

MAGNETIC RESONANCE IMAGING (MRI)
Description
Scanning technique using MRI and not involving ionizing radiation.

Advantages/Disadvantages
Advantages:
- Sensitive and specific
- Safe, does not involve ionizing radiation
- Can visualize pelvic veins, upper extremity veins
- May detect other abnormalities: tumor, Baker's cyst, abscess, lymphadenopathy, superficial thrombophlebitis

Disadvantages:
- Expensive
- Not portable
- Requires specialist interpretation
- Imaging chamber is small, causing claustrophobic reactions in a significant number of patients; some may require sedation or general anesthesia
- May be difficult to obtain in massively obese patients
- Metallic devices secondary to trauma or surgery may not be admissible in the MRI scanning chamber, or may interfere significantly with imaging

Normal
Normal scan.

Abnormal
Any findings suggestive of thrombus, tumor, or other obstructing pathology.

Cause of abnormal result
Venous obstruction due to any cause.

TREATMENT

CONSIDER CONSULT

- If anticoagulation is being considered for possible deep vein thrombosis (DVT), the clinical picture is uncertain, and appropriate diagnostic imaging techniques are not available
- Deep calf thrombosis always needs to be treated promptly with anticoagulants to avoid the risk of propagation
- If arterial insufficiency is suspected and thrombolytic therapy or invasive intervention is contemplated for the purpose of limb salvage
- If an associated pulmonary embolism has already occurred and invasive intervention, such as vena caval filter placement, is being contemplated to prevent further pulmonary embolization

IMMEDIATE ACTION

Immediate action is required:

- In cases of pulmonary embolism, even if the diagnosis of venous thrombophlebitis is not yet established
- In cases of massive thrombosis
- In cases of arterial compromise secondary to venous thrombosis in an extremity

PATIENT AND CAREGIVER ISSUES

Forensic and legal issues

In cases in which immediate action is indicated, it may be necessary for the primary care physician to institute treatment without direct consent from patients who are incapable of giving consent due to psychiatric illness, organic brain disease, disorders of consciousness, medical moribundity, or who are of a minor age.

Impact on career, dependants, family, friends

Chronic debilitation can result either from the direct effects of thrombophlebitis (chronic venous insufficiency, immobility, pain, swelling) or from secondary complications (pulmonary insufficiency from pulmonary embolus, chronic arterial insufficiency, chronic anticoagulation therapy).

Patient or caregiver request

- **Will I need to take blood thinners?** Possibly. Anticoagulants are seldom needed in treatment of superficial thrombophlebitis but are needed for varying periods of time after DVT
- **Do I have to be on blood thinners for the rest of my life?** It is unusual to require lifelong anticoagulation after DVT; long-term anticoagulation may be indicated if you had massive thrombosis or have an inherited or medical condition that predisposes to developing blood clots
- **How life-threatening is thrombophlebitis?** Most cases of thrombophlebitis, when properly diagnosed and treated, resolve without incident. Untreated, thrombophlebitis can lead in a significant number of cases to life-threatening consequences, such as blood clots in the lungs
- **Should I wear special support hose in the future?** While compression stockings are not a first-line therapy for DVT, they may reduce the incidence of postphlebitic syndrome by as much as 50%
- **Are there any foods or beverages I shouldn't eat or drink while being treated for DVT?** Certain foods and beverages can change the effectiveness of oral anticoagulants; alcohol may increase anticoagulant effect, and foods containing vitamin K (e.g. avocados) may decrease the effectiveness of anticoagulants
- **Can I continue to take my herbal supplements along with my regular medication?** Some herbal supplements may contain components that, in conjunction with anticoagulants, can cause dangerous thinning of the blood, resulting in potentially serious bleeding. Others may contain vitamin components or weak hormonal effects that counteract anticoagulant medication or alter how your body metabolizes the medication. Many herbal supplements may be safe, but you should bring all supplements to the attention of your doctor and pharmacist for evaluation before continuing them

Health-seeking behavior

Have you received any advice from a nontraditional healthcare practitioner? Particularly concerning herbal or vitamin supplements that the patient may then take, which can significantly affect pharmacology or metabolism of anticoagulant medications.

MANAGEMENT ISSUES

Goals

Superficial thrombophlebitis:

- Treatment is primarily supportive
- Warm compresses
- Nonsteroidal anti-inflammatory drugs (NSAIDs)
- Watch for signs that superficial thrombosis is extending and may involve deep venous systems

Deep venous thrombophlebitis:

- Anticoagulation to prevent complications such as pulmonary embolism
- Thrombolytics can be considered when arterial compromise results from massive venous thromboembolism to preserve venous valvular function, to decrease the potential for postphlebitic syndrome, and for treatment of pulmonary embolism
- Prophylaxis in patients who are at high risk for primary or recurrent thrombosis

Management in special circumstances

COEXISTING DISEASE

Patients with certain coexisting disease states may be at higher risk for complications from anticoagulation therapy; alternative surgical therapy, such as venous ligation or vena cava filter placement, might be considered ahead of traditional interventions. Such conditions include:

- Disorders complicated by bleeding: tumors, peptic ulcers
- Disorders complicated by increased risk of trauma or falls: uncontrolled seizure disorder, some cases of neurologic compromise
- Disorders requiring chemotherapy that can adversely affect platelet counts
- Primary liver disease

COEXISTING MEDICATION

Medications that may increase predisposition to thrombosis:

- Vitamin K
- Oral contraceptives
- Hormone replacement therapy (HRT)
- Diuretics (including over-the-counter diet and 'waterpills')
- Some herbal supplements: for a list of pharmacologic effects of herbal supplements, refer to the Family Practice Notebook (http://www.fpnotebook.com/PHACh2.htm)

Medications that may increase risk of bleeding:

- NSAIDs
- Aspirin
- Some herbal supplements

Medications that can interfere with the metabolism of anticoagulants and may either prolong or decrease the duration of action:

- Antireflux medications: cimetidine (potentiates), sucralfate (inhibits)
- Cardiac medications: amiodarone, propranolol (potentiate)
- Certain antibiotics, such as nafcillin, rifampin (inhibit), erythromycin, metronidazole, isoniazid (potentiate)
- Aspirin, acetaminophen (may potentiate)
- Barbiturates (inhibit)
- Antifungals: fluconazole, miconazole (potentiate)

A more complete list of warfarin medication interactions has been provided by the Institute for Clinical Systems Improvement: Health Care Guideline (http://www.icsi.org/guide/VTE.pdf; see Appendix D, page 22).

SPECIAL PATIENT GROUPS

Pregnancy is a contraindication to warfarin therapy because of increased risk for bleeding and risk for congenital anomalies. Alternative therapy, such as low-molecular-weight heparin, should be considered.

PATIENT SATISFACTION/LIFESTYLE PRIORITIES

- Anticoagulation can significantly impact on the lifestyle of active patients and may require curtailing of high-risk recreational activities
- Requirements for frequent laboratory evaluation of therapy can significantly impact on lifestyle as well as economics. Lower cost alternatives, such as home test kits, should be considered

SUMMARY OF THERAPEUTIC OPTIONS

Choices

Superficial thrombophlebitis:

- Supportive therapy
- Bed rest with leg elevation
- Warm compresses
- NSAIDs
- Antibiotics may be indicated in cases of superficial thrombophlebitis in which sepsis is a suspected cause. Patients with history of intravenous drug abuse or indwelling venous catheters are particularly at risk. Be aware that septic thrombophlebitis may be a presenting sign of endocarditis. Antibiotic choice is dependent on the organism suspected or cultured from the suspicious site or catheter. Antibiotic treatment would require consultation with a specialist and probably admission to hospital. Septic phlebitis often requires surgical drainage

Deep venous thrombophlebitis, other than calf:

- Anticoagulants (standard therapy): initially unfractionated heparin (UFH) or low-molecular-weight heparin (LMWH). Patients with known heparin-induced thrombocytopenia should not receive UFH or LMWH at any dose. Alternative forms of therapy must be considered. Currently, heparin alternatives should be initiated only in consultation with a specialist and include bivaliruden, hirudin, and danaparoid. Finally, warfarin, overlapping heparin therapy by 4–5 days until full anticoagulant effect of warfarin is achieved. Warfarin would be continued for 3 months in patients with isolated DVT and reversible risk factors, 3–6 months if idiopathic. Studies in patients with associated embolism suggest benefit with longer therapy up to 2 years
- Vena cava plication or filter if anticoagulants are contraindicated or if recurrent embolism in the setting of adequate anticoagulation
- Thrombectomy performed in concert with temporary arteriovenous fistula should be considered with acute iliofemoral thrombosis of <7 days' duration in patients expected to live >10 years
- Thrombolytics (controversial): lytic therapy has been used in patients with extensive acute iliofemoral thrombosis who exhibit vascular compromise. It has been suggested that thrombolytic therapy may decrease the incidence of postphlebitic syndrome, but no long-term randomized studies have been performed. Lytic therapy should be undertaken only in consultation with a specialist. Better results obtained with catheter-based delivery. Agents include streptokinase, urokinase, and tissue plasminogen activator
- After edema subsides following an acute episode of DVT, the patient should be measured for firm, below-knee stocking

Calf thrombophlebitis:

- 20–30% of calf thrombi propagate to the thigh, with increased risk of pulmonary embolism (5–20% incidence with calf thrombi). In addition, isolated calf vein thrombosis has been identified as a cause of embolic stroke via a patent foramen ovale
- Anticoagulants (somewhat controversial): UFH, LMWH, and warfarin are recommended for 3 months if used
- If anticoagulants are not used, then the patient should be followed with serial noninvasive tests to determine whether proximal propagation of clot has occurred

Lifestyle:

- In addition to the treatment options listed above, certain lifestyle measures may reduce the risk of initial or recurrent DVT

Clinical pearl(s)

- Bed rest does not prevent pulmonary emboli. Patients may ambulate with proximal DVT
- As many as 80% of patients with DVT and pulmonary emboli may be managed at home under the supervision of a homecare nurse
- Early aggressive treatment in patients with massive proximal DVT may prevent late venous valve incompetence

Never

- Never institute anticoagulant therapy in an actively bleeding patient
- Never institute anticoagulant therapy in a patient with recent intracranial hemorrhage
- Never institute heparin therapy in a patient with known heparin-induced thrombocytopenia; administration of even small amounts of heparin can lead to catastrophic thrombocytopenia, complicated by massive thrombosis
- Never institute warfarin therapy in patients who are possibly pregnant without consultation with an obstetric specialist
- Extreme caution should be exercised if anticoagulant therapy is considered in patients with recent or imminent surgery, trauma, severe anemia, renal disease, history of gastrointestinal bleeding, active peptic ulcer disease, and liver disease. Specialist consultation is advised

FOLLOW UP

- Baseline and periodic platelet counts should be followed during therapy with UFH or LMWH
- International normalized ratio (INR) values should be determined periodically in patients receiving warfarin therapy; initially 2–3 times per week during the first 2 weeks of therapy, then less frequently (once or twice per month) thereafter, depending on stability of INR
- Serial ultrasound examinations may be useful in two groups of patients: patients with known thrombosis, but contraindication to anticoagulation; and patients with suspicion of calf thrombosis, but initially negative ultrasound
- After therapy for initial episode of idiopathic DVT, work-up for familial hypercoagulable state should be undertaken in consultation with a specialist

Plan for review

Superficial thrombophlebitis:

- Follow up if signs and symptoms do not subside with supportive therapy in 1–2 weeks

Deep venous thrombosis:

- Anticoagulation monitoring after stabilization of therapy at least monthly
- Discontinuation of anticoagulation therapy should be individualized to the patient: 3–6 months in patients with transient risk factors (e.g. immobilization, surgery, estrogen use, trauma); >6 months in patients with idiopathic or medical causes of DVT; 12 months to lifetime in patients with recurrent disease or continued risk factors

- Serial ultrasonographic evaluation in patients with calf thrombosis
- Testing for hypercoagulable conditions 2 weeks after discontinuation of anticoagulants, in consultation with a specialist
- Measure for elastic stockings (firm, below the knee, 30–40mmHg pressure) after edema from initial episode subsides

Information for patient or caregiver

- Anticoagulant therapy for DVT requires meticulous attention to medication and to follow up to evaluate effectiveness of therapy
- Your doctor needs to be informed of any changes in other medications, herbal supplements, or over-the-counter preparations, including antacids, vitamins, antibiotics, and cold remedies before taking them, because they may have serious interactions with anticoagulants
- The primary care physician should be contacted if during the course of therapy any of the following develop: worsening pain or swelling; fever; bloody or dark-colored stools; fatigue or pallor
- The patient should contact an emergency room immediately if any of the following develop: chest pain; shortness of breath, wheezing; changes in consciousness; cyanosis of the lips or fingers; head trauma; bleeding

DRUGS AND OTHER THERAPIES: DETAILS

Drugs

LOW-MOLECULAR-WEIGHT HEPARIN (LMWH)

- Enoxaparin
- Dalteparin
- Tinzaparin (US Food and Drug Administration (FDA) approved, availability pending)

Dose

- Enoxaparin: 1mg/kg subcutaneously twice a day (1.5mg/kg subcutaneously once daily approved for inpatient treatment of DVT)
- Patients with renal failure at half dose: 0.5g/kg subcutaneously twice daily
- Dalteparin: 100U/kg subcutaneously twice daily (effectiveness of once a day dosing of 200U/kg subcutaneously is still controversial)

LMWH should be continued for at least 5 days, and until warfarin is having a therapeutic effect for at least 2 days.

Efficacy

A review of multiple trials comparing therapy of deep venous thrombosis vs UFH showed comparable clinical efficacy of LMWH with reduced cost associated with outpatient treatment. Thromboembolic events can be reduced to 2–5% in patients with adequate anticoagulation treatment, compared with 47% of untreated patients. Morbid events secondary to therapy, such as bleeding or recurrent thromboembolism, are similar to those experienced with treatment with UFH.

Risks/Benefits

Risks

Enoxaparin:

- Use caution with bleeding disorders, renal impairment, gastrointestinal disease, and active peptic ulceration
- Use caution with bacterial endocarditis and hemorrhagic stroke
- Use caution with recent surgery, the elderly, and children

Dalteparin:
- Use caution with renal or hepatic disease, subacute bacterial endocarditis, diabetes mellitus, and severe hypertension
- Use caution with history of gastrointestinal cancer, peptic ulcer disease, active ulceration, gastrointestinal bleeding, and angiodysplastic gastrointestinal disease
- Use caution with bleeding disorders and thrombocytopenia, recent surgery, and retinopathy
- Use caution in the elderly and children

Side-effects and adverse reactions

Enoxaparin:
- Cardiovascular: edema
- CNS: fever, confusion
- Gastrointestinal: altered liver function tests, nausea
- Hematologic: thrombocytopenia, bleeding, anemia
- Skin: irritation, pain

Dalteparin:
- CNS: fever, headache
- Gastrointestinal: vomiting, nausea
- Genitourinary: hematuria, priapism
- Hematologic: hemorrhage, thrombocytopenia, new thrombus formation
- Metabolism: hyperlipidemia, hyperkalemia
- Musculoskeletal: osteoporosis after prolonged treatment
- Respiratory: anaphylactoid reactions, asthma
- Skin: erythema, urticaria, skin necrosis

Interactions (other drugs)

Enoxaparin and dalteparin:
- Angiotensin-converting enzyme (ACE) inhibitors
- Angiotensin II receptor antagonists
- Antiplatelet drugs (clopidogrel, dipyridamole, ticlopidine)
- Glyceryl trinitrate
- NSAIDs (aspirin, diclofenac, ketorolac)

Contraindications

Enoxaparin:
- Active bleeding
- Drug-related thrombocytopenia

Dalteparin:
- Hemophilia and other bleeding disorders
- Thrombocytopenia
- Peptic ulcer
- Severe hypertension
- Recent cerebral hemorrhage
- Severe liver disease

Acceptability to patient
- Subcutaneous dosing allows for initiation of therapy in the outpatient setting, decreasing cost and inconvenience
- No laboratory monitoring of anticoagulation with LMWH is required except in unusual circumstances, decreasing patient expense, inconvenience, and discomfort
- Injection route causes mild-to-moderate temporary discomfort
- Patients or caregivers will require training in drug administration

Follow up plan

Occasionally, monitoring of therapy with LMWH may be needed, for example. in the following circumstances:
- Patients with extensive iliofemoral disease: inpatient clinical monitoring for extension of thrombotic disease

- Patients with significant renal dysfunction: inpatient clinical monitoring for signs of bleeding complications
- Obese patients and those with renal failure need to have anti-Xa level in blood measured 4h after injection

Patient and caregiver information

Patients and/or caregiver will require instruction about administration of subcutaneous injections.

UNFRACTIONATED HEPARIN (UFH)

Heparin.

Dose

Heparin is administered as an intravenous infusion following a bolus dose. Protocols for managing heparin therapy have been shown to achieve therapeutic anticoagulation more rapidly than historic controls.

One example protocol:

- Loading dose: 80U/kg
- Initial maintenance dose: 18U/kg/h
- Measure activated partial thromboplastin time (aPTT) 6h after any dosing change and then every 24h thereafter

Dosage adjustments:

- <35s: 80U/kg bolus, increase infusion by 4U/kg/h
- 35–45s: 40U/kg bolus, increase infusion by 2U/kg/h
- 46–75s: no change
- 75–90s: decrease infusion rate by 2U/kg/h
- 90s: hold infusion for 1h, then decrease infusion rate by 3U/kg/h
- UFH therapy should be continued at least 5 days after initiation of warfarin therapy, and until INR is above 2.0 for two consecutive days

Efficacy

- Similar morbidity and efficacy to LMWH in multiple studies
- Costlier than LMWH when hospital costs of inpatient therapy are considered

Risks/Benefits

Risks:

- Patients may develop 'white clot' syndrome (new thrombus formation)
- Use caution with renal disease and subacute bacterial endocarditis
- Use caution with diabetes mellitus, severe hypertension, history of gastrointestinal cancer and peptic ulcer disease
- Use caution with elderly and children

Side-effects and adverse reactions

- Cardiovascular: shock
- CNS: fever, headache
- EENT: lacrimation, rhinitis
- Gastrointestinal: vomiting
- Genitourinary: hematuria, priapism
- Hematologic: hemorrhage, thrombocytopenia, new thrombus formation
- Metabolic: hyperlipidemia, hyperkalemia
- Musculoskeletal: osteoporosis
- Respiratory: anaphylactoid reactions, asthma
- Skin: cutaneous necrosis, alopecia, erythema, urticaria

Interactions (other drugs)

- ACE inhibitors - Angiotensin II receptor antagonists - Antiplatelet drugs (clopidogrel, dipyridamole, ticlopidine) - Glyceryl trinitrate - NSAIDs (aspirin, diclofenac, ketorolac)

Contraindications

- Hemophilia and other bleeding disorders
- Recent cerebral hemorrhage
- Thrombocytopenia
- Peptic ulcer
- Severe liver disease
- Severe hypertension

Acceptability to patient

- Intravenous infusion requires inpatient monitoring, increasing expense and inconvenience
- Although repeated subcutaneous injections are not necessary, this benefit is offset by requirement of repeated blood draws for laboratory monitoring of anticoagulation

Follow up plan

- Frequent laboratory monitoring of aPTT, as outlined above
- Periodic laboratory monitoring of platelet levels: discontinue heparin if platelet count drops by 30% or to below 100,000/mm^3
- Clinical monitoring for complications of under-anticoagulation (thrombosis) or over-anticoagulation (hemorrhage)

Patient and caregiver information

Therapy will require inpatient care for at least 5 days until warfarin anticoagulation established.

WARFARIN

After initiation of heparin therapy, warfarin should be the treatment goal. Can treat as outpatient with LMWH used as a bridge to warfarin therapy.

Dose

- Initial oral dose of 5mg (less in patients with risk of increased sensitivity to warfarin)
- Dosing adjustments based on INR testing to achieve INR between 2.0 and 3.0
- Loading doses of warfarin are discouraged. Initial doses of 10mg are associated with early over-anticoagulation and are no more effective than 5mg initiating doses in achieving a therapeutic INR within 5 days

Efficacy

- Warfarin combined with heparin is superior to warfarin alone in reducing recurrence rates of DVT
- Warfarin–heparin initiation therapy significantly reduces mortality rates in patients presenting with DVT complicated by pulmonary embolus
- Warfarin–heparin initiation therapy is superior to heparin alone in reducing proximal extension of calf thrombosis

Risks/Benefits

Risks:

- Use caution with infection and trauma, diverticulitis, and renal and hepatic disease
- Use caution with hypertension, congestive heart failure, and tuberculosis
- Use caution with thyroid disease, diabetes mellitus, protein C deficiency, polyarteritis, and vasculitis
- Use caution in the elderly, children, and nursing mothers

Side-effects and adverse reactions

- CNS: fatigue, headache
- EENT: blurred vision
- Gastrointestinal: cramps, diarrhea, vomiting
- Genitourinary: gonadal dysfunction
- Metabolic: altered thyroid, pituitary and adrenal hormones
- Musculoskeletal: weakness
- Skin: contact dermatitis

Interactions (other drugs)

■ Acetaminophen ■ Allopurinol ■ Amiodarone ■ Aminoglutethimide ■ Aspirin (increased risk of bleeding) ■ Azathioprine ■ Barbiturates ■ Bile acid-binding resins ■ Carbamazepine ■ Cephalosporins ■ Chloramphenicol ■ Chloral hydrate ■ Clofibrate ■ Co-trimoxazole ■ Danazol ■ Dextrothyroxine ■ Disulfiram ■ Ethanol ■ Ethchlorvynol ■ Fluconazole ■ Fluorouracil ■ Gemfibrozil ■ Glutethimide ■ Griseofulvin ■ Glucagon ■ Heparin ■ Isoniazid ■ Metronidazole ■ Nalidixic acid ■ Neomycin ■ NSAIDs ■ Oral contraceptives ■ Phenytoin ■ Propafenones ■ Propoxyphene ■ Quinidines ■ Quinolones ■ Rifampin ■ Salicyclates ■ Sertraline ■ Sulfonamides ■ Sulfonylureas ■ Testosterone derivatives

Contraindications

■ Active bleeding ■ Bacterial endocarditis ■ Cerebral hemorrhage ■ Eclampsia ■ Hemorrhagic blood dyscrasias ■ Hemorrhagic tendencies ■ Hypertension ■ Pericarditis ■ Recent surgery presenting heightened risk of bleeding ■ Pregnancy and threatened abortion ■ Hypertension ■ Gastrointestinal ulceration ■ Ulcerative colitis ■ Visceral carcinoma

Acceptability to patient

- Oral dose associated with less discomfort than subcutaneous administration of LMWH
- Periodic laboratory monitoring requires infrequent blood tests
- Decreased expense compared with heparin therapy and any inpatient therapy
- Anticoagulation therapy is associated with increased risk for bleeding from occult gastrointestinal disease or from minor trauma. Patient may have to curtail physical activities that impose a risk for trauma during therapy

Follow up plan

Once therapeutic levels are established, INR should be checked at least twice a week for 2 weeks, then 1–2 times per month thereafter.

Patient and caregiver information

- Anticoagulants are associated with increased risk for bleeding. Patient or caregiver should contact primary care physician if the patient develops signs of bleeding (epistaxis, hemoptysis, blood in the stool, tarry stools) or head trauma
- Warfarin interacts with many prescription and nonprescription preparations, and may have adverse interactions with herbal and over-the-counter pharmaceutics. Dietary components high in vitamin K may decrease the effectiveness of warfarin. The primary physician should be consulted for any additions/changes in prescription, nonprescription, and herbal medications during concomitant warfarin therapy

NONSTEROIDAL ANTI-INFLAMMATORY DRUGS (NSAIDs)

In cases of superficial thrombophlebitis, anti-inflammatory agents (ibuprofen, naproxen) may be helpful in reducing swelling and discomfort.

Dose

- Ibuprofen: 200–800mg orally four times daily, not to exceed 3200mg/day. Doses >1600mg/day may be needed to achieve anti-inflammatory effects
- Naproxen: 250–500mg orally twice daily. May increase to 1.5g/day for limited periods

Efficacy

NSAIDs may be helpful in reducing swelling and discomfort.

Risks/Benefits

Risks:

- All currently available NSAIDs have unwanted effects, especially in the elderly
- Substantial individual variation in clinical response to NSAIDs
- Use caution in renal, cardiac, and hepatic impairment

Benefit: have a range of actions: anti-inflammatory, analgesic, antipyretic.

Side-effects and adverse reactions

- CNS: headache, dizziness
- EENT: tinnitus, decreased hearing
- Gastrointestinal: diarrhea, dyspepsia, nausea, vomiting, gastric bleeding and perforation
- Genitourinary: reversible renal insufficiency, renal disease (high doses over long periods)
- Respiratory: worsening of asthma
- Skin: rashes, urticaria, photosensitivity

Interactions (other drugs)

▪ Antihypertensives (ACE inhibitors, adrenergic neurone blockers, alpha-blockers, angiotensin II receptor antagonists, beta-blockers, clonidine, diazoxide, diuretics, hydralazine, methyldopa, minoxidil, nitroprusside) ▪ Antidysrhythmics (calcium channel blockers, cardiac glycosides) ▪ Antiplatelet agents (clopidogrel, ticlopidine) ▪ Aspirin ▪ Baclofen ▪ Cyclosporine ▪ Corticosteroids ▪ Heparins ▪ Ketorolac ▪ Lithium ▪ Methotrexate ▪ Moclobemide ▪ NSAIDs ▪ Nitrates ▪ Pentoxifylline (oxpentifylline) ▪ Phenindione ▪ Phenytoin ▪ Quinolones ▪ Ritonavir ▪ Sulfonylureas ▪ Tacrolimus ▪ Zidovudine

Contraindications

▪ Pregnancy and breast-feeding ▪ Coagulation defects ▪ Active peptic ulceration

Acceptability to patient

- Relatively inexpensive and readily available
- Over-the-counter preparations may not be covered by insurance
- Generally well tolerated

Follow up plan

Use should be monitored carefully in older patients and patients with renal insufficiency.

Patient and caregiver information

Therapy of superficial thrombophlebitis is primarily supportive: anti-inflammatory medications are indicated for control of discomfort and may reduce inflammation.

Surgical therapy

Deep venous thrombophlebitis: in cases of massive thrombosis or thromboembolism, recurrent thrombosis or thromboembolism on pharmacologically adequate therapy, or in patients in whom anticoagulation or thrombolytic therapy is contraindicated.

VENA CAVA PLICATION OR INFERIOR VENA CAVAL FILTER PLACEMENT

Requires a specialist. Surgical plication of the inferior vena cava or placement of a caval filter may be indicated if:

- Massive thrombosis or thromboembolism has occurred
- Recurrent thrombosis or thromboembolism occurs on pharmacologically adequate anticoagulation
- Anticoagulation therapy is contraindicated
- Patient has severe pulmonary hypertension and will not tolerate the risk of pulmonary embolism

Efficacy

Vena caval filters:

- Most are placed for prophylaxis of pulmonary embolism
- Associated with pulmonary embolism rates of 2.6–3.8% vs up to 50% in untreated patients
- 1–2% mortality rate associated with the procedure
- Do not prevent recurrent DVT (6–32% of patients)
- Inferior vena cava thrombosis occurs in 23–36%
- Appear to be effective in preventing embolism from upper-extremity deep venous thrombosis

Vena caval plication:

- Appears effective in reducing the rate of pulmonary embolism (7.6%)
- Only relatively small series studied

Risks/Benefits

Benefits (vena caval filters):

- Can be placed percutaneously and therefore can be placed under ultrasound guidance in the intensive care unit setting
- Some can be removed at a later time
- Morbidity appears lower than vena caval plication, although no direct comparisons have been made

Acceptability to patient

- Invasive and expensive
- Significant morbidity: leg swelling, recurrent DVT, inferior vena cava thrombosis
- Operative mortality rate of 1–2%

Follow up plan

Routine postsurgical follow up.

Other therapies

COMPRESSION STOCKINGS

After edema subsides following an acute episode of DVT, the patient should be measured for firm, below-knee stocking (providing 30–40mmHg pressure) to control edema that will occur during ambulation and to prevent postphlebitic sequelae of chronic venous insufficiency, such as edema, pain, stasis pigmentation, stasis dermatitis, and stasis ulceration.

Efficacy

- Reduces postphlebitic syndrome following initial episodes of DVT by over 50%
- Used in conjunction with at-home anticoagulation and early mobilization, results in faster resolution of pain and swelling without an increase in rates of pulmonary embolism

Risks/Benefits

Benefit: relatively inexpensive.

Acceptability to patient

- May be uncomfortable to wear and difficult to put on
- Requires measurement and fit specific to patient, which may be inconvenient

LIFESTYLE

To the extent that obesity and sedentary lifestyle contribute to immobilization, weight loss and maintenance of general fitness may reduce the risk of initial or recurrent DVT.

RISKS/BENEFITS

Benefit: weight loss and maintenance of general fitness carries the additional benefit of positive impacts on many other health morbidities.

ACCEPTABILITY TO PATIENT

Both weight loss and a general fitness program are extremely difficult to establish and maintain unless instituted early in life.

OUTCOMES

EFFICACY OF THERAPIES

Superficial thrombophlebitis:

- Uncomplicated superficial thrombophlebitis usually responds to therapy with clinical improvement in 7–10 days
- Outcomes in complicated (septic) superficial thrombophlebitis are related to the underlying and/or secondary morbidities, such as endocarditis

Deep venous thrombophlebitis:

- Within 3 months of institution of anticoagulant therapy, 99% of occluded veins are no longer occluded
- Symptoms persist or worsen despite this in up to one-third of patients, who then may go on to develop recurrent thrombosis or postphlebitic syndrome
- In patients with temporary increased risk of deep venous thrombosis, risk of recurrence is minimal after 3 months of therapy
- Duration of therapy for patients with hypercoagulable states is indefinite, with some authors suggesting lifelong therapy to maintain lower risk of further thromboembolic disease

Review period

6 months.

PROGNOSIS

- Superficial thrombophlebitis: most episodes resolve symptomatically within 2 weeks. Risk of recurrence is dependent on removing underlying causes, such as intravenous drug abuse or sepsis, or removal of indwelling intravenous catheters
- Deep venous thrombophlebitis: with treatment, the vast majority of cases resolve. Untreated, pulmonary embolism occurs in up to 50% of patients. Risk of recurrence persists for years after initial episode and treatment. Thromboembolic complications, including recurrent deep vein thrombosis (DVT), occur in up to 29% of patients. Up to one-third of patients will develop some form of postphlebitic syndrome

Clinical pearl(s)

- Once therapy is under way, a careful historic review for primary coagulopathy and predisposing factors is critical
- In patients without an obvious predisposing factor, arrangements must be made to assess for coagulopathy after anticoagulant therapy is completed. This is often forgotten in clinical practice

Therapeutic failure

Failure of anticoagulation and compression stockings to prevent further thrombosis or thromboembolic events should lead to consideration of referral for surgical intervention, such as vena caval filter placement, to reduce risk of pulmonary embolism.

Recurrence

- Recurrence after discontinuation of anticoagulation should lead to reinstitution of anticoagulation therapy, continuation of compression stockings, and referral to a vascular specialist. If not already done, work-up for hypercoagulable state should be performed, with referral to a coagulation specialist
- Recurrence while on therapeutic anticoagulation is an indication for referral for possible surgical intervention, such as vena caval filter placement

Deterioration

Recurrence of thrombosis, propagation of clot or the occurrence of embolization while on therapeutic anticoagulation, or the development of resistance or reaction prohibiting further use of anticoagulation should prompt referral to a specialist. Consideration should be given to lytic therapy or surgical intervention.

Terminal illness

Treatment of venous thrombosis in the terminally ill patient is directed toward comfort, supportive measures, and prevention of major complications. Late development of venous insufficiency or postphlebitic syndrome is of less concern. When the patient's condition precludes anticoagulation for proximal DVT, consideration should be given to percutaneous vena caval filter placement, a procedure that can be done at the bedside under ultrasound guidance.

COMPLICATIONS

- Postphlebitic syndrome (or post-thrombotic syndrome): develops in up to one-third of patients 6 months or more after acute deep venous thrombophlebitis
- Pulmonary embolism: occurs in up to 50% of untreated patients and about 2% of treated patients
- Paradoxical embolism: a rare complication of thromboembolism in patients with patent foramen ovale. The acutely elevated right heart pressures in the setting of a pulmonary embolus may open a previously insignificant foramen ovale
- Venous insufficiency: can occur after recurrent episodes of deep venous thrombosis
- Hemorrhagic complications of anticoagulation therapy
- Morbidity associated with surgical intervention

CONSIDER CONSULT

- If 'adequate' anticoagulation has been achieved, yet thrombosis recurs, propagates, or embolizes
- If resistance or reaction to anticoagulant drugs develops
- If hemorrhagic complications occur while on anticoagulation
- If deterioration in the patient's clinical condition occurs, such as arterial vascular compromise to the affected limb
- If surgical intervention or lytic therapy is contemplated
- Any patient with DVT who has a history of heparin-induced thrombocytopenia

PREVENTION

Prevention of thromboembolic events, regardless of which of the following clinical situations is involved, should be attempted:

- Prevention of primary events in patients at high risk, such as patients undergoing surgery or with underlying medical conditions or risk factors
- Prevention of recurrence in patients with an episode of thrombophlebitis
- Prevention of catastrophic complications during treatment of thrombophlebitis
- Prevention of postphlebitic syndrome

RISK FACTORS

- **Major surgery:** hip, knee, intra-abdominal or intrathoracic
- **Immobilization:** bed rest for more than 3 days, casting of a lower extremity, congestive heart failure, myocardial infarction, stroke
- **Hypercoagulable state:** genetic susceptibility, pregnancy, thrombocytosis
- **Malignancy:** pancreas, lungs, gastrointestinal, genitourinary, and breast
- **Indwelling venous catheters and infusions**
- **Obesity:** has been shown to increase risk of venous thromboembolism in patients on oral contraceptives
- **Smoking:** has been shown to increase risk of venous thromboembolism in patients on oral contraceptives. Data on other patients inconsistent

MODIFY RISK FACTORS

General:

- Cessation of smoking, weight loss, the use of estrogen or oral contraceptives, and sedentary lifestyle have not been shown directly to decrease risk of venous thrombophlebitis. However, there is indirect evidence that these lifestyle changes may have a positive impact on risk

Perioperative and medical risk factors:

- In patients with medical risk factors for deep venous thrombosis, specific prevention strategies have not been well explored. In patients undergoing certain types of surgery, however, at least 16 randomized controlled trials (RCTs) suggest that perioperative use of compression stockings, intraoperative use of dynamic compression hose, and/or combination therapy with compression stockings and perioperative low-dose heparin therapy significantly reduce the rate of deep venous thrombosis and other thromboembolic phenomena

Guidelines of the American College of Chest Physicians for prevention of thromboembolism include the following recommendations.

General surgery patients:

- Low-risk patient (minor procedure, under 40 years of age, no additional risk factors): early ambulation
- Moderate-risk patient (minor procedure with additional risk factors, or major operations in patients under 40 years of age with no additional risk factors): low-dose unfractionated heparin, low-molecular-weight heparin (LMWH), compression stockings, or intermittent pneumatic compression stockings
- Higher-risk patients (nonmajor surgery, over 40 years of age with additional risk factors): low-dose unfractionated heparin, LMWH, or compression stockings
- Very high-risk patients (multiple risk factors): low-dose unfractionated heparin or LMWH plus compression stockings. In selected patients, postdischarge LMWH or perioperative warfarin should be considered

Gynecologic surgery patients:

- Brief procedure, benign disease: early mobilization only
- Major surgery without additional risk factors: twice-daily low-dose unfractionated heparin, or once-daily LMWH, or intermittent pneumatic compression started just before surgery and continued several days postoperatively
- Extensive surgery for malignancy: three daily doses of low-dose unfractionated heparin alone or combined with compression stockings, or higher-dose LMWH

Urologic surgery patients:

- Transurethral or low-risk procedure: prompt ambulation only
- Major open procedures: low-dose unfractionated heparin, compression stockings, intermittent pneumatic compression, or LMWH
- High-risk patients: compression stockings plus intermittent pneumatic compression, plus low-dose unfractionated heparin or LMWH

Elective hip replacement:

- LMWH (started 12h before surgery, 12–24h after surgery or 4–6h after surgery at half the usual high-risk dose) or adjusted-dose warfarin started preoperatively or immediately after surgery
- Compression stockings might provide additional protection

Elective knee replacement:

- LMWH or adjusted-dose warfarin
- Intermittent pneumatic compression is an alternative
- Low-dose unfractionated heparin is not recommended

Hip fracture surgery:

- LMWH or adjusted-dose warfarin

Other prophylaxis issues for major surgery:

- Optimal duration of anticoagulant prophylaxis for hip or knee surgery is unknown: 7–10 days of prophylaxis is recommended
- Extended LMWH prophylaxis beyond 7–10 days, out of hospital, may reduce the incidence of thromboembolic events, and might be considered for high-risk patients
- Routine duplex ultrasound screening at the time of discharge is not recommended

Neurosurgery:

- Pneumatic intermittent compression stockings with or without elastic compression stockings
- Low-dose unfractionated heparin or postoperative LMWH can be considered
- Combination of compression stockings and anticoagulation may be more effective than either alone

Trauma:

- LMWH, starting treatment as soon as it is safe to do so
- Initial prophylaxis with a mechanical modality (compression or pneumatic intermittent compression stockings)
- In high-risk patients receiving suboptimal prophylaxis, ultrasound screening can be considered
- Inferior vena cava filter in cases where thromboembolism occurs and anticoagulation is contraindicated

Spinal cord injury:

- LMWH
- Low-dose unfractionated heparin, compression stockings, or pneumatic compression stockings are relatively ineffective and not recommended as solo therapy

- Compression stockings may have benefit when used in combination with heparin therapy
- Rehabilitation phase: LMWH or warfarin therapy

Medical conditions:
- Acute myocardial infarction: subcutaneous low-dose unfractionated heparin or intravenous heparin
- Ischemic stroke: low-dose unfractionated heparin, LMWH, or danaparoid. Elastic stockings or intermittent pneumatic compression for cases in which anticoagulation is contraindicated
- Other: low-dose unfractionated heparin or LMWH

Lifestyle and wellness

TOBACCO
- An increased risk of developing venous thromboembolism in patients who are also taking oral contraceptives has been shown
- It is likely that smoking is interrelated with other factors in affecting the risks of venous thromboembolism

DIET

High body mass index (25kg/m^2) was associated in one study with increased risk of venous thromboembolism in oral contraceptive users.

FAMILY HISTORY

A large proportion of patients with idiopathic thrombophlebitis have genetically mediated risk factors for thromboembolism.

DRUG HISTORY
- Estrogens and oral contraceptives have both been implicated as increasing risk of venous thromboembolism
- In a prospective RCT of women receiving hormonal replacement therapy (HRT) versus placebo, women on HRT were 2.8 times as likely as controls to experience venous thrombosis or pulmonary embolism

PREVENT RECURRENCE

- Anticoagulation: instituted to reduce propagation of thrombus and to prevent recurrent thrombosis and potential pulmonary embolus
- Compression stockings and mobilization: demonstrated to reduce recurrence rates of venous thrombosis

Reassess coexisting disease

Although patients with idiopathic thrombophlebitis are at increased risk for developing cancer, no investigations beyond age-appropriate screening are recommended.

INTERACTION ALERT

The American College of Preventive Medicine urges caution and consideration of alternative menopausal therapy (not hormone replacement) in patients with history of thromboembolic disease.

Administration of medications that inhibit the actions of warfarin may have a deleterious effect on reccurrence rates of thrombosis. Such medications include:
- Barbiturates
- Antibiotics, such as rifampin, nafcillin, dicloxacillin
- Sucralfate
- Vitamin K

RESOURCES

ASSOCIATIONS

Institute for Clinical Systems Improvement
Riverview Office Tower
8009 34th Avenue S, Suite 1200
Bloomington, MN 55425
Tel: (952) 814-7060
www.icsi.org

American Heart Association
National Center
7272 Greenville Avenue
Dallas, TX 75231
Tel: 1-800-AHA-USA-1
Tel: 1-800-242-8721
www.americanheart.org

American College of Chest Physicians
3300 Dundee Rd
Northbrook, IL 60062-2348
Tel: (847) 498-1400
www.chestnet.org

KEY REFERENCES

- American College of Chest Physicians Consensus Panel on Antithrombotic Therapy. In: Sixth ACCP Consensus Conference on Antithrombotic Therapy. Chest 2001;119(1 Suppl):22S–38S. Available online: http://www.guidelines.gov/
- Ascher E, Hingorani A, Tsemeklin B, et al. Lessons learned from 6-year clinical experience with superior vena cava Greenfield filters. J Vasc Surg 2000;32:881–7
- Barnt DW, Jordan SC. Anticoagulant drugs in the treatment of pulmonary embolism: a controlled trial. Lancet 1960;i1309–12
- Bernardi E, Prandoni P. The post-thrombotic syndrome. Curr Opin Pulmon Med 2000;6:335–42
- Diagnostic approach to acute venous thromboembolism: Clinical Practice Guideline. Am J Respir Crit Care Med 1999;160:1043–66
- Ebell M. Evaluation of the patient with suspected deep venous thrombosis. J Fam Pract 2001; 50:167–71
- Gould MK. Concise Review: efficacy and cost-effectiveness of low molecular weight heparins in acute deep venous thrombosis. Harrison's Online. New York: McGraw-Hill, 2001. http://www.harrisonsonline.com/
- Haenen JH, Wollersheim H, Jensen MC, et al. Evolution of deep venous thrombosis: a two-year follow up using duplex ultrasound scan and strain-gauge plethysmography. J Vasc Surg 2001;34:649–55
- Raschke RA, Reilly BM, Guidry JR, et al. The weight-based heparin dosing nomogram compared with a 'standard care' nomogram. Ann Intern Med 1993; 119:874–81
- Ridker PM, Hennekens CH, Selhub J, et al. Interrelation of hyperhomocysteinemia, factor V Leiden, and risk of future venous thromboembolism. Circulation 1997;95:1777–82
- Streiff MB. Vena caval filters: a comprehensive review. Blood 2000;45:3669–77
- Vanek VW. Meta-analysis of effectiveness of intermittent pneumatic compression devices with a comparison of thigh high to knee high sleeves. Ann Surg 1998; 64:1050–8

FAQS

Question 1

When the time comes to discontinue anticoagulation, should the medication be tapered or simply discontinued?

ANSWER 1

One randomized controlled trial has shown that there is no difference in recurrence rates when anticoagulation is abruptly discontinued vs tapered withdrawal.

Question 2

Which patients need to be admitted to hospital?

ANSWER 2

Eligible patients must first have an appropriate family and social situation allowing for frequent home nurse visits and careful observation. Eligible patients from a medical perspective include those >18 years old without evidence of pulmonary embolus, active bleeding, deep vein thrombosis (DVT), pain requiring narcotics, or other medical illness requiring hospitalization.

Question 3

How often does a fatal pulmonary embolus occur in patients after treatment begins?

ANSWER 3

In patients treated for DVT, fatal pulmonary embolus occurs in 0.4% during initial therapy and in 0.3% per 100 patient-years after anticoagulation is discontinued. The rate is higher if the initial presentation was for pulmonary embolus: 1.5% during initial therapy and 5.1% after therapy concluded.

Question 4

Who should receive a prophylactic inferior vena caval filter?

ANSWER 4

Patients who, after a first pulmonary embolus, have a high pulmonary artery pressure and in whom a second embolus would likely be fatal. Many centers are also placing filters in high-risk bedridden patients who are poor anticoagulant candidates, such as those with neurologic injury or cancer.

CONTRIBUTORS

Fred F Ferri, MD, FACP
John McB Hodgson, MD, FACC, FSCAI
Benjamin M Scirica, MD

THROMBOTIC THROMBOCYTOPENIC PURPURA

SUMMARY INFORMATION

DESCRIPTION

- A potentially life-threatening hemolytic anemia, characterized by fever, thrombocytopenia, neurologic dysfunction, mild renal dysfunction, and platelet thrombi in the microvasculature
- Clinically similar to hemolytic uremic syndrome (a disease found primarily in children, in which renal failure is more prominent)
- Pathophysiology: the precise cause is unknown. Abnormally large multimers of von Willebrand factor are found in the plasma, usually as a result of decreased activity of von Willebrand factor-cleaving protease (a metalloproteinase). Immunofluorescence studies and the presence of immunoglobulin and complement in arterioles suggest an immunologic etiology
- Treatment of choice is prompt plasmapheresis with plasma replacement

URGENT ACTION

Urgent diagnosis and treatment with plasma is necessary, since the disease is fatal in >90% of untreated patients.

KEY! DON'T MISS!

Any patient with the combination of neurologic dysfunction, thrombocytopenia, and abnormal urinary sediment should be considered a candidate for the diagnosis.

BACKGROUND

ICD9 CODE
446.6 Thrombotic thrombocytopenic purpura

SYNONYMS
- Moschcowitz disease
- TTP
- TTP-HUS

CARDINAL FEATURES
- Fever
- Microangiopathic hemolytic anemia (red blood cell fragments found in the peripheral blood, i.e. schistocytes, helmet cells, burr cells)
- Thrombocytopenia (platelet count is <100,000/mcL, and often <20,000mcL)
- Petechiae and purpura, especially on the lower extremities
- Neurologic dysfunction (including agitation, confusion, disorientation, headache, or, more ominously, coma, seizures, or focal neurologic deficits)
- Renal injury, with nephritic urinary sediment

CAUSES
Common causes
- Gastrointestinal infection with *Escherichia coli* 0157:H7 (verotoxin)
- *Shigella dysenteriae*, serotype 1
- The thienpyridine derivatives, including ticlopidine (an antiplatelet drug used to prevent stroke and coronary stent thromboses) and, less commonly, clopidogrel
- Human immunodeficiency virus (HIV) infection
- Autoimmune diseases, including systemic lupus erythematosus, antiphospholipid antibody syndrome
- Pregnancy

Rare causes
- Drugs such as bleomycin, cyclosporin A, mitomycin C, quinine, valacyclovir, and some oral contraceptives
- Solid tumors, including gastric adenocarcinoma, breast cancer, colon cancer, Kaposi's sarcoma, thymoma, small cell lung cancer
- Bone marrow transplantation

Serious causes
This disease is always serious.

EPIDEMIOLOGY
Incidence and prevalence
Fewer than 1000 cases of thrombotic thrombocytopenic purpura (TTP) are reported each year in the US. A series of about 4500 cases has been compiled by the Centers for Disease Control and Prevention, between 1970 and 1991.

INCIDENCE
0.04–0.004 per 1000. Among pregnant women, the incidence is 0.4 per 1000. Among ticlopidine users, incidence is 0.25–0.7 per 1000.

Demographics
AGE
Can affect individuals of any age.

GENDER

Women are affected 50% more often than men.

RACE

The disease affects all races equally, but some evidence suggests that African-American women have higher mortality from the illness than other patients.

GENETICS

A rare congenital form of the disorder is known, and is associated with familial deficiency of factor H, a protein that regulates complement activation.

GEOGRAPHY

The disease has no defined geographic boundaries.

SOCIOECONOMIC STATUS

TTP may affect individuals of any socioeconomic status. Highest mortality rates are among patients co-infected with HIV.

DIAGNOSIS

DIFFERENTIAL DIAGNOSIS

Sepsis

Any multisystem inflammatory response to overwhelming infection should be considered in the differential diagnosis.

FEATURES

- Fever
- Altered mental status
- Altered organ perfusion, sometimes with renal insufficiency
- Occasionally accompanied by thrombocytopenia, and renal or hepatic dysfunction
- But: usually not accompanied by hemolysis

Vasculitis

Inflammatory dysfunction of small, medium, or large blood vessels in several organs.

FEATURES

- May affect brain, kidneys, liver, colon, testes, joints, and skin
- But: usually not associated with microthrombi or hemolytic anemia

Malignant hypertension

A potentially life-threatening disorder caused by organ damage as a result of severe high blood pressure.

FEATURES

- Often causes lethargy, encephalopathy, seizures and/or myoclonic jerking
- Can produce renal failure
- But: hemolysis is uncommon; and, grade III or IV retinopathy is characteristic of malignant hypertension, not thrombotic thrombocytopenic purpura (TTP)

Autoimmune hemolytic anemias

Destruction of red blood cells by autoantibodies.

FEATURES

- Anemia
- Indirect hyperbilirubinemia
- Elevated lactate dehydrogenase
- But: Coomb's test (the direct antiglobulin test) is positive. In TTP it is negative

Idiopathic thrombocytopenic purpura (ITP)

Autoimmune destruction of circulating platelets.

FEATURES

- Thrombocytopenia
- Petechiae, especially of the lower extremities
- But: typically no evidence of multisystem disease (e.g. no renal, neurologic dysfunction; no anemia as in TTP)

Disseminated intravascular coagulation (DIC)

Systemic illness with simultaneous clotting and bleeding.

FEATURES

- Often associated with sepsis, occasionally with disseminated cancers
- Can produce widespread organ damage, including in brain and kidneys
- Thrombocytopenia is common
- Petechiae and purpura are found
- But: prothrombin time is typically prolonged; fibrinogen levels depleted. These findings are not present in TTP

Pre-eclampsia, eclampsia, and HELLP syndrome

Multiorgan dysfunction, typically in last trimester of pregnancy.

FEATURES

- Neurologic symptoms can include encephalopathy, coma, and seizures
- Elevated blood pressures common
- Renal dysfunction may include hyperalbuminemia, elevated blood urea nitrogen (BUN) and creatinine
- In HELLP syndrome, thrombocytopenia is characteristic
- May be difficult to distinguish clinically from TTP
- But: abnormalities of von Willebrand factor metalloproteinase not present

SIGNS & SYMPTOMS

Signs

- Fever greater than 100°F
- Petechiae or purpura
- Pallor, when anemia is severe
- Jaundice, when hemolysis is brisk
- Tachycardia
- Confusion or disorientation
- Delirium
- Seizures
- Evidence of mild bleeding, e.g. from gastrointestinal or genitourinary tract

Symptoms

- Weakness
- Bleeding from the urinary or gastrointestinal tract
- Pinpoint red rashes, especially around the ankles or lower legs
- Confusion, irritability, seizures
- Loss of consciousness; coma

ASSOCIATED DISORDERS

- Coronary stent placement when treated with prophylactic ticlopidine or clopidogrel
- Carotid artery stenosis, transient ischemic attacks when treated with ticlopidine or clopidogrel

KEY! DON'T MISS!

Any patient with the combination of neurologic dysfunction, thrombocytopenia, and abnormal urinary sediment should be considered a candidate for the diagnosis.

CONSIDER CONSULT

- All patients with TTP should be jointly managed with a hematologist and/or critical care specialist
- Patients should be managed with specialists in plasmapheresis/plasma exchange

INVESTIGATION OF THE PATIENT

Direct questions to patient

- Q **Is there any recent history of bloody diarrhea?** The history may suggest *E. coli* gastroenteritis
- Q **Is there any history of cancer or metastatic cancer?**
- Q **Do you have any history of HIV infection?**
- Q **Has there been any previous use of ticlopidine, chemotherapy, or oral contraceptives?** The history may suggest a drug effect
- Q **Are you pregnant?** The disease is much more common in pregnancy, especially during the peripartum period
- Q **Have you experienced any new onset of seizures or severe neurologic changes?** May suggest microinfarcts in the brain
- Q **Have you had recent coronary stenting?** A cluster of cases has been associated with the procedure, and with drug therapy to maintain stent patency (ticlopidine or clopidogrel)

Examination

- **Evidence of petechiae, especially on the lower extremities?** The finding should suggest thrombocytopenia, and prompt further evaluation
- **Abnormal mental status?** The finding should prompt standard laboratory analysis (complete blood count, chemistries, urinalysis) which may provide clues to the diagnosis

Summary of investigative tests

- Complete blood count
- Examination of peripheral blood smear
- Reticulocyte count
- Urinalysis with microscopic evaluation of urinary sediment
- Blood chemistries (BUN/creatinine)
- Direct antiglobulin test (Coombs' test)
- Lactate dehydrogenase
- Total and indirect bilirubin
- Prothrombin time
- Fibrinogen, fibrin split products, D-dimer
- Biopsy of affected organs
- von Willebrand factor (vWF)-cleaving protease – if available
- Ultra-large vWF multimers – if available

DIAGNOSTIC DECISION

The diagnosis is based on the presence of five clinical findings, some of which may be absent in individual patients:

- Fever
- Thrombocytopenia
- Neurologic dysfunction
- Renal dysfunction
- Petechiae or purpura

CLINICAL PEARL(S)

Each of the individual clinical findings not uncommonly encountered, but the combination of two or more factors, especially in the presence of confirmed thrombocytopenia, must alert the clinician to the possibility of this condition. Petechiae are an important clue to the diagnosis, and should be sought in all patients with the aforementioned clinical findings.

THE TESTS

Body fluids

COMPLETE BLOOD COUNT

Description

Assessment of hemoglobin, hematocrit and platelet counts is crucial to the diagnosis.

Advantages/Disadvantages

- Easy to obtain
- Inexpensive
- Necessary for the diagnosis, and for subsequent assessment of response to therapy

Abnormal

- Majority of patients have a hemoglobin level of less than 10g/dL
- Platelet count can range from 10,000/mcL to 100,000/mcL; most are less than 50,000/mcL
- Keep in mind the likelihood of a false-positive result: anemia and thrombocytopenia are common findings in many more common disorders

Drugs, disorders, and other factors that may alter results

- Pseudothrombocytopenia is a laboratory phenomenon that may result in the reporting of a low platelet count based on the measurement of platelet numbers by an automated counter
- Since pseudothrombocytopenia is caused by the ethylenediamine tetra-acetic acid (EDTA) anticoagulant in the tube of blood, a new blood sample must be obtained in either heparinized or citrated blood, with an automated platelet count performed
- Manual examination of the peripheral blood smear will clarify the diagnosis

EXAMINATION OF PERIPHERAL BLOOD SMEAR

Description

Microscopic evaluation of the appearance of red blood cells and platelets – essential to the diagnosis.

Advantages/Disadvantages

- Easy to obtain
- Inexpensive
- Necessary for the diagnosis, and for subsequent assessment of response to therapy
- Findings may need confirmation by hematologist

Abnormal

Assess for damaged red blood cells, including:

- Schistocytes (red cell fragments)
- Helmet cells
- Burr cells
- Keep in mind the possibility of a false-positive result. The test may be abnormal in other hemolytic anemias

Cause of abnormal result

Microangiopathic hemolytic anemia.

Drugs, disorders, and other factors that may alter results

Schistocytes may be found in patients with may other disorders, such as persons with mechanical heart valves, in whom cells may fragment during intracardiac circulation.

RETICULOCYTE COUNT

Description

- Evidence of active generation of new red blood cells by the bone marrow
- Will be present in all hemolytic anemias, including TTP

Advantages/Disadvantages

- Easy to obtain
- Inexpensive

Abnormal

- Elevated
- Keep in mind the possibility of a falsely abnormal result

Cause of abnormal result

- Keep in mind the probability of a false-positive test result; reticulocyte counts are elevated during recovery from anemia, and in most hemolytic anemias
- In TTP, reticulocytosis results from hemolytic anemia

URINALYSIS WITH MICROSCOPIC EVALUATION OF URINARY SEDIMENT

Description

Search for evidence of proteinuria, hematuria, or white blood cells.

Advantages/Disadvantages

- Easy to obtain
- Inexpensive
- Interpretation of 'active' urinary sediment may need confirmation by a nephrologist, skilled laboratory technician, or pathologist

Abnormal

The urine sediment examination will frequently reveal proteinuria, hematuria, and white blood cells, but may not reflect the severity or time course of the disease. Keep in mind the possibility of a falsely abnormal result.

Cause of abnormal result

Keep in mind the possibility of a false-positive result: nephritic urinary sediments are found in many other disorders, such as pyelonephritis and glomerulonephritis.

BLOOD CHEMISTRIES (BUN/CREATININE)

Description

Determination of serum levels.

Advantages/Disadvantages

- Easy to obtain
- Inexpensive
- Often mildly abnormal in TTP; markedly abnormal (suggesting acute renal failure) in hemolytic uremic syndrome (HUS)

Abnormal

- The BUN elevation frequently reveals evidence of mild azotemia
- Keep in mind the possibility of a falsely abnormal result

Cause of abnormal result

Keep in mind the posibility of a false-positive result; elevations of BUN and creatinine are common in any form of prerenal, intrarenal, or obstructive azotemia.

Drugs, disorders, and other factors that may alter results
- Acute or chronic renal failure
- Corticosteroids (increase BUN levels)
- Tetracyclines (increase BUN levels)
- Large patient with bulky musculature (increases serum creatinine levels)

DIRECT ANTIGLOBULIN TEST (COOMBS' TEST)
Description
Test to assess antibody binding to red blood cell membranes.

Advantages/Disadvantages
- Easy to obtain
- Inexpensive
- If positive, rules out TTP and suggests other causes of hemolytic anemia

Abnormal
The Coombs' test is a qualitative test and is usually positive or negative. If positive, further testing is done to determine the antibody causing the reaction and titration is undertaken to determine the strength. Keep in mind the possibility of a falsely abnormal result.

Drugs, disorders, and other factors that may alter results
Autoimmune hemolytic anemia, rather than TTP.

LACTATE DEHYDROGENASE
Description
Provides evidence of the release of enzymes as a result of red blood cell destruction.

Advantages/Disadvantages
- Easy to obtain
- Inexpensive
- Markedly elevated in TTP (usually >900mg/dL)
- But: is also abnormally high in other forms of hemolysis
- Is followed during management of TTP to assess effect of treatment (should decline with treatment)

Abnormal
- In TTP usually >900mg/dL
- Keep in mind the possibility of a falsely abnormal result

Cause of abnormal result
Hemolysis.

Drugs, disorders, and other factors that may alter results
- May be abnormally high in any hemolytic anemia
- Nonspecifically elevated following injury to many internal organs

TOTAL AND INDIRECT BILIRUBIN
Description
Provides further evidence of red blood cell destruction.

Advantages/Disadvantages
- Easy to obtain
- Inexpensive
- Aids evaluation of jaundice
- Is followed during disease management to assess the effect of treatment

Cause of abnormal result
Hemolysis.

Drugs, disorders, and other factors that may alter results
Elevated serum bilirubin may be found in biliary tract diseases, intrinsic diseases of the liver, and other illnesses of the liver.

PROTHROMBIN TIME
Description
- Provides evidence of coagulopathy
- Also known as Protime or 'PT'

Advantages/Disadvantages
- Easy to obtain
- Inexpensive
- Used to suggest another diagnosis. Abnormalities of coagulation are not found in TTP

Normal
Normal results, in the setting of other typical findings, support the diagnosis of TTP.

Abnormal
Keep in mind the possibility of a falsely abnormal result.

Cause of abnormal result
- Warfarin anticoagulation
- Disseminated intravascular coagulation
- Liver failure or injury
- Sepsis

Drugs, disorders, and other factors that may alter results
Warfarin and related anticoagulants.

FIBRINOGEN, FIBRIN SPLIT PRODUCTS, D-DIMER
Description
These tests are used to determine the presence of a consumptive coagulopathy, such as disseminated intravascular coagulation.

Advantages/Disadvantages
- Easy to obtain
- May require specialized laboratory assays
- Can be used to suggest another diagnosis – results should be normal in TTP

Abnormal
Keep in mind the possibility of a falsely abnormal result.

Cause of abnormal result
Disseminated intravascular coagulation.

Biopsy
BIOPSY OF AFFECTED ORGANS
Description
Tissue biopsies may reveal microthrombi in vasculature.

Advantages/Disadvantages

In general, organ biopsies are not needed to make the diagnosis of TTP, and are not obtained.

Abnormal

Skin, gingivae, and bone marrow biopsies may demonstrate the lesions, but it is difficult to find the hyaline thrombi within arterioles. Autopsy shows the characteristic lesions 50% of the time, and there are many other disorders that can produce similar findings.

Cause of abnormal result

Keep in mind the possibility of a falsely abnormal result.

Special tests

VON WILLEBRAND FACTOR-CLEAVING PROTEASE

Description

A test to determine the presence of a metalloprotein enzyme in the blood that cleaves abnormally large vWF multimers into normal, small subunits.

Advantages/Disadvantages

- Decreased function (or complete absence of activity) of vWF-cleaving protease is characteristic of TTP
- This blood test is available only in referral centers or specialized laboratories

Abnormal

Because the test is rarely performed, keep in the mind the possibility of false-positive and false-negative results.

Cause of abnormal result

Thrombotic thrombocytopenic purpura.

ULTRA-LARGE VWF MULTIMERS

Advantages/Disadvantages

- Blood specimen
- Performed only in very highly specialized laboratories

Abnormal

Keep in mind the possibility of a falsely abnormal result.

Cause of abnormal result

- TTP
- Because the test is rarely performed, keep in mind the possibility of false-positive and false-negative results

IMMEDIATE ACTION
Pending the availability of plasma exchange, fresh frozen plasma should be infused.

MANAGEMENT ISSUES
Goals
- Improvement in neurologic status
- Resolution of renal injury or renal failure
- Normalization of platelet count and hemolytic anemia
- Resolution of elevated lactate dehydrogenase levels

Management in special circumstances
Management protocols generally rely on plasma exchange and infusion, regardless of the underlying condition of the patient or any coexisting diseases. However, in patients who suffer acute renal failure as a result of thrombotic thrombocytopenic purpura (TTP), hemodialysis may be necessary.

SPECIAL PATIENT GROUPS
TTP in pregnancy is managed in standard fashion, with plasma exchange therapy. Outcomes in pregnant patients equal outcomes in other patient groups, and infants born to affected women are typically unaffected by the disease.

SUMMARY OF THERAPEUTIC OPTIONS
Choices
- Plasma exchange therapy is the first choice and is considered the standard of care
- Infusion of fresh-frozen plasma is the second choice, and somewhat less effective
- Third choice is infusion of cryoprecipitate-depleted fraction of fresh-frozen plasma (cryosupernatant). Likely to be highly effective, but more study and more experience is needed. Cryosupernatant is also used for patients refractory to plasma exchange or plasma infusion
- Combination therapy with plasma exchange and cryosupernatant may become treatment of choice in the future
- Corticosteroids are usually given, because an autoimmune mechanism may be involved in the disease, but clinical evidence for efficacy is slight
- Aspirin, dipyridamole, and other antiplatelet drugs are usually given, in an attempt to prevent platelet aggregation, but evidence of efficacy is slight
- Splenectomy is reserved for refractory cases, or for patients who relapse. Evidence for efficacy is largely anecdotal

Clinical pearl(s)
It is essential to initiate therapy as soon as possible, and infusion of fresh-frozen plasma, although less effective than plasma exchange and plasma replacement, should be started if there are anticipated delays.

FOLLOW UP
During treatment the following parameters are followed:
- Hemoglobin, hematocrit (should rise with treatment)
- Platelet count (should rise with treatment)
- Lactate dehydrogenase, indirect bilirubin (should fall with treatment)
- Blood urea nitrogen (BUN), creatinine (should fall with treatment)
- Neurologic status (should improve with treatment)

Plan for review
Affected persons are monitored closely per typical ICU protocols.

Information for patient or caregiver

Most cases of TTP resolve with approximately 1 week or 10 days of plasma exchange.

DRUGS AND OTHER THERAPIES: DETAILS

Drugs

CORTICOSTERIODS

Corticosteroids are often given because an immune mechanism is thought to be involved in the disease. Studies involving steroid therapy are difficult to evaluate as these patients usually receive combinations of interventions. Steroids have not been shown to be of benefit.

Dose

Prednisone:

- Adult: 1–2mg/kg/day orally divided in two to four doses; taper over 2 weeks as symptoms resolve
- Child: 0.05–2mg/kg/day orally; taper over 2 weeks as symptoms resolve

Efficacy

Clinical evidence for efficacy is minimal.

Risks/Benefits

- Corticosteroids can cause mood disorders in the short term, so may contribute to confusion and mental status changes
- Precautions must be taken with associated renal disease
- Overwhelming septicemia if patient has an infection
- Loss of control of blood glucose in those with diabetes
- Use caution in children and the elderly
- Use caution in AIDS, tuberculosis, amebiasis, cerebral malaria, ocular herpes simplex, and live vaccines
- Use caution in diabetes mellitus, glaucoma, hypertension, osteporosis, congestive heart failure
- Prolonged use causes adrenal suppression

Side-effects and adverse reactions

- Side-effects are minimized by short duration of therapy
- Gastrointestinal: dyspepsia, peptic ulceration, esophagitis, oral candidiasis
- Cardiovascular: hypertension, thromboembolism
- Endocrine: adrenal suppression, impaired glucose tolerance, growth suppression in children
- Musculoskeletal: proximal myopathy, osteoporosis
- CNS: insomnia, euphoria, depression, psychosis, seizures
- Skin: delayed healing, acne, striae, fragile skin
- EENT: cataract, glaucoma, blurred vision

Interactions (other drugs)

- Aminoglutethimide
- Antidiabetics
- Barbiturates
- Cholestyramine
- Clarithromycin, erythromycin, troleandomycin
- Colestipol
- Cyclosporine
- Isoniazid
- Ketoconazole
- Nonsteroidal anti-inflammatory drugs (NSAIDs)
- Oral contraceptives
- Rifampin
- Salicylates

Contraindications

- Systemic infection

Acceptability to patient

Patients are generally concerned about the long-term use of steroids due to the large number of common side-effects.

Follow up plan

Follow up for side-effects of medication, and to ensure patient compliance with dosage.

Patient and caregiver information

- Corticosteroids should not be stopped abruptly
- Take with food if there is associated gastrointestinal upset
- Inform patient of the short- and long-term side-effects

ASPIRIN AND DIPYRIDAMOLE

These and other antiplatelet drugs are usually given in an attempt to prevent platelet aggregation and/or consumption.

Studies involving antiplatelet therapy are difficult to evaluate as these patients usually receive combinations of interventions. Antiplatelet agents have not been shown to be of benefit.

Dose

- Aspirin 150–300mg daily (for other indications)
- Dipyridamole 75–100mg four times daily (for other indications)
- The doses for this disorder need to be determined by the clinical situation and should be done so in consultation with a hematologist

Efficacy

There is little evidence regarding efficacy.

Risks/Benefits

- Risk of gastrointestinal bleeding
- Aspirin can cause thrombocytopenia
- Simple dosing regimen allows for better patient compliance
- Use caution in anemia, Hodgkin's disease
- Use caution with gout, hepatic and renal disease
- Use caution with asthma, nasal polyps, nasal allergies
- Use caution with children and teenagers {Reye's syndrome}

Side-effects and adverse reactions

- EENT: hearing loss and tinnitus
- Gastrointestinal: abdominal pain, nausea, dyspepsia, hepatotoxicity
- Hematologic: bleeding disorders, thrombocytopenia
- Respiratory: hyperpnea, asthma
- Skin: angioedema, bruising, rash, urticaria
- CNS: dizziness, headache

Interactions (other drugs)

- Angiotensin-converting enzyme (ACE) inhibitors ■ Acetazolamide ■ Adenosine ■ Antacids ■ Antigout medicines ■ Beta-blockers ■ Corticosteroids ■ Diltiazem ■ Ethanol ■ Griseofulvin ■ Methotrexate ■ Oral anticoagulants ■ Warfarin

Contraindications

- Gastrointestinal bleeding ■ Bleeding disorders
- Hypersensitivity to salicylates, NSAIDs, or tartrazine

Acceptability to patient

Patients may not tolerate gastrointestinal symptoms well.

Follow up plan

Follow up to assess for gastrointestinal side-effects.

Patient and caregiver information

- Take medications with food
- Avoid alcohol ingestion
- Report any gastrointestinal side-effects

Surgical therapy

SPLENECTOMY

Removal of the spleen has been associated with disease remission in many anecdotal reports, especially for patients with refractory or relapsing disease.

Efficacy

- Proof of efficacy is not well established by controlled trials
- Often recommended by experts in the field when other therapies have failed

Risks/Benefits

- Risks of anesthesia
- Major surgery
- Infection
- Postoperative susceptibility to infection with encapsulated microorganisms

Acceptability to patient

May be sought by patients and families when other options have failed.

Follow up plan

Relapses may occur in >10% of patients, but usually respond to therapy.

Other therapies

PLASMA EXCHANGE THERAPY

- Also known as 'plasmapheresis'
- This is an intravenous treatment, by prescription only, usually performed by highly specialized hematologists
- Typical daily exchanges involve the use of 5L of fresh-frozen plasma
- Treatment course is typically 7–10 days
- Variable responses require dosing flexibility (some patients need prolonged treatment)

Efficacy

Reduces mortality rate from 90% to 10%.

Risks/Benefits

- No better options are known or proven
- Can produce volume overload or hypotension
- May cause allergic or anaphylactic reactions
- May activate complement, causing flu-like symptoms, aches, joint pains, chills, etc.
- May be complicated by adverse reactions to catheter placement (bleeding, clotting, organ damage, infections, pneumothorax, etc.)
- May dilute serum concentrations of drugs dissolved in the patient's plasma
- Inability to obtain access to the circulation

Follow up plan

Relapses may occur in >10% of patients, but usually respond to therapy.

Patient and caregiver information

Treatment is performed daily until proof of response is demonstrated.

FRESH-FROZEN PLASMA INFUSION

- A prescription-only treatment, performed by intravenous infusion
- May be performed by primary care and/or emergency medical personnel while awaiting specialty consultation
- Used as a temporizing measure, pending plasma exchange
- Dose is approximately one-third that used in plasma exchange

Efficacy

Efficacy is about half that of plasma exchange.

Risks/Benefits

- In patients with renal dysfunction, may result in volume overload
- By comparison, plasma exchange reduces the risk of volume overload
- May dilute serum concentrations of drugs dissolved in the patient's plasma

Evidence

- In a study by the Canadian apheresis group, plasma infusion alone resulted in about 40% mortality [1]

Follow up plan

Some patients of particular religious persuasions may reject therapy with plasma exchange or plasma infusion.

Patient and caregiver information

Risks, benefits, and alternatives should be described to the patient.

CRYOSUPERNATANT

- Cryoprecipitate-depleted fraction of fresh-frozen plasma (FFP). This is a prescription-only treatment
- Relatively lacking in von Willebrand factor compared with untreated FFP
- Seven or more exchanges are typically performed, usually over a week or more

Efficacy

Has improved remission and survival in patients who are refractory to previous treatment with standard plasma exchange therapy.

Risks/Benefits

- In patients with renal dysfunction, may result in volume overload
- By comparison, plasma exchange reduces the risk of volume overload
- May dilute serum concentrations of drugs dissolved in the patient's plasma

Patient and caregiver information

Risks, benefits, and alternatives should be described to the patient.

OUTCOMES

EFFICACY OF THERAPIES

Plasma exchange therapy decreases the mortality rate from 90% of affected patients with thrombotic thrombocytopenic purpura (TTP) to 10%. In studies of multiple patients, 7–10 days of therapy typically leads to cure or remission. Typical volumes of plasma infused are 45–77 liters of fresh-frozen plasma.

PROGNOSIS

- The majority of treated patients are cured
- Clinical reports from the last 20 years suggest relapse rates varying from 12% to 65%

Therapeutic failure

Infusions of cryosupernatant or splenectomy are reserved for patients who do not respond to plasma infusions or exchange.

Recurrence

Relapse is reported to occur in 12–65% of patients; average about 35%.

Deterioration

- Repeated therapy with plasma exchange or plasma infusion, or
- Cryosupernatant
- Splenectomy

Terminal illness

- Studies by the Centers for Disease Control and Prevention suggest that death caused by TTP is rising in the US despite treatment
- Some of the increased mortality may be associated with occurrence of the disease with HIV infection
- Death from TTP is relatively rare in patients younger than age 20

COMPLICATIONS

- Persistent neurologic dysfunction, in some patients
- Persistent mild renal dysfunction, in some patients
- Relapse, sometimes repeatedly

PREVENTION

Patients previously treated with drugs that have been associated with thrombotic thrombocytopenic purpura should not be treated with those agents in the future.

PREVENT RECURRENCE

Some experiential evidence suggests that splenectomy prevents disease recurrence.

RESOURCES

ASSOCIATIONS

National Organization of Rare Disorders
P.O. Box 8923
New Fairfield, CT 06812-8923
Phone: (203) 746-6518
Fax: (203) 746-6481
Toll-Free: (800) 999-6673
www.rarediseases.org/

KEY REFERENCES

- Furlan M, Robles R, Galbusera M, et al: von Willebrand factor-cleaving protease in thrombotic thrombocytopenic purpura and the hemolytic–uremic syndrome. N Engl J Med 1998;339:1578
- Gordon LI, Kwaan HC. Cancer- and drug-associated thrombotic thrombocytopenic purpura and hemolytic uremic syndrome. Semin Hematol 1997;34:140–7
- Kovacs MJ, Soong PY, Chin-Hee IH. Thrombotic thrombocytopenic purpura associated with ticlopidine. Ann Pharmacother 1993;27:1060–1
- Lara PN Jr, Coe TL, Zhou H, et al. Improved survival with plasma exchange in patients with thrombotic thrombocytopenic purpura–hemolytic uremic syndrome. Am J Med 1999;107(6):573–9

Evidence reference

1 Rock, GA, Shumak KH, Buskard NA, et al. Comparison of plasma exchange with plasma infusion in the treatment of thrombotic thrombocytopenic purpura. N Engl J Med 1991;325:393

FAQS

Question 1

What are the five clinical findings associated with thrombotic thrombocytopenic purpura?

ANSWER 1

Fever, thrombocytopenia, neurologic dysfunction, renal dysfunction, and petechiae or purpura.

Question 2

What novel blood test may help identify the presence of this clinical condition?

ANSWER 2

Identification of ULvWF ('ultra-large von Willebrand factor') multimers.

Question 3

What is the treatment of choice for this condition?

ANSWER 3

Plasmapheresis and plasma exchange.

Question 4

If access to plasmapheresis is limited, or initiation of this treatment modality is delayed, what therapeutic alternative should be considered?

ANSWER 4

Infusion of fresh-frozen plasma.

Question 5
What is the incidence of relapse?

ANSWER 5
>10% (12–65% reported in the medical literature).

CONTRIBUTORS
Gordon H Baustian, MD
Christopher P Cannon, MD
James Orford, MD

VARICOSE VEINS

SUMMARY INFORMATION

DESCRIPTION

- Dilated veins secondary to valvular insufficiency
- Location is usually the lower limbs
- Dull, aching, burning pain common at the site of varicosity
- Symptoms occur after long periods of standing and during warm weather

URGENT ACTION

- Hemorrhage from lower-extremity varicose veins can be fatal without medical intervention
- Sclerotherapy with 1% sodium tetradecyl sulfate (Sotradecol) injected proximally and distally to the site of bleeding, followed by local compression to the rupture, will ablate the vein and halt hemorrhage
- Superficial thrombophlebitis occurs in 20–50% of patients
- Occult deep vein thrombosis is three times more likely in people with varicose veins

KEY! DON'T MISS!

With varicose veins there is an increased risk of deep vein thrombosis, especially for those patients with the complication of superficial thrombophlebitis.

BACKGROUND

ICD9 CODE
454.9 Varicose veins

CARDINAL FEATURES
- Tortuous dilation of superficial veins, usually in the lower extremities
- May be asymptomatic
- Symptoms include dull, aching pain in legs that worsens upon standing and in hot weather
- Extravasation of red blood cells from the veins may result in varicose eczema
- Ulceration of the skin may occur in severe cases or when arterial disease is also present
- Treatment of varicose veins may provide temporary relief of symptoms
- New varicosities often form to replace the old ones

CAUSES
Common causes
- Congenitally absent, or otherwise incompetent, valves in perforator veins that contribute to fluid shift from deep venous system (high pressure) to superficial venous system (low pressure) following pressure gradient
- Thrombophlebitis of deep veins

Contributory or predisposing factors
- Aging
- Standing for long periods
- Pregnancy
- Obesity
- Oral contraceptive use
- Restrictive clothing

EPIDEMIOLOGY
Incidence and prevalence
- Varicose veins affect up to 60% of adults in the US
- This is the most common vascular disease

INCIDENCE
- The exact number of new cases per year has not been determined
- Incidence increases with age
- As the population ages, absolute numbers are expected to increase

Demographics
AGE
- Estimated incidence of varicose veins in the fifth decade of life is 41% for women and 24% for men
- This rises to 72% for women and 43% for men in the seventh decade

GENDER
Female to male 5:1.

GENETICS

There is a familial tendency toward varicose veins. Patients with the following have a tendency to develop varicose veins:

- Marfan's syndrome
- Ehlers–Danlos syndrome
- Distichiasis (double row of eyelashes)

SOCIOECONOMIC STATUS

Occupations that require long hours of standing may contribute to development of varicose veins.

DIFFERENTIAL DIAGNOSIS

The following diseases have similar clinical features to varicose veins.

Intermittent claudication

- Lower limb pain due to atherosclerosis narrowing the arteries
- Stenosis of the peripheral vessels leads to an inability to supply blood to the muscle

FEATURES

- Secondary to arterial disease
- Severe pain on exercise, usually in the calf
- Rest relieves the pain
- Foot pulses may be absent or diminished

Nerve root compression

Compression of the nerve roots of the vertebrae.

FEATURES

- In spinal stenosis, bilateral pain in lower extremities that is exacerbated by standing and walking, and relieved by sitting or leaning forward
- Numbness or weakness in lower extremities
- Congential narrowing of lumbar spinal canal in young patients and chronic disk degeneration and facet joint arthritis in older patients

Deep vein thrombosis

Development of thrombi in the deep veins of the lower limbs or pelvis. The main features of deep vein thrombosis are as follows.

FEATURES

- Rapid onset (over days) of pain and swelling of the lower limb
- Pain with dorsiflexion of ipsilateral foot (Homan's sign)
- Usually discoloration of lower extremity

SIGNS & SYMPTOMS

Signs

- Dilation and tortuosity of superficial veins, usually in the lower extremities
- Ulceration in severe cases
- Pigmented skin at site of varicosity indicating extravasation of red blood cells
- Palpation – shows firm, thickened, vein
- Edema can be present

Symptoms

- Most cases of early disease are asymptomatic
- Cosmetic appearance is often the reason for patients seeking medical care
- Dull aching discomfort in lower extremies
- Exacerbated with standing, restrictive clothing, and hot weather

ASSOCIATED DISORDERS

- Varicose eczema: caused by extravasation of red blood cells. Break down in the skin releasing irritants
- Ulceration: caused by poor healing of eczematous areas. Likelihood of ulceration increases if arterial disease is also present
- Deep vein thrombosis

KEY! DON'T MISS!

With varicose veins there is an increased risk of deep vein thrombosis, especially for those patients with the complication of superficial thrombophlebitis.

INVESTIGATION OF THE PATIENT

Direct questions to patient

- **Q Has there been a recent trauma?** Varicose veins that appear after trauma may be a sign of arteriovenous fistula
- **Q Do you spend many hours in a day on your feet?** Varicose veins are common in people who stand on their feet for long hours
- **Q Do you wear a girdle?** Constrictive clothing can contribute to varicose veins
- **Q Is the leg pain relieved by rest?** Pain associated with varicose veins is usually exacerbated by exercise and relieved by rest and elevation of the involved leg
- **Q Are there areas of pruritus and discoloration on the leg?** Pruritus is associated with varicose eczema and pigment changes; all are associated with varicose veins
- **Q Has there been severe swelling in the affected leg?** This is unusual in varicose veins and implies chronic venous insufficiency or deep vein thrombosis
- **Q Do you take oral contraceptives?** Use of oral contraceptives contributes to varicose veins and increases the risk of deep vein thrombosis

Contributory or predisposing factors

- Standing for long periods
- Wearing constrictive clothing
- Pregnancy

Family history

- **Q Is there a family history of varicose veins?** There may be congenital or hereditary factors in the development of varicose veins.

Examination

- **Visual inspection and palpation of veins will usually confirm the diagnosis**
- **Brodie–Trendelenburg test.** With patient supine, the involved leg is elevated to ensure venous emptying. A tourniquet is placed on the thigh below the saphenofemoral junction to block the superficial veins. The patient stands and venous filling pattern is noted. Normal: veins do not fill within 30s, and there is no rapid refilling with removal of tourniquet. If rapid refilling with removal of tourniquet occurs, suspect incompetent saphenous vein valves. If veins refill rapidly prior to removal of tourniquet, suspect incompetent valves in perforator veins
- **Examine affected extremity for signs of deep vein pathology including: edema, thrombophlebitis, stasis dermatitis, and ulceration**
- **Examine for signs of arterial insufficiency if eczema or ulceration is present.** All pulses in the lower limbs should be palpated

Summary of investigative tests

- Duplex ultrasound: gold standard for assessing venous competence, allows measurement of flow through valves and identification of sources of venous reflux
- Plethysmography: indirect measurement of venous obstruction; readily available in most settings

DIAGNOSTIC DECISION

- Diagnosis is usually clinically evident on visual inspection of tortuous, dilated veins
- Consider deep vein thrombosis if edema is present
- Consider arterial insufficiency when ulceration is present

CLINICAL PEARL(S)

- Distinguish primary varicosities due to incompetent, superficial venous valves from the more serious variety due to incompetent perforator valves or deep venous thrombosis
- Duplex scanning can determine status of deep and perforator systems
- Varicose veins are the most common vascular disorder being described as early as 1550 BC
- Hippocrates discussed their treatment at length 2500 years ago

THE TESTS

Imaging

DUPLEX ULTRASOUND

Description

Duplex ultrasound is considered the imaging method of choice for assessment of varicose veins.

Advantages/Disadvantages

Advantages:

- Venous flow can be directly visualized
- Sources of venous reflux can be identified precisely
- Noninvasive

Disadvantages:

- Expensive
- Accuracy requires experienced sonographer

Normal

In reflux studies, if sum of peak reflux in all veins is <10mL/s, likelihood of skin changes or ulceration is low.

Abnormal

- In reflux studies, if sum of peak reflux in all veins is >10mL/s, likelihood of skin changes or ulceration is high. Extent of change or ulceration cannot be predicted based on values
- Reverse flow of blood following calf muscle compression indicates incompetent vein
- Keep in mind the possibility of a false-positive result

Cause of abnormal result

Venous valvular incompetence.

PLETHYSMOGRAPHY

Description

Plethysmography measures venous obstruction by measuring emptying rate of calf veins when a proximally positioned, inflated pneumatic cuff is deflated.

Advantages/Disadvantages

- Advantages: noninvasive and widely available
- Disadvantage: does not identify anatomically the source of venous reflux

Normal

Changes in blood flow are within normal limits as measured against standard graphs.

Abnormal

- Lower-extremity venous outflow slowed
- Venous capacitance increased

Cause of abnormal result

- Valvular incompetence of vein
- Deep vein thrombosis
- False-positive result can occur

TREATMENT

IMMEDIATE ACTION

- Hemorrhage from lower-extremity varicose veins may be fatal without intervention
- Sclerotherapy with 1% sodium tetradecyl sulfate (Sotradecol) injected proximally and distally to the bleeding site followed by compression at the rupture site will ablate the vein and halt hemorrhage

PATIENT AND CAREGIVER ISSUES

Health-seeking behavior

- **Has the patient waited too long?** Women are more likely to seek early treatment for cosmetic reasons. Progressive enlargement of varicose veins may lead to superficial thrombophlebitis
- **Has the patient tried self-medication/alternative therapy?** Vascular tonics, circulatory stimulants, astringents, anti-inflammatories, and emolients may be recommended as alternative therapies and patient may prefer these to lifestyle changes of weight loss, leg elevation, and compression stockings

MANAGEMENT ISSUES

Goals

- Reduce symptoms of aching, burning, and cramping in legs
- Prevent increase in varicosities
- Prevent eczema and ulceration

Management in special circumstances

- Patients with incompetent valves of the deep and perforator veins are not candidates for vein stripping
- Patients with deep vein obstruction (thrombosis) are not candidates for vein stripping because this may worsen the venous outflow problem
- Pregnant patients should be treated with conservative measures of compression stockings, extremity elevation, and lifestyle changes. Varicose veins may spontaneously recede postpartum

COEXISTING DISEASE

Deep vein obstruction from thrombosis and deep vein insufficiency are contraindications for surgical correction of varicose veins as removal of the offending vein may worsen venous outflow problems.

SPECIAL PATIENT GROUPS

- **Pregnant women:** varicose veins commonly start in the second to third month, increasing in size until the final trimester. Sclerotherapy may be technically difficult and postoperative complications of thrombosis and embolism are serious. Since veins may spontaneously return to normal postpartum, conservative treatment with compression stockings, extremity elevation, and lifestyle changes is recommended
- **Geriatric:** cause is usually degeneration of venous valves but may be chronic venous insufficiency. Conservative therapy is usually preferred to surgical correction

PATIENT SATISFACTION/LIFESTYLE PRIORITIES

- Compliance with above-the-knee compression stockings may be low due to discomfort
- Male patients are often reluctant to wear above-the-knee compression stockings
- In jobs that require standing for long periods of time, conservative therapy that involves rest with lower extremities elevated may be difficult

SUMMARY OF THERAPEUTIC OPTIONS

Choices

- Compression stockings. Use is essential with sclerotherapy. Can also relieve aches in legs when combined with leg elevation
- Sclerotherapy. Injection of 1% to 3% solution of sodium tetradecyl sulfate, or 5% morrhuate sodium. This therapy may be used alone (usually for isolated varicosity) or to supplement surgical stripping
- Ambulatory phlebectomy. Minimally invasive stripping of the veins through narrow incisions
- Surgery. Ligation of saphenous vein or incompetent perforating veins with saphenous vein stripping is used for those who do not obtain symptomatic relief from conservative therapy
- Subfacial endoscopic perforator vein surgery (SEPS) may be useful in advanced cases due to incompetent perforator veins
- External valvular support (EVS). Recent data suggest that use of this surgical procedure renders the venous valves competent using an external constrictor and provides benefit in selected patients. It builds on chronic data showing benefit from open surgical repair of the valves
- Aescin, the active ingredient in horse-chestnut seed appears to restrict edema by reducing the transcapillary filtration of water and protein, and increasing venous tone

Clinical pearl(s)

- Most patients can be managed conservatively with leg elevation and compression stockings
- Surgical therapy with either extensive or selective lower leg stripping offers good long-term results if conservative therapy fails
- Sclerotherapy is less effective than surgery and many patients will not tolerate the required follow up protocol

FOLLOW UP

Plan for review

Follow up to assess effectiveness of conservative or surgical therapy on symptoms.

Information for patient or caregiver

- Compression stockings should be applied before rising in the morning and worn until bedtime
- Avoid long periods of standing or sitting
- Elevate legs whenever possible
- Avoid constricting clothing such as girdles
- Obese patients should be encouraged to start a weight-loss program
- Exercise after sclerotherapy will promote healing

DRUGS AND OTHER THERAPIES: DETAILS

Drugs

SODIUM TETRADECYL SULFATE FOR SCLEROTHERAPY

- Used in sclerotherapy of isolated varicose veins
- Injection into lumen of empty vein causes inflammatory reaction with eventual fibrosis and closing of the lumen

Dose

- 5–20mg (0.5–2mL) of 1% solution for small veins
- 15–60mg (0.5–2mL) of 3% solution for medium to large veins

Efficacy

- Recurrence rate of 29.5% at 3 years, 44% at 10 years
- Success of this procedure is highly dependent upon technique, use of adequate volume and concentration of sclerosant in an empty vein, and compliance with post-treatment venous compression

Risks/Benefits

Risks:

- Allergic reaction to sclerosing agent
- Pain at site
- Chronic swelling

Benefits:

- Outpatient procedure
- No anesthesia required

Side-effects and adverse reactions

- Skin: discoloration at site of injection, chronic swelling if deep vein inadvertently sclerosed, necrosis of tissue if drug extravasated, local pain secondary to inflammatory response, which can be disabling, recurrence of varicosity
- Allergic reaction to sclerosant

Interactions (other drugs)

- Incompatible with heparin

Contraindications

- Known allergy
- Underlying arterial disease
- Women taking oral contraceptives
- Persistent occlusion of deep veins
- Acute superficial thrombophlebitis
- Phlebitis migrans
- Acute cellulitis
- Patients who are bedridden

Evidence

- A systematic review found evidence from randomized controlled trials (RCTs) suggesting that the type of sclerosant, local pressure dressing, and degree and length of compression have no bearing on the efficacy of sclerotherapy in the treatment of varicose veins [1] *Level M*
- An RCT compared sclerotherapy, surgical ligation, and both treatments together in patients with varicose veins and pure, superficial venous incompetence. At 10 years, venous incompetence was present in no patients treated with surgical ligation at the saphenofemoral junction, compared with 18% of patients treated with sclerotherapy. Venous incompetence in the distal venous system was significantly more frequent after sclerotherapy (43.8%) than after combination treatment (16.1%). 36% of patients treated with surgery alone had incompetence of the lower venous system [2] *Level P*

Acceptability to patient

- Outpatient procedure
- May be painful
- Usually needs to be repeated
- Requires compression stockings

Follow up plan

- Assessment for local reaction, extravasation
- Assessment for recurrence of varicosity

Patient and caregiver information

- Sclerotherapy will most likely need to be repeated
- Varicose veins may recur and require further therapy
- Compression stockings required after treatment
- Treatment will not prevent future formation of varicose veins

MORRHUATE SODIUM

- Used in sclerotherapy of isolated varicose veins
- When injected into empty vein, causes inflammation of vein lining and formation of thrombus. Thrombus occludes vein and fibrous tissue forms to obliterate vein

Dose

- 50–100mg (1–2mL of 5% injection) for small to medium veins
- 150–200mg (3–5mL of 5% injection) for larger veins
- Therapy can be repeated every 5–7 days

Efficacy

- Not a permanent treatment but a successful adjunct to venous ligation when used to obliterate remaining varicose veins
- Conflicting evidence exists, with some studies reporting nearly 100% failure and others reporting degrees of success nearing 90%. Success in this procedure is highly dependent upon the practitioner, the amount and concentration of sclerosant used, injection into an empty vein, and adequate post-treatment compression

Risks/Benefits

Risks:

- Allergic reaction
- Local phlebitis

Benefits:

- Outpatient procedure
- No anesthesia required

Side-effects and adverse reactions

- CNS: headache, drowsiness
- Skin: local reactions of burning, cramping, or urticaria, necrosis of tissue if extravasated
- Allergic reaction

Interactions (other drugs)

- No known drug interactions

Contraindications

- Patients who have a known hypersensitivity to the drug or fatty acids of cod liver oil
- Patients with deep vein occlusions
- Acute superficial thrombophlebitis
- Underlying arterial disease
- Varicosities caused by abdominal and pelvic tumors
- Bedridden patients

Acceptability to patient

- Outpatient procedure that may need to be repeated
- Pain at injection site
- Requires compression stockings post-treatment

Follow up plan

Assess for:

- Tissue damage from extravasation
- Infection at site
- Compliance with compression stockings

Patient and caregiver information

- Procedure may need to be repeated
- Need for compliance with compression stockings post-treatment

Surgical therapy

- Indicated in patients with poor results from conservative therapy
- Careful evaluation of venous flow essential prior to surgery
- Contraindicated in patients with deep vein obstruction
- Conservative therapy with compression stockings and elevation preferred in elderly and pregnant patients

AMBULATORY PHLEBECTOMY

- Removal of varicose veins through small punctures made in the skin
- Requires local anesthesia
- Scarring is minimal

Efficacy

- Generally effective but risk of recurrence
- Overall success requires an experienced operator

Risks/Benefits

Risks:

- Bleeding
- Hematoma
- Lymphocele
- Sensory nerve damage
- Chronic foot edema

Benefits:

- Performed as an outpatient procedure
- Requires only local anesthesia
- Small puncture wounds leave little, if any, scar

Acceptability to patient

Outpatient procedure, requires only local anesthesia.

Follow up plan

Follow up to:

- Ensure compliance with postoperative compression stockings
- Evaluate for infection
- Evaluate for recurrent varicose veins

Patient and caregiver information

- Need to wear compression stockings and elevate legs after surgery
- Surgery does not prevent new varicose veins from forming

VEIN STRIPPING

- Removal of varicose veins in operating room through multiple incisions
- Requires general, spinal, or epidural anesthesia

Efficacy

- Good to excellent result in 95% of patients at 5 years
- Good to excellent result in 85% of patients at 10 years
- Key to efficacy is adequate removal

Risks/Benefits
Risks:
- Infection
- Damage to saphenous nerve resulting in neuritis (occurs in one-third of patients)
- Bleeding
- Hematoma
- Lymphocele
- Chronic foot damage

Benefits:
- Complete removal of varicosity leads to low recurrence rates
- Relief of leg pain
- Improved cosmetic appearance
- Prevention of complications of venous stasis including changes in pigmentation, eczema, and ulcers

Acceptability to patient
- Requires hospitalization
- Requires that support stockings be worn for at least 14 days postoperatively when ambulating

Follow up plan
Assessment for postoperative:
- Infection
- Compliance with compression stockings
- Complications of nerve damage

Patient and caregiver information
Surgery does not prevent development of new varicosities.

Complementary therapy
HORSE-CHESTNUT SEED
Efficacy
Appears to restrict edema by reducing the transcapillary filtration of water and protein, and increasing venous tone. An oral dose of 50mg aescin (the active ingredient in horse-chestnut) twice daily gave results equivalent to compression stockings for varicose vein relief.

Risks/Benefits
- Prolongation of prothrombin time is seen with horse-chestnut bark, but not seed
- Horse-chestnut is generally well tolerated with no known toxicities or side-effects
- There have been rare reports of nausea and an isolated case of renal toxicity

Acceptability to patient
Well accepted.

Follow up plan
Standard patient care.

Endoscopic therapy
SUBFACIAL ENDOSCOPIC PERFORATOR VEIN SURGERY
Subfacial endoscopic perforator vein surgery (SEPS) is a new, minimally invasive, technique for patients with advanced venous insufficiency complicated by stasis changes or venous ulcers.

Efficacy

North American registry data show reduced wound infection and more rapid ulcer healing than with traditional surgery.

Other therapies

COMPRESSION STOCKINGS

Efficacy

- Essential adjunct in sclerotherapy. Compression stocking minimizes the size of thrombus formed in vein, and decreases resorption time and the chances of superficial thrombophlebitis occurring
- Combined with leg elevation, it may relieve symptoms of aches in legs for patients unable or unwilling to undergo sclerotherapy or surgical removal
- Aids in healing of venous ulcers

Risks/Benefits

Risk: pain in foot with elevation of leg.

Benefits:

- Decrease in aches and heaviness experienced in affected leg
- After sclerotherapy, decrease in size of thrombus formed with decreased chance of superficial thrombophlebitis

Evidence

A systematic review found that compression was more effective than no compression for the healing of venous leg ulcers [3] *Level M*

Acceptability to patient

- Uncomfortable in warmer climates
- Elderly may have difficulty applying stockings

Follow up plan

- Assess compliance
- Assess fit of stockings

Patient and caregiver information

- Foot cramping may occur with leg elevation, awakening the patient. Pain is relieved by standing
- Compression stocking should be applied before getting out of bed in the morning and worn until bedtime unless otherwise instructed
- Compression stockings should be ordered from a medical supply house that is familiar with fitting them to be assured of correct pressure

LIFESTYLE

Weight loss is recommended to reduce the pressure on lower extremities.

RISKS/BENEFITS

Risk:

- Inadequate nutrition leading to vitamin and mineral deficiencies

Benefits:

- Decreased pressure on lower extremities
- Increased energy
- Increased mobility: ambulation after sclerotherapy promotes healing and stimulates venous return
- Increased self-esteem and confidence

ACCEPTABILITY TO PATIENT

- Difficult to change patterns of eating
- May be difficult to make the connection between weight loss and varicose veins

FOLLOW UP PLAN

Assess for dietary and exercise compliance.

PATIENT AND CAREGIVER INFORMATION

- Increased mobility will assist in healing after sclerotherapy
- Daily walking will assist in venous return

OUTCOMES

EFFICACY OF THERAPIES

- Use of compression stockings and leg elevation should provide relief from symptoms of leg pain and feelings of heaviness in most cases of varicose veins
- Good cosmetic results are obtained with sclerotherapy and vein stripping. Most patients undergoing sclerotherapy and vein stripping will notice a decrease in vein prominence in a few days when post-treatment edema subsides
- The rate of recurrence after treatment is variable

Evidence

- A systematic review found evidence from randomized controlled trials (RCTs) suggesting that the type of sclerosant, local pressure dressing, and degree and length of compression have no bearing on the efficacy of sclerotherapy in the treatment of varicose veins [1] *Level M*
- Sclerotherapy was found to be less effective than a combination of surgical ligation plus sclerotherapy in patients with varicose veins and pure, superficial venous incompetence in one RCT [2] *Level P*
- A systematic review found that compression was more effective than no compression for the healing of venous leg ulcers [3] *Level M*

Review period

- For conservative therapy, review periodically to determine compliance with compression stockings and lifestyle changes
- After sclerotherapy, review periodically to assess efficacy of treatment
- After vein stripping, review periodically to assess venous flow in affected extremity

PROGNOSIS

Varicose veins are usually a chronic condition because treatment does not prevent formation of new varicosities. Lifestyle changes such as weight loss and avoidance of restrictive clothing may help, but this condition remains chronic.

Clinical pearl(s)

- Optimal therapy involves a combined approach with aggressive conservative therapy and appropriately timed surgery
- For conservative treatment failures, combined vein stripping and selective sclerotherapy offers the best long-term chance of success

Therapeutic failure

Failure of conservative therapy or sclerotherapy may lead to surgical referral for vein stripping.

Recurrence

Recurrence of varicose veins after sclerotherapy may lead to surgical referral for vein stripping.

COMPLICATIONS

- Progression of untreated varicose veins may lead to disabling pain
- If venous stasis develops, eczema and varicose ulceration may occur
- With skin ulceration, infection may occur

CONSIDER CONSULT

Surgical referral:

- When conservative measures fail (compression stockings and leg elevation, weight loss, and avoidance of constrictive clothing)
- For cosmetic reasons
- For recurrent superficial thrombophlebitis

PREVENTION

- Keep moving if standing for long periods of time
- Wear compression stockings

RISK FACTORS

- Obesity: puts individuals at risk for varicose veins due to increase in lower-extremity venous pressure
- Activity level: standing or sitting for long periods of time causes venous stasis and increased venous pressure
- Family history: there are indications that varicose veins may have a genetic basis

MODIFY RISK FACTORS

Lifestyle and wellness

DIET

Maintaining ideal weight based on body mass index will help ensure that lower-extremity venous pressure stays within normal limits and that there is no extra stress placed on the veins.

PHYSICAL ACTIVITY

- Maintaining an active lifestyle will ensure that venous return from the lower extremities is brisk, avoiding venous stasis and increased venous pressure that may lead to varicose veins
- Avoiding standing or sitting for long periods of time may also help prevent varicose veins

FAMILY HISTORY

Varicose veins are known to be familial, and thought possibly to have a genetic basis for inheritance, although this has not yet been proven.

PREVENT RECURRENCE

Recurrence of varicose veins after conservative therapy and/or sclerosis therapy varies considerably. Significant recurrence usually occurs within 2 years of original therapy.

ASSOCIATIONS

American College of Phlebology Headquarters
100 Webster Street Suite 101
Oakland, CA 94607-3724
Tel: (510) 834-6500
Fax: (510) 832-7300
http://www.phlebology.org

American Society for Dermatologic Surgery
930 N. Meacham Road
Schaumburg, IL 60173-6016
Tel: (847) 330-9830
Fax: (847) 330-1135
http://www.asds-net.org

KEY REFERENCES

- Brewster DC. Management of peripheral venous disease. In: Goroll AH, May LA, Mulley AG, eds. Primary care medicine. Office evaluation and management of the adult patient. Philadelphia: Lippincott-Raven, 1995, p207–8
- Feied C. Peripheral venous disease. In: Rosen P, Barken R, Danzl DF, et al, eds. Emergency medicine: concepts and clinical practice. St. Louis: Mosby, 1998, p1870–1
- Guidelines of care for sclerotherapy treatment of varicose and telangiectatic leg veins. J Am Acad Dermatol 1996;34(3):523-8
- Little N. Special neurologic problems. In: Rosen P, Barken R, Danzl DF, et al, eds. Emergency medicine: concepts and clinical practice. St. Louis: Mosby, 1999, p2212
- Flye MW. Venous disorders. In: Sabiston DC, Lylerly HK, eds. Textbook of surgery. The biological basis of modern surgical practice, 15th edn. Philadelphia: WB Saunders, 1997, p1581–92
- Braunwald E. Inherited disorders of the circulation. In: Braunwald E, ed. Heart disease: a textbook of cardiovascular medicine, 5th edn. Philadelphia: WB Saunders, 1997, p1677
- Coleman WP. New directions in surgical therapy. Dermatol Clin 1998;16:2;253–9
- Varicose veins: techniques allow outpatient treatment. Mayo Clinic Health Letter, May 1998. Available: http://www.mayohealth.org July 9, 2000
- Weis RA (1998) Radio-frequency endovenous occlusion. Closure technique. Phlebology primer. Available: http://www.phlebology.org July 9, 2000
- McEvoy GK, et al, eds. Sodium tetradecyl sulfate. In: American Hospital Formulary Service Drug Information, 1995, p1269–70
- McEvoy GK et al, eds. Morrhuate sodium. American Hospital Formulary Service Drug Information. Drug information, 1995, p1268–9
- Compression therapy for venous leg ulcers. Drug Ther Bull 2000;38:23–31

Evidence references

1 Tisi PV, Beverley CA. Injection sclerotherapy for varicose veins (Cochrane Review). In: The Cochrane Library, Issue 2, 2002. Oxford: Update Software

2 Belcaro G, Nicolaides AN, Ricci A, et al. Endovascular sclerotherapy, surgery, and surgery plus sclerotherapy in superficial venous incompetence: a randomized 10-year follow-up trial – final results. Angiology 2000;51:529–34. Medline

3 Cullum N, Nelson EA, Fletcher AW, Sheldon TA. Compression for venous leg ulcers (Cochrane Review). In: The Cochrane Library, Issue 2, 2002. Oxford: Update Software

FAQS

Question 1

When should I consider referring a patient for definitive therapy for varicose veins?

ANSWER 1

Referral is indicated after failure of conservative management, for extremely painful varicosities, or for cosmesis.

Question 2

Do all patients with varicose veins need diagnostic tests for confirmation?

ANSWER 2

Not all patients will require tests as outlined in this chapter. Testing should be considered in those patients who are being considered for surgical or sclerotherapy, since incompetence in the perforator or deep vein valves may affect the type of intervention being considered.

Question 3

What conservative measures should be employed in initial management of varicose veins?

ANSWER 3

Initial conservative management involves:

- Limitation of time on feet (elevation of legs allows for draining of pooled venous blood)
- Support stockings (increases venous return to deep system)
- Exercise (lower-extremity muscle tone enhances venous return)
- Weight loss (decreased weight improves fitness and improves venous return)

CONTRIBUTORS

Randolph L Pearson, MD
Jane L Murray, MD
John McB Hodgson, MD, FACC, FSCAI
David A Morrow, MD

VENTRICULAR TACHYCARDIA AND VENTRICULAR FIBRILLATION

SUMMARY INFORMATION

DESCRIPTION

Ventricular tachycardia:

- Most frequently encountered life-threatening arrhythmia, defined as a series of three or more ventricular complexes occurring at a rate of 100–250 beats/min
- Coronary artery disease with myocardial infarction is the most common structural heart disease predisposing to ventricular tachycardia
- Typical symptoms include palpitations, breathlessness, light-headedness, angina, syncope, and cardiac arrest. However, asymptomatic ventricular tachycardia can also occur
- Untreated ventricular tachycardia may degenerate to ventricular fibrillation, resulting in hemodynamic collapse and death
- Sustained ventricular tachycardia (lasting >30s) is life-threatening and requires activation of advanced cardiac life support

Ventricular fibrillation:

- Result of rapid, chaotic, repetitive activation of the ventricles from multiple coalescing and fractionating wave fronts of depolarization
- Associated with disorganized mechanical contraction, hemodynamic failure, and sudden death
- Electrocardiogram reveals irregular and rapid oscillations (250–400 beats/min) of highly variable amplitude without obvious QRS complexes or T waves

URGENT ACTION

Ventricular tachycardia:

- Treatment with immediate synchronized direct-current (DC) cardioversion for sustained ventricular tachycardia with hemodynamic compromise, severe heart failure, or ongoing ischemia or infarction
- Pharmacologic cardioversion with intravenous lidocaine or amiodarone may be attempted in the patient with hemodynamically stable ventricular tachycardia who is under close cardiac monitoring
- Cardiopulmonary resuscitation should begin if there is no pulse
- Initiate advanced cardiac life support
- Immediate transfer to hospital

Ventricular fibrillation:

- Initiate advanced cardiac life support; cardiopulmonary resuscitation and immediate unsynchronized defibrillation is the primary therapy
- Immediate transfer to hospital

KEY! DON'T MISS!

- Ventricular tachycardia can be asymptomatic, particularly when rate of the tachycardia is relatively slow, and baseline hemodynamic function is well preserved
- Hemodynamic stability does not mean that a wide complex tachycardia is supraventricular in origin. Ventricular tachycardia may also be quite hemodynamically stable, but may rapidly deteriorate

ICD9 CODE
427.1 Ventricular tachycardia
427.41 Ventricular fibrillation

SYNONYMS
- Pulseless ventricular tachycardia (ventricular fibrillation)
- Cardiac arrest
- Sudden cardiac death

CARDINAL FEATURES
Ventricular tachycardia:
- Series of three or more ventricular complexes occurring at a rate of 100–250 beats/min, where the origin of activity is within the ventricle
- Wide QRS (usually >120ms), with T-wave polarity opposite that of the major QRS deflection
- Absence of an RS complex in all precordial leads during electrocardiogram (ECG)
- RS interval >100ms in any precordial lead on ECG
- Coronary artery disease with myocardial infarction is the most common structural heart disease predisposing to ventricular tachycardia
- Typical symptoms include palpitations, breathlessness, light-headedness, angina, syncope, and cardiac arrest. However, asymptomatic ventricular tachycardia can also occur
- Untreated ventricular tachycardia may degenerate to ventricular fibrillation, resulting in hemodynamic collapse and death
- Sustained ventricular tachycardia (lasting >30s) is life-threatening and requires activation of advanced cardiac life support and transfer to hospital
- Treatment with immediate synchronized direct-current (DC) cardioversion is the indicated therapy if able to initiate advanced cardiac life support in patients with hemodynamic compromise, severe heart failure, ongoing ischemia, or infarction

Ventricular fibrillation:
- Result of rapid, repetitive activation of the ventricles from multiple coalescing and fractionating wave fronts of depolarization
- Associated with disorganized mechanical contraction, hemodynamic failure, and sudden death
- ECG reveals irregular and rapid oscillations (250–400 beats/min) of highly variable amplitude without obvious QRS complexes or T waves
- Primary therapy is cardiopulmonary resuscitation and immediate defibrillation

CAUSES
Common causes
- Coronary artery disease with myocardial infarction
- Nonischemic cardiomyopathies
- Infiltrative diseases
- Infectious diseases (viral myocarditis, Chagas disease, Lyme disease)
- Congenital myocardial defects (tetralogy of Fallot, pulmonary stenosis)
- Inflammatory diseases that affect the myocardium (systemic lupus erythematosus, rheumatoid arthritis)
- Carbon monoxide poisoning
- Digitalis toxicity (commonly bidirectional ventricular tachycardia)
- Mitral valve prolapse
- Torsade de pointes
- Marfan's syndrome with aortic dissection

- Electrolyte abnormalities (notably of potassium and magnesium)
- Structural, toxic, or metabolic derangement affecting the homogeneity of ventricular repolarization (prolonged QT syndrome)

Contributory or predisposing factors

- Primary and metastatic malignancies that involve the heart muscle
- In the newborn, associated with QT prolongation and Marfan's syndrome
- Surgical repair of congenital heart defect
- Cocaine use
- Alcoholic 'holiday heart'
- Ischemia
- Drugs (quinidine, phenothiazines, tricyclic antidepressants)

EPIDEMIOLOGY

Incidence and prevalence

PREVALENCE

- Nonsustained ventricular tachycardia detected by 24-h ambulatory ECG in older, disease-free people without cardiovascular disease: 2–4%
- Older patients with pre-existing cardiovascular disease: 4–16%
- Ventricular tachycardia and fibrillation is most common within 72h of suffering a myocardial infarction

Demographics

AGE

Prevalence increases with age.

GENETICS

Genetic predisposition for patients with pre-existing cardiomyopathies and prolonged QT syndrome.

SOCIOECONOMIC STATUS

Homes with insufficient ventilation and furnaces in poor condition may contribute to carbon monoxide poisoning, which may cause ventricular tachycardia.

DIFFERENTIAL DIAGNOSIS

Supraventricular tachycardia with aberration

Arrhythmic condition that can present as wide-complex tachycardias owing to rate-dependent aberration of conduction (right or left bundle branch block) or a fixed intraventricular conduction defect.

FEATURES

- No atrioventricular dissociation
- Capture or fusion beats absent
- RS complex present in precordial leads
- RS interval shorter than 100ms in any precordial lead

SIGNS & SYMPTOMS

Signs

Wide complex tachycardia on electrocardiogram (ECG).

Symptoms

- Palpitations
- Breathlessness
- Light-headedness
- Angina
- Syncope
- Loss of consciousness (ventricular fibrillation)
- Note that ventricular tachycardia can be asymptomatic

KEY! DON'T MISS!

- Ventricular tachycardia can be asymptomatic, particularly when rate of the tachycardia is relatively slow, and baseline hemodynamic function is well preserved
- Hemodynamic stability does not mean that a wide complex tachycardia is supraventricular in origin. Ventricular tachycardia may also be quite hemodynamically stable, but may rapidly deteriorate

CONSIDER CONSULT

- Always activate emergency medical system to facilitate transfer to hospital and to begin basic or advanced cardiac life support
- All patients with sustained ventricular tachycardia or ventricular fibrillation should be transferred immediately to hospital and cardiac life support should be initiated immediately
- If ventricular tachycardia is intermittent and not associated with obvious hemodynamic compromise, refer immediately to hospital for evaluation and treatment by cardiologist
- If ventricular tachycardia is sustained and/or associated with hemodynamic compromise, begin cardiopulmonary resuscitation, perform cardioversion/defibrillation if available, and then refer immediately to hospital for continuing emergency management and for evaluation and treatment by a cardiologist

INVESTIGATION OF THE PATIENT

Direct questions to patient

Q What are your symptoms? Typical symptoms in a conscious patient include shortness of breath, palpitations, and light-headedness; some patients can be asymptomatic

Q How long have you been feeling this discomfort? Not typical to have extended periods of tachycardic discomfort as it tends to be episodic

- Q **Have you taken any medication to treat the discomfort? What did you use?** If patient is taking digitalis for heart problems, he/she may have overdosed and triggered a ventricular tachycardia episode
- Q **Have you ever had angina or a heart attack?** Coronary artery disease with myocardial infarction is the most common structural heart disease predisposing to ventricular tachycardia
- Q **Do you have any other heart problems?** Nonischemic cardiomyopathies (either dilated or hypertrophic), congenital myocardial defects, mitral valve prolapse, and torsade de pointes can all predispose to the development of ventricular tachycardia; a previous cardiac arrest is also a risk factor

Contributory or predisposing factors

- Q **Is the patient a heavy drinker of alcohol? If not, has he/she been drinking heavily just prior to start of symptoms?** Alcoholic 'holiday heart' can contribute to ventricular tachycardia
- Q **Is the patient a cocaine user?** This can contribute to ventricular tachycardia
- Q **Does the patient take digitalis?** Ventricular tachycardia may be a sign of digitalis toxicity, e.g. bidirectional ventricular tachycardia. However, patients taking digoxin (for inotropic support) have an underlying cardiomyopathy. The underlying cardiomyopathy is the structural heart disease that predisposes the patient to ventricular tachycardia
- Q **Does the patient have systemic lupus erythematosus, rheumatoid arthritis, or Lyme disease?** All of these conditions can cause cardiovascular complications with ventricular tachycardia. These diseases may lead to cardiomyopathy, which predisposes to ventricular tachycardia
- Q **Does the patient live in a house with an old furnace?** Carbon monoxide poisoning may present with ventricular tachycardia. This is a rare cause of ventricular tachycardia
- Q **Does the patient have Marfan's syndrome?** A cardiac complication of this condition is aortic dissection, which can present as ventricular tachycardia. This is a rare presentation of ventricular tachycardia, unless associated with dissection into a coronary artery or associated with hemodynamic collapse/arrest

Family history

- Q **Do other family members have heart conditions?** There is a genetic component to pre-existing cardiomyopathies and prolonged QT syndrome.

Examination

- **Is there a pulse?** If patient is pulseless, begin cardiopulmonary resuscitation and defibrillate immediately
- **Is the patient hemodynamically stable?** If stable, transfer immediately to hospital
- **Examine the neck if the patient is hemodynamically stable.** Ventricular tachycardia will produce cannon a-waves on jugular venous pulsations caused by atrioventricular asynchrony (right atrium contracting against closed tricuspid valve)
- **Monitor blood pressure.** Ventricular tachycardia will produce a variable blood pressure caused by atrioventricular asynchrony
- **On examination of ECG, is the rhythm ventricular tachycardia?** Patient could be experiencing supraventricular tachycardia with aberrant conduction

Summary of investigative tests

- Definitive test for confirmation of ventricular tachycardia and fibrillation is an ECG. The ECG is critical in determining appropriate acute and chronic therapeutic approach
- If patient is not experiencing ventricular tachycardia or ventricular fibrillation at time of evaluation, but has experienced this in the past, ECG evaluation (using a Holter monitor) with exercise may be indicated

DIAGNOSTIC DECISION

- ECG can make definitive diagnosis of ventricular tachycardia and ventricular fibrillation
- Once patient has been successfully treated for ventricular tachycardia or ventricular fibrillation, a search for the underlying cause using other investigative tests is warranted
- Search for coronary artery disease by cardiac catheterization and evaluation by electrophysiologic testing
- Echocardiography is key to determining the overall systolic function
- If ischemia, medicines, and prolonged QT are excluded, patient should undergo electrophysiologic testing to find a potential focus of the arrhythmia

CLINICAL PEARL(S)

- If patient has a history of myocardial infarction, the chance that a wide-complex tachycardia is ventricular tachycardia is >90%
- Polymorphic ventricular tachycardia is more likely to have ischemic origins
- Monomorphic ventricular tachycardia is more likely to have a fixed lesion (myocardial infarction) as the source of arrhythmia
- Ventricular tachycardia can occur in a patient with a stable blood pressure. The presence of hemodynamic stability does not infer supraventricular tachycardia with aberrant conduction

THE TESTS

Tests of function

ELECTROCARDIOGRAM

Description

- Typical ECG performed in primary care physician's office may be sufficient for diagnosing patients
- ECG using a Holter monitor (with exercise) may be indicated for patients with suspected asymptomatic ventricular tachycardia
- If patient is pulseless, cardiopulmonary resuscitation and cardioversion take priority over performance of ECG

Advantages/Disadvantages

Advantages:

- Does not require referral and is quick, easy, and inexpensive
- Results of standard ECG available immediately
- Often diagnostic

Disadvantages:

- Holter-monitored ECG may be time-consuming and patient may be resistant to wearing the monitoring equipment for 24-h period
- In the patient with intermittent ventricular tachycardia, dysrhythmia may not be detected

Abnormal

Ventricular tachycardia:

- Three or more ventricular complexes occurring at a rate of 100–250 beats/min (origin of activation is within ventricle)
- Wide QRS (usually >120ms)
- T-wave polarity is opposite to that of the major QRS deflection
- Monomorphic ventricular tachycardia has a single QRS morphology throughout the arrhythmia; polymorphic ventricular tachycardia has an ever-changing QRS morphology

Ventricular fibrillation:

- Irregular and rapid oscillations (250–400 beats/min) of highly variable amplitude
- No uniquely identifiable QRS complexes
- No uniquely identifiable T waves

Cause of abnormal result

- Ventricular tachycardia
- Ventricular fibrillation
- Supraventricular tachycardia with aberrant conduction

Drugs, disorders, and other factors that may alter results

- Digitalis toxicity (commonly bidirectional ventricular tachycardia, with two ventricular foci alternating in bigeminal pattern)
- Incorrect application of monitor pads

IMMEDIATE ACTION

Ventricular tachycardia:

- Treatment with immediate synchronized direct-current (DC) cardioversion for sustained ventricular tachycardia with hemodynamic compromise, severe heart failurc, or ongoing ischemia or infarction
- Pharmacologic cardioversion with intravenous lidocaine or amiodarone may be attempted in the patient with hemodynamically stable ventricular tachycardia who is under close cardiac monitoring
- Cardiopulmonary resuscitation (CPR) should begin if there is no pulse
- Initiate advanced cardiac life support
- Immediate transfer to hospital

Ventricular fibrillation:

- Initiate advanced cardiac life support; CPR and immediate unsynchronized defibrillation
- Immediate transfer to hospital

PATIENT AND CAREGIVER ISSUES

Forensic and legal issues

- If patient is received at office of primary care physician (PCP) in pulseless condition, physician will need to treat the patient without consent
- If patient arrives disoriented or with severe angina or syncope, physician may be required to initiate treatment without consent

Impact on career, dependants, family, friends

- Dependants and family members must be made aware of life-threatening nature of condition and should be prepared to act accordingly (conversations with caregivers regarding wills, 'do not resuscitate' orders, and terminal care may be necessary)
- Patients prone to ventricular tachycardia and fibrillation may require intermittent emergency treatment of their condition, with frequent trips to the PCP or emergency room
- Patients may require in-home care if their condition worsens or changes over time

Patient or caregiver request

- **I've heard that drinking too much coffee or caffeine-rich soda will make this worse; is that so?** No. Caffeine ingestion does not increase number or severity of episodes of ventricular tachycardia
- **Does taking aspirin help prevent additional episodes of this kind of heart problem? What about taking aspirin when I'm having an attack?** Preventive treatment with aspirin will not reduce number of tachycardic episodes, nor is aspirin indicated during acute phase of a tachycardic event

Health-seeking behavior

Are you currently taking medication to control your heart disease? Patient should maintain their treatment regimen for pre-existing disease, but PCP should be made aware of any changes to cardiologist's recommended therapeutic plan and cardiologist should be made aware of any incidents reported while patient visits PCP's office.

MANAGEMENT ISSUES

Goals

Without immediate action, ventricular tachycardia can degenerate to ventricular fibrillation and lead to sudden death. Goals are:

- To stabilize a hemodynamically unstable patient and transfer them immediately to hospital
- To stop ventricular tachycardia
- To begin CPR if patient is pulseless

Management in special circumstances

COEXISTING DISEASE

Concomitant illnesses commonly seen with this condition should not have any impact on treatment of sustained ventricular tachycardia with hemodynamic compromise.

COEXISTING MEDICATION

- Concomitant medications commonly used to treat coexisting heart conditions may have an impact on treatment of sustained ventricular tachycardia with hemodynamic compromise
- If patients are currently receiving drugs to treat fluid balance problems or affiliated heart conditions, consideration should be used when designing the medication program after the tachycardic event is stabilized

SPECIAL PATIENT GROUPS

- All patients, no matter their age group, race, possible disability, or possibility of pregnancy, should be treated when the physician diagnoses ventricular tachycardia
- Only exception to this rule is the patient with a terminal illness who has provided the physician with instructions not to perform any life-saving activities if found to be in a potentially life-threatening condition

SUMMARY OF THERAPEUTIC OPTIONS

Choices

Ventricular tachycardia:

- First choice for sustained ventricular tachycardia is immediate synchronized DC cardioversion
- Second choice for hemodynamically unstable ventricular tachycardia is amiodarone and cardioversion, and third choice is lidocaine and cardioversion
- If hemodynamically stable, first choice is pharmacologic cardioversion with intravenous amiodarone and second choice is intravenous lidocaine. Third choice is electrical cardioversion
- Bretylium is still acceptable but is no longer recommended due to a high incidence of side-effects, especially hypotension after resuscitation, and its availability is uncertain
- Magnesium sulfate is given if the patient has hypomagnesemia
- Recurrent sustained ventricular tachycardia should be managed with continuous infusion of an effective antiarrhythmic (e.g. amiodarone, lidocaine, procainamide)

Ventricular fibrillation:

- A cascade of actions is typically required (listed in order of action)
- Confirm airway, breathing, and circulation ('ABC'). If needed, perform CPR until defibrillator is attached. Confirm ventricular fibrillation
- Defibrillate – do not delay until intravenous access can be established
- If fibrillation persists after cardioversion, continue CPR, intubate, and establish intravenous access
- Start treatment with a vasopressor – epinephrine or vasopressin. If vasopressin is used, do not give epinephrine for 10min
- If still in ventricular fibrillation, shock again within 30–60s of first shock whether or not pharmacologic therapy has been started
- If ventricular fibrillation is still present at this point, consider commencing intravenous amiodarone or lidocaine
- After successful defibrillation, continuous intravenous infusion of the successful antiarrhythmic therapy (amiodarone or lidocaine) should be maintained until patient is stabilized
- Primary ventricular fibrillation occurring within first 72h after an acute myocardial infarction usually does not require antiarrhythmic therapy
- Ventricular fibrillation without an identifiable cause requires electrophysiologic testing and possible chronic therapy with either prophylactic antiarrhythmic drugs (amiodarone, sotalol) or implantation of an automatic defibrillator (performed by a specialist)

Never

Do not give epinephrine within 10min of vasopressin therapy.

FOLLOW UP

Once patient is stabilized and is receiving appropriate treatment for the arrhythmia, an attempt to determine true cause of the tachycardic event is indicated.

Plan for review

- The patient needs to be referred to cardiologist for treatment
- Monitor medications prescribed to determine possible drug interactions with other treatments patient is receiving; query patient regarding any unexpected side-effects or difficulties with treatment regimen
- If antiarrhythmia medications appear to lose effectiveness, contact cardiologist for consult regarding treatment changes
- If patient has an indwelling defibrillator, monitor condition of skin around insertion site and query patient regarding possible problems with the device
- Patient with a history of ventricular tachycardia or ventricular fibrillation has come very close to dying; PCP must build a strong relationship with such patients since many factors can increase their predisposition to recurrent ventricular tachycardia or ventricular fibrillation (e.g. use of beta-adrenergic agonists or over-the-counter cough and cold medications, weight loss or gain, electrolyte abnormalities)
- Monitor electrolytes, especially if patient is on diuretic therapy
- Monitor symptoms of ischemia and congestive heart failure, as ventricular arrhythmias occur when these underlying conditions are decompensated

Information for patient or caregiver

- Patient should receive information regarding possible side-effects or drug interactions (antiarrhythmics and alcohol; antiarrhythmics and other medications)
- Patient should receive information about the implanted defibrillator, including what effects would warrant a visit to PCP vs cardiologist
- If patient is in high-risk category for possible future tachycardic or fibrillation events and sudden death, physician should discuss need for 'do not resuscitate' orders or other decisions regarding future treatment options

DRUGS AND OTHER THERAPIES: DETAILS

Drugs

AMIODARONE

- Prolongs action potential duration and effective refractory period
- Produces noncompetitive alpha- and beta-adrenergic inhibition

Dose

- Unstable ventricular tachycardia or ventricular fibrillation: 300mg over 3min by slow intravenous push
- Stable ventricular tachycardia: intravenous loading dose of 150mg intravenously over 10min, followed by infusion at 1mg/min for 6h, then 0.5mg/min
- Repeat 150mg bolus doses may be given if arrhythmia recurs
- If loading dose is given orally, give 200mg three times a day for 1 week, then 200mg twice a day for 1 week, followed by maintenance dose of 200mg once daily

Efficacy

- Effective in treating life-threatening ventricular dysarrhythmias and ventricular fibrillation/pulseless ventricular tachycardia

- Recommended after defibrillation and vasopressors in cardiac arrest with persistent ventricular tachycardia or ventricular fibrillation
- Effective for controlling hemodynamically stable ventricular tachycardia, polymorphic ventricular tachycardia, and wide-complex tachycardia of uncertain origin

Risks/benefits

Risks:

- Long-term therapy is associated with many side-effects
- Should be used only by physicians with access to all methods of treating and monitoring arrhythmias
- Treatment should be initiated in a hospital
- Use caution with thyroid and pulmonary disease
- Use caution with atrioventricular block and bradycardia
- Use caution in electrolyte imbalances
- Owing to the hazards associated with this drug, a decision should be made in each case in regard to whether an implantable defibrillator might be a preferable alternative

Benefits:

- Rapid-acting antiarrhythmic
- Effective in decreasing risk of recurrence
- Preferable to other antiarrhythmics for treatment of ventricular arrhythmias

Side-effects and adverse reactions

- Hypotension with fast infusion
- Prolonged QT
- Long-term use is associated with altered thyroid function, pulmonary fibrosis, hepatitis, corneal microdeposits, peripheral neuropathy and myopathy
- Cardiovascular: congestive heart failure, hypotension, sinoatrial node dysfunction, bradycardia, conduction abnormalities, dysrhythmias
- CNS: headache, ataxia, dizziness, fatigue, tremors, paresthesia, peripheral neuropathy
- EENT: visual disturbances, photophobia, dry eyes
- Gastrointestinal: nausea, vomiting, abdominal pains, constipation, diarrhea, hepatotoxicity, taste abnormalities
- Metabolic: altered thyroid function
- Musculoskeletal: weakness
- Respiratory: cough, dyspnea, pulmonary fibrosis
- Skin: contact dermatitis, rashes, itching, angioedema

Interactions (other drugs)

▪ Antiretroviral protease inhibitors ▪ Antiarrhythmics (flecainide, digoxin, dofetilide, procainamide, quinidine, beta-blockers, calcium-channel blockers) ▪ Cevimeline ▪ Cholestyramine ▪ Cisapride ▪ Cyclosporine ▪ Dextromethorphan ▪ Fentanyl ▪ Fosphenytoin ▪ Gatifloxacin, grepafloxacin, moxifloxacin, sparfloxacin ▪ Inhalation anesthetics ▪ Irbesartan ▪ Phenothiazines ▪ Phenytoin ▪ Pimozide ▪ Sirolimus ▪ Tramadol ▪ Tricyclic antidepressants ▪ Warfarin

Contraindications

▪ Atrioventricular block ▪ Hypotension ▪ Hypersensitivity ▪ Pregnancy ▪ Severe sinus node disease with bradycardia ▪ Syncope

Acceptability to patient

Patients may have some problems with side-effects/adverse reactions.

Follow up plan

- In the acute setting, the patient requires continuous electrocardiogram (ECG) monitoring
- Monitor electrolyte levels, liver and thyroid function every 6 months
- Monitor for CNS symptoms
- Question the patient for any drug side-effects

Patient and caregiver information

- If amiodarone is used for long-term prophylactic therapy the patient must be made aware of the side-effects and be encouraged to see their doctor for regular follow up every 6 months
- Most patients taking long-term amiodarone develop corneal microdeposits which may affect night vision. Patients should see their doctor if they develop visual problems such as difficulty driving at night
- Amiodarone contains iodine and can affect thyroid function. Regular blood tests to check thyroid function are required
- Amiodarone can lead to changes in the lungs such as pulmonary fibrosis, pnuemonitis, and alveolitis. Patient should see their doctor if they develop progressive shortness of breath or a persistent cough
- Amiodarone can affect liver function. Patient should see their doctor if they develop jaundice or a tender abdomen
- Amiodarone may lead to myopathy and neuropathy. The patient should see their doctor if they develop any neurologic symptoms such as numbness, tingling, or persistent muscle aches

EPINEPHRINE

- Stimulates alpha-, $beta_1$- and $beta_2$-adrenergic receptors
- Effects on vasculature are dose dependent: small doses produce vasodilation and large doses produce vasoconstriction
- Use in ventricular tachycardia or ventricular fibrillation is an off-label indication

Dose

- For ventricular fibrillation or pulseless ventricular tachycardia give initial dose of 1.0mg by intravenous bolus
- May be repeated every 3–5min
- Can increase dose if no response, choosing between the following regimens: intermediate dose of 2–5mg intravenous bolus; escalating 1 to 3 to 5mg intravenous bolus; or 0.1mg/kg as an intravenous bolus
- Epinephrine may be given intravenously, or via an endotracheal tube if no intravenous access is established

Efficacy

When ventricular fibrillation persists without documented interruption by electric countershock, administration of epinephrine may increase peripheral vasoconstriction, thereby increasing critical organ perfusion and facilitating a subsequent defibrillation attempt.

Risks/benefits

Risks:

- Excessive activity from epinephrine can cause other life-threatening cardiac reactions (tachydysrhythmia, hypertension, myocardial ischemia, stunned heart syndrome)
- Use caution in the elderly
- Use caution in patients who are breast-feeding
- Use caution in cardiovascular disease, hypertension
- Use caution in thyrotoxicosis and hyperthyroidism
- Effects on vasculature are dose dependent

Benefit: may be life saving.

Side-effects and adverse reactions

- Cardiovascular: hypertension, palpitations, myocardial ischemia, myocardial infarction, tachydysrhythmia
- CNS: headache, tremor, subarachnoid hemorrhage (in overdosage), anxiety, dizziness, cold extremities
- Gastrointestinal: nausea and vomiting

Interactions (other drugs)

▪ Alpha$_2$-adrenoceptor stimulants ▪ Antidepressants (monoamine oxidase inhibitors [MAOIs] and tricyclics) ▪ Antipsychotics ▪ Beta-blockers ▪ Doxapram ▪ Oxytocin

Contraindications

▪ Local anesthesia of fingers and toes ▪ General anesthesia with halogenated hydrocarbons or cyclopane ▪ Labor ▪ Cardiac dysrhythmias ▪ Coronary insufficiency ▪ Angle-closure glaucoma ▪ Organic brain damage

Acceptability to patient

With implied or definitive patient consent in an emergency situation, patient comfort and side-effects are not a concern in a situation of cardiac resuscitation.

Follow up plan

- Patient needs continuous monitoring of ECG, blood pressure, and heart rate
- Examine fundi for evidence of increased intracranial pressure, after patient is stabilized

LIDOCAINE

- Decreases depolarization, automaticity, and excitability in the ventricles during diastolic phase without involvement of autonomic system
- Despite its long history of use, it is now considered a second-line treatment after amiodarone for acute events

Dose

- In hemodynamically stable ventricular tachycardia, 1.0–1.5mg/kg intravenously as an initial bolus
- In ventricular fibrillation and pulseless ventricular tachycardia, if arrhythmia continues after cardioversion and vasopressors, 1.0–1.5mg/kg intravenously as an initial bolus
- 0.5–0.75mg/kg can be given as an additional bolus for refractory arrhythmias
- If effective, consider a continuous infusion at 1–4mg/min. If arrhythmia reappears, a small bolus (0.5mg/kg) may be given, together with an increase in the infusion rate (up to 4mg/min)
- Reduce dose in elderly patients and in those with liver impairment (usual bolus dose followed by half the maintenance infusion dose)

Efficacy

Considered a second-line treatment after amiodarone for ventricular tachycardia and fibrillation.

Risks/benefits

Risks:

- Use caution in children and the elderly
- Use caution in inflammation, sepsis, and shock
- Use caution in severe liver disease, cardiac conditions, or respiratory impairment
- Use caution in methemoglobinemia

Benefits:

- May be life saving
- Rapid acting (immediate onset of effect with intravenous dose administration)
- Lidocaine is easier to administer than amiodarone but is less effective
- Lidocaine has fewer short-term side-effects but has no proven short- or long-term efficacy in cardiac arrest

Side-effects and adverse reactions

- Cardiovascular: dysrhythmias, cardiac depression, changes in blood pressure, bradycardia
- CNS: convulsions, confusion, respiratory depression
- Gastrointestinal: nausea, vomiting
- Respiratory: respiratory depression
- Skin: hypersensitivity reactions, burning, stinging, urticaria
- True allergy is rare – may see local skin reaction

Interactions (other drugs)

- Antiarrhythmics
- Cimetidine
- Diuretics
- Propranolol
- Suxamethonium

Contraindications

- Ophthalmic use
- Heart block
- Septicemia
- Spinal anesthesia
- Do not use in the ear
- True lidocaine allergy

Acceptability to patient

May save the patient's life.

Follow up plan

- Continuous ECG and blood pressure monitoring during infusion
- Check for signs of toxicity (muscle twitching, seizures, change in mentation, bradycardia)
- Monitor blood levels

Patient and caregiver information

As drug is administered intravenously in the office or hospital setting, there are no issues with regard to dose administration or long-term side-effects.

PROCAINAMIDE

- Acts to decrease myocardial excitability, contractility, conduction velocity, and increases threshold potential of ventricle
- Not the first-line agent for ventricular tachycardia or fibrillation

Dose

- For ventricular tachycardia give in intravenous increments of 20mg/min until arrhythmia is controlled, hypotension occurs, QRS complex is prolonged by 50% from its original duration, or a total dose of 17mg/kg has been administered
- If effective, may follow with a maintenance intravenous infusion of 2mg/min (range 1–4mg/min)

Efficacy

Effective in treating life-threatening ventricular dysarrhythmias.

Risks/benefits

Risks:

- Use caution in tartrazine or sulfide sensitivity
- Use caution in myasthenia gravis, dental disease
- Use caution in patients who are breast-feeding
- Use caution in renal dysfunction or hepatic impairment
- Use caution in history of idiopathic systemic lupus erythematosus
- Use caution in congestive heart failure and following myocardial infarction
- Need to infuse procainamide slowly to avoid significant hypotension. This side-effect limits its use in truly life-threatening arrhythmias

Benefits:

- May be life saving
- Rapid acting

Side-effects and adverse reactions

- Gastrointestinal: nausea, diarrhea, vomiting, abdominal pain, bitter taste
- Cardiovascular: myocardial depression, heart failure, hypotension, ventricular arrhythmias, second-degree heart block, PR and QT prolongation, torsade de pointes, angioedema
- Hematologic: neutropenia, agranulocytosis, bone marrow depression, agranulocytosis, thrombocytopenia
- CNS: dizziness, confusion, psychosis, headache, hallucinations
- Lupus erythematosus-like syndrome with prolonged therapy

Interactions (other drugs)

- Amiodarone ■ Antiarrhythmics ■ Antidepressants (tricyclic) ■ Antihypertensives ■ Captopril ■ Cimetidine ■ Ethanol ■ Muscle relaxants ■ Neostigmine ■ Ofloxacin ■ Phenothiazines ■ Pimozide ■ Pyridostigmine ■ Sotalol ■ Thioridazine ■ Trimethoprim

Contraindications

- Ejection fraction <45% ■ Prolonged QT ■ Heart block ■ Hypotenison ■ Digitalis toxicity ■ Torsade de pointes ■ Pre-existing cytopenia or bone marrow depression ■ Intramuscular injections

Acceptability to patient

Usually high as it may be life saving.

Follow up plan

- ECG should be monitored continuously during administration for evidence of overdose (widening of QRS complex or QT prolongation)
- Blood pressure must be monitored continuously during administration since procainamide can cause significant hypotension
- Blood levels should be monitored in patients with significant renal impairment and those receiving a constant infusion of >3mg/min for longer than 24h

Patient and caregiver information

As drug is administered intravenously in the office or hospital setting, there are no issues with regard to dose administration or long-term side-effects.

VASOPRESSIN

- Reacts with V1 receptors in peripheral arteries to stimulate vasoconstriction
- Useful alternative to epinephrine, especially after prolonged resuscitation
- This is an off-label indication

Dose

Seek specialist advice.

Efficacy

When ventricular fibrillation persists without documented interruption by electric countershock, administration of vasopressin promotes peripheral vasoconstriction, thereby improving critical organ perfusion during CPR.

Risks/benefits

Risks:

- Use caution in thyroid, cardiac, vascular, or renal disease
- Use caution in epilepsy, migraine, asthma, or polyuria
- Use caution in the elderly and children
- Use caution in pregnancy and breast-feeding
- Can cause water intoxication

Benefits:

- May be life saving
- Rapid clinical effect

Side-effects and adverse reactions

- Gastrointestinal: nausea, vomiting, abdominal pain, diarrhea, flatulence
- Genitourinary: uterine contractions
- Cardiovascular: hypertension, sinus bradycardia, myocardial infarction, angina, dysrhythmias, atrioventricular block
- CNS: headache, dizziness, confusion, flushing, tremor
- Skin: sweating, pallor, urticaria, injection site reaction
- Metabolic: hyponatremia

Interactions (other drugs)

- Antidepressants (tricyclic) ▪ Carbamazepine ▪ Chlorpropamide ▪ Clofibrate ▪ Epinephrine ▪ Ethanol ▪ Fludrocortisone ▪ Heparin ▪ Lithium ▪ Morphine

Contraindications

- Peripheral vascular disease ▪ Chronic nephritis ▪ Coronary artery disease

Acceptability to patient

Usually highly acceptable due to the life-threatening arrythmia.

Follow up plan

Monitor blood pressure and heart rate.

Patient and caregiver information

As drug is administered intravenously in the office or hospital setting, there are no issues with regard to dose administration or long-term side-effects.

SOTALOL

- Nonselective beta-blocker
- Blocks cardiac muscle receptors along with bronchial and vascular receptors, inhibiting chronotropic, inotropic, and vasodilator responses to beta-adrenergic stimulation

Dose

- Initial oral dose of 80mg orally twice a day; can be increased to 240–320mg/day, adjusting dose every 2–3 days
- Some patients may require up to 480–640mg/day

Efficacy

- May prevent recurrent ventricular tachycardia and fibrillation – especially useful as adjunctive therapy in patients with a defibrillator
- Some data suggest that there is uncertain efficacy in treating ventricular tachycardia and fibrillation with sotalol and that it should be avoided
- Other data suggest that sotalol may be effective. Use of sotalol is controversial but may still be indicated in certain patient populations (e.g. those with existing defibrillators)

Risks/benefits

Risks:

- Do not withdraw sotalol treatment abruptly
- Use caution in hyperthyroidism, renal impairment
- Use caution in electrolyte imabalance
- Use caution in vasospastic angina and pheochromocytoma
- Use caution in surgery
- Negative inotropic effect may worsen heart failure
- Proarrhythmic, especially where QT interval prolonged and/or potassium level low; risk of torsade de pointes
- May aggravate obstructive airways disease
- Can mask hypoglycemic symptoms – important for patients with diabetes
- Peripheral vascular disease symptoms may be aggravated

Benefits:

- May be life saving
- No pharmacokinetic drug–drug interactions
- Entirely renally excreted

Side-effects and adverse reactions

- Gastrointestinal: nausea, vomiting, diarrhea, constipation
- Cardiovascular: beta-blockers must not be withdrawn suddenly in coronary heart disease – may precipitate myocardial infarction; sinus bradycardia, angina, palpitations, QT prolongation, proarrhythmic events, torsade de pointes, peripheral vasoconstriction
- CNS: fatigue, dizziness, sleep disturbances
- Respiratory: dyspnea, bronchospasm
- Metabolic: hyperglycemia
- Skin: rashes, exacerbation of psoriasis
- Hematologic: blood cell dyscrasias

Interactions (other drugs)

■ Alpha-blockers and agonists ■ Antacids ■ Antiarrhythmics (amiodarone, adenosine, disopyramide, procainamide, quinidine, dofeltilide, lidocaine, flecainide ■ Antidepressants (tricyclic and possibly MAOIs) ■ Astemizole ■ Calcium channel blockers ■ Cevimeline ■ Cimetidine ■ Cisapride ■ Clarithromycin, erythromycin, and fluoroquinolones ■ Clonidine ■ Cocaine ■ Digoxin ■ Diuretics ■ Hypoglycemic agents ■ Insulin ■ Liothyronine ■ Neostigmine, physostigmine ■ Neuroleptics ■ Nonsteroidal anti-inflammatory drugs ■ Phenothiazines ■ Pimozide ■ Reserpine ■ Tacrine ■ Terbutaline ■ Terfenadine ■ Theophylline

Contraindications

■ **Sinus bradycardia** ■ **Sick sinus syndrome** ■ **Second- or third-degree atrioventricular block** ■ **QT prolongation syndromes** ■ **Heart failure** ■ **Hypokalemia** ■ **Cardiogenic shock** ■ **Bronchospastic disorders and asthma** ■ **Raynaud's disease or peripheral vascular disease**

Acceptability to patient

Usually high due to the life-threatening nature of the condition.

Follow up plan

- Provide ongoing cardiac monitoring
- Adjust dose according to response

MAGNESIUM SULFATE

- Affects smooth and skeletal muscle contractility, increases membrane potential, prolongs atrioventricular conduction, and increases absolute refractory period. These effects result in a 'cardioprotective' environment for the myocardium
- May be useful in specific situations, e.g. torsade de pointes or severe hypomagnesemia
- Off-label indication

Dose

- Seek specialist advice for dosage
- May use: intravenous infusion of 1–2g over 60s
- Constant infusion of 0.5–1g/h recommended if the magnesium successfully treats the dysrhythmia

Efficacy

Beneficial in the treatment of intractable ventricular tachycardia and fibrillation.

Risks/benefits

Risks:

- Parenteral magnesium therapy may cause abnormally high levels of magnesium in the plasma, which may lead to respiratory depression. (A preparation of calcium, such as the gluconate or gluceptate, should be at hand for intravenous administration as an antidote)
- Administer with caution if flushing and sweating occurs
- When barbiturates, narcotics, or other hypnotics (or systemic anesthetics) are to be given in conjunction with magnesium, their dosage should be adjusted with caution because of additive CNS depressant effects of magnesium
- Use caution in patients with serious impairment of renal function

Benefits:

- Very fast action (almost instantaneous)
- Duration of action is 30min

Side-effects and adverse reactions

- Cardiovascular: hypotension, circulatory collapse, and cardiac and CNS depression
- CNS: flushing, sweating
- Respiratory: respiratory depression (most life-threatening effect)

Interactions (other drugs)

■ **Barbiturates (additive CNS depressant effects of magnesium)** ■ **Narcotics (additive CNS depressant effects of magnesium)** ■ **Hypnotics (additive CNS depressant effects of magnesium)** ■ **Calcium (may antagonize effects of magnesium)**

Contraindications

- Magnesium sulfate should not be administered parenterally in patients with heart block or myocardial infaction ▪ Pregnancy category C ▪ Breast-feeding ▪ Safety and efficacy in children have not been established

Acceptability to patient

Usually highly acceptable due to the life-threatening risks of the condition.

Follow up plan

- Monitor for possible drug interactions while patient is receiving magnesium
- Check levels

Patient and caregiver information

As drug is administered intravenously in the office or hospital setting, there are no issues with regard to dose administration or long-term side-effects.

Other therapies

DIRECT-CURRENT CARDIOVERSION – SYNCHRONIZED

- Transthoracic application of a brief current pulse synchronized in time to the QRS complex
- Indicated for stable ventricular tachycardia, supraventricular tachycardia, and stable wide complex tachycardia of unclear etiology
- For stable ventricular tachycardia, initial cardioversion with 50J may be used, after the patient is sedated
- For unstable wide complex tachycardia, initial cardioversion with 200J is performed. Subsequently, 300J then 360J may be delivered. If further cardioversion is needed, 360J should be delivered as per Advanced Cardiac Life Support (ACLS) protocol

Efficacy

For stable ventricular tachycardia, supraventricular tachycardia, or stable wide complex tachycardia of unclear etiology, synchronized DC cardioversion is successful in restoring sinus rhythm in >90% of patients with recent-onset ventricular tachycardia.

Risks/benefits

Risks:

- May trigger ventricular fibrillation
- Painful and distressing to awake patients – if patient is hemodynamically stable and awake, intravenous sedation may be administered prior to cardioversion of ventricular tachycardia

Benefits:

- Life-saving procedure
- Can be performed in the PCP's office as part of advanced cardiac life support for hemodynamically unstable patients

Acceptability to patient

Highly acceptable as it is a life-saving procedure.

Follow up plan

Patient will immediately be transferred to hospital for continued medical care.

Patient and caregiver information

Reassure patient and caregiver that cardioversion has stabilized the heart condition, but that ongoing monitoring is required in hospital.

DEFIBRILLATION

- Therapeutic process of choice if patient is in unresponsive ventricular fibrillation (use unsynchronized shock) or pulseless ventricular tachycardia (use synchronized shock)
- Defibrillation with 200J is performed initially. Subsequent defibrillations are with 300J then 360J. If further defibrillations are necessary, 360J are utilized, as per ACLS protocol

Efficacy

Effective in terminating ventricular fibrillation.

Risks/benefits

Benefits:

- Life-saving procedure
- Can be performed in PCP's office as part of ACLS for hemodynamically unstable patients

Follow up plan

Following resuscitation and defibrillation to stabilize the patient in ventricular fibrillation, patient should be referred immediately to hospital for evaluation by cardiologist.

Patient and caregiver information

Reassure patient and caregiver that defibrillation has stabilized the heart condition, but that the patient needs to be monitored in hospital for evaluation of further treatment needs.

OUTCOMES

EFFICACY OF THERAPIES

- Both ventricular tachycardia and fibrillation carry a high mortality; only 16% of patients with an out-of-hospital sudden cardiac arrest survive to discharge
- An initial rhythm of ventricular fibrillation predicts a worse survival than ventricular tachycardia, probably because it signifies a longer period of pulselessness

Review period

- Once patient is released from hospital and returns to primary physician's care, evaluation of treatment efficacy and monitoring of possible drug side-effects should be performed on a routine basis with regular scheduled return visits
- Electrolytes should be monitored, especially in patients given diuretic therapy
- The primary care physician should monitor the patient for symptoms of coronary artery disease or decompensated congestive heart failure

PROGNOSIS

- Inhospital risk of recurrent cardiac arrest is relatively low and arrhythmias account for only 10% of inhospital deaths after successful prehospital resuscitation. However, overall mortality during hospitalization is 50%
- Long-term prognosis post-hospitalization (with medical or surgical treatment) is high, with 95% of patients still alive at 5 years. However, this value decreases with increasing severity of patients' underlying conditions (multiple vessel disease, history of heart failure)

Clinical pearl(s)

- In a patient with previous myocardial infarction, treat a wide complex tachycardia as ventricular tachycardia until proven otherwise
- In a hemodynamically stable patient, sedation should be given prior to cardioversion
- In a hemodynamically unstable patient, emergent cardioversion should be performed
- All patients with ventricular tachycardia and ventricular fibrillation require immediate transfer to a hospital and referral to an electrophysiologist
- Chances of successful resuscitation decrease dramatically when ventricular tachycardia deteriorates to ventricular fibrillation

Recurrence

- Among survivors of out-of-hospital cardiac arrest not associated with acute myocardial infarction, risk of recurrent arrest is 30% at 1 year and 45% at 2 years after initial incident, with high mortality associated with recurrence
- Patients with recurrent ventricular tachycardia or ventricular fibrillation may require surgical implantation of an automatic cardioverter–defibrillator device which monitors patient's heart rhythm for possible arrhythmic events. If an event occurs, a defibrillation is triggered to try to overdrive pace of ventricular tachycardia, thereby breaking arrhythmia circuit
- Recurrent ventricular tachycardia and fibrillation refractory to therapy should prompt transplant evaluation if suitable

Terminal illness

- Recurrent ventricular tachycardia and fibrillation refractory to therapy should prompt plans for palliative care
- Any new treatments may be palliative in nature, reducing any pain patient is experiencing or stabilizing severe cardiac complications

COMPLICATIONS

- Patients with history of ventricular tachycardia and fibrillation may be prone (with medication being used to treat these conditions) to drug–drug interactions and fluid-balance complications (owing to diuretics)
- Psychologic complications, with depression and fear of death are most common
- Some patients with indwelling defibrillators experience psychologic stress regarding their need for the device; in addition, the firing of an internal defibrillator may be a traumatic experience for patients

CONSIDER CONSULT

- Referral to a defibrillator support group for problems adjusting to having an indwelling defibrillator device
- Referral to hospice care and support may be indicated if patient's illness is terminal

PREVENTION

MODIFY RISK FACTORS

Lifestyle and wellness

TOBACCO

- Patients at risk of general coronary artery disease should discontinue use of tobacco products, including cigarettes, cigars, pipes, and chewing tobacco
- Smoking is a major risk factor for developing heart disease, which is a major cause of ventricular tachycardia and ventricular fibrillation

ALCOHOL AND DRUGS

- Patients at risk for sudden cardiac death should reduce alcohol consumption and avoid recreational drug use
- Heavy alcohol consumption can cause cardiomyopathy which is a risk factor for ventricular tachycardia and ventricular fibrillation
- One glass of wine (especially red) or beer every day reduces the risk of coronary artery disease

DIET

Patients at risk for sudden cardiac death should modify their diets to reduce fat and red meat, and increase fruit, vegetables, and fish.

PHYSICAL ACTIVITY

Patients at risk for coronary artery disease should maintain regular physical activity programs with an emphasis on cardiovascular exercise.

FAMILY HISTORY

- Patients with a family history of sudden cardiac death and coronary artery disease are at risk and should take lifestyle preventive measures
- Diseases that contribute to heart disease, including hyperlipidemia, hypertension, diabetes, and others, are familial

DRUG HISTORY

- Drugs that can interfere with antiarrhythmic medications should be substituted with those that do not cause reactions
- Patients taking over-the-counter or alternative medications should inform their primary care physician to ensure they are not using something contraindicated for their underlying cardiovascular condition

SCREENING

ELECTROCARDIOGRAM

- Evaluation of patients at possible risk due to family history or other conditions should undergo an electrocardiogram (ECG) evaluation at their annual physical examination
- Those at highest risk may need to have a 24-h Holter monitor, echocardiogram, and a stress test performed

Cost/efficacy

- Cost of ECG is not significant and may be a standard procedure at annual physical for at-risk patients
- Holter monitor, echocardiogram, and stress test are costly but can identify those patients with early signs of ventricular tachycardic episodes

PREVENT RECURRENCE

Prevention of second episodes, which are associated with high mortality, is of significant concern; current recommendation for preventive intervention is use of an implantable cardiac defibrillator.

RESOURCES

ASSOCIATIONS

American Heart Association
National Center
7272 Greenville Avenue
Dallas, TX 75231
Tel: (800)-AHA-USA1 (800) 242-8721
www.americanheart.org

KEY REFERENCES

- Guidelines 2000 for cardiopulmonary resuscitation and emergency cardiovascular care. Circulation 2000:102(Suppl I):1–370
- Atkins DL, Dorian P, Gonzalez ER, et al. Treatment of tachyarrhythmias. Ann Emerg Med 2001;37(Suppl 4):S91–109
- Strobel JS, Epstein AE. Large clinical trials in the management of ventricular arrhythmias. Applying group results to individual cases. Cardiol Clin 2000;18:337–56
- Kudenchuk PJ, Cobb LA, Copass MK, et al. Amiodarone for resuscitation after out-of-hospital cardiac arrest due to ventricular fibrillation. N Engl J Med 1999;341:871–8
- Levine JH, Massumi A, Scheinman MM, et al. Intravenous amiodarone for recurrent sustained hypotensive ventricular tachyarrhythmias. Intravenous Amiodarone Multicenter Trial Group. J Am Coll Cardiol 1996;27:67–75

FAQS

Question 1

In a patient with previous myocardial infarction and wide complex tachycardia, what is the most likely rhythm diagnosis?

ANSWER 1
Ventricular tachycardia.

Question 2

What is the most common structural heart disease that predisposes patients to ventricular tachycardia?

ANSWER 2
Previous myocardial infarction.

Question 3

When should patients with ventricular tachycardia be referred to a specialist?

ANSWER 3
Immediately. All patients with ventricular tachycardia – both nonsustained and sustained – should be referred to a cardiac electrophysiologist.

Question 4

When should patients with ventricular fibrillation be referred to a specialist?

ANSWER 4
Immediately. All patients who survive an episode of ventricular fibrillation should be referred to a cardiac electrophysiologist.

Question 5

What screening tests should be used in patients with previous myocardial infarction to help predict risk for ventricular tachycardia?

ANSWER 5

A 24-h Holter monitor and echocardiogram.

CONTRIBUTORS

Russell C Jones, MD, MPH
Kara J Quan, MD
Benjamin M Scirica, MD

WOLFF–PARKINSON–WHITE SYNDROME

SUMMARY INFORMATION

DESCRIPTION

- An abnormal electrical pathway connecting the atria and ventricles that bypasses the atrioventricular node. It may create a circuit that facilitates tachycardias, including paroxysmal supraventricular tachycardia, atrial fibrillation, and atrial flutter
- These rhythms may cause hemodynamic compromise, syncope, or, rarely, cardiac arrest
- Identifiable on the electrocardiogram by a cluster of findings: short PR interval, 'delta wave' at the beginning of the QRS complex, and ST-T wave anomalies
- May be treated by catheter ablation of the atrioventricular bypass tracts. Alternatives include drug therapy or surgical ablation of the bypass tract

URGENT ACTION

Treat poorly tolerated tachycardias with urgent electrical cardioversion; for example patients with:

- Hypotension with impaired perfusion of vital organs
- Syncope
- Cardiac arrest

KEY! DON'T MISS!

- Persons with Wolff–Parkinson–White syndrome and very short R-R intervals during tachycardias have the greatest risk of sudden death
- During episodes of atrial fibrillation, the atria may pace the ventricles at abnormally high speeds, resulting in ventricular fibrillation

BACKGROUND

ICD9 CODE

426.7 Wolff–Parkinson–White syndrome

SYNONYMS

- Pre-excitation syndrome
- WPW syndrome
- Accessory pathways syndrome

CARDINAL FEATURES

- Abnormal electrical connections between the atria and the ventricles, which may conduct electrical energy to or from the ventricles and produce tachyarrhythmias
- PR interval lasting less than 120ms (often less than 100ms)
- Abnormally wide QRS complex, with an initial deflection that has an abnormal slope (a 'slurred' onset of the QRS – the so-called 'delta wave'). The delta wave represents the fusion of electrical impulses descending the atrioventricular node and the accessory pathway simultaneously
- ST-T wave abnormalities, characterized by deflections that are directed negatively with respect to the direction of the dominant QRS deflection

CAUSES

Common causes

An anomalous electrically conducting path between the atria and ventricles ('bundle of Kent') is the most common cause of Wolff–Parkinson–White syndrome.

Rare causes

Accessory electrically conductive path between the atria and the His bundle ('atriohisian pathway'; the so-called 'Lown–Ganong–Levine' syndrome).

Serious causes

Wolff–Parkinson–White syndrome is on occasion found in patients with other structural heart defects including:

- Cardiomyopathies
- Ebstein's anomaly
- Mitral valve prolapse
- Ventricular septal defect

EPIDEMIOLOGY

Incidence and prevalence

PREVALENCE

- Average: about 1.5 cases per year per 1000 population
- Reported range: 0.1–3.0 per 1000

Demographics

AGE

- More common in young persons than in the elderly (usually found in first, second, or third decade of life)
- Incidence may decline with age as a result of loss of conduction over the accessory pathway

GENDER

More common in males than females.

RACE
Affects all races equally.

GENETICS
May be transmitted occasionally in an autosomal-dominant manner.

GEOGRAPHY
The condition does not cluster geographically.

SOCIOECONOMIC STATUS
Affects persons of all socioeconomic classes.

DIFFERENTIAL DIAGNOSIS
Lown–Ganong–Levine Syndrome
- Short PR interval
- QRS complex is of normal duration, and no delta wave is present

FEATURES
Clinically demonstrable tachycardias rarely occur in association with this abnormality on the surface electrocardiogram.

SIGNS & SYMPTOMS
Signs
- During tachycardias, heart rate is typically greater than 150 beats/min, and may be regular (if paroxysmal supraventricular tachycardia or atrial flutter) or irregular (if atrial fibrillation)
- Between episodes and in asymptomatic patients, no signs or symptoms may be present
- When poorly tolerated, the condition may present with loss of consciousness, pulmonary rales, signs of shock, or frank cardiac arrest (pulselessness, apnea)

Symptoms
Evidence of Wolff–Parkinson–White syndrome may be an asymptomatic finding on the static electrocardiogram. The syndrome may produce intermittent symptoms in patients during tachycardias including:
- Palpitations
- Dizziness, light-headedness
- Difficulty breathing
- Chest pain
- Presyncope
- Syncope
- Frank cardiac arrest

ASSOCIATED DISORDERS
Associated, in a small percentage of patients with:
- Ebstein's anomaly
- Ventricular septal defect
- Mitral valve prolapse
- Cardiomyopathies
- Other rare congenital defects

KEY! DON'T MISS!
- Persons with Wolff–Parkinson–White syndrome and very short R-R intervals during tachycardias have the greatest risk of sudden death
- During episodes of atrial fibrillation, the atria may pace the ventricles at abnormally high speeds, resulting in ventricular fibrillation

CONSIDER CONSULT
- Patients with recurrent or refractory symptomatic arrhythmia due to an accessory atrioventricular bypass tract should be referred for expert opinion in medical centers with electrophysiologists for consideration of the role of medical vs invasive treatment options
- Asymptomatic patients with the characteristic electrocardiographic features of Wolff–Parkinson–White syndrome, and coexistent structural or functional cardiac disease, may also benefit from prompt referral, especially (and most importantly) those with a family history of sudden cardiac death

INVESTIGATION OF THE PATIENT

Direct questions to patient

- Q Do you have episodes of rapid or irregular heartbeating?
- Q Have these episodes ever caused you to faint?
- Q Do you have difficulty breathing or chest pain when your heart races?
- Q Have you ever had an electrocardiogram before? Were you told it was abnormal?
- Q Have you ever been told you have 'WPW' or 'Wolff–Parkinson–White syndrome'? Many patients will recall the name of the syndrome only if prompted
- Q Does anyone in your family have a history of sudden cardiac arrest at an early age?

Contributory or predisposing factors

- Q Physical or psychosocial stress
- Q Some stimulant drugs
- Q Excessive use of caffeinated beverage

Family history

Family history of cardiac arrhythmia, and especially sudden cardiac death.

Examination

- Tachycardia
- Hypotension
- Evidence of structural cardiac defects

Summary of investigative tests

- Electrocardiogram (ECG): during tachycardias, and after cardioversion. The ECG is essential to the diagnosis – it identifies an abnormally shortened PR interval, and the presence of the delta wave

The following tests may be performed by a specialist to establish or confirm the diagnosis:

- Continuous cardiac monitoring, during tachycardias. All patients with rapid irregular heartbeats should be monitored continuously so that rapid interventions can be made if the heart rhythm changes or degenerates
- Holter monitoring: should be used to establish the presence of arrhythmias in patients with a history of frequent, symptomatic palpitations or syncope
- Cardiac event monitoring: should be used to establish the presence of arrhythmias in patients with a history of rare or occasional palpitations or syncope
- Exercise stress testing: may sometimes be used to establish the effect of exercise on the generation of cardiac rhythm disturbances
- Electrophysiologic testing: performed by a specialist

DIAGNOSTIC DECISION

The features of the surface ECG are used to identify patients with Wolff–Parkinson–White syndrome.

THE TESTS

Other tests

ELECTROCARDIOGRAM (ECG)

Description

- Monitoring electrodes are placed in conventional positions, on the arms, legs, and across the precordium
- Rhythm strips and standard 12-lead recording are obtained

Advantages/Disadvantages

- Easy to obtain
- Inexpensive
- Provides definitive evidence of preexcitation (shortened PR interval, delta wave) when electrical impulses conduct to the ventricles simultaneously through the accessory pathway and the atrioventricular node
- Complications of the procedure are extraordinarily rare

Normal

- A normal PR interval is 0.12–0.20s long
- The normal QRS complex lasts less than 0.12s, and typically less than 0.10s. The initial deflection of the QRS complex has a steep slope

Abnormal

- In Wolff–Parkinson–White syndrome the PR interval is typically less than 0.12s, and the QRS complex is wider than 0.12s. The initial deflection of the QRS complex has a slope that is distinctly different ('slurred') from the upslope or downslope of the rest of the QRS
- Keep in mind the possibility of a falsely abnormal (false-negative) result: in some patients with Wolff–Parkinson–White syndrome, the accessory tract is concealed and not evident on the surface ECG

Cause of abnormal result

Pre-excitation of the ventricles by the anomalous electrical tract.

Drugs, disorders, and other factors that may alter results

Many drugs, including antiarrhythmic agents, can alter conduction through the atrioventricular node or the accessory electrical pathway, and influence the ECG appearance of Wolff–Parkinson–White syndrome.

TREATMENT

IMMEDIATE ACTION

Hypotensive patients, or persons with shock, syncope, chest pain, or congestive heart failure, should be treated with urgent electrical cardioversion.

MANAGEMENT ISSUES

Goals

Goals of treatment are:

- To eliminate or manage palpitations and symptomatic tachycardia
- To eliminate episodes of syncope or near-syncope
- To reduce the risk of sudden death

Management in special circumstances

- Some volatile anesthetics (e.g. the 'fluranes') alter conduction over accessory atrioventricular pathways, and may need to be used judiciously during surgery on patients with Wolff–Parkinson–White syndrome
- There is a risk of sudden deterioration or death in patients who present with wide complex tachycardias if they are treated with verapamil

COEXISTING MEDICATION

Many patients with Wolff–Parkinson–White syndrome are treated with antiarrhythmic drugs, such as digoxin, procainamide, and verapamil. Care should be taken to avoid adverse drug interactions and drug toxicities caused by many of these agents that may have a narrow therapeutic index.

SPECIAL PATIENT GROUPS

- Over-40s with Wolff–Parkinson–White syndrome: organic and structural heart disease is more prevalent than in younger patients. Some experts have reported a higher incidence of syncope and cardiac arrest in this age group during arrhythmias
- Infants: in infants who present with Wolff–Parkinson–White syndrome, congenital cardiac defects, such as Ebstein's anomaly or ventricular septal defect, are common. Infants with structural heart defects and Wolff–Parkinson–White syndrome often have multiple accessory pathways
- Pregnancy: some obstetricians have reported an increased rate of arrhythmias in their pregnant patients with Wolff–Parkinson–White syndrome. In this population, the use of antiarrhythmic drugs must be carefully weighed against the risk of teratogenic side-effects

PATIENT SATISFACTION/LIFESTYLE PRIORITIES

- Wolff–Parkinson–White syndrome patients with a history of syncope should be restricted from driving, in accordance with local or state governmental protocols
- Some occupational choices should be discouraged in symptomatic patients with Wolff–Parkinson–White syndrome (e.g. piloting aircraft)
- The participation of athletes with Wolff–Parkinson–White syndrome in organized sports is controversial. Medicolegal realities dictate that patients with Wolff–Parkinson–White syndrome (whether symptomatic or not) be referred to cardiologists for consideration of exercise stress testing or electrophysiologic testing before sports participation

SUMMARY OF THERAPEUTIC OPTIONS

Choices

Chronic management:

- If patients have only an ECG tracing of Wolff–Parkinson–White syndrome and no history of palpitations, syncope, or arrhythmia, then they do not necessarily require therapy

- If the patient does have a history of palpitations, syncope, or arrhythmia, then they should be referred to a cardiologist for consideration of treatment with catheter ablation (or in some rare cases surgical ablation) or medical therapy
- Catheter ablation is a reasonable option for the management of recurrent or refractory tachyarrhythmia associated with Wolff–Parkinson–White syndrome
- Surgical ablation of accessory pathways may be necessary in intractable cases
- Chronic therapy with some atrioventricular nodal blocking agents can be recommended in some patients to decrease the propensity for paroxysmal supraventricular tachycardia. Agents such as oral verapamil or beta-blockers (e.g. sotalol) can be considered. Digoxin has variable effects on conduction in the accessory pathway, and is generally not recommended

Antiarrhythmic agents considered for the chronic management of Wolff–Parkinson–White syndrome:
- Verapamil (calcium channel blocker, class IV antiarrhythmic)
- Quinidine (class Ia antiarrhythmic)
- Flecainide (class Ic antiarrhythmic)
- Amiodarone (class III antiarrhythmic)
- Sotalol (beta-blocker)

There are no formal studies on the effects of exercise, dietary restrictions, or the use of on patients with Wolff–Parkinson–White. Nonetheless, it is prudent to recommend that patients institute certain lifestyle changes, such as avoiding excessive use of alcohol, stimulants, or illicit drugs.

Acute management of supraventricular tachycardia:
Immediate hospital referral.

Never

- Never treat a patient with a wide complex tachycardia with intravenous verapamil as this may result in sudden death or other forms of severe cardiac decompensation in this setting
- Never treat a patient with Wolff–Parkinson–White syndrome who presents with atrial fibrillation or flutter with intravenous digoxin, verapamil, or lidocaine. These drugs may increase the rate of ventricular response and produce cardiac decompensation (e.g. ventricular fibrillation)

FOLLOW UP

Most antiarrhythmic agents used to manage Wolff–Parkinson–White syndrome will require regular follow-up to determine drug levels or clinically evident side-effects.

Plan for review

Patient follow up will typically include monitoring of symptoms and recording of a 12-lead ECG.

Information for patient or caregiver

- It is important that patients take their medications precisely as prescribed
- Many patients will prefer the simplicity and effectiveness of ablation therapy instead of medication use; this option should be carefully explained to patients, because the risk of side-effects with chronic use of antiarrhythmic drugs is considerable
- Use of tobacco should always be discouraged, but there is no known link between tobacco use and Wolff–Parkinson–White syndrome
- Excessive use of alcohol, or use of stimulant drugs (such as cocaine, methamphetamine) should be discouraged in Wolff–Parkinson–White syndrome
- There are no known effects of specific food groups on patients with Wolff–Parkinson–White syndrome
- Before engaging in high-level physical activity, persons with Wolff–Parkinson–White syndrome may benefit from exercise stress testing. There are no known adverse or beneficial effects of high-level exercise on the disorder
- Stimulant use (e.g. pseudoephedrine, ephedra, ma huang) should be limited

DRUGS AND OTHER THERAPIES: DETAILS

Drugs

VERAPAMIL

Calcium channel blocker. Class IV antidysrhythmic.

Dose

120–480mg daily in divided doses, orally.

Efficacy

Can slow conduction of orthodromic impulses (i.e. in paroxysmal supraventricular tachycardia, electrical signals that descend via the atrioventricular node, and then return to the atria through accessory pathways).

Risks/Benefits

- May trigger ventricular fibrillation in some patients
- The vasodilatory effects of verapamil may cause hemodynamic complications in patients with a substantial outflow gradient or markedly elevated pulmonary pressure

Use caution:

- With congestive heart failure and hypotension
- With renal and hepatic disease
- With Duchenne's muscular dystrophy
- In children
- In acute phase of myocardial infarction
- In beta-blocker therapy

Side-effects and adverse reactions

- Gastrointestinal: nausea, constipation, vomiting, abdominal pain
- CNS: dizziness, flushing, headache, fatigue
- EENT: tinnitus
- Genitourinary: impotence, nocturia, polyuria, gynecomastia
- Cardiovascular: tachycardia, bradycardia, palpitations, congestive heart failure, atrioventricular block, hypotension, peripheral edema
- Skin: rash

Interactions (other drugs)

■ Antidysrhythmics (amiodarone, digoxin, disopyramide, dofetilide, encainide, flecainide, procainamide, quinidine) ■ Antihypertensives (particularly alpha- and beta-blockers) ■ Antivirals ■ Aspirin ■ Azole antifungals ■ Barbiturates ■ Benzodiazepines ■ Buspirone ■ Calcium ■ Carbamazepine ■ Cardiac glycosides ■ Cimetidine ■ Cisapride ■ Clarithromycin, erythromycin ■ Cyclosporine, tacrolimus ■ Dantrolene ■ Diclofenac ■ Doxorubicin ■ Ethanol ■ Fentanyl ■ General and local anesthetics ■ Grapefruit juice ■ Histamine H_2 antagonists ■ Imipramine ■ Lithium ■ Neuromuscular blockers ■ Phenytoin ■ Rifampin ■ Seratonin-selective reuptake inhibitors (SSRIs) ■ Statins ■ Theophylline

Contraindications

Should not be used in patients with Wolff–Parkinson–White syndrome and wide complex atrial fibrillation (antidromic conduction) due to risk of ventricular fibrillation. Also contraindicated in: ■ Cardiogenic shock ■ Second- or third-degree heart block ■ Severe heart failure, history of heart failure ■ Hypotension ■ Pregnancy ■ Sick sinus syndrome ■ Porphyria

Acceptability to patient

Often less well accepted than catheter ablation.

Patient and caregiver information
Common side-effects of verapamil use (constipation, edema, fatigue) should be reviewed with patients.

QUINIDINE
Quinidine sulfate immediate-release tablets.

Dose
Initially 200–300mg orally every 6–8h. Can be increased to 600mg every 6h if indicated based on serum quinidine concentrations.

Risks/Benefits
- Use caution in congestive heart failure
- Use caution in asthma or fever, as these may mask quinidine hypersensitivity
- Use caution in hepatic or renal disease
- Use caution in pregnancy and breast-feeding

Side-effects and adverse reactions
- Gastrointestinal: nausea, vomiting, diarrhea, anorexia, bitter taste, esophagitis, abdominal pain, hepatotoxicity
- Cardiovascular: ECG changes, ventricular tachycardia, hypotension, syncope, sinus bradycardia
- CNS: cinchonism (tinnitus, headache), dizziness, vertigo, confusion, depression
- Hematologic: hemolysis, thrombocytopenia, agranulocytosis, aplastic anemia
- EENT: visual and hearing disturbances
- Skin: rashes, pruritus, photosensitivity, urticaria, exfoliative dermatitis, macropapular rash

Interactions (other drugs)
■ Antacids ■ Antiarrhythmics (digoxin, amiodarone, ibutilide, procainamide, propafenone, dofeltilide, disopyramide, verapamil) ■ Anticoagulants ■ Antidepressants (tricyclic) ■ Antihypertensive agents ■ Barbiturates and primidone ■ Cimetidine ■ Cisapride ■ Codeine ■ Coumarins ■ Diltiazem ■ Diuretics ■ Erythromycin ■ Itraconazole ■ Kaolin ■ Mefloquine ■ Methadone ■ Muscle relaxants ■ Nelfinavir ■ Neostigmine, pyridostigmine ■ Neuromuscular blockers ■ Nifedipine ■ Phenothiazines ■ Phenytoin ■ Pimozide ■ Quinolones ■ Quinupristin/dalfopristin ■ Rifamycins ■ Ritonavir ■ Sotalol ■ Timolol ■ Tramadol

Contraindications
■ Atrioventricular block ■ Conduction disorders associated with digitalis therapy, digitalis toxicity ■ Severe intraventricular conduction defects, left bundle branch block, or ventricular ectopy ■ Hypotension ■ Myasthenia gravis

FLECAINIDE
Class IC antidysrhythmic.

Dose
- 50mg orally every 12h. Can be increased by 50-mg increments twice daily over 4 days until desired response is achieved
- Maximum daily dosage: 300mg/day

Risks/Benefits
- Use caution in hepatic or renal impairment
- Use caution in respiratory depression
- Use caution in patients under 18 years old
- Use caution in myasthenia gravis
- Use caution in pregnancy and breast-feeding

Side-effects and adverse reactions
- Gastrointestinal: nausea, vomiting, diarrhea, constipation, flatulence, abdominal pain, taste changes, dry mouth
- Cardiovascular: angina, palpitations, edema, ventricular tachycardia, sinus bradycardia, QT prolongation, torsade de pointes, proarrhythmic effect
- CNS: headache, dizziness, fatigue, asthenia, tremor, vertigo, somnolence, anxiety, insomnia, depression
- EENT: visual impairment, tinnitus
- Genitourinary: impotence, urinary difficulties, loss of libido
- Hematologic: leukopenia, thrombocytopenia
- Skin: rashes, pruritus, urticaria

Interactions (other drugs)
■ Acetazolamide ■ Antacids ■ Antiarrhythmics (amiodarone, verapamil) ■ Antidepressants (tricyclic) ■ Beta-blockers ■ Cimetidine ■ Diuretics ■ Fluoxetine ■ Quinine ■ Ritonavir

Contraindications
■ Heart failure ■ Recent myocardial infarction, history of myocardial infarction and either asymptomatic ventricular ectopics or asymptomatic non-sustained ventricular tachycardia ■ Atrioventricular block, bundle branch block ■ Sick sinus syndrome ■ Cardiogenic shock ■ Frequent premature ventricular contractions

AMIODARONE
Class III antidysrhythmic.

Dose
- Doses for amiodarone must be individualized. Close monitoring of the patient is advised during the loading dose; this is usually carried out in a hospital setting
- Loading dose: 800–1600mg/day required for 1–3 weeks, followed by a reduction to 600–800mg/day for 1 month
- Maintenance dose: 200–600mg/day. Maintenance dose is determined according to antiarrhythmic effects, Holter recordings, programmed electrical tolerance, and patient tolerance

Risks/Benefits
- Should be used only by physicians with access to all methods of treating and monitoring arrhythmias
- Treatment should be initiated in hospital
- Use caution with thyroid and pulmonary disease
- Use caution with atrioventricular block and bradycardia
- Use caution in electrolyte imbalances
- Withdraw any concurrent antiarrhythmic therapy
- Due to the long half-life of amiodarone, any further antiarrhythmic therapy should not be initiated until 2 weeks after the discontinuation of amiodarone therapy

Side-effects and adverse reactions

- Gastrointestinal: nausea, vomiting, abdominal pains, constipation, diarrhea, hepatotoxicity, taste abnormalities
- Cardiovascular: congestive heart failure, hypotension, sinoartial node dysfunction, bradycardia, conduction abnormalities, dysrhythmias
- Respiratory: cough, dyspnea, pulmonary fibrosis
- CNS: headache, ataxia, dizziness, fatigue, tremors, paresthesia, peripheral neuropathy
- EENT: visual disturbances, photophobia, dry eyes
- Metabolic: altered thyroid function
- Musculoskeletal: weakness
- Skin: contact dermatitis, rashes, itching, angioedema

Interactions (other drugs)

■ Antiretroviral protease inhibitors ■ Antiarrhythmics (flecainide, digoxin, dofetilide, procainamide, quinidine, beta-blockers, calcium channel blockers) ■ Cevimeline ■ Cholestyramine ■ Cisapride ■ Cyclosporine ■ Dextromethorphan ■ Fentanyl ■ Fosphenytoin ■ Gatifloxacin, grepafloxacin, moxifloxacin, sparfloxacin ■ Inhalation anesthetics ■ Irbesartan ■ Phenothiazines ■ Phenytoin ■ Pimozide ■ Sirolimus ■ Tramadol ■ Tricyclic antidepressants ■ Warfarin

Contraindications

■ Atrioventricular block ■ Hypotension ■ Hypersensitivity ■ Pregnancy ■ Severe sinus node disease with bradycardia ■ Syncope

SOTALOL

Beta-blocker.

Dose

- Initial dose: 80mg twice daily, orally
- Dose may be increased to 120–160mg twice daily (adjusted gradually allowing 2–3 days between increases)

Efficacy

Use to terminate paroxysmal supraventricular tachycardia (not atrial fibrillation with wide QRS complexes).

Risks/Benefits

- Do not withdraw sotalol treatment abruptly
- Use caution in hyperthyroidism
- Use caution in electrolyte imbalance
- Use caution in renal impairment
- Use caution in vasospastic angina and pheochromocytoma
- Use caution in surgery
- Use caution in diabetes mellitus

Side-effects and adverse reactions

- Gastrointestinal: nausea, vomiting, diarrhea, constipation
- Cardiovascular: sinus bradycardia, angina, palpitations, QT prolongation, proarrhythmic events, torsade de pointes, peripheral vasoconstriction
- CNS: fatigue, dizziness, sleep disturbances
- Respiratory: dyspnea, bronchospasm
- Metabolic: hyperglycemia
- Skin: rashes, exacerbation of psoriasis
- Hematologic: blood cell dyscrasias

Interactions (other drugs)

■ Alpha-blockers and agonists ■ Antacids ■ Antiarrhythmics (amiodarone, adenosine, disopyramide, procainamide, quinidine, dofeltilide, lidocaine, flecainide) ■ Antidepressants (tricyclic and possibly monoamine oxidase inhibitors) ■ Astemizole ■ Calcium channel blockers ■ Cevimeline ■ Cimetidine ■ Cisapride ■ Clarithromycin, erythromycin, and fluoroquinolones ■ Clonidine ■ Cocaine ■ Digoxin ■ Diuretics ■ Hypoglycemic agents ■ Insulin ■ Liothyronine ■ Neostigmine, physostigmine ■ Neuroleptics ■ Nonsteroidal anti-inflammatory drugs ■ Phenothiazines ■ Pimozide ■ Reserpine ■ Tacrine ■ Terbutaline ■ Terfenadine ■ Theophylline

Contraindications

■ Sinus bradycardia ■ Sick sinus syndrome ■ Second- or third-degree atrioventricular block ■ QT prolongation syndromes ■ Heart failure ■ Hypokalemia ■ Cardiogenic shock ■ Bronchospastic disorders and asthma ■ Raynaud's disease or peripheral vascular disease

Acceptability to patient

Generally well tolerated.

Follow up plan

Most patients treated acutely will be referred for follow up with a cardiologist.

Patient and caregiver information

Watch for excessively slow pulse (rate less than 55 beats/min), wheezing, or other difficulty breathing, excessive fatigue, sexual or erectile dysfunction, palpitations, syncope.

Surgical therapy

SURGICAL ABLATION OF ACCESSORY PATHWAYS

Surgery to excise accessory electrical pathways is rarely needed, because catheter ablation techniques are highly effective and generally well tolerated. After mapping or locating the accessory pathway, it is surgically divided or frozen ('cryoablation').

Efficacy

Typically more than 90% effective in abolishing arrhythmias caused by the accessory pathway.

Risks/Benefits

- More invasive than catheter ablation techniques
- Recovery from the procedure is more prolonged than with catheter ablation, and more likely to be complicated, although reported complication rates are low
- Occasionally results in complete atrioventricular block
- Rarely causes death

Acceptability to patient

Most patients prefer the less invasive option of catheter ablation.

Follow up plan

Follow up includes assessment of effectiveness by cardiac surgeon, consultation with cardiologists, and monitoring symptoms and surface ECG.

Patient and caregiver information

- Sternal wound care may be needed postoperatively
- Lifting of objects weighing more than 5–10 pounds will be restricted during the first 6 weeks after surgery
- Patients should immediately report any problems with difficulty breathing, chest pain, palpitations, arrhythmias, fevers, poor wound healing, or presyncope or syncope

Other therapies

CATHETER ABLATION OF ACCESSORY BYPASS TRACT(S)

- Specially designed catheters are inserted into the chambers of the heart to locate and then obliterate electrical conduction on the accessory pathway
- Usually the procedure is performed with bursts of radiofrequency energy (range 4–20 times). Less often, direct electrical current is used

Efficacy

This procedure is highly effective and may eliminate arrhythmia in more than 90% of patients.

Risks/Benefits

Risks

- Bleeding
- Infection
- Damage to blood vessels or intracardiac structures
- Complete heart block (need for pacemaker implantation)
- Stimulation of adverse heart rhythms
- Death

Benefit: immediate ablation of the bypass tract with cure.

Acceptability to patient

Usually preferred by patients relative to the alternatives, for example:

- Long-term management with antiarrhythmic drugs (may cause serious side-effects)
- Cardiac surgery (more invasive)

Follow up plan

Follow up examination by a cardiologist. Occasionally the syndrome may recur following ablation.

Patient and caregiver information

- Patients should be aware that complete heart block and the need for permanent pacemaker implantation are important, although infrequent complications of the procedure
- Duration of the procedure is typically 2–3h
- With radiofrequency catheter ablation, general anesthesia is unnecessary
- With direct-current catheter ablation, general anesthesia is required

LIFESTYLE

There are no formal studies on the effects of exercise, dietary restrictions, or the use of alcohol, stimulants, or illicit drugs on patients with Wolff–Parkinson–White syndrome. Nonetheless it is prudent to recommend that patients avoid excessive use of:

- Caffeinated drinks
- Decongestants (such as pseudoephedrine)
- Some stimulating herbal remedies (such as ma huang – 'ephedra')
- Cocaine, methamphetamines, crank, crack, or other illicit drugs that may trigger tachycardic heart rhythms

OUTCOMES

EFFICACY OF THERAPIES

In more than 90% of patients, catheter ablation of anomalous pathways between the atria and the ventricles is immediately effective in eliminating Wolff–Parkinson–White syndrome.

PROGNOSIS

- An unknown percentage of patients with Wolff–Parkinson–White syndrome first present in ventricular fibrillation/sudden death
- The vast majority of those who present with asymptomatic ECG abnormalities, or other arrhythmias, are successfully managed

Clinical pearl(s)

Consider Wolff–Parkinson–White syndrome in a patient complaining of 'palpitations' without a considerable or excessive use of caffeinated beverages or use of stimulants.

Therapeutic failure

- Failed treatments (catheter ablation, surgery) are usually repeated
- Success after second intervention is likely

Recurrence

Wolff–Parkinson–White syndrome that recurs after radiofrequency catheter ablation can sometimes be successfully treated with re-ablation, surgical interruption of the accessory pathway(s), or drug therapies.

COMPLICATIONS

- Many people have characteristic but asymptomatic abnormalities of the surface ECG and no complications. They do not need referral, special medications or procedures, or unusual follow up
- Patients with tachycardias may have presyncope, syncope, fatigue, depression, congestive heart failure, or sudden death

PREVENTION

RISK FACTORS

Patients without accessory pathways will not develop them as a result of behaviors, diet, excesses, etc.

MODIFY RISK FACTORS

SCREENING

There is no evidence that random screening for the disorder (e.g. with mass use of electrocardiography in schools or childhood assessments) would be beneficial or cost-effective.

RESOURCES

ASSOCIATIONS

The American College of Cardiology
Heart House
9111 Old Georgetown Road
Bethesda, MD 20814-1699
Tel: (800) 253-4636 or (301) 897-5400
Fax: (301) 897-9745
http://www.acc.org

National Organization for Rare Disorders, Inc. (NORD)
P.O. Box 8923
New Fairfield, CT 06812-8923
Telephone: (203) 746-6518
Fax: (203) 746-6481
Toll free: (800) 999-6673
http://www.rarediseases.org

KEY REFERENCES

- Guirandon GM, Guiraudon CM, Klein GJ, et al. Operation for the Wolff–Parkinson–White syndrome in the catheter ablation era. Ann Thorac Surg 1994;57:1084–88
- Hogenhuis W, Stevens SK, Wang P, et al. Cost-effectiveness of radiofrequency ablation compared with other strategies in Wolff–Parkinson–White syndrome. Circulation 1993; 88:II437–46
- Jackman WM, Wang X, Friday KJ, et al. Catheter ablation of accessory atrioventricular pathways (Wolff–Parkinson–White syndrome) by radiofrequency current. N Engl J Med 1991;324:1605–11

FAQS

Question 1

What are the characteristic abnormalities of the surface electrocardiogram of patients with Wolff–Parkinson–White syndrome?

ANSWER 1

Short PR interval (<0.12s), prolongation of the QRS complex (>0.12s) and a delta wave.

Question 2

Should asymptomatic patients with abnormalities of the static surface electrocardiogram be referred for specialist opinion?

ANSWER 2

No. Specialist opinion is not necessary if the patient is asymptomatic and there is no family history of sudden cardiac death or clinical evidence of structural or functional cardiac disease.

Question 3

What is the appropriate immediate treatment for an episode of hemodynamically unstable tachyarrhythmia?

ANSWER 3

Immediate electrical cardioversion. If the pathways are known, and an electrophysiologist is available, the patient may benefit from immediate ablation – if stable.